BIOMATERIALS

A Basic Introduction

QIZHI CHEN • GEORGE THOUAS

BIOMATERIALS

A Basic Introduction

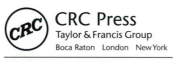

CRC Press
Taylor & Francis Group
Boca Raton London New York

CRC Press is an imprint of the
Taylor & Francis Group, an **informa** business

CRC Press
Taylor & Francis Group
6000 Broken Sound Parkway NW, Suite 300
Boca Raton, FL 33487-2742

© 2015 by Taylor & Francis Group, LLC
CRC Press is an imprint of Taylor & Francis Group, an Informa business

No claim to original U.S. Government works

Printed and bound in India by Replika Press Pvt. Ltd.

Printed on acid-free paper
Version Date: 20140514

International Standard Book Number-13: 978-1-4822-2769-7 (Hardback)

Library of Congress Cataloging-in-Publication Data

Chen, Qizhi, 1963- author.
    Biomaterials : a basic introduction / Qizhi Chen and George Thouas.
    p. ; cm.
    Includes bibliographical references and index.
    Summary: "Biomaterials is a multidisciplinary subject, involving materials science, engineering, cell biology, and medicine. This textbook therefore provides an appropriate balance between depth and broadness of coverage, sufficient to enable understanding of the most important concepts and principles at the right level by students from a wide academic spectrum. This project has been developed from extensive lecture notes created by Dr. Chen in the teaching of biomaterial at Monach U, since 2008."--Provided by publisher.
    ISBN 978-1-4822-2769-7 (alk. paper)
    I. Thouas, George, author. II. Title.
    [DNLM: 1. Biocompatible Materials. 2. Bioengineering--methods. 3. Prostheses and Implants. QT 37]

R856
610.28--dc23
    2014017882

Visit the Taylor & Francis Web site at
http://www.taylorandfrancis.com

and the CRC Press Web site at
http://www.crcpress.com

CONTENTS

PART I
Biomaterials Science

Contents

Contents

Contents

Contents

Contents

Contents

PART II
Medical Science

Contents

Contents

Contents

Contents

Contents

Contents

PART III
Evaluation and Regulation of Medical Devices

Chapter 20

Contents

Contents

PREFACE

Biomaterials refers to subtype materials, which are defined mainly by their medical applications as synthetic tissue implants. In the past two decades, rapid growth has been witnessed in the fields of science and engineering and toward production of biomaterial-based components. Despite this fact, only a few textbooks on biomaterial science are available and designed for undergraduate' training. *Biomaterials: An Introduction* by Park and Lakes was first published in 1979. The successive second and the third editions were published in 1992 and 2007, respectively. Up to 2004, this was the only commercially available textbook on biomaterials until a multiauthored textbook, *Biomaterials Science: An Introduction to Materials in Medicine*, edited by B. D. Ratner, A. S. Hoffman, F. J. Schoen, and J. E. Lemons came into the market. To date, however, Park and Lakes' book remains the only commercially available biomaterials textbook that is suitable for undergraduate students.

In addition, this textbook has been developed from my lecture notes prepared during my teaching of biomaterials in universities. The book is easy to study and provides a substantial introduction to fundamental science relating to biomaterials, such as materials science, biology, and medicine, among others. The book is designed efficiently to serve the needs of junior students (typically at second year level majoring in any natural sciences or engineering). It begins by introducing basic concepts and principles and critically analyzes the important properties of biomaterials. Gradually, the book presents students with an opportunity to build up skills and knowledge that will enable them to select and design biomaterials used in medical devices.

APPROACH

Biomaterials is a multidisciplinary subject that involves materials science, engineering, cell biology, and medicine. Covering all the aspects involved in these subjects in a comprehensive and timely manner is often a daunting task; this textbook, however, provides the reader with an appropriate balance between the depth and breadth of the topics covered. The book is equally simple and sufficient, enabling students to understand the most important biomaterials and bioengineering concepts and principles at various levels within the broad academic spectrum. This approach has been derived from my many years of experience in a multidisciplinary research environment.

I, a physicist-turned-biomedical engineer, have had the privilege to developed the most relevant knowledge and skills of life science, most of which nonmedical students should possess in order to appreciate the study of biomedical science. In addition, having worked closely with cell biologists, physicians and surgeons, I was able to develop an understanding that medical professionals can best grasp the concepts and principles of biomaterial science and engineering when the discussions use their own technical terminologies and jargon.

The other crucial aspect of the book is its organic combination of the principles of materials science and medical sciences in a unique and comprehensive way that most biomaterial books have not achieved. Moreover, there are more general and closely related concepts and principles among materials science, engineering, and medical science; nonetheless, these are always considered separate disciplines and often described using different terminologies. This textbook makes an introduction of the properties and principles of biomaterials from the perspective of clinical applications. In this sense, *materials* students can enjoy new information that has not been given in any of the traditional science course books; similarly, *medical* students are enabled to easily understand the concepts and principles of materials science. Furthermore, the book covers aspects of biomedical science from a materials point of view. This approach enables students majoring in materials science or engineering to equally understand the fundamentals of biometric materials' behavior at their respective biological levels for any given application. Medical students also earn the privilege of obtaining fresh information that is seldom found in any traditional medical program. I, therefore, believe that this concept would be of great significance to students both in the biomedical and bioengineering disciplines.

Consequently, the textbook is based on philosophical teachings that have been perfected over the years through observations and experiments in engineering schools. Learning is thus achieved primarily in the relevant context. It is imperative for students to view the relevant applications of materials relative to their daily livelihood. The book is tailored to bridge the gap between a student's mind and the knowledge found in the subject, hence making the learning process relevant. Besides, effective learning is mostly achieved through analogy, by comparing various features of biomaterial science. Students pursuing this program are many, majoring in different disciplines. The students are, therefore, well placed to understand the principles and concepts of the nonmajored discipline if the new information is discussed relative to their majored discipline.

ORGANIZATION

The textbook has been organized into three parts. Part I discusses biomaterials, Part II medical science, and Part III discusses evaluation and regulation of medical devices. Part I commences with an overview on engineering and materials science, then proceeds to focus on the definitions of biomaterials and biocompatibility, concluding with a summary of these subjects. Subsequently, Chapters 4 through 11 provide specific emphasis on metallic, ceramic, polymeric, and composite biomaterials. Part II begins with an overview of medical science vis-a-vis materials science (Chapter 12).

Chapters 13 through 18 describe anatomy, histology, and cell biology, respectively. The objective of these chapters, therefore, is to highlight health issues and diseases where biomaterials can easily find medical applications. The interactions between the biomaterials and the living body constitute the last chapter (Chapter 19) of Part II. In Part III, the penultimate chapter of the book, Chapter 20, evaluates medical devices while the final chapter, Chapter 21, looks into their respective regulations.

ACKNOWLEDGMENTS

I take this opportunity to recognize and appreciate the support I received from my coauthor Dr. George Thouas, without whom I would not have been able to complete the book. My deep gratitude goes to my family members. Special thanks go to my son Thomas Robert Cuvelier, who constantly showed his true love by asking me simple questions throughout the journey—"Mom, which chapter are you writing?" His purely innocent face and the sparklingly bright eyes gave me the strength and morale to write each chapter with enthusiasm and confidence.

Qizhi Chen
Melbourne, Victoria, Australia

AUTHORS

Qizhi Chen earned her PhD in biomaterials from Imperial College London in 2007. She is currently an academic in the Department of Materials Engineering at Monash University. Previously she was employed by the National Heart and Lung Institute London and the University of Cambridge. She has produced more than 100 peer-reviewed journal articles and book chapters and has attracted more than $5 million in research grants from numerous government research councils. Dr. Chen's research interests broadly cover polymeric, ceramic, metallic, and composite biomaterials for application in biomedical engineering. Her teaching interests include physics and various topics of materials science and engineering, in addition to biomaterials.

George Thouas graduated with a master's degree in biomedical sciences at Monash University, Melbourne, where he also earned his PhD in the same area in 2006. As an academic researcher, he specialized in developmental biology and reproductive medicine, with a focus on cellular metabolism and mitochondrial function. He has also spent a major part of his career working in bioengineering research, enabling interdisciplinary projects in bioreactor design, medical devices, and novel biomaterials, with applications in tissue engineering and regeneration. Dr. Thouas has produced more than 50 publications, including peer-reviewed journal articles, book chapters, patents, and conference proceedings.

PART I

BIOMATERIALS SCIENCE

CHAPTER 1

BIOMATERIALS SCIENCE AND ENGINEERING

LEARNING OBJECTIVES

After a careful study of this chapter, you should be able to do the following:

1. Understand the scope of materials science and engineering.
2. Appreciate the multilevel structures in materials and the critical level that classifies materials into metallics, ceramics, and polymers.
3. Be very familiar with three crystalline structures: FCC, BCC, and HCP, in iron, cobalt, titanium, and their alloys.
4. Briefly describe the properties of the aforementioned three types of materials and the common issue of each type.
5. Describe the definitions of biomedical materials, biomaterials, and biological materials.
6. Describe the definition of biocompatibility.

1.1 MATERIALS SCIENCE AND ENGINEERING

It is common to subdivide the discipline of materials science and engineering into two subdisciplines: *materials science* and *materials engineering*. To understand the boundary and relationship of these two subdisciplines, let us start by looking into materials around us and question why we use materials. The world is comprised of materials that play essential roles in virtually all aspects of our everyday life. Our houses are built from stone, concrete, steel, and glass materials; our clothing is produced from natural (e.g., cotton) or synthetic (e.g., nylon) polymers, and even the food we produce is composed of biological polymers. Human beings are also composed of complex biological materials, derived from raw materials in the environment we occupy.

We select a material (e.g., glass) for a specific application (e.g., window) because the material has a special property (e.g., transparency) that satisfies our needs (e.g., day light). In essence, the properties of any material are determined by its structure. The discipline *materials science* is concerned with the study of relationships

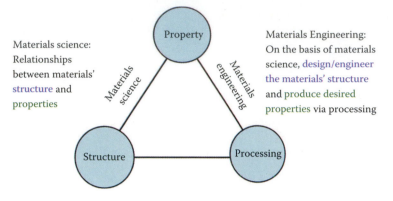

Figure 1.1
The interrelationship between structure, properties, and processing depicted as a schematic illustration.

between structure and property of materials (Figure 1.1). However, raw materials generally possess unsatisfactory properties and seldom meet the demands of applications. Hence, we seek to change the structure of natural materials so that they can provide us with desired properties and perform expected functions. *Materials engineering* is all about how to design and manipulate the structure of a material to produce desired properties via processing (Figure 1.1). Historically, it is the large amount of experimental work in materials engineering that led to the establishment of materials science. Nowadays, it is materials science that guides the innovation in materials engineering.

1.2 MULTILEVELS OF STRUCTURE AND CATEGORIZATION OF MATERIALS

Condensed materials (i.e., liquids and solids) exhibit structure on more than one length scale (Figure 1.2):

- Atomic structure (i.e., the structure within an atom)
- Lattice structure (i.e., the agglomeration network of atoms)
- Microscopic structure (e.g., defects and grain boundary, which can only be viewed under microscopes)
- Macroscopic (bulk) structure (e.g., deformation and fracture, which can be viewed by the naked eye)

The atomic structure determines the nature of chemical bonds at the lattice level, which in turn produces the specific properties of the material. The types of chemical bonds are listed in Figure 1.3, and the major characteristics of chemical bonds are summarized in Table 1.1. It is the structure at the atomic and molecular lattice levels that primarily defines material properties and classifies most solid matter into three basic types: metallic, ceramic, and polymeric. Metallic bonding forms metals and alloys, with single or multiple elements arranged in geometric lattices, surrounded by electrons. Either ionic or rigid covalent (electron shared) bonding can result in brittle ceramics (e.g., NaCl and diamond). In polymers, rotational covalent bonds between atoms

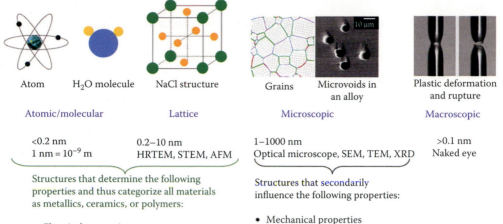

| Atom | H_2O molecule | NaCl structure | Grains | Microvoids in an alloy | Plastic deformation and rupture |

| Atomic/molecular | Lattice | Microscopic | Macroscopic |

<0.2 nm
1 nm = 10^{-9} m   0.2–10 nm
HRTEM, STEM, AFM   1–1000 nm
Optical microscope, SEM, TEM, XRD   >0.1 nm
Naked eye

Structures that determine the following
properties and thus categorize all materials
as metallics, ceramics, or polymers:

Structures that secondarily
influence the following properties:

- Chemical properties
- Electrical properties
- Magnetic properties
- Optical properties
- Thermal properties
- Mechanical properties

- Mechanical properties

Figure 1.2
Multilevel structures of materials and primarily related properties.

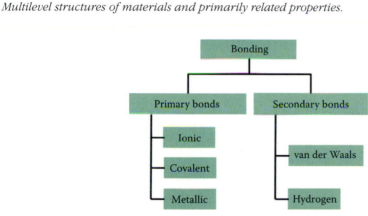

Figure 1.3
Types of atomic and molecular bonding.

produce flexible, long molecules, and the molecular chains are glued together by secondary chemical bonds, such as hydrogen and/or van der Waals bonding.

Crystallographic structure refers to a unique arrangement of atoms or molecules in a solid. The arrangement can be either regular (*crystal*) or random (*glass*). The most frequently occurring crystalline structures in metals include *face-centered cubic* (FCC) (Figure 1.4a), *body-centered cubic* (BCC) (Figure 1.4b), and *hexagonal closely packed* (HCP) (Figure 1.4c). FCC and HCP are the most closely packed structures, with a packing fraction (the volume fraction of space occupied by atoms) being 74%. BCC is secondarily densely packed, with a packing fraction being 68%. To demonstrate these three-dimensional (3D) crystal structures with a see-through effect, atoms or molecules are often represented by a small point. The structure formed by all these points is known as a *lattice* structure. Remember that the actual arrangements of atoms are as

Table 1.1
Characters of Chemical Bonds in Various Substances

Bonding Type	Substance	Length (nm)	Bonding Energy (kJ/mol)	Melting Point (°C)	Directionality/ Electron Location
Metallic	Hg	0.264	68	−39	Nondirectional/ Free
	Al	0.242	314	660	
	Fe	0.264	406	1538	
	W	0.324	849	3410	
Covalent	Si	0.222	450	1410	Directional/ locally shared
	C (Diamond)	0.145	713	>3550	
Ionic	NaCl	0.236	640	801	Nondirectional/ transferred
	MgO	0.175	1000	2800	
Hydrogen	NH_3	0.285	35	−189	Directional/ localized
	H_2O	0.197	51	−101	
van der Waals	Ar	0.376	7.7	−78	Nondirectional/ localized
	Cl_2	0.350	31	0	

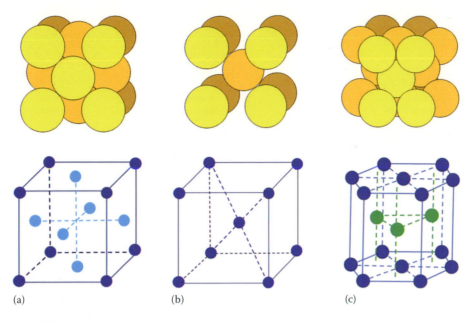

(a)   (b)   (c)

Figure 1.4
The three most common crystalline (lattice) structures in metals. Students should be very famil-iar with these three structures, as iron-, cobalt-, and titanium-based alloys, three predominant metallic implant materials used in orthopedics, are in these three structures. (a) Face-centered cubic (FCC) examples: γ-Fe (austenitic) and β-Co (austenitic); (b) body-centered cubic (BCC) examples: α-Fe (ferrite) and β-Ti; (c) hexagonal closely packed (HCP) examples:α-Ti and α-Co.

close as those in the first row of Figure 1.4, rather than as apparently separated as those in the second row. The lattice diagrams are invented simply for ease in studying 3D crystallographic structures.

Microscopic structure refers to various defects existing in lattices (Figure 1.5), including the following:

- Vacancies and their aggregation (i.e., microvoids). A *vacancy defect* is a lattice site from which an atom is missing.
- Alloying (substitutional or interstitial) atoms and their precipitates (second-phase particles). A *substitutional defect* is an impurity atom that occupies a regular atomic site in the crystal structure. An *interstitial defect* is an atom that occupies a site in the crystal structure at which there is usually not an atom.
- Dislocations (i.e., line defects). A *dislocation* is a linear defect around which some of the atoms of the crystal lattice are misaligned.
- Stacking faults (planar defects). A *stacking fault* is an interruption in the stack-ing sequence of the crystal structural planes.
- Grain boundaries and phase interfaces. A *grain boundary* is the interface between two grains (also called crystallites) in a polycrystalline material. A *phase interface* is the boundary between two phases in a multiphase material.
- Microvoids and microcracks.

These defects can be categorized, according to their geometric dimensions, into point, line, area/planar, and volume/3D defects, as listed in Figure 1.6. Microstructures have significant influences on mechanical properties (typically, ultimate tensile

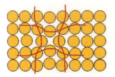
Vacancies:
vacant atomic sites

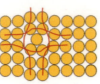
Self interstitials:
extra atoms

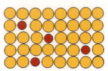
Impurities:
substitutional

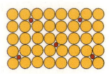
Impurities:
interstitial

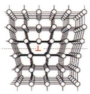
Dislocations

Grain boundaries

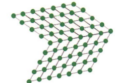
Twinning boundaries

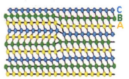
Stacking faults

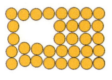
Microvoids

Microcracks

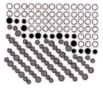
Phase interfaces

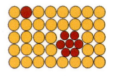
Second phase precipitates

Figure 1.5
Schematic microstructures of various defects.

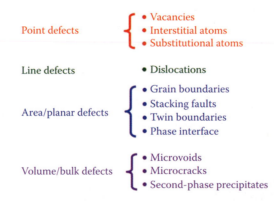

Point defects
{
• Vacancies
• Interstitial atoms
• Substitutional atoms

Line defects
• Dislocations

Area/planar defects
{
• Grain boundaries
• Stacking faults
• Twin boundaries
• Phase interface

Volume/bulk defects
{
• Microvoids
• Microcracks
• Second-phase precipitates

Figure 1.6
Categorization of defects in solid materials.

strength and elongation at break), but not on physical properties (e.g., Young's modulus, electromagnetic and optical properties). Nonetheless, their impacts on mechanical properties are limited within each type of material such that in general, a modification in microstructures will not change one material into any other of the main material types.

Macroscopic/bulk structures are the results of the performance of a material, which can be used to indicate the relationships between structures and properties and reveal the mechanisms of intended or unexpected performance.

1.3 FOUR CATEGORIES OF MATERIALS

As mentioned earlier, solid materials have been grouped into three basic classifications: metals, ceramics, and polymers. This scheme is primarily based on chemical makeup and bonding, that is, the structures at the atomic and lattice levels. Most materials fall into one distinct grouping or another. In addition, there is a fourth type of material, the composites. These materials are primarily physical combinations of two or more of the aforementioned three basic materials classes. This section provides a brief description of each in terms of representative characteristics and biomedical applications, aiming to highlight the most common and critical issues of each material type.

1.3.1 Metallics

Materials in this category are composed of one or more metallic elements (e.g., Fe, Ni, Al, Cu, Zn, and Ti), and often also nonmetallic elements (e.g., C, N, and O) in relatively small amounts. Atoms in metals and their alloys are arranged in a very orderly manner. Metallic bonding is found in metals and their alloys, and a simple model has been established for this chemical bonding, described as follows. The valance electrons of metallic atoms are delocalized and form an electron cloud, in which metal ions are embedded; metallic bonding is the electrostatic attractive forces between the negatively charged electron cloud and the positively charged metal ions (Table 1.1). In other words, the free electrons act as a *glue* to hold the metal ion cores. Metallic bonding is typified by conduction valence electrons and a nondirectional character.

Some characteristic behaviors of metallic materials can be interpreted by the nature of metallic bonding. Metals are good conductors of both electricity and heat, as a result of their free valence electrons (Figure 1.7a). In contrast, ionically and covalently bonded materials are typically electrical and thermal insulators, due to the absence of large numbers of free electrons. The nondirectional nature of metallic bonding gives metal

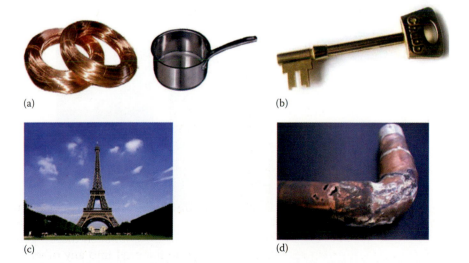

(a) (b)

(c) (d)

Figure 1.7
(a) Conductive (electrically and thermally). (b) Tough (combined strength and ductility). (c) Strong and ductile. (d) Corroded. (a–c) Typical properties of metals and alloys and related applications; (d) the most common issue of metallic materials, corrosion.

atoms (Hg is an exception) the capacity to compact closely and to slide past each other without causing permanent rupture. Locally, bonds can easily be broken and replaced by new ones after the deformation. This gives rise to the typical mechanical properties of metals: ductility and toughness. The application of keys (Figure 1.7b) requires the material to have a satisfactory combination of ductility and strength, which cannot be provided by either polymers or ceramics. The former are plastic but soft, the latter are strong but brittle. *Toughness* is a property quantifying the combination of strength and ductility. The excellent toughness of Fe-based alloys ensures the mechanical safety of structures like the Eiffel Tower (Figure 1.7c).

However, the conduction valence electrons in metals also impart metals and alloys with corrosion (Figure 1.7d). Corrosion is a common problem for metals and alloys in wet and/or salty environments, such as sea, earth, circulated water, damp atmospheres, or living tissue. Metal atoms react spontaneously with oxygen, hydrogen protons, and ionic salts over time to form metal oxides, which form micro- and macrostructural defects in the bulk metal. Body tissue fluids provide an aggressive environment to metallic implants, as they contains all three of these reactive elements (oxygen, hydrogen protons, and ionic salts). Hence, corrosion of alloys is the most serious issue during the long-term performance of a permanently implanted metallic material. As a matter of fact, corrosion resistance of metallic implant materials determines the long-term success of a metallic implant. This issue will be discussed in greater detail in Chapter 2. Figure 1.8 demonstrates four examples of medical applications of metallic materials.

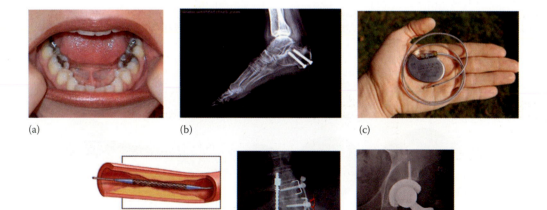

(a) (b) (c)

(d) (e) (f)

Figure 1.8
Medical applications of alloys. (a) Tooth filling made of amalgam. (b) Fixation screw made of stainless steel. (c) Pacemaker case made of a Ti alloy. (d) Self-expandable coronary stent made of TiNi. (e) Harrington rod, a spinal corrective device, made of stainless steels. (f) Total hip replacement prosthesis made of a Co alloy. (d: Modified graphic from the WikimediaCommons, http:// commons.wikimedia.org/produced by the National Institutes of Health.)

1.3.2 Ceramics

The term *ceramics* encompasses a variety of inorganic compounds of metallic and nonmetallic elements, including oxides (e.g., Al_2O_3, SiO_2, and ZrO_2), nitrides (e.g., Si_3N_4), carbides (e.g., SiC), and various salts (e.g., $NaCl$ and $Ca_3(PO_4)_2$). Some elements, such as carbon or silicon, are considered ceramics as well. Ceramic materials may be fully crystalline, partially crystalline, or fully amorphous (i.e., glass) in structure. Traditionally, the definition of ceramics was restricted to inorganic crystalline materials, as opposed to the noncrystalline glasses; this definition is still widely used in practice. Nowadays, the definition of ceramics is expanded to include amorphous glass materials, which are called noncrystalline ceramics.

In ceramics, atoms are bonded covalently (e.g., oxides, nitrides and carbides, diamond and silicon), and/or ionically (e.g., salts). Covalent bonds between identical atoms (as in silicon) are nonpolar, that is, electrically uniform, while those between unlike atoms are polar, that is, one atom is slightly negatively charged and the other is slightly positively charged. This partial ionic character of covalent bonds increases with the difference in the electronegativities of the two atoms.

Covalent and ionic bonds are typified by localized valence electrons and a lack of tolerance to lattice deformation, which are responsible for the characteristic behaviors of ceramics. Ceramics are generally electrical and thermal insulators (Figure 1.9a,b) because of the absence of large numbers of conduction electrons. The delocalization of electrons also makes ceramics inert and thus resistant to chemical and electrochemical (i.e., corrosive) attack, as compared to metallic materials. Many ceramics are indeed relatively inert, at room temperature, under dry atmosphere, over long time intervals (Figure 1.9c). However, with increasing temperature, specific chemical composition

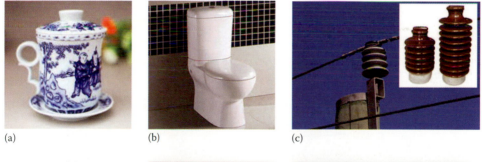

(a) (b) (c)

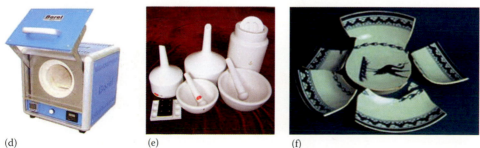

(d) (e) (f)

Figure 1.9
Typical properties of ceramics and related applications. (a) Thermal insulators. (b) Inert (resistant to corrosion). (c) Electrical insulators. (d) Thermally stable (furnace chamber). (e) Hard (resistant to wearing and friction). (f) Brittle.

(e.g., bioactive ceramics) or environment (e.g., body fluid), the propensity to degradation could be considerable. The strong ionic and covalent bonding (indicated by high bonding energy and high melting point) makes many ceramics (e.g., ZrO_2) thermally stable and thus an ideal choice of material to work at high temperature (Figure 1.9d), compared with metals and alloys.

Mechanically, ceramics are typically rigid and hard (Figure 1.9e), which are also attributed to their strong chemical bonds. Ceramics are generally much more brittle (Figure 1.9f) than metals and can have stiffness (modulus of elasticity) and strength similar to metallic materials, particularly in compression. But in a tensile or bending test, they are likely to fail at a much lower applied stress. The reason for this is twofold. First, the surfaces of ceramics nearly always contain microcracks, which magnify the applied stress (called stress concentration). Second, ionic and covalent bonds each lack tolerance to lattice deformation. The covalent bonding lacks tolerance to the deviation in directionality. Covalent bonds themselves are directional, meaning that atoms so bonded prefer specific orientations relative to one another. Any deviation from this specific direction is forbidden. Ionic bonding lacks tolerance in terms of neighboring, which means that atoms prefer to neighbor with oppositely charged atoms. If the correct directionality or neighboring is disturbed by deformation (Figure 1.10), there will be a huge tension (energy) increase locally such that the separation of atoms (i.e., fracture) is the only path to release the energy. This explains the brittle fracture behavior of ceramics. While advances in materials engineering have transformed a few formerly brittle ceramics into materials tough enough to withstand engine environments, brittleness issues remain with the majority of ceramics.

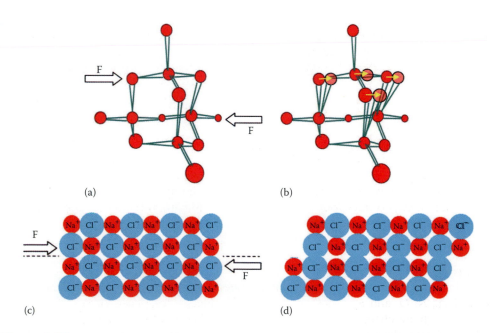

(a) (b) (c) (d)

Figure 1.10
Schematic illustration showing that covalently and ionically bonded ceramics lack tolerance of deformation in their lattice structures. (a) Diamond structure (C, Si, Ge). (b) Forbidden directionality of diamond lattice. (c) NaCl structure. (d) Forbidden neighboring of NaCl lattice.

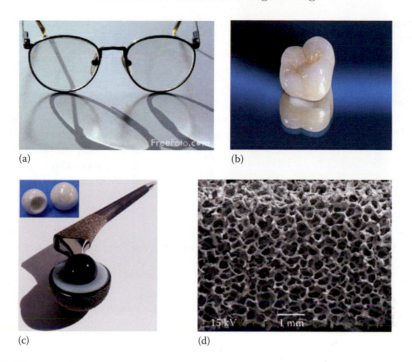

(a) (b)

(c) (d)

Figure 1.11
Medical applications of ceramics. (a) Corrective glasses. (b) Implantable teeth made of Al_2O_3. (c) Al_2O_3 head of total hip prosthesis (note: the stem is made of an alloy). (d) Bioglass-ceramic bone scaffold.

In addition to those representative applications illustrated in Figure 1.9, ceramics have also found applications in the field of biomedical devices, such as corrective glasses, implantable teeth, ceramic bone fillers, and heads of total hip prostheses (Figure 1.11).

1.3.3 Polymers

The terms *polymer* and *polymeric material* encompass very broad classes of compounds, both natural and synthetic, organic (mostly) and inorganic (e.g., sol–gel-derived SiO_2, a sol–gel polymer), with an extraordinary variety of properties. They play ubiquitous roles in everyday life, from those of familiar synthetic plastics, rubbers and resins used in day-to-day work and home life, to the natural biological polymers fundamental to biological structure and function (Figure 1.12). Some of the common and familiar synthetic polymers are polyethylene (PE), nylon, poly(vinyl chloride) (PVC), polycarbonate (PC), polystyrene, and silicone rubber. In this book, we use the term *polymer* to refer to organic polymers.

Chemically, polymers are based on carbon, hydrogen, and other nonmetallic elements (e.g., N, O, and Si). These materials are typically composed of very large molecules, which are chain- or network-like with a backbone of carbon atoms. The atoms within polymer chains are covalently bonded. Long chains are physically associated with each other, intertwining and entangling. Neighboring chains are also chemically bonded with each other, via either secondary weak bonding (such as in thermoplastics) or primary covalent bonding (cross-linking, such as in rubbers and resins). Although the

13

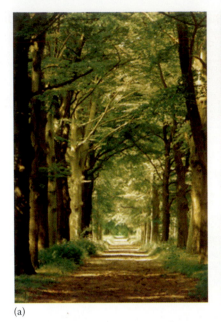

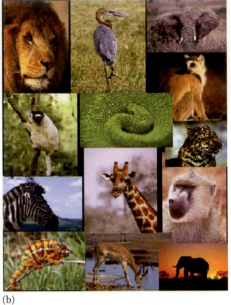

(a)   (b)

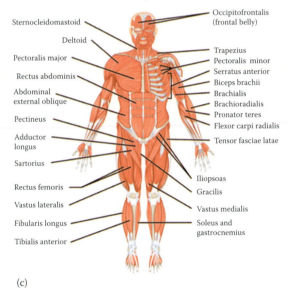

(c)

Figure 1.12
Naturally occurring polymers. (a) Plants (b) Animals (c) Human. (c: From the WikimediaCommons, http://commons.wikimedia.org/.)

σ covalent bond between the backbone atoms is strong and directional, it is also free to rotate about the bonding axis. This rotation freedom allows a polymer chain to bend, twist, coil, and kink.

In general, polymers are relatively inert chemically and unreactive in a large number of environments due to the lack of free electrons. This is the scientific reason for white pollution, referring to the massive amount of inert material (such as disposable plastic grocery bags provided in supermarkets), rather chemically active contaminants

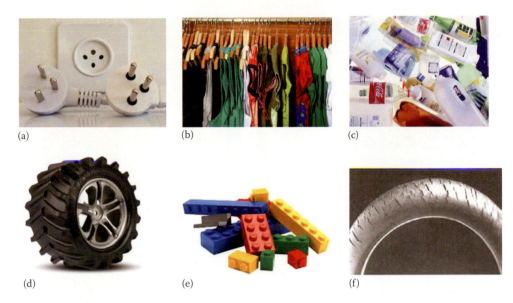

Figure 1.13
(a) Plastic plug and socket. (b) Soft and light clothes. (c) Plastic containers (PE). (d) Elastic tire. (e) Rigid Lego™. (f) Oxidation-induced cracks in medical tubing. (a–e) Typical properties of polymers and related applications; (f) the most common issue of polymeric materials, thermal instability and oxidization.

in the environment. Moreover, polymers generally have low electrical conductivity (Figure 1.13a) and are nonmagnetic. Mechanically, polymers are very dissimilar to the metallic and ceramic materials. Many polymers are very soft and compliant due to the flexibility of polymer chain (Figure 1.13b). If the association between neighboring polymer chains is physical tangling and/or secondary weak chemical bonding, the polymers can be extremely ductile and pliable (plastic) such that they can easily be formed into complex shapes (Figure 1.13c). If polymer chains are bonded via covalent bonding, the cross-linking produces either elastic rubbers or rigid polymers, depending on the degree of cross-links. A low degree of cross-links gives rise to flexible rubber (Figure 1.13d), and highly cross-linked polymers are relatively rigid and hard (Figure 1.13e). One major drawback to the polymers is their tendency to soften and/or decompose at modest temperatures, or to degrade (or age) via oxidation or hydrolysis over a long time interval in ambient conditions. Polymer oxidation has caused accidents involving medical devices (Figure 1.13f). Figure 1.14 illustrates a few applications of polymers as medical devices.

1.3.4 Composites

A *composite* is composed of two or more constituent materials of the three basic classes, that is, metallics, ceramics, and polymers. The design goal of a composite is to achieve a combination of properties that is not displayed by any single material alone, with the advantages of each of the component materials being incorporated and the disadvantages being minimized. A large number of synthetic composite types exist, which are classified according to the combination of metals, ceramics, and polymers, as listed as in Table 1.2. White tooth fillings and artificial

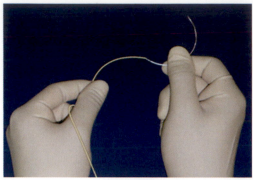
(a)

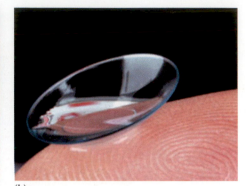
(b)

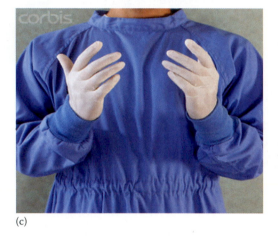
(c)

Figure 1.14
Medical applications of polymers. (a) Degradable surgical suture. (b) Contact lens. (c) Medical gloves.

Table 1.2
Classification of Composites

Polymer–matrix composites (PMC)
    Metal-reinforced
    Ceramic-reinforced
Metal–matrix composites (MMC)
    Ceramic-reinforced
Ceramic–matrix composites (CMC)
    Ceramic fiber–reinforced

bone pastes/cements (Figure 1.15) are typical medical applications of synthetic composites. There are also a few naturally occurring composites, such as wood and bone (Figure 1.16). Bone is a polymer-based ceramic-reinforced composite, where the protein molecule collagen is the polymer, and calcium phosphate hydroxyapatite, $Ca_{10}(PO_4)_6(OH)_2$, is the ceramic.

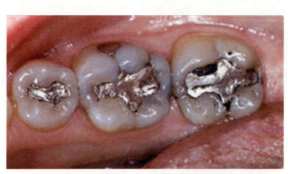

Traditional metallic filling

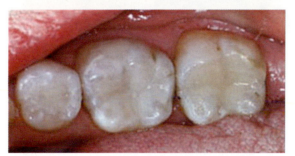

Composite white filling

(a)

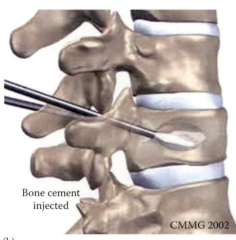

Bone cement
injected

CMMG 2002

(b)

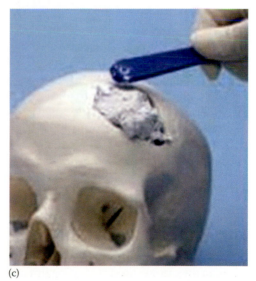

(c)

Figure 1.15
Medical applications of composite bone cement. (a) White tooth filling. (b) Bone cement to treat diseased spines. (c) Bone paste to repair damaged skulls.

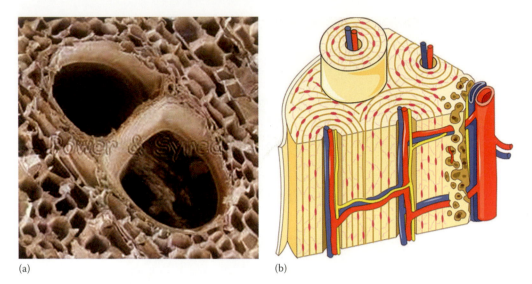

(a)   (b)

Figure 1.16
Naturally occurring composites. (a) Wood, a composite of cellulose and lignin; in porous wood such as balsa, air can be considered a third component. (b) Bone, a composite of polymer (collagen protein) and ceramic (calcium phosphate hydroxyapatite).

1.4 DEFINITIONS OF BIOMATERIALS, BIOMEDICAL MATERIALS, AND BIOLOGICAL MATERIALS

Before defining biomaterials, let us look at a few applications of biomaterials (Figure 1.17). The common feature of these applications is that these biomaterials are used in intimate contact with living body tissue. In the scientific field of biomaterials, a biomaterial is defined as "a substance that has been engineered to take a form which, alone or as part of a complex system, is used to direct, by control of interactions with components of living systems, the course of any therapeutic or diagnostic procedure." In most cases, a *biomaterial* is any *biocompatible* material, natural or man-made, that is used to replace or assist part of an organ or its tissue, while in *intimate contact with living tissue*. The prefix *bio* of biomaterials refers to *biocompatible*, rather than *biological* or *biomedical* as misunderstood by many people intuitively.

However, the term *biomaterial* is used within different definition boundaries in the scientific and legal communities. In the legal field, medical devices are defined as "any instrument, apparatus, implement, machine, appliance, implant, in vitro reagent or calibrator, software, material or other similar or related articles, intended by the manufacture to be used, alone or in combination, for human beings for one or more of the specific purposes of diagnosis, prevention, monitoring, treatment, investigation, supporting or sustaining life, control of conception, and disinfection of medical devices," and a biomaterial is defined as a component of a medical device [1]. In this textbook, the term *biomedical material* is used to represent a component of any biomedical device applied either *with* or *without* intimate contact with living tissue, and

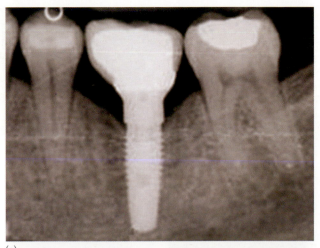

(a)

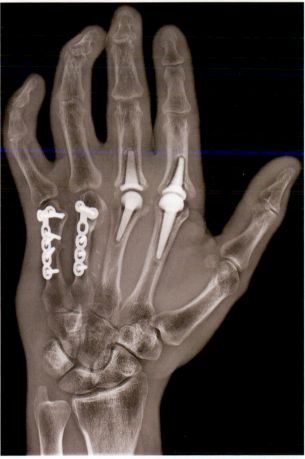

(b)

Figure 1.17
Four applications of biomaterials. (a) Tooth implants (Ti alloys). (b) Artificial finger joint (polyethylene).

(Continued)

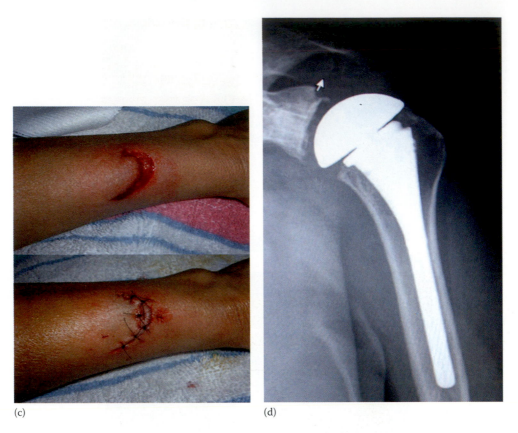

(c)   (d)

Figure 1.17 (Continued)
Four applications of biomaterials. (c) Surgical suture (polyesters). (d) Total shoulder replacement (alloys).

the definition of *biomaterials* prevalent in the scientific community is used to describe biocompatible materials used *with* intimate tissue contact.

According to the aforementioned definition, the materials used for contact lenses (Figure 1.18a) and total hip replacement (Figure 1.18c) are biomaterials, whereas those used for corrective eyewear (Figure 1.18b) and artificial leg prostheses (Figure 1.18d) are biomedical devices, typically not dealt with in the scientific field of biomaterials.

A biomaterial can be either synthetic or naturally occurring, such as bone and cotton. In general, we refer to naturally occurring materials as *biological materials*. Figure 1.19 demonstrates the definition boundaries of *biomedical materials*, *biomaterials*, and *biological materials*.

1.5   BIOCOMPATIBILITY

Since a biomaterial is designed to be used in intimate contact with living tissue, it is essential that the implanted material does not cause any harmful effects to host tissues and organs. Williams [2] suggests that biocompatibility refers to the ability to perform

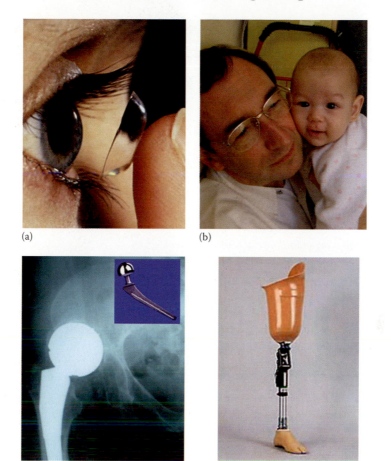

(a)   (b)

(c)   (d)

Figure 1.18

A graphical depiction of biomaterials and nonbiomaterials used in medical devices. Contact lenses (a), corrective eyewear (b), total hip-joint replacements (c), and a whole-leg prostheses (d) are considered as medical devices; however, (a) and (c) are examples of biomaterials, whereas (b) and (d) are constructed from biomedical materials, but usually of no concern to the scientific field of biomaterials.

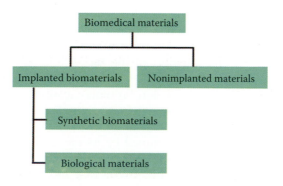

Figure 1.19

The definition boundaries of biomedical materials, biomaterials, and biological materials.

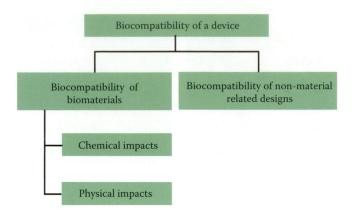

Figure 1.20
Contributors to the biocompatibility of a medical device.

with an appropriate host response in a specific application. The requirements for this biocompatibility are complex and strict, varying with specific medical applications. A material used satisfactorily in orthopedic surgery may be inappropriate for cardiovascular applications because of its thrombogenic properties. Biocompatibility of biomaterials is further classified according to their ability to induce cell or tissue death (cytotoxicity), to induce cancer formation (carcinogenicity), to damage genes (mutagenicity), to induce immune responses (pyrogenicity and allergenicity), or to induce blood clotting (thrombogenicity). Taking all of these types of biocompatibility problems into account, a universally prevalent definition of biocompatibility has been provided by the US Food and Drug Administration (FDA) [1], to the effect that the material induces no measurable harm to the host. Put simply, *no harm to the host body defines biocompatibility.*

Therefore, the biocompatibility of a medical device covers both the compatibility of the materials used and how the device has been engineered (e.g., geometric, mechanical, and/or electrical properties) (Figure 1.20). Indeed, many clinical failures of joint replacements, for example, are due to suboptimal mechanics of the device, rather than problems of the materials properties [3]. These nonmaterial issues are beyond the scope of this book. For our purposes, the biocompatibility of implant materials includes not only the chemical interactions of the implanted material with the host physiological system (e.g., corrosion of alloys, oxidation of polymers, and toxicities of metal ions) but the physical impact of the implanted material on the surrounding tissues (mechanical properties of the material), though the former is the common and primary concern of material biocompatibility. In general, chemical impact is the foremost aspect of the biocompatibility evaluation on new biomaterials.

In this book, we confine our discussion on biocompatibility to the chemical interactions of materials with the biological system and physical interactions based on the mechanical properties of the biomaterial. Within this concept, the chemical impact of an implant biomaterial is directly determined by its inertness in a biological environment and the performance of released species, including ions and molecules. The mechanical properties of an implant biomaterial are more relevant to the complex dynamic features of the tissue structure. Ideally, both aspects of material biocompatibility are engineered in parallel.

Table 1.3
Major Characteristics of Four Materials Types

	Metallic	Ceramic	Polymeric	Composite
Characters of chemical bonding	Metallic bonding	Ionic bonding	Covalent bonding within molecular chain	Physical mixture
	Delocalized electrons	Localized electrons	Localized electrons	
	Nondirectional	Nondirectional	Directional	
		Zero tolerance to wrong atomic neighboring	Rotational	
		Covalent bonding Localized electrons Directional	Secondary weak bonds between chains	
Typical properties	Conductive Tough Ductile and strong	Nonconductive Inert (corrosion resistant) Thermally stable Strong and hard	Nonconductive Inert Soft, flexible Plastic or elastic	Combination of component materials
Major problems	Corrosion	Brittle	Thermally unstable Oxidation (aging)	Expensive processing

1.6   CHAPTER HIGHLIGHTS

1. *Materials science* is the study of relationships between structures and properties. *Materials engineering* is all about designing and engineering materials' structures to produce desired properties via processing.
2. The structures at the atomic and molecular lattice levels determine properties and divide all materials into metallics, ceramics, or polymers.
3. Three common lattice (crystallographic) structures: FCC, BCC, and HCP (Figure 1.4).
4. Major characters of chemical bonds and representative properties of four materials types (Table 1.3).
5. *Biomaterial* is any biocompatible material, which is used to replace or assist part of an organ or its tissue, while in intimate contact with living tissue. *Biomedical material* represents a component of any biomedical device applied with or without intimate contact with living tissue. *Biological material* refers to a naturally occurring material.
6. No harm to the host body defines *biocompatibility*.

ACTIVITIES

1. Become familiar with the societies and organizations of materials science and engineering. http://guides.lib.udel.edu/content.php?pid=163409&sid=1730512.
2. Visit *American Society for Testing and Materials (ASTM)*: http://www.astm.org/.
3. Visit *ASM International*, formerly known as the American Society for Metals: http://www.asminternational.org/.

SIMPLE QUESTIONS IN CLASS

1. Which level of microstructure categorizes materials into metallic, ceramic, and polymer?
   a. Structure associated with grain size
   b. Length of molecular chains in materials
   c. Chemical bonding between atoms and/or molecules
   d. Microstructure associated with various defects
2. What is the most common issue associated with metallic materials?
   a. Corrosion
   b. Nonconductivity
   c. Brittleness
   d. Hardening
3. What is the most common issue associated with ceramic materials?
   a. Corrosion
   b. Nonconductivity
   c. Brittleness
   d. Hardening
4. What is the most common issue in the application of polymeric materials?
   a. Softness
   b. Nonconductivity
   c. Brittleness
   d. Oxidation
5. Which of the following descriptions is true for the definition of biocompatibility?
   a. The ability to heal an injured or diseased organ or tissue.
   b. The capacity to encourage damaged tissue to regenerate.
   c. It is not about therapeutic performance. A material is considered to be biocompatible, as long as it has no harm on the host body.
   d. Therapeutic function.
6. Which material in the following medical devices is a biomaterial in the scientific community of biomaterials?

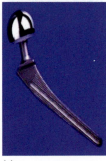
(a)

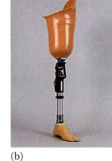
(b)

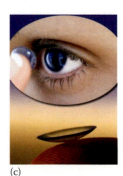
(c)

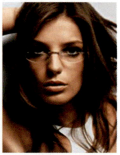
(d)

PROBLEMS AND EXERCISES

1. Describe the typical properties of metals, ceramics, and polymers and the common issue of each type of materials. Explain the structural mechanisms behind each common issue.

2. Calculate the atomic packing fraction (or called factor) of FCC, BCC, and HCP structures of pure metals.
3. What is a dislocation? List five more microscopic defects in bulk materials. Which of the following properties are most sensitive to dislocation structures in materials?
   a. Young's modulus
   b. Yield strength
   c. Conductivity
   d. Transparency
4. Discuss the following three questions:
   a. Why are door keys always made of metal, rather than ceramics or polymers?
   b. What properties of metals make them the choice of materials of door keys?
   c. Among many metals, why are copper alloys better than Fe-alloys for the application of keys? (Tip: you need to discuss this question from both materials science and economic points of view.)
5. Define biomaterials, biomedical materials, and biological materials.
6. Give two pairs of new examples (different from those used in Chapter 1) of materials used in medical devices, one of each pair being a biomaterial of interest to the biomaterials scientific community and the other nonbiomaterial but biomedical material. The two examples of each pair must be used in the treatments for the clinical issues of the same organs or tissues (e.g., contact lens and glasses). You are encouraged to search on the Internet, and you may use images to illustrate and refer to the figures with a short description.

BIBLIOGRAPHY

References

1. Von Recum, A.F., *Handbook of Biomaterials Evaluation: Scientific, Technical and Clinical Testing of Implant Materials*, 2nd edn. London, U.K.: Taylor & Francis, 1999.
2. Williams, D., *Definitions in Biomaterials: Proceedings of a Consensus Conference of the European Society for Biomaterials*, Chester, England, March 3–5, Elsevier, 1986.
3. D'Angelo, F., L. Murena, E. Vulcano, G. Zatti, and P. Cherubino, Seven to twelve year results with Versys ET cementless stem. A retrospective study of 225 cases. *Hip International*, 2010;**20**:81–86.

Websites

ASM International (formally known as American Society for Metals) is the society for materials scientists and engineers. http://www.asminternational.org/portal/site/www/.
http://www.pearson-studium.de/books/3827370597/cd01/Gallery/Images/Crystal.htm.
The Food and Drug Administration: Medical Devices http://www.fda.gov/MedicalDevices/default.htm.

Further Readings

Callister, W.D., *Materials Science and Engineering*, 7th edn. New York: John Wiley & Sons, Inc., 2007, Chapters 1–4.
Davis, J.R. (ed.), Chapter 1: Overview of biomaterials and their use in medical devices. In *Handbook of Materials for Medical Devices*. Materials Park, OH: ASM International, 2003.

Park, J. and R.S. Lakes, Chapter 1: Introduction. *Biomaterials: An Introduction*, 3rd edn. New York: Springer, 2007.

Ratner, B.D., A.S. Hoffman, F.J. Schoen, and J.E., Lemons. *Biomaterials Science: An Introduction to Materials in Medicine*, 2nd edn. London, U.K.: Elsevier Academic Press, 2004, Chapters 1–2.

Von Recum, A.F., *Handbook of Biomaterials Evaluation: Scientific, Technical and Clinical Testing of Implant Materials*, 2nd edn. London, U.K.: Taylor & Francis, 1999.

CHAPTER 2

TOXICITY AND CORROSION

LEARNING OBJECTIVES

After a careful study of this chapter, you should be able to do the following:

1. Describe the concept of trace elements and understand their biological roles and toxicities.
2. Predict the corrosion tendency of metals in body fluid using galvanic series.
3. Describe the corrosive nature of body fluid.
4. Read Pourbaix diagrams.
5. Predict the possible events when metals are immersed in the body fluid using galvanic series and Pourbaix diagrams.
6. Describe the strategies to minimize corrosion/toxicity of metallic implants in the body.

2.1   ELEMENTS IN THE BODY

As highlighted in Chapter 1, a biomaterial must be nontoxic to the host body. A simple strategy to be nontoxic is to be nonreactive under biological conditions (bioinert). In reality, no material is completely inert in a living body over a reasonable period of time. Sooner or later, ions or small molecules will be released from implants, introducing foreign body effects on the functional living (physiological) system. In the selection of nontoxic materials, an immediate thought may be those chemicals and elements naturally existing in the body. Hence, let us look at our body first.

Most of the human body is made up of water, H_2O, with cells containing 65–90 wt.% water. In a baby's body, there is approximately 75%–80% water. As an individual grows older, this percentage reduces to approximately 60%–65% for men and 50%–60% for women. Therefore, it is not surprising that most of a human body's mass is oxygen and carbon. A list of elements commonly found in the human body is given in Table 2.1. Approximately 96% of the weight of the body results from the elements oxygen, carbon, hydrogen, and nitrogen, which are the building blocks of both water

Table 2.1
Elements in the Human Body

Element	O	C	H	N	Ca	P	K	S	Na	Cl	Mg	Trace Element
Wt.%	65.0	18.5	9.5	3.3	1.5	1.0	0.4	0.3	0.2	0.2	0.1	<0.01
At.%	25.5	9.5	63.0	1.4	0.31	0.22	0.06	0.05	0.3	0.03	0.1	<0.01

and proteins. The rest (~4%) of the mass of the body exists largely either in bone and teeth as minerals (Ca, Mg, and P) or in blood and extracellular fluid as major electrolytes (Na, K, and Cl) (Table 2.2).

In addition, there are a number of elements that are needed in extremely low quantities (<0.01%) for the proper growth, development and physiology of the body. These elements are referred to as *trace elements* or *micronutrients*, a list that is continually increasing (Table 2.3).

Table 2.2
Macro Elements and Their Primary Roles in the Human Body

Macro Elements	Roles
O, C, H, N	In water and the molecular structures of proteins
Ca	Structure of bone and teeth; role in cell signaling, metabolism, tissue maintenance
P	Structure of bone and teeth. Required for ATP, the energy carrier in animals.
Mg	Important in bone structure. Deficiency results in tetany (muscle spasms) and can lead to a calcium deficiency.
Na	Major electrolyte of blood and extracellular fluid. Required for maintenance of pH and osmotic balance, nerve and muscle function.
K	Major electrolyte of blood and intracellular fluid. Required for maintenance of pH and osmotic balance, nerve and muscle function.
Cl	Major electrolyte of blood and extracellular and intracellular fluid. Required for maintenance of pH and osmotic balance.
S	Element of the essential amino acids methionine and cysteine. Contained in the vitamins thiamine and biotin. As part of glutathione, it is required for detoxification. Poor growth due to reduced protein synthesis and lower glutathione levels potentially increasing oxidative or xenobiotic damage are consequences of low sulfur and methionine and/or cysteine intake.

Table 2.3
List of Known Trace Elements in the Human Body[a]

Barium	Cobalt	Lithium	Strontium
Beryllium	Copper	Manganese	Tungsten
Boron	Iron	Molybdenum	Zinc
Caesium	Fluorine	Nickel	
Chromium	Iodine	Selenium	

[a] *These elements are all toxic at high levels.*

2.2   BIOLOGICAL ROLES AND TOXICITIES OF TRACE ELEMENTS

Trace elements are essential for the proper growth, development, and maintenance of the health and normal function of the body. Too little trace elements will result in diseases, even leading to morbidity and death. Figure 2.1 illustrates four trace-element-deficiency diseases: anemia, osteoporosis, thyroid imbalance, and premature graying of hair, which are due to deficiency in iron, boron, iodine, and copper, respectively. The primary biological functions of some trace elements are summarized in Table 2.4.

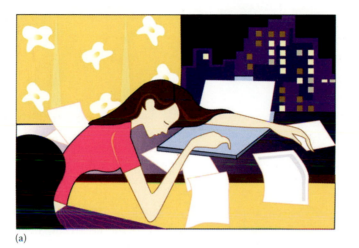

(a)

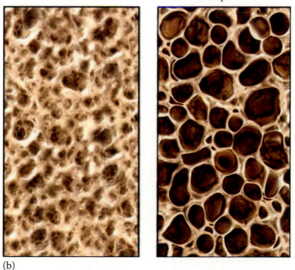

Normal bone   Osteoporosis

(b)

Figure 2.1
(a) Iron-deficiency anemia; (b) boron-deficiency osteoporosis;   *(Continued)*

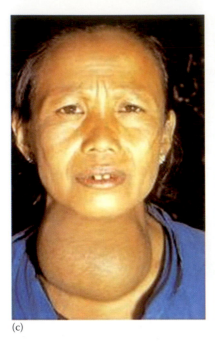
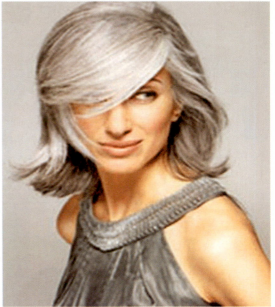

(c)   (d)

Figure 2.1 (Continued)
(c) thyroid gland enlargement caused by iodine deficiency; and (d) premature hair graying due to lack of copper.

However, an excessive level of any trace element in the body will cause adverse effects on its physiology. Nickel, chromium, and cobalt, for example, are a major cause of contact dermatitis. Table 2.5 lists the percentage of population who suffer from metal allergies.

The toxicity of nickel, chromium, and cobalt also causes internal diseases. Cobalt-containing dust, for example, caused lung diseases in workers of the metallurgical industry. In 1966, the addition of cobalt compounds to stabilize beer foam in Canada caused cardiomyopathy, which came to be known as beer drinker's cardiomyopathy. The carcinogenicity of chromate dust was known as early as 1890, when the first publication described the elevated cancer risk of workers in a chromate dye company. Table 2.6 lists the primary toxicities of some trace elements due to an excessive level. The nontoxicity (i.e., biocompatibility) of the pure metals used in metallic biomaterials and their alloys are compared in Figure 2.2.

In summary, many metal elements are required by the human body as micronutrients. However, it is also important to bear in mind that these trace elements are all toxic at levels higher than required, especially if they are not cleared properly.

2.3 SELECTION OF METALLIC ELEMENTS IN MEDICAL-GRADE ALLOYS

The toxicity of a metallic biomaterial stems from the toxicity of the released metal ions and associated compounds. In principle, nontoxic elements should be selected as alloying elements, when it comes to developing a new biomedical implant

Table 2.4
Some Trace Elements and Their Primary Roles in the Human Body

Trace Elements	Biological Roles	Trace-Element-Deficiency Diseases
Fe	Contained in heme groups of hemoglobin and myoglobin which are required for oxygen transport in the body, as well as many other metabolic enzymes and Fe-S proteins. Part of the cytochrome p450 family of enzymes.	Anemia is the primary consequence of iron deficiency.
Cu	Contained in enzymes of the ferroxidase system which regulates iron transport in the blood and facilitates release from storage.	Copper deficiency can result in anemia and premature hair graying.
Mn	Major component of the mitochondrial antioxidant enzyme manganese superoxide dismutase.	Manganese deficiency can lead to improper bone formation and reproductive disorders.
I	Required for production of thyroxine which plays an important role in metabolic rate.	Deficient iodine intake can cause goiter, an enlarged thyroid gland.
Zn	Important for reproductive function due to its role in FSH (follicle stimulating hormone) and LH (leutinizing hormone). Important in prostate gland health.	Zinc deficiency can lead to diarrhea, wasting of body tissues and anorexia.
Se	Contained in the antioxidant enzyme glutathione peroxidase and heme oxidase.	Human deficiency causes cardiomyopathy and is known as Keshan's disease.
Co	Contained in vitamin B_{12}.	Cobalt deficiency can lead to vitamin B_{12} deficiency with anemia.
Mo	Contained in the enzyme xanthine oxidase. Required for the excretion of nitrogen in uric acid in birds.	Molybdenum deficiency, a rare human disease, can lead to accumulation of toxic levels of sulfite and neurological damage.
Cr	A cofactor in the regulation of sugar levels.	Chromium deficiency may cause hyperglycemia (elevated blood sugar) and glucosuria (glucose in the urine).
F	Bones and teeth, with apatites.	Dental problems if not enough.

Table 2.5
Metal Sensitivity

	Percent Metal-Sensitive (%)
General population	10
Patients with stable total joint replacements	25
Patients with loose total joint replacements	60

Table 2.6

Toxicities of Some Trace Elements in the Human Body

Trace Elements	Toxicities
Fe	Excess iron levels can enlarge the liver, may provoke diabetes and cardiac failure. The genetic disease hemochromatosis results from excess iron absorption. Similar symptoms can be produced through excessive transfusions required for the treatment of other diseases.
Cu	Excess copper levels cause liver malfunction and are associated with genetic disorder Wilson's disease.
Mn	An excess of manganese can lead to poor iron absorption.
I	Excessive iodine intake can cause goiter (an enlarged thyroid gland).
Zn	An excess of zinc may cause anemia or reduced bone formation.
Se	An excess of selenium can lead to selenosis.
Co	An excess may cause cardiac failure.
Mo	An excess can cause diarrhea and growth reduction.
Cr	Elevated levels of some forms of chromium, such as Cr(VI), can be carcinogenic.
F	Bone brittleness and increased risk of fracture.

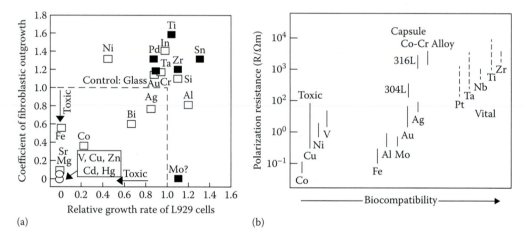

Figure 2.2

(a) Cytotoxicity of some pure metals. (b) The relationship between polarization resistance and biocompatibility of pure metals, cobalt–chromium alloy, and stainless steels.

material. It follows that materials using elements that naturally occur in the body are likely to be more compatible than elements naturally excluded by the body. Hence, trace elements including Fe, Co, Mo, Cr, Zn, Mn, and W should be given priority in the selection of alloy elements. However, trace elements are all toxic at levels higher than required. As such, their use must be combined with high corrosion resistance design.

Nonetheless, there are also a number of metal elements that are virtually nontoxic, with unknown biological roles in the body. The excellent biocompatibility of these elements, which include Zr, Ti, Nb, Ta, Pt, Ag, and Au, is due to their high stability (i.e., superb resistance to corrosion) in physiological environments. Hence, these elements are also frequently used in medical-grade, especially titanium-based, alloys. Since the 1990s, an increasing number of new metallic implant materials have been developed using these inert elements, such as β-titanium (Ti-Mo-Zr-Fe) and magnesium (Mg-Nd-Zn-Zr) alloys.

In short, chemical impacts (i.e., systemic toxicity) of a metallic material on the host body are directly determined by its corrosion resistance. Hence, improving the biocompatibility of metallic biomaterials is best achieved by the minimization of corrosion. The rest of this chapter is devoted to the corrosion behaviors of metals and the strategies to minimize corrosion (and thus toxicity) of implant biomaterials.

2.4 CORROSION OF METALS

2.4.1 Why Do Metals Corrode?

The lowest free energy state of many metals in an oxygenated and hydrated environment is in the form of a metal oxide, which is the natural state of elements in ores. After a series of processing steps (Figure 2.3), the metal elements in final products are no longer in the lowest free energy state. During the service of a metallic implant, which is typically in an oxygenated and hydrated environment, metal elements will always tend to revert to their natural form as ores, a process called *corrosion*.

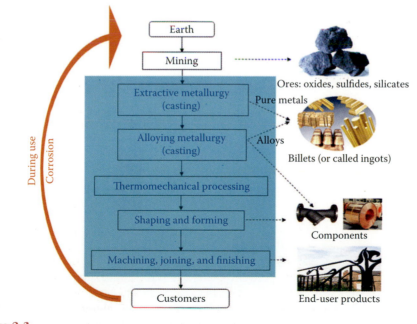

Figure 2.3
Processing of metals.

2.4.2   Corrosion Tendencies of Dissimilar Metals: Electrode Potentials

Corrosion occurs when metal atoms give away electrons and become positive ions. The metal ions go into solution or combine with oxygen or other species in solution to form a compound that flakes off or dissolves. To reiterate, the ionization of metal atoms is the first step of corrosion.

Different atoms have different tendencies to be ionized. Assume we place a piece of magnesium and copper in a beaker of pure water (Figure 2.4). With the magnesium plate, the magnesium atoms will tend to shed electrons and go into solution as magnesium ions, and the electrons will be left behind on the magnesium. The negatively charged magnesium will be closely surrounded by a layer of positive ions in the solution. Concurrently, some of magnesium ions could reclaim their electrons and reattach to the metal. A dynamic equilibrium will be established when the rate at which ions leave the surface is exactly equal to the rate at which they join it again. At the equilibrium state, there will be a constant negative charge on the magnesium, and a constant number of magnesium ions present in the solution around it. The same process will happen with the copper plate as well. However, copper is less reactive than magnesium and has a lesser tendency to release ions. At an equilibrium state, there will be less charge on the copper, and fewer copper ions in solution. Hence, at the equilibrium state, the magnesium plate will be more negatively charged than the copper one.

The difference in electric potentials across a metal/solution interface is commonly referred to as an *electrode potential*. Theoretically, the electrode potential can be measured as voltage and used to indicate the tendency of electrons to flow away, that is, the tendency of the metal to be ionized. Unfortunately, that voltage, that is, the *absolute* value of electrode potential, is impossible to measure. Practically, we measure the *relative* electrode potential. That is, we measure the electrode potential versus a standard reference electrode. The hydrogen electrode is universally accepted as the primary standard, against which all electrode potentials are compared in their standard states, which is unit activity (~1 M) for ions and 1 atm pressure for gases at 25°C. Under these standard conditions, the electrode potential of hydrogen is arbitrarily defined as $E^0 = 0.000$ V. In addition to this standard hydrogen electrode (SHE), saturated calomel electrode (SCE) is another widely used reference electrode, based on mercury.

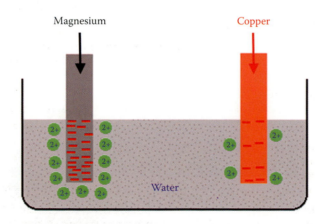

Figure 2.4
Electrical double layer (EDL) around metals in pure water, showing that an electrode potential exits across the metal/solution interface.

By measuring electrode potentials relative to the SHE, a series of (relative) standard electrode potentials have been measured for metals immersed in their own ions at unit activity (Table 2.7). This standard electrode potential series is also known as the standard electrochemical series or the *electromotive force series* (emf). The electrode potential series defines the corrodibility of metals. The lower the standard electrode potential value of a metal, the higher is the corrosion tendency of that metal. In another words, metals near the top of the emf series are less prone to corrosion. Metals located near the positive end of the emf series are referred to as "noble" metals, while metals near the negative end of the emf scale are called "active" metals.

Table 2.7
Standard Electrode Potentials at 25°C

Reaction	E^0 (V vs. SHE)
$Au^{3+} + 3e^- \rightarrow Au$	+1.498 noble
$Pt^{2+} + 2e^- \rightarrow Pt$	+1.18 ↑
$Pd^{2+} + 2e^- \rightarrow Pd$	+0.951
$Hg^{2+} + 2e^- \rightarrow Hg$	+0.851
$Ag^+ + e^- \rightarrow Ag$	+0.800
$Cu^+ + e^- \rightarrow Cu$	+0.521
$Cu^{2+} + 2e^- \rightarrow Cu$	+0.342
$2H^+ + 2e^- \rightarrow H_2$	0.000
$Pb^{2+} + 2e^- \rightarrow Pb$	−0.126
$Sn^{2+} + 2e^- \rightarrow Sn$	−0.138
$Mo^{3+} + 3e^- \rightarrow Mo$	−0.200
$Ni^{2+} + 2e^- \rightarrow Ni$	−0.257
$Co^{2+} + 2e^- \rightarrow Co$	−0.28
$Cd^{2+} + 2e^- \rightarrow Cd$	−0.403
$Fe^{2+} + 2e^- \rightarrow Fe$	−0.447
$Ga^{3+} + 3e^- \rightarrow Ga$	−0.549
$Ta^{3+} + 3e^- \rightarrow Ta$	−0.6
$Cr^{3+} + 3e^- \rightarrow Cr$	−0.744
$Zn^{2+} + 2e^- \rightarrow Zn$	−0.762
$Nb^{3+} + 3e^- \rightarrow Nb$	−1.100
$Mn^{2+} + 2e^- \rightarrow Mn$	−1.185
$Zr^{4+} + 4e^- \rightarrow Ze$	−1.45
$Hf^{4+} + 4e^- \rightarrow Hf$	−1.55
$Ti^{2+} + 2e^- \rightarrow Ti$	−1.630
$Al^{3+} + 3e^- \rightarrow Al$	−1.662
$U^{3+} + 3e^- \rightarrow U$	−1.798
$Be^{2+} + 2e^- \rightarrow Be$	−1.847
$Mg^{2+} + 2e^- \rightarrow Mg$	−2.372
$Na^+ + e^- \rightarrow Na$	−2.71
$Ca^{2+} + 2e^- \rightarrow Ca$	−2.868
$K^+ + e^- \rightarrow K$	−2.931 ↓
$Li^+ + e^- \rightarrow Li$	−3.040 active

Source: Vanysek, P., in *CRC Handbook of Chemistry and Physics*, D.R. Lide, ed., CRC Press, Boca Raton, FL, 2001, pp. 8–21.

While appreciating the indicative role of standard electrode potentials, one must bear in mind the following limitations of the *emf* series [2]:

1. The emf series applies to pure metals in their own ions at unit activity. This set of conditions is important in the development of the concept of electrode potentials, but these conditions are quite restrictive and are not those found in most practical situations. Although the electrode potential for a metal immersed in a solution of its ions at concentrations other than unit activity can be calculated based on its standard electrode potential (at unit activity) by the Nernst equation, there is still the restriction in the emf series that the solution contains cations of only the metal of interest.
2. The relative ranking of metals in the emf series is not necessarily the same (and is usually not the same) in other aqueous solutions (such as physiological fluids, seawater, groundwater, sulfuric acid). Thus, the emf series cannot be used reliably to predict the corrosion tendencies of coupled metals in other environments.
3. The emf series applies to pure metals only and not to metallic alloys.
4. The relative ranking of metals in the emf series gives corrosion tendencies (subject to the restrictions mentioned earlier) but provides no information on corrosion rates.

Any metal or alloy placed in a corrosive environment has its own electrode potential, called the *corrosion potential* E_{corr}. The *galvanic series* (in seawater) is an ordered listing of experimentally measured corrosion potentials in natural seawater for both pure metals and alloys. Note that the electrode potentials in the galvanic series in Figure 2.5 are measured relative to a saturated calomel electrode (SCE), whereas standard electrode potentials are always referred to as the standard hydrogen electrode (SHE). The conversion between the electrode potentials measured against the two reference electrodes is given by the following:

$$E \text{ vs. SHE} = E \text{ vs. SCE} + 0.242 \tag{2.1}$$

In principle, the galvanic series for seawater should not be used to predict corrosion tendencies in solutions that vary in composition, such as HCl solution, which is strongly acid. The use of the galvanic series in seawater is more appropriate for similar aqueous solutions, in terms of acidity and ionic species. For instance, the galvanic series in seawater may be applied (with some caution) to the behavior of metals and alloys used for joint replacements in the human body [2]. This is because a commonly used simulated physiological fluid known as Ringer's solution contains a mixture of dissolved NaCl, KCl, and $CaCl_2$ (~0.12 M sodium/0.13 M chlorides). Thus, body fluids and Ringer's solution can be considered a dilute version of seawater (~0.54 M sodium, 0.47 M chlorides). So, the galvanic series for seawater can be used as a first approximation, although data in Ringer's solution itself should be used if available. As per the standard electrode potential series, any galvanic series gives no information about corrosion rates, but only about corrosion tendencies [2].

2.4.3   Factors Affecting Electrode Potentials

Actual electrode potentials are affected by several variables including (1) the nature of the metal, (2) the chemical nature of the aqueous solution, (3) the presence of oxide

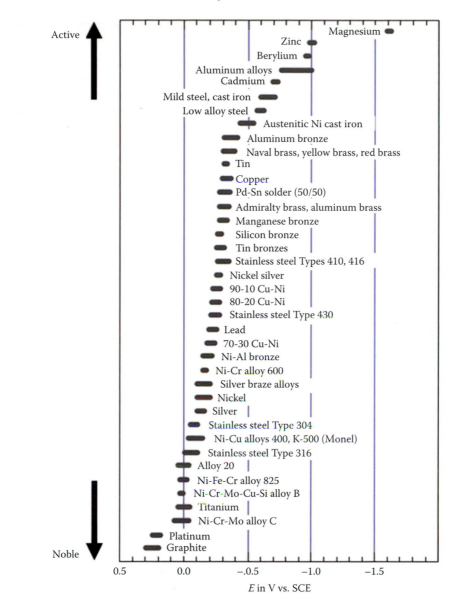

Figure 2.5

The galvanic series in seawater. (Redrawn from LaQue, F.L.: Marine Corrosion, Chapter 6. 1975. Copyright Wiley-VCH Verlag GmbH & Co. KGaA, New York. Reproduced with permission.)

films on the metal surface, (4) the presence of adsorbed gases on the metal surface, and (5) the presence of mechanical stress on the metal [3].

2.4.4 Galvanic Corrosion

When two dissimilar metals are immersed in an electrolyte and electrically connected, one metal corrodes preferentially to another, a process called Galvanic corrosion. In Galvanic corrosion, the anodic metal will have a higher corrosion rate in the couple than in the freely corroding (uncoupled) condition. Galvanic corrosion is usually not a desired occurrence. It can be minimized by the following methods [5]:

1. Select combinations of metals as near to each other as possible in the galvanic series.
2. Insulate the contact between dissimilar metals whenever possible.
3. Apply organic coatings, but coat both members of the couple or coat only the cathode. Do not coat only the anode, because if a defect (holiday) develops in the organic coating, an accelerated attack will occur because of the unfavorable effect of a small anode area and a large cathode area.
4. Avoid the unfavorable area effect of having a small anode coupled to a large cathode.
5. Install a third metal which is anodic to both metals in the galvanic couple ("sacrificial" anode).

2.4.5 Corrosion Possibility of a Metal under Different Conditions: Pourbaix Diagrams

In the freely corroding (uncoupled) condition, corrosion possibility of a metal can be predicted by its thermodynamically stable state under specific *electric potential* applied on the metal and the pH value of the environment. Note: the actual electric potential of a metal is not necessarily its electrode potential, as you can apply an electric potential to a metal using an external electric power supply.

To illustrate the stable (equilibrium) states for a given metal at various conditions of electric potential and pH, Marcel Pourbaix developed a useful potential–pH diagram, called a Pourbaix diagram (Figures 2.6 and 2.7). Pourbaix diagrams are phase diagrams for corrosion scientists, to illustrate all possible equilibrium (i.e., stable) states of a metal element over the entire range of pH and electric potential values in an aqueous environment. More specifically, these diagrams indicate certain regions of potential and pH where the metal undergoes corrosion, and other regions of potential and pH where the metal is protected from corrosion. Pourbaix diagrams are available for over 70 different metals [6].

Pourbaix diagrams are typically produced for standard conditions, that is, room temperature (25°C) and 1 atm. For the construction of a Pourbaix diagram, students can refer to the textbooks and websites provided on the reading list for this chapter. The goal of this section is to learn how to read a Pourbaix diagram, which you will practice as a biomaterial engineer.

In a Pourbaix diagram, the horizontal axis is the pH value of the aqueous environment, and the vertical axis is the equilibrium electric potential applied on the metal. Figure 2.6 is the Pourbaix diagram of water, and the meanings of the two lines (a) and (b), and three regions are summarized below the figure. These basic oxidation/reduction reactions for aqueous systems can be superimposed on a Pourbaix diagram of a metal, together showing under what conditions a metal will corrode. Figure 2.7a is the Pourbaix diagram of copper superimposed by the water reactions. Figure 2.7b illustrates three featured regions of the copper Pourbaix diagram: corrosion, passivation, and immunity. In the blue or gray regions, Cu^{2+} or CuO_2^{2+} ions are stable respectively, which means that copper tends to form soluble ions, that is, tends to corrode, under the conditions of these two regions. In the yellow region, a thin oxide or hydroxide layer forms on the copper surface, which can protect the metal from anodic dissolution.

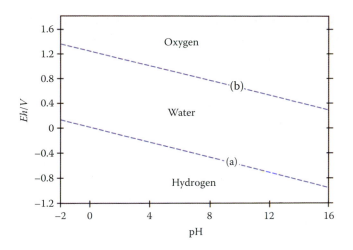

Figure 2.6
Pourbaix diagram of water.
Two lines:
Below line (a)—water is unstable and must decompose to H_2
Above line (a)—water is stable and any H_2 present is oxidized to H^+ or H_2O
Above line (b)—water is unstable and must oxidize to give O_2
Below line (b)—water is stable and any dissolved O_2 is reduced to H_2O
Three regions:
Upper: H_2O electrolyzed anodically to O_2
Lower: H_2O electrolyzed cathodically to H_2
Middle: H_2O stable and will not decompose

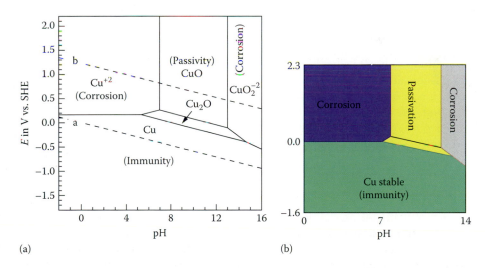

(a)   (b)

Figure 2.7
Pourbaix diagram of copper. (a) The Pourbaix diagram of copper superimposed by diagram for water. (b) Three regions: corrosion, passivation, and immunity. (From the WikimediaCommons, http://commons.wikimedia.org/.)
In regions where
- *Cu^{2+} or CuO_2^{2-} ion is stable, corrosion is possible*
- *Copper oxide Cu_2O or copper hydroxide $Cu(OH)_2$ is stable, passivity is possible*
- *Cu is stable, thermodynamically immune to corrosion*

39

Table 2.8
How to Read a Pourbaix Diagram

	Interpretations
Vertical lines	Separate species that are in acid/alkali equilibrium
Nonvertical lines	Separate species at redox equilibrium
Horizontal lines	Separate redox equilibrium species not involving hydrogen or hydroxide ions
Diagonal lines	Separate redox equilibrium species involving hydrogen or hydroxide ions
Dashed lines	Enclose the practical region of stability of the aqueous solvent to oxidation or reduction, i.e., the region of interest in aqueous systems; outside this region, it is the water that breaks down, not the metal
Redox equilibria	Where oxidation and reduction could equally occur and are completely reversible
Any point of the diagram	The most thermodynamically stable form of the metal can be found for any given potential and pH

This process is called passivation. However, oxide will itself also corrode under certain conditions. In the green region, the copper atom itself is stable, which means that copper is immune from any forms of corrosion under the conditions of the green region. More reading details are summarized in Table 2.8.

Figure 2.8 demonstrates four Pourbaix diagrams of metals, including silver (Ag), iron (Fe), copper (Cu), and titanium (Ti). When no external electric potential is applied to a metal, as in the scenario of a metallic implant in the body (fluid), the working conditions of the metal are the *corrosion potential E_{corr}* of the metal in the body fluid and the pH value of the body. For the electric potential, we use the corrosion potential E_{corr} in seawater as the first approximation (Figure 2.5). As for pH value, the body fluids are nearly neutral, with pH value 7.2–7.4. However, the pH value of body fluid can vary in certain tissues, and change dramatically in tissue that has been injured or infected. In *a wound it can be as low as 3.5 due to severe inflammation. In an infected wound the pH can increase to 9.0.* Table 2.10 also gives a brief estimation of possible events of these four pure metals in the body, which reveals that iron would tend to corrode in a wound site due to severe inflammation. Silver is immune from corrosion, and titanium could be passivated.

Pourbaix diagrams provide a first guide as to the corrosion behavior of a given metal. Despite their usefulness, however, Pourbaix diagrams are subject to several important limitations, as follows [2]:

1. Equilibrium is assumed. (But in practical cases, the actual conditions may be far from equilibrium.)
2. Pourbaix diagrams give no information on actual corrosion rates.
3. Pourbaix diagrams apply to single elemental metals only and not to alloys.
4. Passivation is ascribed to all oxides or hydroxides, regardless of their actual protective properties. Corrosion may sometimes proceed by diffusion of ions through oxide films, a process which is ignored in the construction of the diagrams.
5. Pourbaix diagrams do not consider localized corrosion by chloride ions.
6. Conventional Pourbaix diagrams apply to a temperature of 25°C.

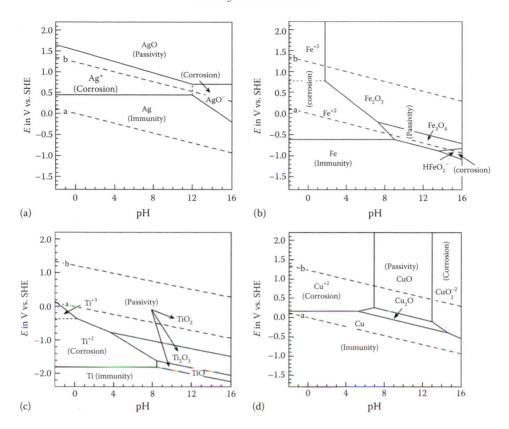

Figure 2.8
Pourbaix diagrams of silver (Ag), iron (Fe), titanium (Ti), and copper (Cu). (a) E_{corr} = −0.12 V (SCE) = 0.122 V (SHE). When pH = 3.5, 7.4 or 9.0, Ag is stable. Immunity is possible. (b) E_{corr} = −0.466 V (SCE) = −0.224 V (SHE) [7], when pH = 3.5 or 7.4, Fe^{+2} is stable, Corrosion is possible; when pH = 9.0, Fe_2O_3 is stable, Passivity is possible. (c) E_{corr} = 0 V (SCE) = 0.242 V (SHE), when pH = 3.5, 7.4 or 9.0, TiO_2 is stable, Passivity is possible. (d) E_{corr} = −0.3 V (SCE) = −0.058 V (SHE), when pH = 3.5 or 7.4, Cu is stable, Immunity is possible. When pH = 9.0, Cu_2O is stable, Passivity is possible.

2.5 ENVIRONMENT INSIDE THE BODY

To thoroughly understand the corrosion behaviors of metallic implants, we must first look at the nature of aqueous conditions within the tissue. Inside the human body, the environment is physically and chemically different from the ambient environment. Consequently, a metal that performs well (is inert or passive) in the air may suffer a severe corrosion in the body. As a matter of fact, the most corrosion-resistant stainless steels typically cause chronic allergy and toxic reactions in the host body, which are only diagnosed after a sufficiently long time postimplantation.

Moreover, different parts of the body have different pH values and oxygen concentrations. An implant that performs well in one region of the body may suffer an unacceptable amount of corrosion in another, due to acidic erosion and oxidation. As mentioned before, these body fluids are nearly neutral, with pH value 7.2–7.4 at 37°C.

Table 2.9

Ionic Concentrations (mM) of Human Blood Plasma

Ion	Human Tissue Fluid	Human Blood Plasma
Na^+	142.0	142.0
HCO_3^-	4.2	27.0
K^+	5.0	5.0
HPO_4^{2-}	1.0	1.0
Mg^{2+}	1.5	1.5
Cl^-	147.8	103.0
Ca^{2+}	2.5	2.5
SO_4^{2-}	0.5	0.5

However, the pH value of body fluid can vary in pH during normal and healing states (e.g. uninjured skin is slightly acidic).

Corrosion is also accelerated by aqueous ions, as commonly seen for metals in ambient air near coastal areas. Under normal conditions, most human body fluids contain around 0.9% saline, solutions of mostly Na^+, Cl^-, and other trace ions (Table 2.9), as well as amino acids and a range of soluble proteins. There is also trace debris and cellular material that can result in focal adhesions onto implants. Combined with fluctuations in ionic strength in relation to high blood pressure, or due to ion deposits, the human body presents an aggressive and variable environment for any implant.

Furthermore, the internal partial pressure of oxygen is about one quarter of atmospheric oxygen pressure. While less reactive in terms of oxidation, lower oxygen actually accelerates corrosion of metallic implants by slowing down the formation of protective passive oxide films on the metal surfaces once an implant is broken or removed. Ideally, corrosion resistance should be such that the release of metal ions from a metallic implant will be minimized in the harshest conditions of the body, and remain at a satisfactorily low level over a long service period (more than 30 years) under normal physiological conditions.

2.6 MINIMIZATION OF TOXICITY OF METAL IMPLANTS

The minimization of toxicity of metallic implants involves alloy design, galvanic corrosion control, and careful surgical procedure. These are summarized in Table 2.10.

Table 2.10

Strategies to Minimize Toxicities of Metallic Implants

1. Select corrosion-resistant materials
   - Use appropriate metals (inert or trace elements of the body).
   - Design alloys to minimize corrosion.
2. Avoid dissimilar metals
   - Avoid implantation of different types of metal in the same region.
   - In the manufacturing process, provide matched parts from the same batch of the same variant of a given alloy.
3. Avoid surface damage
   - In surgery avoid contact between metal tools and the implant, unless special care is taken.

2.7 CHAPTER HIGHLIGHTS

1. Most metal elements exist in the body as *trace elements*. Trace elements can be tolerated by the body in minute amounts, but cannot be tolerated in large amounts.
2. *Corrosion resistance* stands in the first place of consideration in the design of metallic biomaterials, in alignment with the requirement of nontoxicity of biomaterials.
3. The *galvanic series* for seawater can be used as a first approximation to predict corrosion tendencies of dissimilar metals in the body fluid.
4. Corrosion, passivity, and immunity regions of *Pourbaix diagrams*.
5. The body fluids are nearly neutral, with pH value 7.2–7.4. However, the pH value of body fluid can vary, especially in tissue that has been injured or infected. In a wound it can be as low as *3.5* due to severe inflammation. In an infected wound the pH can increase to *9.0*.
6. Strategies to minimize toxicities of metallic implants:
   - Select/design corrosion-resistant materials
   - Avoid using dissimilar metals in one implant
   - Avoid surface damage

LABORATORY PRACTICE 1

- Measure *corrosion potential* E_{corr} of Ti, Ti-6Al-4V, 316L stainless steel, and Mg in simulated body fluid and standard tissue culture medium.

SIMPLE QUESTIONS IN CLASS

1. "Biocompatible" means that a material
   a. Must biologically support and foster living tissues
   b. Must be biologically harmless
   c. Should be biologically nutritious to cells, tissue, or organs
   d. Bioactive
2. Which of the following elements is a trace element in the body?
   a. Hydrogen
   b. Magnesium
   c. Carbon
   d. Zinc
3. Are the following statements true (T) or false (F)?
   a. Since trace elements are native to the body, they are always more biocompatible than those that are nonnative.____
   b. Since trace elements are essential to maintain normal functions of the body, they can be used in medical devices without caution.____
   c. Most trace elements can be tolerated by the body in minute amounts, but cannot be tolerated in large amounts.____
   d. Elements that are nonnative to the body should not be considered in the development of any biomaterials.____

4. What is the first consideration in the design of new metallic biomaterials?
   a. Easy to process and thus low cost
   b. Mechanical properties
   c. Specific functional properties, such as transparency, conductivity, etc.
   d. Biocompatibility
5. Which of the following data can best predict the corrosion tendency of a series of metals in the body fluid?
   a. Corrosion potentials in tissue culture medium
   b. Standard electrode potential series
   c. Galvanic series
   d. Corrosion potentials in water
6. Which of the following strategies would not minimize corrosion of metallic implants?
   a. Use inert elements.
   b. Use metals of the passivation mechanism.
   c. Use the same alloys regardless of batches.
   d. Avoid surface damage.

PROBLEMS AND EXERCISES

1. The Pourbaix diagram of manganese is given in the following. Mark each zone with corrosion, passivation, or immunity.

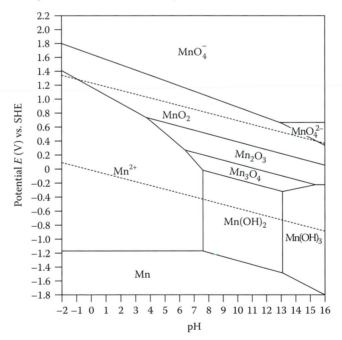

2. Fill the blanks in the following description:
   The pH value can change in tissue that has been injured or infected.
   a. Normal tissue fluid has a pH of about
   b. In a wound it can be as low as
   c. In an infected wound the pH can increase to

3. Search on the Internet (Google, PubMed, and Web of Science are recommended) and find the pH values of the following organs of the body:
   a. Stomach
   b. Lung
   c. Liver
   d. Small intestine
4. Search on the Internet (Google, PubMed, and Web of Science are recommended) for the electrode potential of Co or Co-based alloys in seawater. Use this electrode potential as the first approximation to predict the corrosion potential of Co in the body, based on the following Pourbaix diagram of Co. Analyze what could happen if a cobalt prosthesis is exposed to the aforementioned three anatomical environment in Exercise 3 and cite the reference properly.

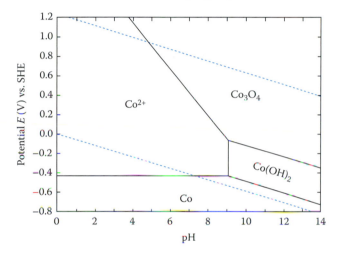

5. Read the corrosion potential of magnesium on Figure 2.5. The Pourbaix diagram of magnesium is given in the following. Analyze the corrosion tendency of this metal in normal body fluid.

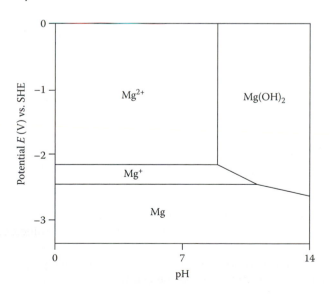

6. Compare the relative location of the following pairs of metals in the emf series and in the galvanic series for seawater.
   a. Zinc and chromium (use 316 stainless steels for chromium in the galvanic series for seawater)
   b. Platinum and titanium
   c. Nickel and silver
   d. Titanium and aluminum (use aluminum alloys for aluminum in the galvanic series for seawater)
   What does the relative position of these various pairs of metals tell you about the use of the emf series to predict possible galvanic corrosion in seawater?
7. Avoid surface damage of metallic implants is strongly advised to orthopedists in surgical operations. Explain the reason behind this clinical good practice.
8. What long-term toxic effects could be caused by the release of nickel and chromium ions?
9. Although magnesium is a macroelement in the body, what disease could be introduced by a long-term overdose of magnesium in the body?
10. Search on the Internet and identify at least two trace elements that are not included in Table 2.4. Describe their biological roles in maintaining health, and their toxicity if overdosed.

ADVANCED TOPIC: BIOLOGICAL ROLES OF ALLOYING ELEMENTS

Aluminum

Aluminum is a naturally abundant element but has little known function in the human body. Despite its acute toxicity only in very high doses, public awareness of chronic aluminum toxicity, especially its links to neurological problems [116], has increased, due to its use in domestic cookware.

Aluminum is involved in the causality of several diseases. By competing with calcium for absorption, increased amounts of dietary aluminum may contribute to the reduced skeletal mineralization (osteopenia) observed in infants. Aluminum is also associated with altered function of the blood–brain barrier [117] and brain neurotoxicity [118]. Like other metals, aluminum toxicity is also a major problem in people with kidney disease [119]. Aluminum intolerance also causes contact dermatitis, digestive disorders, vomiting, or other symptoms. There are concerns that excessive exposure to aluminum may increase the risk of breast cancer and Alzheimer's disease [120–122], although the use of aluminum cookware has not been shown to lead to aluminum toxicity in general and there is no scientific consensus regarding whether or not aluminum exposure could directly increase disease risk.

Calcium

Calcium is the most abundant mineral and mainly stored in bones and teeth. Other diverse biological roles in the human body include blood clotting and coactivation and stabilization of enzymes [139–141]. Compared with other metals, the calcium ion and its compounds have very low toxicity. This is not surprising given the high natural abundance of calcium compounds in the body. Calcium poses few serious clinical problems, with kidney stones being the most common side effect, and local tissue calcification sometimes occurring around dead or dying tissue. Acute calcium poisoning is rare, although excessive consumption of calcium carbonate supplements can potentially cause renal failure [142,143]. Consumption of more than 10 g/day of $CaCO_3$ (= 4 g Ca) raises the risk of developing milk–alkali syndrome [144].

Chromium

Chromium in the Body as a Trace Element   Chromium is a member of the transition metals in group 6, having an electronic configuration of $4s^13d^5$. As a trace element, chromium is a cofactor in the regulation of sugar levels in blood. Chromium deficiency may cause hyperglycemia (elevated blood sugar) and glucosuria (glucose in the urine). Hence, chromium concentrations in blood, plasma, serum, or urine may be measured to monitor for safety in exposed individuals [8–10].

Toxicity of Chromium   Among a range of possible oxidation states of chromium, the Cr^{3+} and Cr^{6+} states are the most common forms, with the toxicity depending on the oxidation state of the metal. Water-insoluble trivalent chromium (III) compounds and chromium metal are not classified to be a health hazard, while the toxicity and carcinogenic properties of hexavalent chromium (VI) have been well documented [11–13]. The carcinogenicity of chromate dust was known as early as 1890, when the first publication described the elevated cancer risk of workers in a chromate dye company [14–16]. Chromium salts (chromates), which are often used to manufacture leather products, paints, cement, mortar, and anticorrosives, are also the cause of allergic reactions in some workers. Contact with products containing chromates can lead to allergic contact dermatitis and irritant dermatitis, resulting in ulceration of the skin (chrome ulcers) [17,18]. This skin disease is often found in workers that have been exposed to strong chromate solutions in electroplating, tanning, and chrome-producing manufacturers [19–21]. An actual litigation conducted in 2009 on hexavalent chromium release into drinking water was used as the plot of 2010 biographical film *Erin Brockovich*.

Chromium, as well as nickel, is received into the body via the lungs [22], oral intake [23], skin contact [13], and implants [8]. In the body, chromium (VI) is reduced to chromium (III) in the blood before it enters the cells. The chromium (III) is excreted from the body via urine. In vitro studies have indicated that high concentrations of chromium (III) in the cell can lead to DNA damage [24–27]. The acute toxicity of chromium (VI) is due to its strong oxidative properties. After it reaches the bloodstream, it damages the kidneys, liver, and blood cells through oxidation reactions, resulting in hemolysis, which causes renal and liver failure [11,12]. The lethal dose for chromium (VI) ranges between 50 and 150 mg/kg [28]. The World Health Organization–recommended maximum chromium (VI) is 0.05 mg/L [29–31].

Cobalt

Cobalt in the Body as a Trace Element   Cobalt is an essential trace element found principally in the maturation of human and animal red blood cells as a constituent of vitamin B_{12} (cyanocobalamin). Vitamin B_{12} exists with two types of alkyl ligand: methyl and adenosyl. *Methylcobalamin* promotes methionine synthesis. Methionine supply ultimately influences DNA synthesis [73]. *Deoxyadenosylcobalamin* performs a key role in the energy metabolism of ruminants by facilitating the metabolism of propionate, which is an important precursor of glucose in ruminants [74]. Changes in lipid [75] and amino acid metabolism [76] during cobalt deficiency have been reported. In short, vitamin B_{12} plays a critical role in the extraction of energy from proteins and fats. Cobalt deficiency causes metabolic deficiencies and poor conception rates.

Toxicity of Cobalt   Being an essential trace element, cobalt can also cause serious adverse health effects at high exposure levels [77,78]. Like chromium and nickel, cobalt is received into the body via the lungs, oral intake, by skin contact, and from implant release products. The median lethal dose (LD_{50}) value for soluble cobalt salts has been estimated to be between 150 and 500 mg/kg. Hence, for a 100 kg person, the LD_{50} would be about 20 g [79,80]. In 1966, the addition of cobalt compounds to stabilize beer foam in Canada caused cardiomyopathy, which came to be known as beer drinker's cardiomyopathy [81]. After nickel and chromium, cobalt is a major cause of contact dermatitis [82]. The toxicity of cobalt-containing dust also caused interstitial lung disease in workers of the metallurgical industry [83].

   With hip replacements made of cobalt alloys, there is in general a local release of metallic particles, and in some individuals there is a hypersensitivity reaction that causes more severe damage to the tissues in the immediate vicinity of the prosthesis [84]. Cobalt toxicity has been reported to contribute to the pathology of systemic and neurological symptoms in some patients with metal-on-metal hip prostheses after 4–5 years of implantation [85]. The symptoms include painful muscle fatigue and cramping, dyspnea, inability to perform simple motor tasks, decline in cognitive function, memory difficulties, severe headaches, and anorexia [85]. It has been recommended that health care providers other than orthopedic specialists be aware that patients with a cobalt implant are at risk for cobalt poisoning, and might present with cardiac or some of the listed neurologic symptoms [77,78,86].

Copper

Copper is another essential trace element present in human and animal tissue [146,149]. The human body contains copper at a level of about 1–3 mg/kg of body mass [150,151]. Copper is absorbed in the gut and then transported to the liver [152,153]. After processing in the liver, copper is distributed to other tissues. Copper is mainly carried by ceruloplasmin in blood. Copper is absorbed in the body normally about 1 mg/day in the diet and excreted from the body, with some ability to excrete some excess copper via bile, which carries extra copper out of the liver [154]. Excessive copper levels in the body have been linked to neurodegenerative diseases including Alzheimer's, Menkes, and Wilson's diseases [155]. Studies have revealed that serum levels with either high copper and low magnesium or concomitance of low zinc with either high copper or low magnesium can both increase the mortality risk for middle-aged men [156].

Iron

Iron in the Body as a Trace Element   Iron is a necessary trace element found in almost all living organisms, ranging from primitive bacteria to humans. Iron is present in all cells in the human body, and has several vital functions. Many cellular enzymes vital to life contain iron, such as those that oxidize food nutrients to produce energy [1]. Iron is also an essential component of hemoglobin, an iron-containing protein in blood that binds and carries oxygen to the tissues from the lungs. Iron is absorbed into the body via oral intake, and its deficiency is one of the most common nutritional deficiencies. Too little iron can interfere with these vital functions and lead to morbidity and death. The direct consequence of iron deficiency is iron-deficiency anemia [2].

Toxicity of Iron   Large amounts of iron released from metallic implants can cause excessive levels of iron in the blood. High blood levels of free ferrous iron react with peroxides to produce free radicals, which are highly reactive and can damage DNA, proteins, lipids, and other cellular components. Iron typically damages cells in the heart and liver, which can cause significant adverse effects, including coma, metabolic acidosis, shock, liver failure, adult respiratory distress syndrome, long-term organ damage, and even death if left untreated [3–5]. Iron accumulates in the brain of those with Alzheimer's and Parkinson's diseases [6]. Humans experience iron toxicity above 20 mg of iron/kg of body mass, and 60 mg/kg is considered a lethal dose [7].

Magnesium

Magnesium is needed for more than 300 biochemical reactions in the body. At the biochemical level, magnesium is involved in energy metabolism and protein synthesis, maintains normal muscle and nerve function, supports a healthy immune system, and keeps bones strong. Magnesium also helps regulate blood sugar levels and promotes normal blood pressure, playing important roles in preventing and managing disorders such as hypertension, cardiovascular disease, and diabetes [135,136]. Dietary magnesium is absorbed in the small intestines and is excreted through the kidneys [135,136]. The kidneys are efficient at excreting excess magnesium and it is unlikely that the mineral will accumulate to toxic levels, although there is a risk of renal dysfunction with an overdose of magnesium. A high intake of magnesium can compete with calcium, and lead to impairment of its absorption [137]. Symptoms of magnesium overload include diarrhea, difficulty breathing and depression of the central nervous system, causing muscle weakness, lethargy, sleepiness, or even hyperexcitability [138].

Manganese

Manganese is an essential trace mineral, which plays a number of roles in cellular systems as cofactors for metalloenzymes, including oxidases and dehydrogenases, DNA and RNA polymerases, kinases, decarboxylases, and sugar transferases [145,146]. In humans, excessive exposure to Mn has been reported to induce "Manganism," which is a neurological disorder similar to Parkinson's disease [147,148].

Molybdenum

Molybdenum in the Body as a Trace Element   Molybdenum is an essential trace element for a number of enzymes important to cellular metabolism. The most important enzymes that require molybdenum are sulfite oxidase, xanthine oxidase, and aldehyde oxidase. Sulfite oxidase catalyzes the oxidation of sulfite to sulfate, necessary for metabolism of sulfur amino acids. Sulfite oxidase deficiency or absence leads to neurological symptoms and early death. Xanthine oxidase catalyzes oxidative hydroxylation of purines and pyridines, including conversion of hypoxanthine to uric acid. Aldehyde oxidase oxidizes purines, pyrimidines, and pteridines, and is also involved in nicotinic acid metabolism. Low dietary molybdenum leads to low urinary and serum uric acid concentrations and excessive xanthine excretion [87].

The human body contains about 0.07 mg of molybdenum per kilogram of weight [88], with higher concentrations occurring in the liver and kidneys, and lower concentrations in the vertebrae. Molybdenum is also present within human tooth enamel and may help prevent its decay [89]. Dietary molybdenum deficiency has been associated with increased rates of esophageal cancer in a geographical band from China to Iran [90], possibly due to low soil levels that end up in crops. Compared to the United States, which has a greater supply of molybdenum in the soil, people living in deficient areas have about 16 times greater risk for esophageal squamous cell carcinoma [90].

Toxicity of Molybdenum Molybdenum is much less toxic than many other metals (e.g., Co, Cr, and Ni) of industrial importance. Molybdenum does not constitute a hazard to human beings either in trace concentrations occurring naturally, because of environmental pollution, or from exposure to higher concentrations encountered in industrial processes and applications [87,91,92]. Nevertheless, molybdenum dusts and fumes generated by mining or metal working can be toxic with chronic exposure. Low levels of prolonged exposure can cause irritation to the eyes and skin. Direct inhalation or ingestion of molybdenum and its oxides should be avoided. Hence, precautions are recommended to avoid repeated exposure of humans to molybdenum compounds, especially in dusts and fumes of molybdenum metal and molybdenum trioxide powders [91,93,94].

Acute toxicity has not been reported in humans, such as accidental deaths due to molybdenum poisoning in industry. However, studies on rats show a median lethal dose (LD_{50}) as low as 180 mg/kg for some molybdenum compounds. There is virtually no chronic toxicity data for molybdenum in humans, but animal studies have shown that chronic ingestion of more than 10 mg/day of molybdenum can cause diarrhea, growth retardation, infertility, low birth weight, and gout, also affecting the lungs, kidneys, and liver [91,95]. Chronic exposure to molybdenum and its compounds is blamed for some symptoms including fatigue, headaches, and joint pains [91,94,96].

Studies on the concentrations of chromium, cobalt, and molybdenum in patients with metal-on-metal total hip replacement and hip resurfacing arthroplasty showed that the level of molybdenum in serum is generally low, compared with Cr and Ni [97,98]. So far, no data are reported on systemic toxicity of molybdenum, with regard to metallic implants.

Nickel

Nickel in the Body as a Trace Element The biological role of nickel as an essential trace element was recognized in the 1970s [32,33]. Nickel exists in urease, an enzyme that assists in the hydrolysis of urea. In blood, nickel is mainly bound to the albumin fraction, but also to some other proteins of serum [34]. Most of the nickel is eliminated into urine (90%). The concentrations of nickel in human tissues are estimated to be (mg/kg of dry weight): 173 in lung, 62 in kidney, 54 in heart, 50 in liver, 44 in brain, 37 in spleen, and 34 in pancreas [35].

Nickel deficiency has been found to have a number of deleterious effects and result in pathological consequences in goats, rats, and chicks, including reduced growth, weight loss, increased perinatal mortality [36], skin changes (pigmentation and parakeratosis), and uneven hair development [37]. Animals with nickel deficiency have been found to have impaired metabolism of iron, fats, glucose, and glycogen [38,39]. Nickel deficiency interferes with the incorporation of calcium into the skeleton and decreases the length/width ratios of chick tibias and femurs. It also suppresses the activity of enzymes in the heart, liver, and kidneys, leading to the degeneration of cardiac and skeletal muscle [37,38,40–43].

Toxicity and Carcinogenicity of Nickel   Similar to chromium, the toxicology of nickel was initially revealed by contact-allergy-related dermatitis, causing itchy and red skin due to its use in ear-piercing [44,45]. The amount of nickel allowed in products that come into contact with human skin is regulated by the European Union, and nickel has been previously recognized as one of the most important allergens by the American Contact Dermatitis Society [46]. In the United States, the minimal risk level of nickel and its compounds is set to 0.2 $\mu g/m^3$ for inhalation during 15–364 days [47,48]. Diseases caused by the toxicology of nickel include [49] acute pneumonitis from inhalation of nickel carbonyl [50], chronic rhinitis, and sinusitis from inhalation of nickel aerosols, cancers of nasal cavities and lungs in nickel workers, and [49] dermatitis and other hypersensitive reactions from cutaneous and parental exposures to nickel alloys [51].

The toxicity and carcinogenesis are related to certain nickel-containing compounds rather than pure Ni^{2+} ions. Nickel sulfide fume and dust are known to be carcinogenic [52]. Nickel carbonyl, $[Ni(CO)_4]$, is an extremely toxic gas. Inhaled Ni_3S_2 caused adenomas and carcinomas of the lungs in rats, but nickel oxide did not [53]. In the body, Ni^{2+} ions may cross the cell membrane using the Mg^{2+} ion transport mechanism. Once Ni^{2+} is inside the cell, it binds to cytoplasmic ligands and it does not accumulate in the cell nucleus at the concentrations needed to have a genetic effect [54,55]. In addition, soluble Ni^{2+} is rapidly cleared in the body. Hence, there is no direct efficient delivery of Ni^{2+} to the target site within the cell nucleus to cause carcinogenic effects in the body [53].

A mechanism by which a nickel compound may be harmful is due to its ability to cross cell membranes (endocytosis). Some of the characteristics of nickel compounds that increase their ability to be endocytosed include its crystalline nature, negative surface charge, 2–4 μm range particle size, and low solubility [56]. Ni_3S_2, which shows low solubility in vivo, may act by this mechanism [57]. When the nickel compound particles are endocytosed by target cells, the endocytic vesicles are acidified by fusion with lysosomes and Ni^{2+} is released. Deleterious changes, such as the formation of oxygen radicals and subsequent DNA damage can occur, a known mechanism for initiating tumorigenesis [58,59].

Experiments have shown that nickel is harmful to cultured bone cells, but to a lesser level than cobalt or vanadium [60]. Tests have shown cobalt, nickel, and chromium to have a potential for carcinogenicity [61]. Pure nickel implanted intramuscularly or inside bone has been found to cause severe local tissue irritation and necrosis [62,63]. Malignant fibrous histiocytomas or fibrosarcomas are also associated with the ability to retain nickel [64]. Released metal ions due to the corrosion of the implants can also migrate into distant organs, and are more readily able to cross cell membranes. Systemic toxicity may be caused by the accumulation, processing, and subsequent reaction of the host to corrosion products [65–67]. When high-dose nickel salts were injected into mice, accumulation of nickel was observed in the liver, kidney, and spleen, causing local deleterious effects [68]. Increased nickel concentrations have also been found in tissues adjacent to stainless steel implant materials (116 and 1200 mg/L) as well as in some distant organs [65,69]. Other factors, such as infection and mechanical damage (wearing/friction), may further encourage nickel release, raising the concentration retained local to the implant site [70–72].

Niobium

While niobium has little known biological roles in humans, some niobium-containing compounds are toxic, including niobates and niobium chloride, two chemicals that are water soluble [123]. One recent study actually found niobium to be one of the more toxic metal ions, along with cobalt, tested for their ability to induce DNA damage and cause immune cell death [124]. As more information becomes available, this element should be treated with care, especially when several alloying elements are used.

Silver

Silver has no known biological roles, and possible health effects of silver are a disputed subject [131–133]. Although silver itself is nontoxic, most silver salts are, and some may be carcinogenic [134]. Silver ions can bind to sulfur groups in intermolecular bonds in some biomolecules.

Tantalum

Pure tantalum has excellent resistance to corrosion in a large number of acids, most aqueous solutions of salts, organic chemicals, and in various combinations and mixtures of these agents. The corrosion resistance of tantalum is approximately the same as that of glass. Tantalum has no known biological role [125], and is nontoxic. Compounds containing tantalum are rarely encountered in the natural environment. Tantalum is among the most biocompatible metals used for implantable devices [126]. There is some evidence linking tantalum to local sarcomas [127] and toxicity of its oxide to alveolar cells.

Titanium

Titanium is not found in the human body, and does not play any known biological role in the human body [105], and is nontoxic even in large doses. When quantities of up to 0.8 mg of titanium were ingested by humans on a daily basis, most titanium was found to pass through without being digested or absorbed [106]. Titanium implants are not rejected by the body, and generally make good physical connections with the host bone. In vitro, titanium can however inhibit osteogenic differentiation of mesenchymal stem cells [107] and may cause genetic alterations in connective tissue [108]. Titanium particles also have size-specific biological effects on white blood cells in vivo [109].

Tungsten

Tungsten (atomic number 74) is chemically very similar to molybdenum (atomic number 42). However, the biological role of tungsten has only recently been discovered in prokaryotes, but not as yet in eukaryotes [99,100]. Tungsten is insoluble in water and only very slightly soluble in nitric and sulfuric acids. The toxicity of tungsten is very low; however, implantable materials made from this metal degrade very rapidly in the body, and remain in the serum, probably as tungsten particles [101]. Despite this, no ill-effects were observed in patients given 25–80 g powdered tungsten metal by mouth as a substitute for barium in radiological examinations [102]. Moreover, the fact that patients can rapidly recover both from seizures and renal failure while high levels of tungsten persisted for several weeks in the patient's serum and urine suggests that there was no causal relation between the tungsten and toxicity. The excretion of tungsten is very rapid with a biological half-life of a few hours for soft tissues [102]. Directly implanted tungsten also showed very low toxicity, even though significant levels could be detected after implantation [103]. While the potential health effects of tungsten remain to be fully defined, some researchers recommend caution [104].

Vanadium

Vanadium plays a less defined biological role in the human body [110,111], and can have both negative and positive cellular responses [109], with toxicity mainly from its compounds such as oxides [112]. Animal trials show that oral or inhalation exposures to vanadium and vanadium compounds result in cancer formation, and various adverse effects on the respiratory system, blood parameters, liver, neurological system, and other organs [113,114]. There is lack of reports on the toxicity of vanadium as alloying elements in Ti alloy implants, although a case study has suggested a possible link between vanadium release and failed implants [115].

Zinc

Zinc, as a trace mineral in the human body, is also essential for hundreds of biological enzymes, and transcription factors that are often coordinated with amino acids [157]. Zn is less detrimental than Mn, Al (see Advanced Topics and Chapter 5), and Cu, because Zn is readily absorbable by biological functions within the cell [157]. Like Ca, excessive amounts of Zn have the potential to be corrosive in nature if ingested [158]. In a biological system, zinc (Zn^{2+}) ions can form $ZnCl_2$, which has been shown to damage parietal cells lining the stomach.

Zirconium

Zirconium, which exists in the body at only 1 mg on average, does not play a natural biological role in humans. The daily intake of zirconium is approximately 50 µg. Short-time exposure to zirconium powder can cause irritation, and inhalation of zirconium compounds can cause skin and lung granulomas. Persistent exposure to zirconium tetrachloride results in increased mortality in rats and guinea pigs and a decrease of blood hemoglobin and red blood cell in dogs [128–130]. Nonetheless, zirconium metal exhibits the highest biocompatibility of all metals in the body (Figure 2.2), and zirconium compounds are of low toxicity.

BIBLIOGRAPHY

References for Text

1. Vanysek, P., Revision of tables of electrochemical series, In *CRC Handbook of Chemistry and Physics*, D.R. Lide, ed. Boca Raton, FL: CRC Press, 2001, pp. 8–21.
2. McCafferty, E., *Introduction to Corrosion Science*. New York: Springer Science Business Media, LLC, 2010. doi:10.1007/978-1-4419-0455-3_6.
3. Akimov, G.V., Electrode potentials, *Corrosion*, 1955;**11**:477t.
4. LaQue, F.L., *Marine Corrosion*. New York: John Wiley, 1975, Chapter 6.
5. Fontana, M.G. and N.D. Greene, *Corrosion Engineering*. New York: McGraw-Hill, 1978, p. 37.
6. Pourbaix, M., *Atlas of Electrochemical Equilibria in Aqueous Solutions*. Houston, TX: National Association of Corrosion Engineers, 1974.
7. Heldtberg, M., I.D. MacLeod, and V.L. Richards, Corrosion and cathodic protection of iron in seawater: A case study of the *James Matthews* (1841). *Proceedings of Metal 2004*, National Museum of Australia Canberra ACT, Canberra, Australian Capital Territory, Australia, October 4–8, 2004.

Websites

http://www.corrosion-doctors.org/Definitions/galvanic-series.htm.
http://en.wikipedia.org/wiki/Allergen_of_the_Year.
National Association of Corrosion Engineers (NACE), International, the Corrosion Society. http://www.nace.org/home.aspx.
The *Journal of Trace Elements in Medicine and Biology*, http://www.sciencedirect.com/science/journal/0946672X.

References for Advanced Topic

1. Lippard, S.J. and J.M. Berg, *Principles of Bioinorganic Chemistry*. Mill Valley, CA: University Science Books, 1994.
2. Umbreit, J., Iron deficiency: A concise review. *American Journal of Hematology*, 2005;**78**(3):225–231.
3. Cheney, K. et al., Survival after a severe iron poisoning treated with intermittent infusions of deferoxamine. *Journal of Toxicology-Clinical Toxicology*, 1995;**33**(1):61–66.
4. Abdelmageed, A.B. and F. Oehme, A review of the biochemical roles, toxicity and interactions of zinc, copper and iron. 3. Iron. *Veterinary and Human Toxicology*, 1990;**32**(4):324–328.
5. Hoppe, J.O., G.M.A. Marcelli, and M.L. Tainter, A review of the toxicity of iron compounds. *American Journal of the Medical Sciences*, 1955;**230**(5):558–571.
6. Brar, S. et al., Iron accumulation in the substantia nigra of patients with Alzheimer disease and parkinsonism. *Archives of Neurology*, 2009;**66**(3):371–374.
7. Esteve, C., E. Alcaide, and R. Urena, The effect of metals on condition and pathologies of European eel (*Anguilla anguilla*): In situ and laboratory experiments. *Aquatic Toxicology*, 2012;**109**:176–184.
8. Tsuchiya, T. et al., A method to monitor corrosion of chromium-iron alloys by monitoring the chromium ion concentration in urine. *Materials Transactions*, 2002;**43**(12):3058–3064.
9. Denizoglu, S. and Z.Y. Duymus, Evaluation of cobalt, chromium, and nickel concentrations in plasma and blood of patients with removable partial dentures. *Dental Materials Journal*, 2006;**25**(2):365–370.
10. Meacham, S.L. et al., Whole blood concentrations of minerals, including chromium and boron, were obtained from a population of indigenous horses in Southern Nevada. *FASEB Journal*, 2003;**17**(4):A706–A706.

11. Dayan, A.D. and A.J. Paine, Mechanisms of chromium toxicity, carcinogenicity and allergenicity: Review of the literature from 1985 to 2000. *Human and Experimental Toxicology*, 2001;**20**(9):439–451.

12. Rudolf, E., A review of findings on chromium toxicity. *Acta Medica (Hradec Kralove). Supplementum Universitas Carolina, Facultas Medica Hradec Kralove*, 1998;**41**(1):55–65.

13. Barceloux, D.G., Chromium. *Journal of Toxicology-Clinical Toxicology*, 1999;**37**(2):173–194.

14. Langard, S., 100 years of chromium and cancer—A review of epidemiological evidence and selected case-reports. *American Journal of Industrial Medicine*, 1990;**17**(2):189–215.

15. Stearns, D.M. and K.E. Wetterhahn, Are high valent chromium species the ultimate carcinogens in chromate-induced cancer? *Abstracts of Papers of the American Chemical Society*, 1996;**212**:208-INOR.

16. Becker, N., Cancer mortality among arc welders exposed to fumes containing chromium and nickel—Results of a third follow-up: 1989–1995. *Journal of Occupational and Environmental Medicine*, 1999;**41**(4):294–303.

17. Blair, J., Chrome ulcers—Report of twelve cases. *Journal of the American Medical Association*, 1928;**90**:1927–1928.

18. Colomb, D., H. Perrot, and A.J. Beyvin, Ulcers in a person working with chromium. *Bulletin de la Societe francaise de dermatologie et de syphiligraphie*, 1969;**76**(1):130–131.

19. Mahto, A. and B. De Silva, 'Leather sofa dermatitis' due to contact allergy to chrome: An unusual cause of eczema in a child. *British Journal of Dermatology*, 2009;**161**:126–127.

20. Hansen, M.B. et al., Quantitative aspects of contact allergy to chromium and exposure to chrome-tanned leather. *Contact Dermatitis*, 2002;**47**(3):127–134.

21. Kim, M.H. et al., Prurigo pigmentosa from contact allergy to chrome in detergent. *Contact Dermatitis*, 2001;**44**(5):289–292.

22. Rosenman, K.D. and M. Stanbury, Risk of lung cancer among former chromium smelter workers. *American Journal of Industrial Medicine*, 1996;**29**(5):491–500.

23. Dubey, C.S., B.K. Sahoo, and N.R. Nayak, Chromium (VI) in waters in parts of Sukinda chromite valley and health hazards, Orissa, India. *Bulletin of Environmental Contamination and Toxicology*, 2001;**67**(4):541–548.

24. Oliveira, S.C.B. and A.M. Oliveira-Brett, In situ evaluation of chromium-DNA damage using a DNA-electrochemical biosensor. *Analytical and Bioanalytical Chemistry*, 2010;**398**(4):1633–1641.

25. Nickens, K.P., S.R. Patierno, and S. Ceryak, Chromium genotoxicity: A double-edged sword. *Chemico-Biological Interactions*, 2010;**188**(2):276–288.

26. Burkhardt, S. et al., DNA oxidatively damaged by chromium(III) and H_2O_2 is protected by the antioxidants melatonin, N-1-acetyl-N-2-formyl-5-methoxykynuramine, resveratrol and uric acid. *International Journal of Biochemistry and Cell Biology*, 2001;**33**(8):775–783.

27. Rudolf, E. and M. Cervinka, Trivalent chromium activates Rac-1 and Src and induces switch in the cell death mode in human dermal fibroblasts. *Toxicology Letters*, 2009;**188**(3):236–242.

28. Berry, W.J. et al., Predicting the toxicity of chromium in sediments. *Environmental Toxicology and Chemistry*, 2004;**23**(12):2981–2992.

29. AlSaleh, I.A., Trace elements in drinking water coolers collected from primary schools, Riyadh, Saudi Arabia. *Science of the Total Environment*, 1996;**181**(3):215–221.

30. Al-Saleh, I. and I. Al-Doush, Survey of trace elements in household and bottled drinking water samples collected in Riyadh, Saudi Arabia. *Science of the Total Environment*, 1998;**216**(3):181–192.

31. Segura-Munoz, S.I. et al., Heavy metals in water of drinking fountains. *Archivos Latinoamericanos de Nutricion*, 2003;**53**(1):59–64.

32. Ryhanen, J., *Biocompatibility Evaluation of Nickel-Titanium Shape Memory Metal Alloy*. Oulu, Finland: Oulu University Linrary, 1999.

33. Sigel, A., H. Sigel, and R.K.O. Sigel (eds.), *Nickel and Its Surprising Impact in Nature: Metal Ions in Life Sciences*, Vol. 2. Chichester, U.K.: John Wiley & Sons, Chichester, UK, 2007.

34. Nielsen, J.L., O.M. Poulsen, and A. Abildtrup, Studies of serum-protein complexes with nickel using crossed immunoelectrophoresis. *Electrophoresis*, 1994;**15**(5):666–671.

35. Rezuke, W.N., J.A. Knight, and F.W. Sunderman, Reference values for nickel concentrations in human-tissues and bile. *American Journal of Industrial Medicine*, 1987;**11**(4):419–426.
36. Anke, M. et al., Nickel—An essential element. *IARC Scientific Publications*, 1984;(53):339–365.
37. Szilagyi, M., M. Anke, and I. Balogh, Effect of nickel deficiency on biochemical variables in serum, liver, heart and kidneys of goats. *Acta Veterinaria Hungarica*, 1991;**39**(3–4):231–238.
38. Nielsen, F.H. et al., Nickel influences iron-metabolism through physiologic, pharmacologic and toxicologic mechanisms in the rat. *Journal of Nutrition*, 1984;**114**(7):1280–1288.
39. Stangl, G.I. and M. Kirchgessner, Effect of nickel deficiency on fatty acid composition of milk and adipose tissue of rats. *Trace Elements and Electrolytes*, 1996;**13**(3):117–122.
40. Nielsen, F.H. et al., Nickel deficiency in rats. *Journal of Nutrition*, 1975;**105**(12):1620–1630.
41. Nielsen, F.H. et al., Nickel deficiency and nickel-rhodium interaction in chicks. *Journal of Nutrition*, 1975;**105**(12):1607–1619.
42. Stangl, G.I. and M. Kirchgessner, Effect of nickel deficiency on various metabolic parameters of rats. *Journal of Animal Physiology and Animal Nutrition*, 1996;**75**(3):164–174.
43. Stangl, G.I. and M. Kirchgessner, Nickel deficiency alters liver lipid metabolism in rats. *Journal of Nutrition*, 1996;**126**(10):2466–2473.
44. Santucci, B. et al., Nickel dermatitis from cheap earrings. *Contact Dermatitis*, 1989;**21**(4):245–248.
45. Gaul, L.E., Dermatitis from metal spectacles—Demonstration of nickel and copper compounds from corrosion of earpieces. *Archives of Dermatology*, 1958;**78**(4):475–478.
46. http://en.wikipedia.org/wiki/Allergen_of_the_Year.
47. Kawamoto, T. et al., Historical review on development of environmental quality standards and guideline values for air pollutants in Japan. *International Journal of Hygiene and Environmental Health*, 2011;**214**(4):296–304.
48. Hughes, K. et al., Nickel and its compounds—Evaluation of risks to health from environmental exposure in Canada. *Environmental Carcinogenesis and Ecotoxicology Reviews-Part C of Journal of Environmental Science and Health*, 1994;**12**(2):417–433.
49. Coogan, T.P., D.M. Latta, E.T. Snow, and M. Costa, Toxicity and carcinogenicity of nickel compounds, *Crit Rev Toxicol*, 1989;**19**(4):341–384.
50. Ashman, R.B. et al., Mechanical testing of spinal instrumentation. *Clinical Orthopaedics and Related Research*, 1988;**227**:113–125.
51. Sunderman, F.W., Review of metabolism and toxicology of nickel. *Annals of Clinical and Laboratory Science*, 1977;**7**(5):377–398.
52. Zhao, J. et al., Occupational toxicology of nickel and nickel compounds. *Journal of Environmental Pathology Toxicology and Oncology*, 2009;**28**(3):177–208.
53. Oller, A.R., M. Costa, and G. Oberdorster, Carcinogenicity assessment of selected nickel compounds. *Toxicology and Applied Pharmacology*, 1997;**143**(1):152–166.
54. Abbracchio, M.P., J. Simmonshansen, and M. Costa, Cytoplasmic dissolution of phagocytized crystalline nickel sulfide particles—A prerequisite for nuclear uptake of nickel. *Journal of Toxicology and Environmental Health*, 1982;**9**(4):663–676.
55. Abbracchio, M.P. et al., The regulation of ionic nickel uptake and cytotoxicity by specific amino-acids and serum components. *Biological Trace Element Research*, 1982;**4**(4):289–301.
56. Sunderman, F.W. Jr., Physicochemical and biological attributes of nickel compounds in relationship to carcinogenic activities. *Journal of UOEH*, 1987;**9**(Suppl.):84–94.
57. Dunnick, J.K. et al., Comparative carcinogenic effects of nickel subsulfide, nickel-oxide, or nickel sulfate hexahydrate chronic exposures in the lung. *Cancer Research*, 1995;**55**(22):5251–5256.
58. Klein, C.B., K. Frenkel, and M. Costa, The role of oxidative processes in metal carcinogenesis. *Chemical Research in Toxicology*, 1991;**4**(6):592–604.
59. Klein, C.B. et al., Senescence of nickel-transformed cells by an x-chromosome—Possible epigenetic control. *Science*, 1991;**251**(4995):796–799.
60. Yamamoto, A., R. Honma, and M. Sumita, Cytotoxicity evaluation of 43 metal salts using murine fibroblasts and osteoblastic cells. *Journal of Biomedical Materials Research*, 1998;**39**(2):331–340.

61. Hayes, R.B., The carcinogenicity of metals in humans. *Cancer Causes and Control*, 1997;**8**(3):371–385.
62. Martz, C.D. et al., Use and abuse of metal implants. *Canadian Medical Association Journal*, 1967;**96**(9):568.
63. Laing, P.G., A.B. Ferguson, and E.S. Hodge, Tissue reaction and trace element concentration in rabbit muscle exposed to metallic and non-metallic implants. *Journal of Bone and Joint Surgery. American Volume*, 1965;**A47**(5):1102.
64. Takamura, K. et al., Evaluation of carcinogenicity and chronic toxicity associated with ortho-pedic implants in mice. *Journal of Biomedical Materials Research*, 1994;**28**(5):583–589.
65. Bergman, M., B. Bergman, and R. Soremark, Tissue accumulation of nickel released due to electrochemical corrosion of non-precious dental casting alloys. *Journal of Oral Rehabilitation*, 1980;**7**(4):325–330.
66. Lugowski, S.J. et al., Release of metal-ions from dental implant materials in vivo—Determination of Al, Co, Cr, Mo, Ni, V, and Ti in organ tissue. *Journal of Biomedical Materials Research*, 1991;**25**(12):1443–1458.
67. Ishimatsu, S. et al., Distribution of various nickel compounds in rat organs after oral-admin-istration. *Biological Trace Element Research*, 1995;**49**(1):43–52.
68. Pereira, M.C., M.L. Pereira, and J.P. Sousa, Evaluation of nickel toxicity on liver, spleen, and kidney of mice after administration of high-dose metal ion. *Journal of Biomedical Materials Research*, 1998;**40**(1):40–47.
69. Michel, R. and J. Zilkens, Studies on presence of metal traces in tissue surrounding A.O. angle plates, based on neutron-activation analysis. *Zeitschrift fur Orthopadie und ihre Grenzgebiete*, 1978;**116**(5):666–674.
70. Hierholzer, S. et al., Increased corrosion of stainless-steel implants in infected plated frac-tures. *Archives of Orthopaedic and Trauma Surgery*, 1984;**102**(3):198–200.
71. De Souza, R.M. and L.M. De Menezes, Nickel, chromium and iron levels in the saliva of patients with simulated fixed orthodontic appliances. *Angle Orthodontist*, 2008;**78**(2):345–350.
72. Bruce, I. and C.E. Swanson, Metal ion levels in patients with stainless steel spinal instru-mentation. *Spine*, 2007;**32**(18):1963–1968.
73. Kennedy, D.G. et al., Cobalt—Vitamin B-12 deficiency and the activity of methylmalonyl CoA mutase and methionine synthase in cattle. *International Journal for Vitamin and Nutrition Research*, 1995;**65**(4):241–247.
74. Kennedy, D.G. et al., Rumen succinate production may ameliorate the effects of cobalt-vitamin-B-12 deficiency on methylmalonyl CoA mutase in sheep. *Journal of Nutrition*, 1991;**121**(8):1236–1242.
75. Stangl, G.I., F.J. Schwarz, and M. Kirchgessner, Moderate long-term cobalt-deficiency affects liver, brain and erythrocyte lipids and lipoproteins of cattle. *Nutrition Research*, 1999;**19**(3):415–427.
76. Stangl, G.I., F.J. Schwarz, and M. Kirchgessner, Amino acid changes in plasma and liver of cobalt-deficient cattle. *Journal of Animal Physiology and Animal Nutrition*, 1998;**80**(1):40–48.
77. Tower, S.S., Arthroprosthetic cobaltism associated with metal on metal hip implants. *British Medical Journal*, 2012;**344**:e430.
78. Tower, S.S., Arthroprosthetic cobaltism: Neurological and cardiac manifestations in two patients with metal-on-metal arthroplasty a case report. *Journal of Bone and Joint Surgery. American Volume*, 2010;**92A**(17):2847–2851.
79. Kobayashi, M. and S. Shimizu, Cobalt proteins. *European Journal of Biochemistry*, 1999;**261**(1):1–9.
80. Donaldson, J.D. and D. Beyersmann, Cobalt and cobalt compounds. In *Ullmann's Encyclopedia of Industrial Chemistry 2005*, V.A. Welch, K.J. Fallon, and H.P. Gelbke, eds. Weinheim, Germany: Wiley-VCH, 2005.
81. Barceloux, D.G. Cobalt. *Journal of Toxicology-Clinical Toxicology*, 1999;**37**(2):201–216.
82. Basketter, D.A. et al., Nickel, chromium and cobalt in consumer products: Revisiting safe levels in the new millennium. *Contact Dermatitis*, 2003;**49**(1):1–7.

83. Lison, D., Human toxicity of cobalt-containing dust and experimental studies on the mechanism of interstitial lung disease (hard metal disease). *Critical Reviews in Toxicology*, 1996;**26**(6):585–616.

84. Jones, D.A. et al., Cobalt toxicity after McKee hip arthroplasty. *Journal of Bone and Joint Surgery. British Volume*, 1975;**57**(3):289–296.

85. Mao, X., A.A. Wong, and R.W. Crawford, Cobalt toxicity—An emerging clinical problem in patients with metal-on-metal hip prostheses? *Medical Journal of Australia*, 2011;**194**(12):649–651.

86. Tower, S.S., Cobalt toxicity in two hip replacement patients. Bulletin No. 14, Division of Public Health, State of Alaska Epidemiology, Anchorage, AK, 2010. http://www.epi.alaska.gov/.

87. Turnlund, J.R., Molybdenum metabolism and requirements in humans. *Molybdenum and Tungsten: Their Roles in Biological Processes*, 2002;**39**:727–739.

88. Pazzaglia, U.E. et al., Cobalt, chromium and molybdenum ions kinetics in the human body: Data gained from a total hip replacement with massive third body wear of the head and neuropathy by cobalt intoxication. *Archives of Orthopaedic and Trauma Surgery*, 2011;**131**(9):1299–1308.

89. Curzon, M.E.J., J. Kubota, and B.G. Bibby, Environmental effects of molybdenum on caries. *Journal of Dental Research*, 1971;**50**(1):74–77.

90. Taylor, P.R. et al., Prevention of esophageal cancer—The nutrition intervention trials in linxian, China. *Cancer Research*, 1994;**54**(7):S2029–S2031.

91. Barceloux, D.G., Molybdenum. *Journal of Toxicology-Clinical Toxicology*, 1999;**37**(2):231–237.

92. Coughlan, M.P., The role of molybdenum in human-biology. *Journal of Inherited Metabolic Disease*, 1983;**6**:70–77.

93. Molybdenum toxicity. *Nutrition Reviews*, 1960;**18**(2):54–56.

94. Liber, K., L.E. Doig, and S.L. White-Sobey, Toxicity of uranium, molybdenum, nickel, and arsenic to *Hyalella azteca* and *Chironomus dilutus* in water-only and spiked-sediment toxicity tests. *Ecotoxicology and Environmental Safety*, 2011;**74**(5):1171–1179.

95. Anke, M. et al., The biological and toxicological importance of molybdenum in the environment and in the nutrition of plants, animals and man—Part V: Essentiality and toxicity of molybdenum. *Acta Alimentaria*, 2010;**39**(1):12–26.

96. Vyskocil, A. and C. Viau, Assessment of molybdenum toxicity in humans. *Journal of Applied Toxicology*, 1999;**19**(3):185–192.

97. Witzleb, W.-C. et al., Exposure to chromium, cobalt and molybdenum from metal-on-metal total hip replacement and hip resurfacing arthroplasty. *Acta Orthopaedica*, 2006;**77**(5):697–705.

98. Antoniou, J. et al., Metal ion levels in the blood of patients after hip resurfacing: A comparison between twenty-eight and thirty-six-millimeter-head metal-on-metal prostheses. *Journal of Bone and Joint Surgery. American Volume*, 2008;**90A**:142–148.

99. Kletzin, A. and M.W.W. Adams, Tungsten in biological systems. *FEMS Microbiology Reviews*, 1996;**18**(1):5–63.

100. Smart, J.P., M.J. Cliff, and D.J. Kelly, A role for tungsten in the biology of *Campylobacter jejuni*: Tungstate stimulates formate dehydrogenase activity and is transported via an ultra-high affinity ABC system distinct from the molybdate transporter. *Molecular Microbiology*, 2009;**74**(3):742–757.

101. Peuster, M. et al., Dissolution of tungsten coils does not produce systemic toxicity, but leads to elevated levels of tungsten in the serum and recanalization of the previously occluded vessel. *Cardiology in the Young*, 2002;**12**(3):229–235.

102. Lison, D., J.P. Buchet, and P. Hoet, Toxicity of tungsten. *Lancet*, 1997;**349**(9044):58–58.

103. Peuster, M., C. Fink, and C. von Schnakenburg, Biocompatibility of corroding tungsten coils: In vitro assessment of degradation kinetics and cytotoxicity on human cells. *Biomaterials*, 2003;**24**(22):4057–4061.

104. Witten, M.L., P.R. Sheppard, and B.L. Witten, Tungsten toxicity. *Chemico-Biological Interactions*, 2012;**196**(3):87–88.

105. Pais, I. et al., Titanium as a new trace-element. *Communications in Soil Science and Plant Analysis*, 1977;**8**(5):407–410.

106. Yaghoubi, S., C.W. Schwietert, and J.P. McCue, Biological roles of titanium. *Biological Trace Element Research*, 2000;**78**(1–3):205–217.

107. Wang, M.L. et al., Direct and indirect induction of apoptosis in human mesenchymal stem cells in response to titanium particles. *Journal of Orthopaedic Research*, 2003;**21**(4):697–707.

108. Coen, N. et al., Particulate debris from a titanium metal prosthesis induces genomic instability in primary human fibroblast cells. *British Journal of Cancer*, 2003;**88**(4):548–552.

109. Kumazawa, R. et al., Effects of Ti ions and particles on neutrophil function and morphology. *Biomaterials*, 2002;**23**(17):3757–3764.

110. Koval'skii, V.V. and L.T. Rezaeva, The biological role of vanadium in ascidia. *Uspekhi Sovremennoi Biologii*, 1965;**60**(1):45–61.

111. Daniel, E.P. and E.M. Hewston, Vanadium—A consideration of its possible biological role. *American Journal of Physiology*, 1942;**136**(5):0772–0775.

112. Altamirano-Lozano, M.A., M.E. Roldan-Reyes, and E. Rojas, Genetic toxicology of vanadium compounds. *Vanadium in the Environment, Pt 2: Health Effects*, 1998;**31**:159–179.

113. Rhoads, L.S. et al., Cytotoxicity of nanostructured vanadium oxide on human cells in vitro. *Toxicology In Vitro*, 2010;**24**(1):292–296.

114. Ress, N.B. et al., Carcinogenicity of inhaled vanadium pentoxide in F344/N rats and B6C3F(1) mice. *Toxicological Sciences*, 2003;**74**(2):287–296.

115. Moretti, B. et al., Peripheral neuropathy after hip replacement failure: Is vanadium the culprit? *Lancet*, 2012;**379**(9826):1676–1676.

116. Verstraeten, S.V., L. Aimo, and P.I. Oteiza, Aluminium and lead. Molecular mechanisms of brain toxicity. *Archives of Toxicology*, 2008;**82**(11):789–802.

117. Banks, W.A. and A.J. Kastin, Aluminum-induced neurotoxicity—Alterations in membrane-function at the blood-brain-barrier. *Neuroscience and Biobehavioral Reviews*, 1989;**13**(1):47–53.

118. Yokel, R.A., The toxicology of aluminum in the brain: A review. *Neurotoxicology*, 2000;**21**(5):813–828.

119. Kerr, D.N.S. et al., Aluminum intoxication in renal-disease. *Ciba Foundation Symposia*, 1992;**169**:123–141.

120. Darbre, P.D., Metalloestrogens: An emerging class of inorganic xenoestrogens with potential to add to the oestrogenic burden of the human breast. *Journal of Applied Toxicology*, 2006;**26**(3):191–197.

121. Darbre, P.D., Environmental oestrogens, cosmetics and breast cancer. *Best Practice and Research Clinical Endocrinology and Metabolism*, 2006;**20**(1):121–143.

122. Ferreira, P.C. et al., Aluminum as a risk factor for Alzheimer's disease. *Revista Latino-Americana de Enfermagem*, 2008;**16**(1):151–157.

123. Downs, W.L. et al., Toxicity of niobium salts. *American Industrial Hygiene Association Journal*, 1965;**26**(4):337–346.

124. Caicedo, M. et al., Analysis of metal ion-induced DNA damage, apoptosis, and necrosis in human (Jurkat) T-cells demonstrates Ni^{2+}, and V^{3+} are more toxic than other metals: Al^{3+}, Be^{2+}, Co^{2+}, Cr^{3+}, Cu^{2+}, Fe^{3+}, Mo^{5+}, Nb^{5+}, Zr^{2+}. *Journal of Biomedical Materials Research. Part A*, 2008;**86A**(4):905–913.

125. Black, J., Biological performance of tantalum. *Clinical Materials*, 1994;**16**(3):167–173.

126. Metallic materials. In *Handbook of Materials for Medical Devices*, J.R. Davis, ed. ASM International, Materials Park, OH, 2003, pp. 21–50.

127. Oppenheimer, B.S. et al., Carcinogenic effect of metals in rodents. *Cancer Research*, 1956;**16**(5):439–441.

128. Martins, A.S.B., P.M.F.C. Fresco, and M.J. Pereira, Toxicity of zirconium on growth of two green algae. *Fresenius Environmental Bulletin*, 2007;**16**(8):869–874.

129. Delongeas, J.L. et al., Toxicity and pharmacokinetics of zirconium oxychlorure in the mouse and in the rat. *Journal de Pharmacologie*, 1983;**14**(4):437–447.
130. McClinton, L.T. and J. Schubert, The toxicity of some zirconium and thorium salts in rats. *Journal of Pharmacology and Experimental Therapeutics*, 1948;**94**(1):1–6.
131. Raskin, R.B., Toxicity of silver amalgam: Fact or fiction. *The New York State Dental Journal*, 1984;**50**(9):587.
132. Gorsuch, J.W. and S.J. Klaine, Toxicity and fate of silver in the environment. *Environmental Toxicology and Chemistry*, 1998;**17**(4):537–538.
133. Call, D.J. et al., Toxicity of silver in water and sediment to the freshwater amphipod *Hyalella azteca*. *Environmental Toxicology and Chemistry*, 2006;**25**(7):1802–1808.
134. Hemati, S. et al., Topical silver sulfadiazine for the prevention of acute dermatitis during irradiation for breast cancer. *Supportive Care in Cancer*, 2012;**20**(8):1613–1618.
135. Pleshchitser, A.L., Biological role of magnesium. *Clinical Chemistry*, 1958;**4**(6):429–450.
136. Torshin, I.Y. and O.A. Gromova, The biological roles of magnesium. In *Magnesium and Pyridoxine: Fundamental Studies and Clinical Practice*. New York: Nova Science Publisher, New York, 2009, pp. 1–17.
137. Stahlmann, R., Magnesium-related skeletal toxicity of quinolones. *Journal of Antimicrobial Chemotherapy*, 2001;**47**:11–12.
138. Kim, W.S., Magnesium toxicity and its use for prediction of calcium deficiency in apple fruit before harvest. In *Mineral Nutrition and Fertilizer Use for Deciduous Fruit Crops*, J.M.L.M.E. Val, ed. Leuven, Belgium: ISHS, International Society for Horticultural Science, 1997, pp. 358–359.
139. Williams, R.J.P., Calcium: The developing role of its chemistry in biological evolution. In *Calcium as a Cellular Regulator*, E. Carafoli and C. Klee, eds. New York: Oxford University Press, 1999, pp. 3–27.
140. Laborit, H. et al., Biological and therapeutic role of calcium salts in anesthesiology, artificial hibernation and surgical therapeutics. *Anesthesie et Analgesie*, 1955;**12**(3):593.
141. Ambard, L. and F. Schmid, On the biological role of the salts of calcium. *Comptes rendus des seances de la Societe de biologie et de ses Filiales*, 1928;**98**:1220–1222.
142. Hovda, K.E. et al., Renal toxicity of ethylene glycol results from internalization of calcium oxalate crystals by proximal tubule cells. *Toxicology Letters*, 2010;**192**(3):365–372.
143. Zhang, J.G. and W.E. Lindup, Role of calcium in cisplatin-induced cell toxicity in rat renal cortical slices. *Toxicology In Vitro*, 1996;**10**(2):205–209.
144. Bailey, C.S. et al., Excessive calcium ingestion leading to milk-alkali syndrome. *Annals of Clinical Biochemistry*, 2008;**45**:527–529.
145. Nasolodin, V.V., Biological role of manganese and the prevention of its deficiency in the human body. *Voprosy Pitaniia*, 1985(4):3–6.
146. Artamonov, V.S., The role of bio-elements (copper and manganese) in improving biological value of the human milk. *Pediatriia akusherstvo i ginekologiia*, 1968;**5**:43–46.
147. Lebda, M.A., M.S. El-Neweshy, and Y.S. El-Sayed, Neurohepatic toxicity of subacute manganese chloride exposure and potential chemoprotective effects of lycopene. *Neurotoxicology*, 2012;**33**(1):98–104.
148. El-Sayed, Y., M. Lebda, and M. El-Neweshy, Neurohepatic toxicity of manganese exposure and chemoprotective effects of lycopene. *Toxicology Letters*, 2012;**211**:S145–S145.
149. Elbowicz-Waniewska, Z., Biological role of copper compounds. *Polski Tygodnik Lekarski (Warsaw, Poland: 1960)*, 1968;**23**(23):882–884.
150. The minerals we need. The human body and a sturdy building have many elements—that is, minerals—in common, including calcium, iron, potassium, copper, molybdenum, and zinc. Both are built to last. *Harvard Women's Health Watch*, 2003;**10**(9):6–7.
151. Carrel, R. et al., The accumulation of the base metals (copper, zinc, and mercury) in the human body. *Pennsylvania Dental Journal*, 1978;**45**(3):14–16.

152. Wacker, W.E.C. et al., Relation of copper to ceruloplasmin activity and zinc to malic and lactic dehydrogenase activity in acute myocardial infarction. *Journal of Clinical Investigation*, 1956;**35**(6):741–742.

153. Adelstein, S.J., T.L. Coombs, and B.L. Vallee, Metalloenzymes and myocardial infarction.1. Relation between serum copper and ceruloplasmin and its catalytic activity. *New England Journal of Medicine*, 1956;**255**(3):105–109.

154. Bremner, I. et al., Effects of dietary copper supplementation of rats on the occurrence of metallothionein-i in liver and its secretion into blood, bile and urine. *Biochemical Journal*, 1986;**235**(3):735–739.

155. Abdelmageed, A.B. and F.W. Oehme, A review of the biochemical roles, toxicity and interactions of zinc, copper and iron. 2. Copper. *Veterinary and Human Toxicology*, 1990;**32**(3):230–234.

156. Leone, N. et al., Zinc, copper, and magnesium and risks for all-cause, cancer, and cardiovascular mortality. *Epidemiology*, 2006;**17**(3):308–314.

157. Abdelmageed, A.B. and F.W. Oehme, A review of the biochemical roles, toxicity and interactions of zinc, copper and iron. 1. Zinc. *Veterinary and Human Toxicology*, 1990;**32**(1):34–39.

158. Salga, M.S. et al., Acute oral toxicity evaluations of some zinc(II) complexes derived from 1-(2-salicylaldiminoethyl)piperazine Schiff bases in rats. *International Journal of Molecular Sciences*, 2012;**13**(2):1393–1404.

Further Readings

Berg, J.M., J.L. Tymoczko, and L. Stryer, *Biochemistry (Molecular Biology)*, 5th edn. New York: W.H. Freeman and Company, 2002, Chapter 1.

Chapter 4: Corrosion of metallic implants and prosthetic devices. In *Handbook of Materials for Medical Devices*, Davis, J.R. ed.. Materials Park, OH: ASM International, 2003.

Groover, R.E., J.A. Smith, and T.J. Lennox Jr., Electrochemical potentials of high purity metals in sea water, *Corrosion*, 1972;**28**:101.

Kruger, J. In *Equilibrium Diagrams: Localized Corrosion*, R.P. Frankenthal and J. Kruger eds. Pennington, NJ: The Electrochemical Society, 1984, p. 45.

McCafferty, E., *Introduction to Corrosion Science*. New York: Springer Science+Business Media, LLC, Dordrecht, the Netherlands, 2010. doi:10.1007/978-1-4419-0455-3_6.

Pourbaix, M., *Atlas of Electrochemical Equilibria in Aqueous Solutions*. Houston, TX: National Association of Corrosion Engineers, 1974.

CHAPTER 3

MECHANICAL PROPERTIES OF BIOMATERIALS

LEARNING OBJECTIVES

After a careful study of this chapter, you should be able to do the following:

1. Describe mechanical properties of general importance.
2. Describe two special mechanical working conditions: fatigue and stress-corrosion environment.
3. Describe mechanical working conditions of the leg.
4. Understand and describe fatigue properties of materials.
5. Describe aseptic loosening due to wearing of orthopedic implants.

3.1 ROLE OF IMPLANT BIOMATERIALS

It is important to note at the early stage of a biomaterials course that the use of bio-materials as medical implants is primarily aimed at the recovery of physical, especially mechanical, functions of injured or diseased organs or tissues. The application of biomaterials lies in the fact that besides physical support, biomaterials have no other biological functions.

Although all organs and their tissues have biological functions, some of them primarily perform a physical (including mechanical) function, and the loss of their other biological aspects can be tolerated. It is in these types of organs or their tissues that biomaterials find major applications. For example, in the skeletal system, the function is largely mechanical such that orthopedists can use metal implants to restore the mechanical function of damaged bones. The heart, although a vital organ of the body,

63

is actually a mechanical pump that moves blood throughout the blood vessels. This explains why artificial hearts, for example, pacemakers, have been widely and successfully applied to improve quality of life in heart failure patients worldwide. Blood vessels (arteries and veins) are hollow, elastic tubes that transport blood throughout the entire body. Hence, the function of the blood vessel is primarily also of a physical nature, which could be replaced by artificial tubes. In short, implant biomaterials are used to recover lost physical, especially mechanical, functions of the host body. Therefore, from the clinical application point of view, mechanical properties of bulk materials are the second-most important aspect of biomaterials, following biocompatibility.

3.2   MECHANICAL PROPERTIES OF GENERAL IMPORTANCE

In general, the mechanical working conditions of implant biomaterials are very complicated in the body, and mechanical properties under special conditions must be considered. This topic will be discussed in great detail in Section 3.7. Nevertheless, special mechanical properties (e.g., fatigue) are always closely correlated and thus can be predicted by their mechanical properties of general importance, which typically include Young's modulus E, yield strength σ_y, ultimate tensile strength (UTS) or ultimate compressive strength (UCS), fracture toughness, and elongation at break (Figures 3.1 and 3.2). Among these five properties, Young's modulus is the only one that is nonsensitive to microstructures (Figure 1.5) and is primarily determined by the chemical bonding between atoms and/or molecules (Figure 1.3), whereas the other four properties are all sensitively influenced by microstructures.

For most metallic materials, elastic deformation persists only to strains of ~0.5%. The transition from elastic to plastic is a gradual one for most metals, and it is technically tricky to determine the yield point. In practice, the yield stress is determined using the stress 0.2% strain offset method (Figure 3.1). At room temperature and tensile loading conditions, ceramics, regardless of whether they are crystalline or noncrystalline

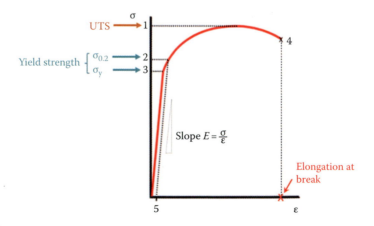

Figure 3.1
A typical stress–strain curve of metallic material under static fixed loading conditions. For ceramic materials.

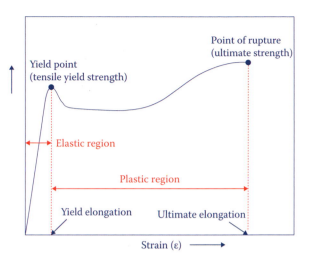

Figure 3.2
A typical stress–strain curve of thermoplastics under static fixed tensile loading conditions.

(i.e., glassy), almost always fracture before any plastic deformation can occur. That is to say, ceramics almost fracture at point 3 of Figure 3.1. Some metallic materials and many thermoplastics exhibit stress–strain curves with the so-called yield point phenomenon. At the upper yield point, plastic deformation is initiated followed by a drop in stress (Figure 3.2). Elastomeric polymers, on the other hand, deform elastically to large strains, typically >100%, and rupture after limited plastic deformation occurs. These five mechanical properties of selected metallic, ceramic, and polymeric biomaterials are listed in Table 3.1.

3.3   HARDNESS

Another mechanical property that is important to medical implants (such as the head in a total hip replacement) is hardness, which is a measure of a material's resistance to wear and friction, the form of localized plastic deformation. Hardness, which is not a well-defined material property, has been quantitatively measured using various techniques, with Rockwell and Britnell hardness tests being the two most common methods. The scale of Rockwell hardness is designated by the symbol HR, and the Britnell harness number is marked by HB. Since both tensile strength and hardness are indicators of a metal's resistance to plastic deformation, the hardness of the material is roughly proportional to its tensile strength [1]:

$$\text{Tensile strength}\left(\text{MPa}\right) = 3.45 \times \text{HB},$$

$$\text{Tensile strength}\left(\text{psi}\right) = 500 \times \text{HB}.$$

(3.1)

Hardness is also roughly proportional to its yield strength (Figure 3.3a) and Young's modulus (Figure 3.3b). Hence, materials of high Young's moduli generally demonstrate good resistances to wear.

Table 3.1
Mechanical Properties of Selected Implant Materials and Biological Tissues

Materials	Young's Modulus, E (GPa)	Yield Strength, σ_y (MPa)	Ultimate Tensile (T) or Compressive (C) Strength (MPa)	Fracture Toughness (K_{IC} or J_{IC})	Elongation at Break (%)
316L stainless steel	200	200–700	500–900 (T)	~100 (MPa $\sqrt{m}$)	10–50
Orthinox	200	400–1550	700–1,700 (T)	~100 (MPa $\sqrt{m}$)	20–35
CoCrMo alloys	240	450–1500	600–1,600 (T)	~100 (MPa $\sqrt{m}$)	10–30
Ti alloys	105–125	350–1050	600–1,100 (T)	~80 (MPa $\sqrt{m}$)	5–50
Al_2O_3	380–420	N.A.[a]	4,000–4,500 (C)	3–6 (MPa $\sqrt{m}$)	0.1–0.3
Hydroxyapatite	~100	N.A.	~50 (T) >400 (C)	~1.0 (MPa $\sqrt{m}$)	0.1–0.3
Polyethylene (PE)	0.8–1.6	20–30	40–50 (T)	90 (MPa $\sqrt{m}$)	350–550
Poly(methyl methacrylate) (PMMA)	3.0–3.5	60	35–80 (T)	1.0 (MPa $\sqrt{m}$)	2–55
Poly(lactic acid) (PLA)	3–15	30–60	30–80 (T)	3–5 (MPa $\sqrt{m}$)	2–60
Skin	5–40	N.A.	30 (T)	30–70 (kJ/m²)	~100
Cortical bone	10–30	100–120	130–150 (T)	6–12 (MPa $\sqrt{m}$)	3

[a] *Not applicable.*

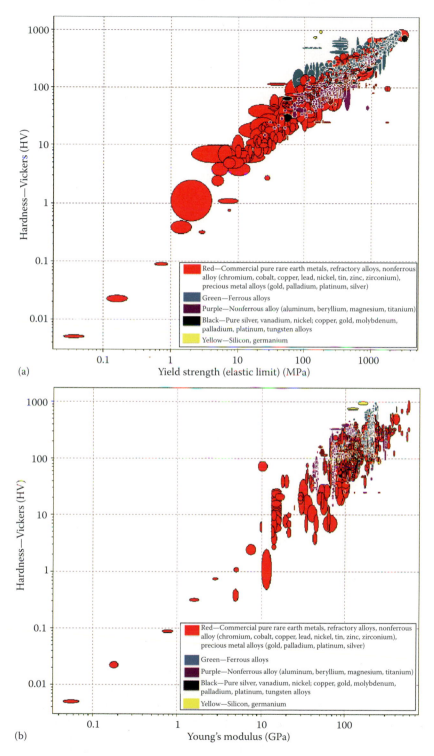

Figure 3.3
Relationships between the hardness, yield strength and Young's modulus of materials. (a) Hardness vs yield strength of materials. (b) Hardness vs Young's modulus of materials.

3.4 ELASTICITY: RESILIENCE AND STRETCHABILITY

In addition to the five mechanical properties depicted in Section 3.2, elasticity is the most important property for elastomeric materials, including synthetic elastomers and many biological tissues.

When a material is described as *elastic*, it is implied that it can recover from deformation when a force is applied to it. The mechanical work required to deform the object is stored as strain energy, which can be recovered when the force is removed [1]. *Resilience* is the capacity of a material to absorb energy when it is deformed elastically and, upon unloading, to have this energy recover. In other words, resilience is the maximum energy per unit volume that can be *elastically* stored.

For materials that have a yield point, resilience is quantitatively described by the *modulus of resilience*, W_y, which is the strain energy per unit volume required to stress a material from an unloaded state *up to the yield point* [1]:

$$W_{yield} = \int_0^{\varepsilon_y} \sigma \cdot d\varepsilon. \tag{3.2}$$

For elastomeric materials that virtually have no yield point, quantitative resilience can be better described by the *coefficient of restitution*, *R*, which is represented by the ratio of the two areas under the loading and recovering curves in the elastic region of the stress–strain curve (Figure 3.4) [2]:

$$R = \frac{W_{unload}}{W_{Load}}. \tag{3.3}$$

Theoretically, all *solid* materials are elastic within their elastic deformation limits, before the maximal elastic strain is reached, and beyond which deformation is irreversible (plastic). In practice, however, an object is often described as *more elastic* if it can recover its shape from larger deformation strains. Hence, the generic term *elastic* is often taken to mean stretchable, like a rubber band, with stretchability of a material defined by the elongation at break (i.e., the maximal strain at rupture). Ideally, *a full description of elasticity of any material should include both its measured resilience and rupture elongation values.*

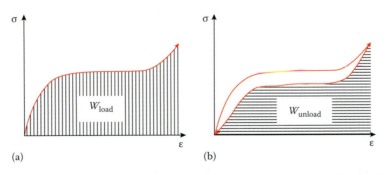

(a)   (b)

Figure 3.4
Examples of curves for stress (σ) versus strain (ε) during loading and unloading of an elastic material. (a) The work done during loading (W_load) and (b) unloading (W_unload) is expressed as the integral area under the curves. Unlike Young's modulus (σ/ε), resilience is represented by the ratio of W_load to W_unload (Equation 3.3) for a given material.

3.5 MECHANICAL PROPERTIES TERMS USED IN THE MEDICAL COMMUNITY

In the medical research community, researchers have developed a separate set of terms for describing the mechanical properties of tissues and biomolecules such as proteins. These terms are not always necessarily understandable by materials science and engineering researchers, and vice versa, and are more likely to be within the domain of biophysics and biomechanics. Table 3.2 outlines the two sets of terms used in the field of materials engineering or medical science.

3.6 FAILURE

The failure of materials is always an undesired event. Hence, understanding the reasons behind a failure is always important. The fracture mechanism of a material varies with its working conditions, based on which the fracture properties of materials are named, such as fatigue properties (cyclic loading), creep properties (at elevated temperature), stress corrosion cracking (SCC), and so on. Although these fractures appear complicated and vastly different, the fundamental mechanism is the same, that is, the breakage of chemical bonding between atoms or molecules. Among these failure forms, fatigue and SCC frequently occur in medical implants. Hence, this section is focused on an introduction to the fundamental concepts of these two topics.

3.6.1 Fatigue

Fatigue is the progressive structural damage that occurs when a material is subjected to cyclic loading. In general, cyclic loading will promote material damage

Table 3.2
Terms Describing Mechanical Properties of Proteins

Materials Properties	Equivalent Term Used in Medical Community	Units
Young's modulus, E	Stiffness	N m^{-2}
Ultimate tensile strength (stress at fracture, σ_{max})	Strength	N m^{-2}
Toughness	Toughness	
Energy-to-break		J m^{-3}
Work of fracture		J m^{-2}
Strain at rupture, ε_{max}	Extensibility or stretchability	No units
Resilience	Spring efficiency	%
Fatigue lifetime	Durability	Number of cycles to failure
Energy storage capacity, W	Spring capacity	J kg^{-1}

Source: Gosline, J. et al., *Philos. Trans. R. Soc. Lond. B Biol. Sci., 357, 121, 2002.*

more efficiently than static loading. Under static loading conditions, a material will only undergo permanent (plastic) deformation when the externally applied stress is higher than the yield stress limit (i.e., yield strength σ_y) of the material, and fracture can occur only when the applied stress reaches the tensile stress limit (i.e., UTS) of the material (Figure 3.1). However, when a material is subjected to a cyclic loading, it can fracture far below its UTS, and even below the yield strength of the material. As such, a fatigue failure is of the brittle type, which takes place with very little observable plastic deformation and minimal absorption of energy. Generally speaking, brittle fractures are more dangerous than ductile fractures because they occur abruptly under normal service conditions with little or no warning prior to rupture. Indeed, medical devices manufactured from any material expected to survive millions of cyclic deformations over their lifetime require scrutiny of the fatigue and fracture resistance, with fatigue fracture being the major cause of premature failure in biomedical implants.

Theoretically, a structurally perfect material (free of defects) would not suffer fatigue. In the real world, no materials are perfect, and fatigue usually initiates at a defect that acts as a stress concentration. Imperfections can arise from nonhomogeneity in microstructure (e.g., impurities, second phase particles, and grain boundaries) (Figure 1.5), manufacturing defects of the metallic component (e.g., holes and welds), or surface imperfections (scratches, sharp fillets, notches, and pits) from machining operations. Stress concentrates locally to these imperfect sites when the material is subjected to external loading. As a result, there is a fluctuating stress field inside the material. The internal stress field always increases proportionally to the external load. When the external load increases to a certain level, stress concentration can escalate to permanent defects, such as dislocations and microcracks (Figure 1.5) that cannot be removed by unloading. Instead, the defects either accumulate in number or grow in size during the process of cyclic loading. Eventually, a progressively growing crack develops under normal service conditions until the final catastrophic failure. Among these imperfections, defects on surfaces are the most dangerous. As a matter of fact, the crack associated with fatigue failure almost always initiates (or nucleates) on the surface of a component at some point of stress concentration.

One specific fatigue mechanism is associated with dislocations. Assume we have a piece of material free of macroscopic or microscopic discontinuities, but having microstructural defects, such as second phase particles and grain boundaries. For these structure defects, students can refer to Figure 1.5. When a low external load is applied to the material and the fluctuating stress field is well below the yield strength of the material, no dislocations will be produced, and thus, no structural damage will take place under this load. However, when the external load increases to a certain value (a threshold) at which the highest point of the fluctuating stress field approaches the material yield strength, dislocations will be produced locally (Figure 3.5). The number of dislocations produced by a single loading may not be so large as to cause visible damage. However, dislocations, which are permanent defects, can accumulate during the process of repeated loading. After thousands of loadings, the accumulated dislocations can develop into a microcrack, which can subsequently grow in size and lead to the final rupture of the working component. To reiterate, the fluctuating stresses inside a material due to the structural inhomogeneity of the material may lead to the initiation and growth of a crack, which, upon reaching a critical size, leads to complete fracture.

Fatigue properties of a material are commonly characterized by an *S-N curve*, also known as a *Wöhler curve* (Figure 3.6). This is a graph of the magnitude of a

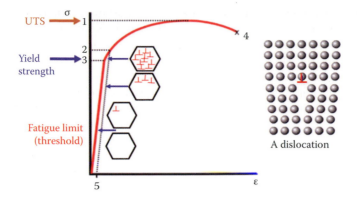

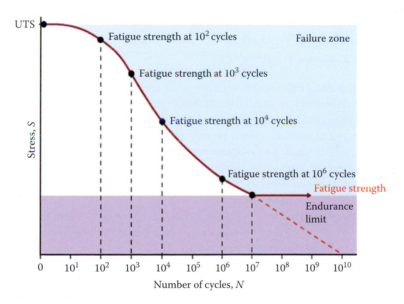

Figure 3.5

Theoretically, dislocation movement and increment occurs only when a perfectly homogeneous material is subjected to a stress of the yield strength or higher. In reality, no materials are absolutely homogeneous. More or less, dislocations are involved locally at stress-concentrated regions when the nominal stress is still lower than the yield strength. However, if a cyclic applied stress is sufficiently low, lower than a threshold such that virtually no dislocations are invoked, then fatigue will not happen. This threshold defines the fatigue limit.

Figure 3.6

S–N curves, where S represents magnitude of a cyclic stress, and N is the number of cycles to failure.

cyclic stress (S) against the logarithmic scale of cycles to failure (N). When considering Figure 3.6, it makes sense that the higher the external stress (S) is, the more the dislocations produced by a single load would be, and thus a lower number (N) of cyclic loads would be needed to accumulate dislocations toward failure. *Fatigue limit* or *endurance limit* refers to the maximal amplitude (or range) of cyclic stress that can be applied to a material without causing fatigue failure, regardless of how many cycles it is loaded. Most nonferrous alloys do not have a fatigue limit, in that the *S-N* curve continues its downward trend at increasingly greater *N* values. Thus, fatigue will ultimately occur regardless of the magnitude of the stress [1]. For these materials, the number of 10^7 cycles has been widely used as the *infinitely* large number of cycles, and the stress level at which failure will occur at 10^7 cycles is called *fatigue strength.*

The fatigue mechanisms described earlier explain why fatigue strength sensitively varies with the microstructure of materials, surface quality of products, and service conditions (e.g., load vectors, cyclic frequency, wearing, and corrosion environment). Nevertheless, generic relationships exist between the fatigue strength, UTS, yield strength, and Young's modulus of materials, which provide us with a very useful guide in the selection and design of materials for a good overall fatigue resistance. The fatigue strength is lineally proportional to UTS (Figure 3.7a):

$$\sigma_{fatigue} \approx 0.5 \ \sigma_{UTS}. \tag{3.4}$$

Since UTS is roughly proportional to the yield strength (Figure 3.7b) and Young's modulus (Figure 3.7c), fatigue strength and UTS are also roughly proportional to the yield strength and Young's modulus. In principle, materials of UTS, Young's modulus, and high yield strength tend to have excellent fatigue resistance.

3.6.2   Stress Corrosion Cracking

Stress corrosion cracking (SCC) is an unexpected sudden brittle failure of normally ductile or tough metals subjected to a tensile stress in a mild corrosive environment. SCC is induced by the synergistic influence of tensile stress (mechanical force) and a corrosive environment (chemical action), which is only mildly corrosive to the metal otherwise. In other words, neither the stress nor the corrosion conditions alone can cause failure, but in combination they are more likely to contribute to SCC. In essence, fracture of a material is a process of breakage of chemical bonding between atoms. Chemical bonds can be broken mechanically (tensile stretch), chemically (corrosion), or jointly (i.e., SCC). With the assistance of chemical action (i.e., corrosion) on a metallic material, the mechanical stress needed to break a chemical bond can be well below the tensile stress limit (i.e., UTS). In practice, cracking from stress corrosion has been shown to occur under a stress much lower than UTS, such as occurring in an implant with residual stresses. Like fatigue failure, SCC is of a brittle type. It can lead to unexpected sudden failure of normally ductile metals subjected to a tensile stress well below the yield strength of the material.

SCC typically occurs in stainless steels that work in a chloride-rich medium. In these situations, Cl^- or OH^- ions are key environmental species that cause SCC in stainless steels. Although the mechanisms of SCC are not fully understood, we do know that diffusion of Cl^- ions from a surrounding solution into a material (Figure 3.8) is the critical step. Since diffusion is always faster in a loosely packed structure than in a densely packed structure, FCC (closely packed) is much less susceptible to SCC than BCC (loosely packed). This explains why the presence of the BCC structured phase makes steels more susceptible to SCC, compared with the FCC structured (austenitic) steels. For this reason, Ni, an FCC stabilizing element (Figure 3.9), is widely used in stainless steels to effectively reduce the incidence of SCC.

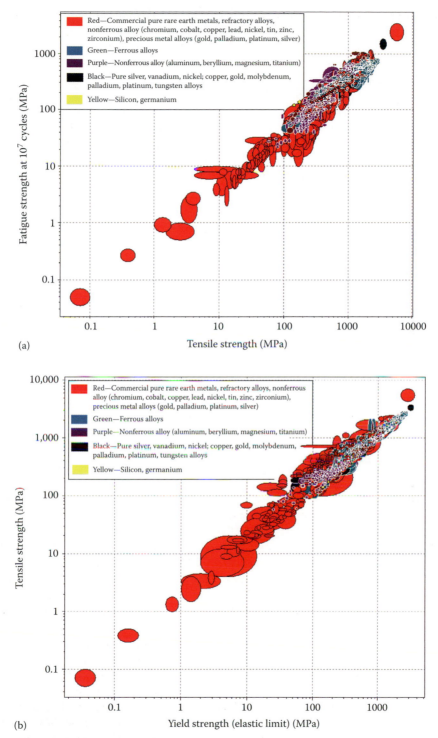

Figure 3.7
Relationships between the fatigue strength, ultimate tensile strength (UTS), yield strength, and Young's modulus of metallic materials. (a) Fatigue strength vs ultimate tensile strength of metallic materials. (b) Ultimate tensile strength vs yield strength of metallic materials. (Continued)

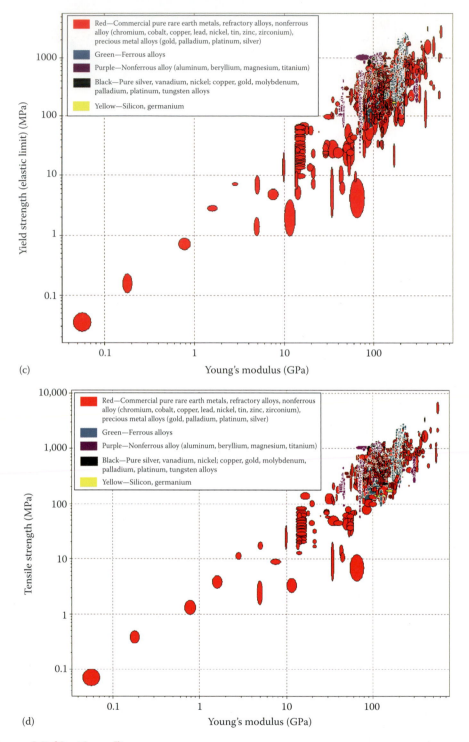

Figure 3.7 (Continued)

Relationships between the fatigue strength, ultimate tensile strength (UTS), yield strength, and Young's modulus of metallic materials. (c) Yield strength vs Young's modulus of metallic materials. (d) Ultimate tensile strength vs Young's modulus of metallic materials.

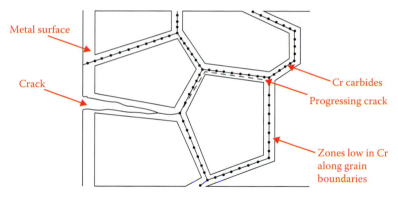

Figure 3.8
Mechanisms of SCC under the attack of Cl⁻ ions.

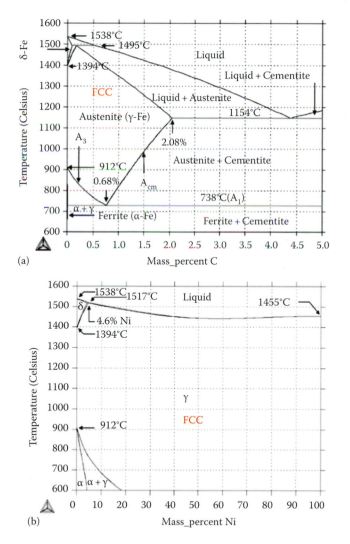

Figure 3.9
Phase diagrams of Fe–C and Fe–Ni systems. (a) F–C phase diagrams and (b) Fe–Ni phase diagrams.

3.7 ESSENTIAL MECHANICAL PROPERTIES OF ORTHOPEDIC IMPLANT BIOMATERIALS

In order to serve safely and appropriately at load-bearing sites for a long period of time without rejection, a metallic implant should possess the following essential characteristics:

1. No toxicity (equivalent to *excellent corrosion resistance*)
2. Suitable mechanical strength
3. High wear resistance
4. Osseo-integration ability (including bone bonding)

The fundamental science of corrosion of metals has been provided in Chapter 2. The present section is aimed to provide a generic introduction to the remaining three requirements of orthopedic implant biomaterials, and related fundamental concepts. The properties of specific alloys (stainless steels, CoCr-based alloys, and Ti alloys) will be described in Chapter 4.

3.7.1 Mechanical Working Environments of Implants in the Body

In Chapter 2, we discussed that when it comes to the selection of nontoxic materials, our immediate thought is to utilize those elements and compounds that naturally occur in the body. Likewise, in the design of mechanical requirements of biomaterials, a first step may be to understand the mechanical working conditions of implants. Hence, let us look at our body again.

3.7.1.1 Fatigue The mechanical working conditions within the human body are complex. Human beings normally walk several thousand steps a day at a rate of 1 Hz. As such, skeletal bone implants such as artificial hip joints, knee joints, spinal fixations, plates, and wires suffer from fatigue due to cyclic loading. In the case of total hip replacements (Figure 1.8f), the loading stress level is several times higher than that of the patient body weight. This is because when the hip joint is located out of the perpendicular alignment of the body weight, the balance between body weight and muscular strength pivots on only one leg. Loading stress on the leg during this motion is estimated to be ~50 MPa on average, when a load of five times of the body weight is applied to the cross section of the stem of a total hip prosthesis [3]. Under this average loading, according to finite element analysis, the maximal tensile stress in a total hip replacement in the body is around 200 MPa in the stem, and ~300 MPa in the neck (Figure 3.10). This is a conservative estimation, under the assumption that patients with hip implants would not jump or run. This value could be higher in practical situations, such as jumping, running, falling down, stepping down, carrying heavy loads on one side, so on.

With the increase of human life span, total hip replacements are expected to serve for 20 years. Assuming that a person walks 2×10^3 steps, the total number of steps over 20 years is estimated to be 2000 × 365 day × 20 years ≈ 1×10^7 cycles (Table 3.3). Cyclic stress also occurs in dental implants during chewing motion and in nonosseous tissue implants, such as pacemaker electrodes in response to myocardial activity.

As discussed previously, cyclic loading will promote material damage more efficiently than static loading. Hence, the most important mechanical requirement on

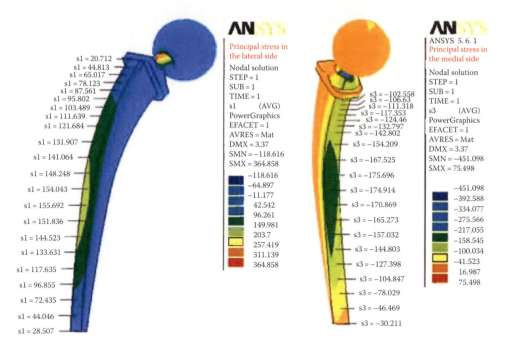

Figure 3.10

The principal stress contours, in MPa, in the hip prosthesis. The maximal tensile stress is around 200 MPa in the stem, and ~300 MPa in the neck. (From El-Shiekh, H.E.D.F., Finite element simulation of hip joint replacement under static and dynamic loading, PhD thesis, Dublin City University, Dublin, Ireland, 2002.)

Table 3.3
Fatigue Mechanical Working Conditions of Some Implants

Implants	Loading Strength	Loading Frequency (Hz)	Expected Total Number of Loading over the Lifetime of a 65-Year-Old Patient (i.e., 20 Years Implantation)
Joints	Compression ~50 MPa	1	10^7
	Bending 200–300 MPa		
Pacemaker	Not available	1	10^9
Tooth fillings	Not available	1	10^7

a biomaterial used in orthopedic implants for load-bearing sites is strength against fatigue. In total hip replacements, the stem material is expected to maintain physical integrity after being loaded to ~300 MPa for ~1×10^7 times.

3.7.1.2 Fretting Fatigue and Corrosion Fretting Fatigue The mechanical working conditions of orthopedic implants are frequently complicated by concurrent cyclic stress and friction, a scenario called *fretting fatigue*. Fretting fatigue is attributed to cyclic friction stress superimposed onto the plain fatigue stress. When fretting fatigue occurs, a foreign body is statically pressed to the surface of the specimen to which cyclic stress is applied. Fretting occurs as a result of relative movement with small amplitudes, which may occur between adjacent contacting surfaces of components. This results in the production of oxide debris and fresh metal surfaces. Visible damage is found even when the amplitude of slip is as little as 10^{-4} mm. A crack initiates at the contact site and it soon propagates before it finally breaks. Artificial hip joints, bone plates, and wires are likely to suffer from fretting fatigue [3].

Fatigue can also be complicated by concurrent corrosion. Inside the living body, the surface wear of metallic materials leads to successive release of metal ions, metallic compounds, and debris. The release of these products into the areas surrounding an implant may provoke toxicity in local tissues or organs. The necrosis (cellular death) of these injured tissues tends to acidify the surrounding environment, which can become very corrosive to the implant. When fatigue occurs along with corrosion, it is known as *corrosion fatigue*. Fretting fatigue with corrosion is thus known as *fretting corrosion fatigue*. Metallic implant biomaterials tend to be damaged by corrosion fatigue or fretting corrosion fatigue in the human body. In short, the interior of the living body is a mechanically, as well as chemically, harsh environment for metallic materials.

3.7.2 Wear of Joints

Wear is an inevitable problem in any joint replacements, no matter what materials are used. The low wear resistance or high friction coefficient of a joint system results in implant loosening. Although not fully understood, a frequent incident caused by wearing damage is *aseptic loosening* (Figure 3.11), which occurs when a large amount of tiny microscale particles are generated around a joint replacement. While a joint replacement performs its intended biomechanical function very well initially, a gradual increase in the amount of particles occurs over long-term wear, attracting cells of the immune system (called macrophages) that recognize and engulf the particles as foreign bodies, just as they do with bacteria. This is a natural defense mechanism (the *foreign body* response). However, the same particles tend to kill macrophages after ingestion. As a result, dying macrophages break down and release enzymes and metabolites which are acidic and cause severe acidification in the surrounding microenvironment. It is these enzymes, acidic chemicals, ions, and cellular debris that contribute to the erosion of both the implant and bone. There are also concerns over the adverse reactions to systemic distribution of metal wear particles and ions due to the toxicities of most alloying elements, as discussed in Chapter 2. In brief, wear debris causes severe adverse responses, whereby a revision surgery is likely to be required.

The wear resistance of a material is closely controlled by its hardness, which is roughly proportional to its yield strength, Young's modulus, and tensile strength. Hence, materials of high values in these three mechanical strengths generally demonstrate good resistances to wear. Alternatively, wear resistance of an implant can also be improved by surface modification or treatment. Zr-based alloys, for example, can be oxidized at 500°C to form a hard zirconia coating, which imparts excellent wear resistance.

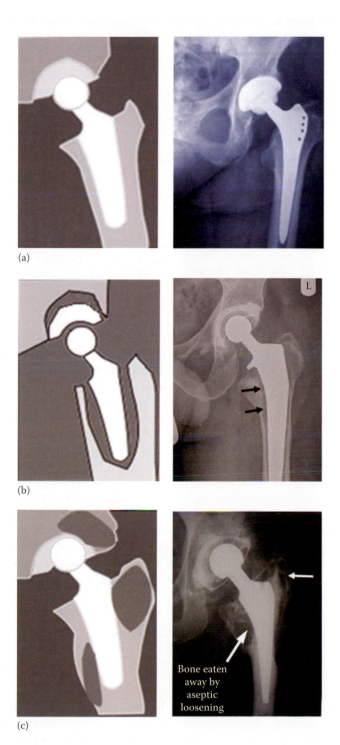

(a)

(b)

(c)

Figure 3.11

Aseptic loosening. (a) Stable prosthesis. (b) Linear osteolysis. (c) Expansile osteolysis.

3.7.3   Osseo-Integration

While high fatigue strength, excellent corrosion resistance, and wear resistance are the key properties that determine the longevity of permanent orthopedic implants in human bodies, the ability of an implant to bond with host bone is another fundamental requirement of permanent implants in orthopedics. *Osseo-integration* is a term that describes the bonding process of an implant with bone. The incapability of an implant surface to join with the adjacent bone and other tissues due to micromotions will cause the formation of fibrous tissue around the implant and promote loosening of the prosthesis. Therefore, it is essential for an implant to have an appropriate surface to integrate well with surrounding bone to prevent osteolysis. Materials (especially surface) chemistry, surface roughness, and surface topography are all factors that need to be considered for good osseo-integration.

Nevertheless, the bone-bonding process is not desired in the applications of temporary devices, such as internal fixation or traction devices. In these applications, the devices are removed after healing has taken place, and any bonding of the device to the host bone would complicate the removal surgery and cause further damage to the attached bone.

3.8   CHAPTER HIGHLIGHTS

1. The use of biomaterials as medical implants primarily helps the recovery of physical, especially mechanical, functions of injured or diseased organs or tissues.
2. Mechanical properties of general importance include Young's modulus E, yield strength σ_y, ultimate tensile strength (UTS) or ultimate compressive strength (UCS), fracture toughness, and elongation at break. Young's modulus is the only one that is not sensitive to microstructures.
3. Hardness is a measure of a material's resistance to wearing and friction, the form of localized plastic deformation. The hardness of the material is roughly proportional to its mechanical strength.
4. A full description of elasticity of a material should include both its measured resilience and rupture elongation values.
5. Resilience is the capacity of a material to absorb energy when it is deformed elastically and, upon unloading, to have this energy recover. In other words, resilience is the maximum energy per unit volume that can be *elastically* stored. For materials that have a yield point, resilience is quantitatively described by the modulus of resilience, W_y:

$$W_{\text{yield}} = \int_{0}^{\varepsilon_y} \sigma \cdot d\varepsilon$$

For elastomeric materials that virtually have no yield point, quantitative resilience can be better described by the coefficient of restitution, R:

$$R = \frac{W_{\text{unload}}}{W_{\text{load}}}$$

6. Fatigue is the progressive structural damage that occurs when a material is subjected to cyclic loading. In general, cyclic loading will promote material damage more efficiently than static loading. A fatigue failure is of the brittle type, and thus very dangerous.

7. Fatigue limit or endurance limit refers to the maximal amplitude (or range) of cyclic stress that can be applied to a material without causing fatigue failure, regardless of how many cycles it is loaded. For materials that do not have a fatigue limit, the number of 10^7 cycles is typically used as the *infinitely* large number of cycles, and the stress level at which failure will occur at 10^7 cycles is called *fatigue strength*.

8. The fatigue strength of a material is roughly linearly proportional to its mechanical strength, including Young's modulus E, yield strength σ_y and UTS:

$$\sigma_{\text{fatigue}} \approx 0.5\ \sigma_{\text{UTS}}.$$

9. Since hardness and fatigue strength of a material are both roughly proportional to its Young's modulus, yield strength, and UTS, materials of high UTS, Young's modulus, and high yield strength tend to have excellent resistance to both wearing and fatigue.

10. SCC is induced by the synergistic influence of tensile stress (mechanical force) and a corrosive environment (chemical action), which is only mildly corrosive to the metal otherwise. An SCC failure is also of the brittle type, and thus very dangerous.

11. Cyclic loading is the typical mechanical working condition of orthopedic implants in the body, and corrosion fretting bending fatigue is the major failure type in total hip replacements.

12. In total hip replacements, the stem material is expected to maintain physical integrity after being loaded to $\sim$300 MPa for $\sim 1 \times 10^7$ times.

13. The low wear resistance or high friction coefficient of a joint system results in implant loosening, a mechanism called aseptic loosening.

ACTIVITIES

1. Become familiar with the Medical Devices and Database pages of US Food and Drug Administration (FDA) and read "Class 2 Recall Accolade TMZF Plus Hip Stem" on the website of FDA: http://www.accessdata.fda.gov/scripts/cdrh/cfdocs/cfres/res.cfm?id=99392.

2. Visit http://www.matweb.com/, which is an excellent website providing mechanical properties of synthetic materials and biological tissues, such as bone.

SIMPLE QUESTIONS IN CLASS

1. The role of implant materials is primarily
   a. To biologically support organ or tissue regeneration
   b. To enhance cell proliferation
   c. To help the recovery of physical, especially mechanical, functions of injured or diseased organs or tissues
   d. To improve the biological function of diseased organs or tissues
2. Which of the following properties is nonsensitive to microstructures?
   a. Rupture elongation (or called elongation at break)
   b. Young's modulus
   c. Ultimate strength
   d. Fracture toughness
3. Hardness and fatigue strength of a material are NOT proportional to its
   a. Fracture toughness
   b. Yield strength
   c. Young's modulus
   d. Tensile strength
4. A full description of elasticity of a material should include both
   a. Elastic modulus and maximal elastic elongation
   b. Resilience and maximal elastic elongation
   c. Elastic modulus and yield strength
   d. Yield strength and plastic stretchability
5. Which of the following mechanical properties is of concern with regard to orthopedic implant biomaterials?
   a. Fatigue
   b. Creep
   c. Wear
   d. Elasticity
6. Aseptic loosening refers to implant loosening
   a. Due to the implant sterilization
   b. Due to the surgical sterilization process
   c. Due to the release of large wearing debris that kill cells that attempt to remove them
   d. Due to osteoporosis

PROBLEMS AND EXERCISES

1. In Table 3.1, the yield strength is not applicable (N.A.) for ceramics and skin. Explain the reasons.
2. The tensile engineering stress–strain curve of an alloy is given in the following.
   a. What is the yield strength at a strain offset of 0.002?
   b. What is the ultimate tensile strength?
   c. What is the elongation at break?

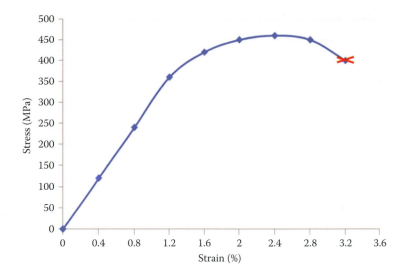

3. The stress–strain curve of a material is given in the following. Determine the $\sigma_{0.2}$ and $\varepsilon_{0.2}$. Calculate the *modulus of resilience* of the material.

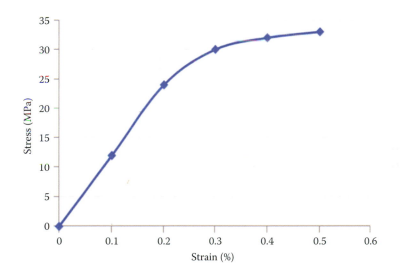

4. The loading and unloading stress–strain loop of a material is given in the following. Calculate
   a. The *modulus of resilience* of the material
   b. The total energy stored in the material at the end of the loading process
   c. The elastic energy released at the end of the unloading process
   d. The plastic energy stored in the material at the end of the cycle
   e. Resilience

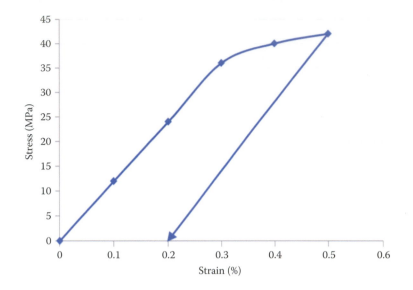

5. Explain why fatigue and SCC failures are much more dangerous than ductile rupture.

6. What is stress corrosion cracking (SCC)? Which element in the body is the key factor that causes SCC of 316L stainless steel implants?

7. SCC typically occurs in stainless steels that work in a chloride-rich medium. In these situations, Cl⁻ or OH⁻ ions are key environmental species that cause SCC in stainless steels. Would SCC occur in a hip replacement implant that is made of a martensitic or ferrite stainless steel? Explain your answer.

8. What is fretting fatigue? What is corrosion fatigue? And what is fretting corrosion fatigue?

9. What is the difference between fatigue limit (or endurance limit) and fatigue strength?

10. Predict, based on the data provided in Table 3.1, which materials could very likely have a good resistance to both wearing and fatigue? Explain your answers.

BIBLIOGRAPHY

References

1. Callister, W.D., *Materials Science and Engineering,* 7th edn. New York: John Wiley & Sons, Inc. 2007, Chapter 6.
2. Gosline, J., M. Lillie, E. Carrington, P. Guerette, C. Ortlepp, and K. Savage, Elastic proteins: Biological roles and mechanical properties. *Philosophical Transactions of the Royal Society of London. Series B, Biological Sciences*, 2002;**357**:121–132.
3. Sumita, M., T. Hanawa, I. Ohnishi, and T. Yoneyama, Failure processes in biometallic materials. In *Comprehensive Structural Integrity*, Vol 9. I. Milne, R. O. Ritchie, and B. Karihaloo, (Eds.), London, U.K.: Elsevier Science Ltd, 2003, pp. 131–167.
4. El-Shiekh, H.E.D.F., Finite element simulation of hip joint replacement under static and dynamic loading, PhD thesis, Dublin City University, Dublin, Ireland, 2002.

Websites

http://orthoinfo.aaos.org/.
http://teamwork.aaos.org/ajrr/default.aspx.
http://www.fda.gov/default.htm.
http://www.fda.gov/MedicalDevices/default.htm.
http://www.njrcentre.org.uk/njrcentre/default.aspx.

Further Readings

Callister, W.D., Characterization of materials. In *Materials Science and Engineering*, 7th edn. New York: John Wiley & Sons, Inc., 2007, Chapters 3 and 4.

Mazzocca, A.D. et al. Principles of internal fixation, In *Skeletal Trauma*. Browner, B.D., J.B. Jupiter, A.M. Levine, P.G. Trafton, and C. Krettek (eds). Chapter 4, W.B. Saunders Co, Philadelphia PA, USA, an imprint of Elsevier, 2009.

Park, J. and R.S. Lakes, Chapter 5: Metallic implant materials. In *Biomaterials: An Introduction*, 3rd edn. Hayton, J. and K. Santor, New York: Springer, 2007.

Wagner, M.A. and R. Frigg, In *Skeletal Trauma*. Browner, B.D., J.B. Jupiter, A.M. Levine, P.G. Trafton, and C. Krettek (eds). Chapter 5, W.B. Saunders Co, Philadelphia PA, USA, an imprint of Elsevier, 2009.

CHAPTER 4

METALLIC BIOMATERIALS IN ORTHOPEDIC IMPLANTS

LEARNING OBJECTIVES

After careful study of this chapter, you should be able to do the following:

1. Describe the corrosion-resistant mechanisms of stainless steels, CoCrMoNi alloys, and Ti alloys.
2. Describe the application principles of stainless steels, CoCrMoNi alloys, and Ti alloys.
3. Describe the advantages and disadvantages of stainless steels, CoCrMoNi alloys, and Ti alloys.
4. Select metallic materials for medical devices.
5. Describe the stress-shielding effect.

4.1   DEVELOPMENT OF METALLIC BIOMATERIALS

The use of metallic materials for medical implants can be traced back to the nineteenth century, leading up to the era when the metal industry began to expand during the Industrial Revolution. The development of metallic implants was primarily driven by the demands for new approaches to bone repair, typically internal fracture fixation of long bones. However, almost no attempts of implanting metallic devices such as spinal wires and bone pins made from iron, gold, or silver were successful, until Lister's aseptic surgical technique was implemented in the 1860s. Since then, metallic materials have become the most predominant in orthopedic surgery, playing a major role in most orthopedic devices, including temporary devices (e.g., bone plates, pins, and screws) and permanent implants (e.g., total joint replacements). For a detailed historic retrospective on the development of total joint replacements, readers can refer to the Advanced Topic in Chapter 6. Concurrently, metals also found applications in dental and orthodontic practice, including tooth fillings and roots. Recently, increasing research effort in metallic biomaterials has been invested in the application of the non-conventional reconstructive surgery of hard tissues/organs, such as the application of NiTi shape memory alloys as vascular stents and the development of new magnesium-based alloys for bone tissue engineering and regeneration.

Despite the large number of metals and metal alloys that are able to be produced in industry, only a few are biocompatible and capable of long-term success as an implant material. These form components in the vast majority of orthopedic medical devices available commercially and can be categorized in the following four groups based on the matrix alloying element (Table 4.1): (iron-based) stainless steels, cobalt-based alloys, titanium-based alloys, and miscellaneous others (e.g., NiTi and alloys of Mg and Ta).

A variety of medical implants made of the metallic materials in the first three groups have been approved by the US Food and Drug Administration (FDA)* and are routinely used in orthopedic practice. Figures 4.1 and 4.2 depict some of the typical clinical

Table 4.1
Four Categories of Metallic Biomaterials and Their Primary Applications as Implants

Type	Primary Utilizations[a]	Status of Applications
Stainless steels	1. Temporary devices (fracture plates, screws, hip nails, etc.) (Class II)	FDA approved and routinely applied
	2. Total hip replacements (Class II)	
Co-based alloys	3. Total joint replacements (wrought alloys) (Class II)	FDA approved and routinely applied
	4. Dentistry castings (Class II)	
Ti-based alloys	5. Stem and cup of total hip replacements with CoCrMo or ceramic femoral heads (Class II)	FDA approved and routinely applied
	6. Other permanent devices (nails, pacemakers) (Class III)	
Miscellaneous others		
NiTi	1. Orthodontic dental archwires (Class I)	FDA approved
	2. Vascular stents (Class III)	FDA approved
	3. Vena cava filter (Class II)	FDA approved
	4. Intracranial aneurysm clips (Class II)	FDA approved
	5. Contractile artificial muscles for an artificial heart (Class III)	Research
	6. Catheter guide wires (Class II)	FDA approved
	7. Orthopedic staples (Class I)	FDA approved
Mg	Biodegradable orthopedic implants (Class III)	Animal trial
Ta	8. Wire sutures for plastic surgeons and neurosurgeons (Class III)	FDA approved
	9. A radiographic marker (Class II)	FDA approved

[a] *Class I–III are defined in Table 21.2 in Chapter 21.*

* *FDA approves medical devices, rather than any materials.*

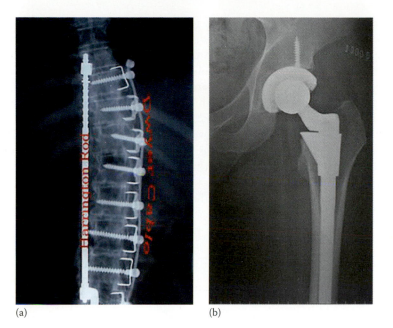

(a)   (b)

Figure 4.1
(a) Harrington rod is a stainless steel surgical device. (b) The stem of a total hip replacement (THR) is made from one of the following three alloys: stainless steel, cobalt-based, or titanium-based alloys. (From Tom, E., Adolescent (Idiopathic) Scoliosis, 2010, http://drerrico.com/html/idiopathic.html.)

application scenarios. The materials of the last group have recently been developed because of their unique material properties (such as the shape memory of NiTi and the degradability of Mg) that could potentially meet more specialized tissue requirements, depending on intrinsic tissue requirements (Figure 4.2). However, some medical implants made with these newly developed alloys are not FDA-approved yet, primarily due to the significant issues associated with biocompatibility, the principal requirement for the clinical application of any biomedical implant. Clinical applications and current status of the four classes of metallic biomaterial are summarized in Table 4.1. This chapter is devoted to the orthopedic metallic implant materials, that is, stainless steels, cobalt-based alloys, and titanium-based alloys. The last group (miscellaneous others) is the topic of Chapter 5.

4.2 STAINLESS STEELS

Stainless steel is the generic name for a number of iron-based alloys that contain a high percentage (11–30 wt.%) of chromium and varying amounts of nickel. Stainless steels can be categorized into two groups: the chromium and chromium–nickel types, according to chemical composition. Alternatively, they can also be grouped into four families based on the lattice structure (Figure 1.4) of the alloys: martensitic (BCC), ferritic (BCC), austenitic (FCC), or duplex (austenitic plus ferritic), as listed in Table 4.2. Except for the duplex type, each of the other three groups of stainless steels finds applications in medical devices. The superb hardness of martensitic

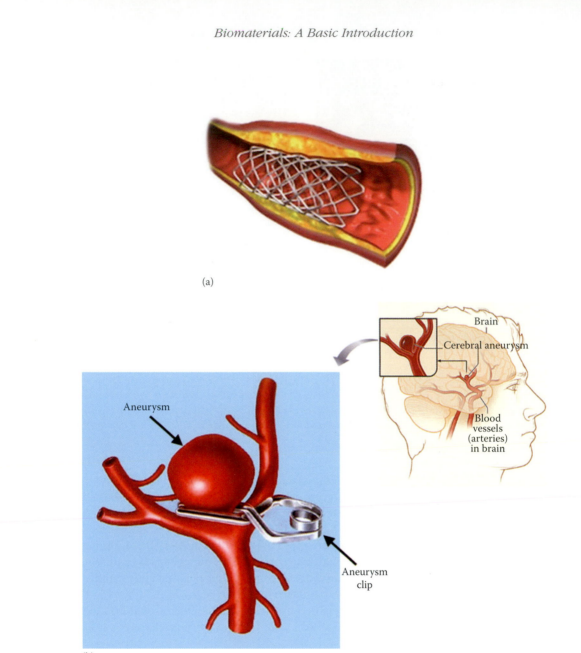

(a)

(b)

Figure 4.2

(a) Vascular stent and (b) aneurysm clip, which are made from NiTi alloy. Clipping is a surgical procedure performed to treat a balloon-like bulge of an artery (known as an aneurysm). As an aneurysm grows, it becomes thinner and weaker. It can become so thin that it ruptures, releasing blood into the spaces around the brain—called a subarachnoid hemorrhage (SAH). A tiny clip can be placed across the neck of the aneurysm to stop or prevent an aneurysm from bleeding. (Produced by KimvdLinde, http://illumin.usc.edu/assets/media/391/v_220pxHipreplacement-232x400.jpg.)

Table 4.2

Four Categories of Stainless Steels and Typical Medical Applications

Material Type	Application Grade	Examples
Martensitic	Dental and surgical instruments	Bone curettes, chisels and gouges, dental burs, dental chisels, curettes, explorers, root elevators and scalers, forceps, hemostats, retractors, orthodontic pliers, and scalpels
Ferritic	Very limited surgical instruments	Solid handles for instruments, guide pins, and fasteners
Austenitic[a]	A large number of nonimplantable medical devices	Cannulae, dental impression trays, guide pins, hollowware, hypodermic needles, steam sterilizers, storage cabinets and work surfaces, and thoracic retractors
	Many temporary implants	Fracture plates, fixing screws, hip nails, etc.
	Total hip replacements	Stem of total hip replacements
Duplex	Not yet applied in the biomedical field	

[a] *The focus of Section 4.2.*

stainless steels makes them ideally suited for dental and surgical instruments. Ferritic stainless steels find very limited applications in medical devices. Austenitic stainless steels are applied in various nonimplantable or implantable medical devices where good corrosion resistance and moderate or high strength is required. These applications often require a material that is easily formed into complex shapes. However, *only austenitic (FCC) stainless steels are used for implants*, so these materials will form the focus of this section.

4.2.1 Corrosion Resistance of Stainless Steels

The minimum percentage of chromium (Cr) in stainless steel is ~11 wt.%, the amount needed to prevent the formation of rust in unpolluted atmosphere. In addition to chromium, nickel (Ni), molybdenum (Mo), and manganese (Mn) are three other major alloying elements in medical-grade stainless steels. These elements all contribute to increase the corrosion resistance of the matrix element iron, except for manganese, which is added to improve the workability of steel at high temperatures by the formation of a high melting sulfide. Table 4.3 lists the compositions of 316 (ASMT F138) stainless steel and its variants, which have been widely used in temporary devices following bone trauma (such as fracture plates, screws, and hip nails) and in permanent implants (such as total hip replacements).

4.2.1.1 Chromium (Passivity) Under normal physiological conditions, pure iron is subject to corrosion, as indicated by the Pourbaix diagram of iron (Figure 2.8b). The 316 type stainless steel has a corrosion potential E_{corr} around −0.1 (SCE) = +0.142 (SHE) in a saline solution (Figure 2.5). Using this E_{corr} as the first approximation in body fluid, the stable state of chromium is Cr_2O_3 (pH = 7.2–74) according to Figure 4.3. Indeed, the chromium in stainless steel has a great affinity for oxygen, which allows the formation of an invisible chromium-rich oxide film (~2 nm thick) on the surface of the steel, which is adhesive and promotes self-healing in the presence of oxygen.

Table 4.3

Compositions of 316 (ASTM F138) Stainless Steel and Variants (wt.%)

ASTM Code/UNS No of Stainless Steels	Cr	Ni	Mo	Mn	Si	Cu	N	C	P	S
F138/S31673	17.00–19.00	13.00–15.00	2.25–3.00	2.00	0.75	0.50	0.10	0.030	0.025	0.010
F1314/S20910	20.50–23.50	11.50–13.50	4.00–6.00	2.00–3.00	0.75	0.50	**0.20–0.40**	0.030	0.025	0.010
F1586/S31675 (Orthinox)	19.50–22.00	9.00–11.00	2.00–4.25	2.00–3.00	0.75	0.25	**0.25–0.50**	0.08	0.025	0.010
F2229/S29108	19.00–23.00	**0.10**	**21.00–24.00**	0.50–1.50	0.75	0.25	**>0.90**	0.08	0.03	0.010

Source: Davies, J.R. (ed.), Mettalic materials, in Handbook of Materials for Medical Devices, Materials Park, OH, ASM International, 2003, pp. 21–50.

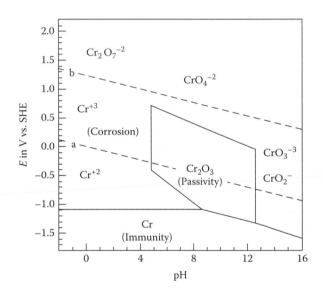

Figure 4.3
Pourbaix diagrams of chromium in water. 316 stainless steels have corrosion potentials E_{corr} around −0.1 (SCE) = +0.142 (SHE) in seawater, which is similar to body fluid of pH = 7.2. In such environments, the stable state of chromium is as the oxide Cr_2O_3. Hence, passivity is possible.

4.2.1.2 Nickel (Passivity and FCC Structure Formation)

Further improvement in corrosion resistance, as well as a wide range of mechanical properties, is achieved by the addition of nickel. Nickel is the main alloying element that stabilizes the formation of a closely packed structure (face-centered cubic = FCC, austenite) in iron, which enhances corrosion resistance. An alloy in a closely packed structure always shows a better corrosion resistance than its loosely packed counterpart, principally because the chemical bonds in a closely packed structure are stronger than those of the same atoms in a loosely packed structure. Nickel also contributes to increase corrosion resistance by the formation of protective nickel oxide (NiO) films on the surface of the alloys.

4.2.1.3 Molybdenum (Carbide Formation and Minimization of Pitting Corrosion) The addition of some other alloying elements may enhance resistance to specific corrosion mechanisms or develop desired mechanical and physical properties. For example, in addition to enhancing corrosion resistance, with a resultant strengthening passive film, the use of molybdenum further increases resistance to pitting corrosion caused by chromium carbide formation.

Pitting corrosion is a form of highly localized corrosion that leads to the formation of small holes in metals. The thermodynamic reason for pitting corrosion is that small depassivated areas become anodic, while the remaining vast area becomes cathodic.

In chromium steels, chromium has a strong affinity with carbon, leading to the formation of carbides in carbon-rich regions, typically grain boundaries. The precipitation of chromium carbide (Cr_3C_2, Cr_7C_3, and $Cr_{23}C_6$) results in the depletion of chromium and thus the depassivation of the small regions around chromium carbides (Figure 4.4). Consequently, the corrosion resistance of the steel surrounding the chromium carbides is reduced. The addition of molybdenum, which has a strong tendency to form carbides as well, can effectively trap carbon by forming molybdenum carbides and thus reduce the level of chromium carbide formation. The chemistry of 316L stainless steel and variants is designed to maximize the pitting corrosion resistance. It should be noted that it is also necessary to decrease the carbon content to improve corrosion resistance, although carbon contributes to increasing the strength of steels.

4.2.1.4 Nitrogen (Enhance Resistance to Pitting and Crevice Corrosion) *Crevice corrosion* refers to corrosion occurring in a confined space, to which the access of the surrounding fluid is limited. The mechanism of crevice corrosion in passivatable alloys (e.g., stainless steels) exposed to chloride-rich body fluids is gradual acidification of the environment inside the crevice, leading to the appearance of highly aggressive local conditions that gradually destroy the passivity. Crevice corrosion is encountered frequently between the underside of a bone screw head and the countersunk area of the bone plate. It starts with the depletion of oxygen in the crevice. While the anodic reaction continues in the crevice, the oxygen concentration is not readily replenished by the fluids outside the crevice. Meanwhile, smaller chlorine ions diffuse into the

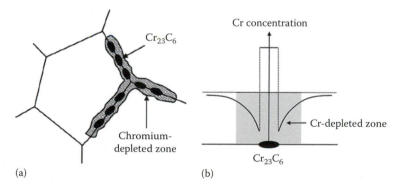

(a)   (b)

Figure 4.4
Schematic illustration showing the mechanism of how the formation of chromium carbides along a grain boundary leads to depletion of chromium: (a) formation of chromium carbides along grain boundaries; (b) depletion of chromium along a grain boundary due to the formation of chromium carbides.

crevice, drawn there by the metal ions being released by the anodic reaction. The pH in the crevice region thus decreases, causing accelerated metal oxidation.

Nitrogen is soluble in a relatively high content in closely packed structured (austenitic) stainless steels and stabilizes the austenitic structure of iron. It can be used as a substitute for nickel in those variants of 316L (Table 4.3) to increase mechanical strength as well as to enhance resistance to pitting and crevice corrosion. In 1998, high-nitrogen ASTM F1586 (i.e., Orthinox) came into use as a stem material in total hip replacements. More recently, nickel-free, austenitic steels with high nitrogen concentration (ASTM F2229) have also been developed for medical use.

4.2.1.5 Metallurgical Processing Routes That Enhance Corrosion Resistance   In addition to the aforementioned alloying chemistry, special production routes such as vacuum melting, vacuum arc remelting (VAR), or electroslag refining are required to produce implant-grade stainless steels. The vacuum melting step improves the cleanliness of the process, such that the quantity and size of nonmetallic inclusions are minimized and the pitting and crevice corrosion resistance are maximized in the steels produced. Type 316L is a vacuum-melted variant of the standard type 316 composition. Finally, passivity of stainless steel implants is enhanced by nitric acid passivation before the implant is sterilized and packaged for delivery to a medical facility.

4.2.1.6 Stress Corrosion Cracking   While corrosion resistance (including pitting and crevice corrosion) of stainless steels has been improved by the alloying chemistry and metallurgical processing mentioned earlier, the form of corrosion known as stress corrosion cracking (SCC) (Section 3.6.2) cannot be prevented by the aforementioned methods. As discussed in Chapter 3, SCC is an unexpected sudden brittle failure of normally ductile or tough metals subjected to a tensile stress in a mild corrosive environment. SCC frequently occurs in stainless steels that work in a chloride-rich medium, where the diffusion of Cl^- or OH^- ions is believed to play a critical role in SCC failure. Hence, caution must be taken in the applications of implants made from stainless steel, as body fluid is both aqueous and chloride-rich. Since diffusion is always slower in a densely packed structure than in a loosely packed structure, FCC (closely packed) is much less susceptible to SCC than BCC (loosely packed). Today, ferrite (BCC structured) stainless steels have limited applications in medical devices, and duplex (FCC matrix with the second BCC structured phase) stainless steels have yet to make an impact in the biomedical field. Only austenitic (FCC) stainless steels are used for orthopedic implants.

4.2.1.7 Summary   The corrosion resistance of iron-based stainless steels is primarily achieved by alloying chemistry, with the inclusion of chromium, nickel, molybdenum, and nitrogen. These elements protect steels via different mechanisms. Chromium, which plays a primary role in the corrosion resistance of steels, forms a protective chromium-oxide film on the surface of the steels (passivity). Nickel enhances corrosion resistance through two mechanisms: the formation of the closely packed FCC structure and the contribution of an oxide film on the surface (passivity). Molybdenum, which has a strong tendency to form molybdenum carbide, minimizes pitting by decreasing chromium carbide formation. Similarly to nickel, nitrogen enhances resistance to pitting and crevice corrosion by stabilizing the closely packed FCC structure.

Although the success of stainless steels makes these alloys widely accepted as such, they are not completely *stain-proof*. This is especially true in corrosive human body fluids, with pitting corrosion, crevice corrosion, and corrosion fatigue being frequently

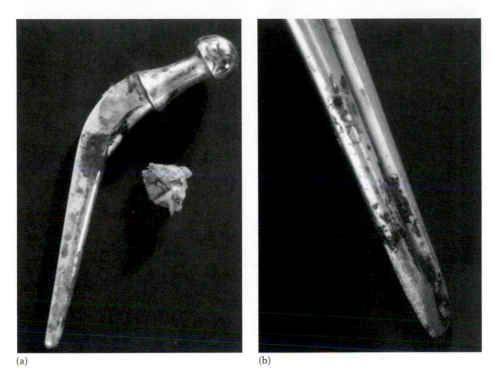

(a)   (b)

Figure 4.5
(a) Corrosion scale on a Charnley stainless steel stem and (b) pitting and corrosion of a Müller stainless steel stem after implant removal. (Reprinted from Biomaterials, 19(1–3), Walczak, J., Shahgaldi, F., and Heatley, F., In vivo corrosion of 316L stainless-steel hip implants: Morphology and elemental compositions of corrosion products, 229–237, 1998, Copyright 1998, with permission from Elsevier.)

reported in the application history of 316L stainless steels implants (Figure 4.5). Stainless steels can also suffer from SCC, in a chloride-rich medium, especially at highly stressed regions in the body. The high-nitrogen variants of 316 composition (e.g., Orthinox) have much more satisfactory resistance to corrosion in the body.

4.2.2   Biocompatibility of Stainless Steels

Since the Iron Age around 1200 BC, when the people first mastered iron metallurgy, containers made of iron have been used in preparing and keeping food in kitchens. This suggests that elemental iron has relatively no impact on human health. In confirmation of this, and scientific study on the toxicity of metal ions has recently classified iron as the safest of several metals in a rank of toxicity:

cobalt > vanadium > nickel > chromium > titanium > iron.

As listed in Table 4.3, the major alloying elements in 316L stainless steel (ASTM F138) and variants are chromium, nickel, molybdenum, and manganese, in addition to the matrix element iron. For the toxicity of these elements, readers can refer to the appropriate Advanced Topics at the end of Chapter 2.

The use of stainless steel in medical implants started in the 1930s, when cytotoxicity evaluation standards had not yet been established. Hence, there is almost no literature focusing on the biocompatibility of stainless steels both in vitro and in vivo from this period. The reasonably good biocompatibility of this alloy was recognized by the early clinical success of total hip replacements in the 1960s and 1970s. Stainless steel has since been used as a control material in many subsequent studies. More detailed review will be given in the context of NiTi alloys (Chapter 5). In general, stainless steel shows good biocompatibility, but to a less satisfactory level than CrCrMo alloys or Ti alloys due to its greater corrosion rates. The systemic toxicity and carcinogenicity of released nickel and chromium are the major related concerns.

4.2.3   Mechanical Properties of Implant-Grade Stainless Steels

As mentioned in Chapter 3, most mechanical properties (e.g., yield strength, fatigue strength, UTS, and elongation at break) vary not only with alloy type (i.e., alloy chemistry) but with processing conditions (i.e., microstructure). The elastic (Young's or shear) modulus is an exception, which is determined by the alloy type rather than its microstructure (Table 3.1). Austenitic stainless steels for implants are all wrought alloys, that is, they are fabricated by forging (cold/hot working) and machining. Figure 4.6 demonstrates three manufacture processes: casting, wroughting/forging, and annealing. When a forged metal becomes hard, the annealing treatment can make it softer. A summary of microstructure-sensitive mechanical properties of type 316L stainless steel and variants is provided in Table 4.4. The high-nitrogen variants (cold-worked F1314, F1586, and F2229) are stronger than the original 316 composition (cold-worked F138).

The fatigue strength of F138 stainless steels is typically between 300 and 400 MPa in air, or 200 and 300 MPa in a biological aqueous solution. Considering that the stem in total hip replacements in the body is subject to a maximal loading of ~300 MPa (Figure 3.9), 316L stainless steels are not sufficiently reliable in terms of fatigue properties. The wear resistance of 316L stainless steel is also relatively poor, and wear debris leading to allergic reaction in surrounding tissue is another reason to restrict their application in permanent implants at load-bearing sites.

As described in Section 3.6.1, fatigue crack initiation is frequently correlated to the presence of surface imperfections on metals. With stainless steels in saline solutions, corrosion pits frequently act as stress raisers and thus preferential sites for fatigue crack initiation. Hence, adding elements such as molybdenum and nitrogen, which improve the pitting corrosion resistance of stainless steels, is an effective way of improving the corrosion fatigue resistance of stainless steel implants. This is the rationale behind the development of F1586 (Orthinox) and F2229 (Table 4.3). The fatigue strength of these two alloys is typically around 500 MPa in physiological environments, well above the maximal loading stress value of hip stems in the body.

4.2.4   Application Principles of Stainless Steels in Orthopedics

The features of corrosion, fatigue, and SCC in stainless steels define their medical application principles. First, failures due to corrosion, fatigue, and SCC in the body do not happen in a short time, but rather after a long service period that is typically of several months to years. Hence, 316L stainless steels can be used in temporary devices (e.g., the nail in Figure 4.7a). In these applications, the devices are removed after healing has taken place. Indeed, the low cost of 316L steels has maintained their application in a large number of short-term temporary devices, such as internal

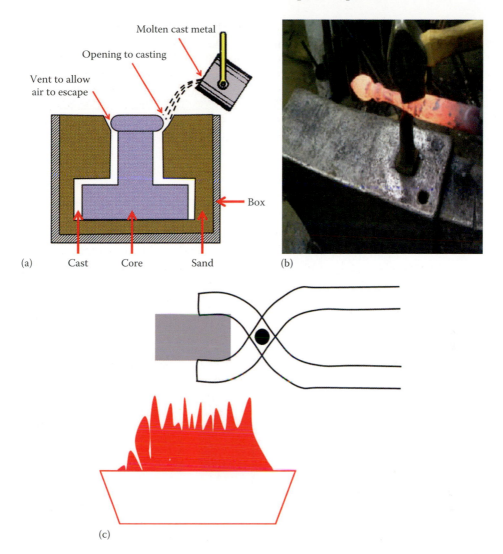

Figure 4.6

Three processing methods of materials, casting, wroughting, and annealing: (a) Casting: shaping by pouring a liquid material into a mold, which contains a hollow cavity of the desired shape, and then the liquid solidifies. (b) Wroughting/forging: materials are wrought or forged into shape with tools. Forged iron means the metal was shaped under heat, that is, hot-worked; wrought iron means shaped cold with a machine, that is, cold-worked. (c) Annealing: heating up to soften a work-hardened metal. Work hardening is caused by the increase in dislocations, which can be removed by heat during annealing.

fracture fixation and traction devices for the spine, bone screws, bone plates, intra-medullary nails and rods (Figure 4.8).

Second, if a loading stress is lower than the fatigue and SCC strength of the alloy, fatigue and SCC will virtually never happen. Hence, stainless steels have been used in permanent implants for shoulders (Figure 4.7b), as the loading stresses at these lightly stressed regions are generally lower than the fatigue and SCC strength of 316L stainless steels. However, the same grade of stainless steel (fatigue strength being ~300 MPa) is

Table 4.4

Mechanical Requirements for 316L (ASTM F138) and Variants in Bar

Steels	Conditions	UTS, min/MPa	Yield Strength (0.2%) (min/MPa)	Elongation in 4D, min (%)
F138	Annealed	490	190	40
	Cold-worked	860	690	12
F1314	Annealed	690	380	35
	Cold-worked	1035	862	12
F1586	Annealed	740	430	35
(Orthinox)	Cold-worked	1000	700	20
F2229	Annealed	931	586	52
	Cold-worked 10%	1062	786	37
	Cold-worked 20%	1262	952	25
	Cold-worked 30%	1496	1227	19
	Cold-worked 40%	1731	1551	12

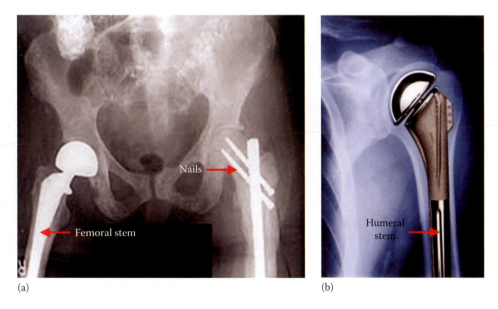

(a)   (b)

Figure 4.7

Application principles of stainless steels: (a) 316L stainless steel can be used in hip nails (temporary device), but not in the total hip replacement (THR) on the left side. Orthinox is now used in the femoral stem of THRs. (b) 316L stainless steel has been used as the humeral stem in total shoulder replacements (TSRs), which is a lightly stressed region. However, due to its poor long-term resistance to corrosion, the stainless steel is now replaced by a titanium alloy Ti-6Al-4Nb in TSR.

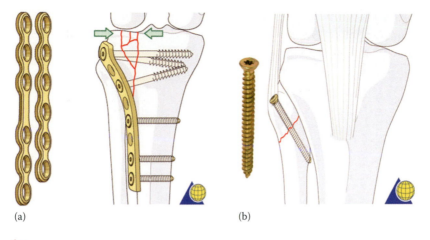

(a)   (b)

Figure 4.8
Temporary devices made of 316 type stainless steels. (a) Fracture plates; (b) fixing screws. (From www2.aofoundation.org. Copyright by AO Foundation, Davos, Switzerland. Reprinted with permission.)

not recommended to be used in permanent implants at load-bearing sites such as hip, knee, and ankle joints, because the loading stresses at these highly stressed regions in the body* are in the order of 300 MPa.

In contrast, Orthinox is less susceptible to either fatigue or SCC in the body at these highly stressed regions due to its improved resistance to pitting and crevice corrosion and mechanical strength, compared with the 316L alloy. According to the 8th National Joint Registry Annual Report (UK) in 2011, the top two Orthinox hip stem brands, Exeter V40 and Charnley, occupied approximately 60% and 10% of the market in the United Kingdom, respectively [3]. Table 4.5 lists various implantable device applications for stainless steels.

To summarize, stainless steels remain popular for implant applications because of their lower cost, accepted biocompatibility, and toughness. However, 316L stainless steel implants are often degraded due to pitting, crevices, corrosion fatigue, wearing, fretting corrosion, and SCC in the body, which restrict their application in permanent implants at heavy load-bearing sites. Nowadays, 316L stainless steel is predominant in a large number of temporary devices. Nevertheless, the leading role of stainless steel as stem materials in permanent hip prostheses has been maintained by the application of high-nitrogen stainless steels.

4.2.5 Critical-Sized Defects

One may question what happens to the holes left behind in the bone after a temporary device is removed. The healing ability of such defects is size-dependent. Generally speaking, the organs of the body have an ability to regenerate and recover when

---

* A "high stress in the body" described by a surgeon is relatively lower than a "high stress in an engineering structure" described by an engineer.

Table 4.5

Medical Applications of Stainless Steels

Materials	Devices	Applications
Type 316L stainless steel	Bone screws and pins	Internal fixation of diaphyseal fractures of cortical bone, metaphyseal and epiphyseal fractures of cancellous bone; screws comprised of hexagonal or Philips recess driving head, threaded shaft, and self-tapping or nonself-tapping tip
Type 316L stainless steel	Onlay bone plates	Internal fixation of shaft and mandibular fractures: thin, narrow plate with slots or holes for retaining screws
Type 316L stainless steel	Blade and nail bone plates	Internal fixation of fracture near the ends of weight-bearing bones: plate and nail, either single unit or multicomponent
Type 316L stainless steel	Intramedullar bone nails	Internal fixation of long bones: tube or solid nail
Orthinox stainless steel	Total joint prostheses	Replacement of total joints with metal and plastic components (shoulder, hip, knee, ankle, and great toe): humeral, femoral (hip and knee), talus, and metatarsal components
Type 316L stainless steel	Wires	Internal tension band wiring of bone fragments or circumferential cerclage for comminuted or unstable shaft fractures
Type 316L stainless steel	Harrington spine instrumentation	Treatment of scoliosis by the application of correction forces and stabilization of treated segments: rod and hooks
Types 316 and 316L stainless steel	Mandibular wire mesh prostheses	Primary reconstruction of partially resected mandible
Types 304, 316, and 316L stainless steel	Sutures	Wound closure, repair of cleft lip and palate, securing of wire mesh in cranioplasty, mandibular and hernia repair and realignment, tendon and nerve repair
Types 316 and 316L stainless steel	Stapedial prostheses for middle ear repair	Replacement of nonfunctioning stapes: various types comprised of wire and piston or wire and cup piston (synthetic fluorine-containing resin/stainless steel piston, platinum and stainless steel cup piston, and all stainless steel prostheses)
17–7PH, 17–7PH (Nb), PH-15–7Mo, and types 301, 304, 316, 316L, 420, and 431 stainless steel	Neurosurgical aneurysm and microvascular clips	Temporary or permanent occlusion of intracranial blood vessels; tension clips of various configurations, ~2 cm (0.8 in.) or less in length and constructed of one piece or jaw, pivot, and spring components (similar and dissimilar compositions)

Material	Device	Application
Stainless steel wire formed in a zigzag configuration of 5–10 bends	Self-expanding stent	Treatment of tracheobronchial stenosis, tracheomalacia, and air collapse following tracheal reconstruction: 0.457 mm (0.018 in.)
Stainless steel	Balloon-expandable stent	Dilation and postdilation support of complicated vascular stenosis (experimental)
Type 316 stainless steel	Hydrocephalus drainage valve	Control of intercranial pressure: one-way valve
Type 304 stainless steel	Trachea tube	Breathing tube following tracheotomy and laryngectomy: tube-within-a-tube construction
Type 316 stainless steel, with spring steel diaphragm	Electronic laryngeal prosthesis system	Electromagnetic voicing source following total laryngectomy: implanted unit comprised of subdermal transformer, rectifier pack, and transducer encased in type 316 stainless steel, with spring steel diaphragm
Types 304, 316, and 316L stainless steel	Electrodes and lead wires	Anodic, cathodic, and sensing electrodes and lead wires: intramuscular stimulation, bone growth stimulation, cardiac pacemaker (cathode), electromyography (EMG), electroencephalogram (EEG), and lead wires in a large number of devices
Stainless steel	Arzbaecher pill electrode	Atrial electrocardiograms: swallowed sensing electrode of short metal tubing segments forced over plastic tubing
Type 316L stainless steel	Cardiac pacemaker housing	Hermetic packaging of electronics and power source: welded capsule
Types 316 and 316L stainless steel	Wire mesh	Inguinal hernia repair, cranioplasty (with acrylic), orthopedic bone cement restrictor
Types 304 and 316 stainless steel	Retention pins for dental amalgam	Retention of large dental amalgam restorations: cemented, friction lock, and self-threading pins, placed ~2 mm (0.08 in.) within dentin with ~2 mm (0.08 in.) exposed
Types 304 and 316 stainless steel	Preformed endodontic post and core	Restoration of endodontically treated teeth: post fixed within root canal preparation, with exposed core providing a crown foundation
Type 304 stainless steel	Preformed dental crowns	Restoration for extensive loss of tooth structure in primary and young permanent teeth: preformed shell
Types 302, 303, 304, and 305 stainless steel	Fixed orthodontic appliances	Correction of malocclusion by movement of teeth: components include bands, brackets, archwires, and springs
Stainless steel	Percutaneous pin bone fixation	External clamp fixation for fusion of joints and open fractures of infected nonunions: external frame supporting transfixing pins

(Continued)

Table 4.5 (Continued)
Medical Applications of Stainless Steels

Materials	Devices	Applications
Stainless steel	Variable capacitance transducer	Measurement of pressure on sound: metal diaphragm, mounted in tension
Stainless steel	Variable resistance transducer	Measurement of respiratory flow: metal arms supporting wire strain gage
Stainless steel	Intrauterine device (IUD)	Contraception: stainless steel (Majzlin spring, M-316, M device), stainless steel and silicone rubber (Comet, M-213, Ypsilon device), stainless steel and natural rubber (K S Wing IUD), stainless steel and polyether urethane (Web device)
Stainless steel	Intrauterine pressure-sensor case	Protective shroud for transducer
Stainless steel	Osmotic minipump	Continuous delivery of biologically active agents: implanted unit comprising elastomeric reservoir, osmotic agent, rate-controlling membrane, and stainless steel flow moderator and filling tube
Stainless steel	Radiographic marker	Facilitation of postoperative angiography of bypass graft: open circle configuration of 25 gage suture wires
Stainless steel	Butterfly cannula	Intravenous infusion
Stainless steel	Cannula	Coronary perfusion: silicone rubber reinforced with an internal wire spiral
Stainless steel	Acupuncture needle	Acupuncture: 0.26 mm (0.01 in.) diameter × 5–10 cm (2–4 in.) length needles
Steel and stainless steel	Limb prostheses, orthoses, and adaptive devices	Substitution, correction, support, or aided function of movable parts of the body, and technical aids not worn by the patient: components such as braces, struts, joints, and bearings of many items

Source: Davies, J.R. (ed.), Metallic materials, in Handbook of Materials for Medical Devices, Materials Park, OH, ASM International, 2003, pp. 21–50.

102

they are diseased or injured; however, regeneration can only occur at a limited scale. A *critical-sized defect* (CSD) is defined as the minimal defect that cannot heal without medical manipulation, regardless of how much time it is given to heal. When natural healing is almost impossible, medical devices are needed. If the sizes of defects, such as the holes of screws, are smaller than the CSD of human bones, they can heal spontaneously after the temporary device is removed, typically by gradual osteoblast infiltration and subsequent ossification.

4.2.6   Current Issues and Challenges

Being used as a short-term device (from several months to several years) does not guarantee absence of a failure in stainless steel. There have been premature failures of 316L stainless steels reported in orthopedic implants (Figure 4.9). The time of failure varies from several months to several years after implantation. Failure analysis of 316L implants has revealed that the fractures appear to be due to fatigue failure, with implants showing very poor surface finishing and fatigue cracking initiated at sites of machining imperfections and crevice corrosion. Hence, the fatigue failure of 316L stainless steel implants can be prevented by a quality surface finishing and treatment (e.g., nitriding), which is primarily a quality-control issue, rather than a challenge in materials science and engineering.

A more significant issue is that there have been premature fractures of Orthinox steel reported in the stems of hip implants (Figure 4.10), with a ~10% incidence. The fracture positions in these cases are always around the middle of the stem, which is

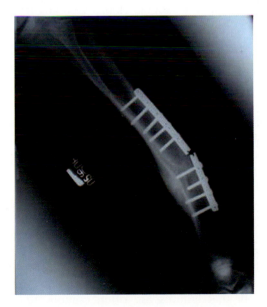

Figure 4.9
Radiographic image of a failed stainless steel implant inside a patient. (Reprinted from Int. J. Fatig., 29(6), Niinomi, M., Fatigue characteristics of metallic biomaterials, 992–1000, 2007, Copyright 2007, with permission from Elsevier.)

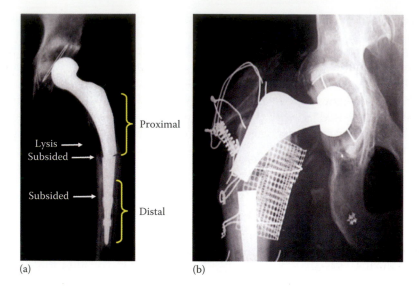

(a)   (b)

Figure 4.10
(a) Stem fracture after 8.6 years. Endosteal bone lysis surrounds the proximal half of the stem. The stem has subsided 1.6 cm, partly within the cement, together with the distal cement mantle. (From Røkkum, M. et al., Acta Orthopaedica, 66(5), 435. Copyright 1995, Informa Healthcare.) (b) Fractured Exeter stem after 3 years. (From van Doorn, W.J. et al., Acta Orthop. Scand., 73(1), 111. Copyright 2002, Informa Healthcare.)

the most highly stressed region (Figure 3.9). The examinations of fracture surfaces have revealed that the cause of failure is fatigue. Hence, bending fatigue is the major cause of stem fracture of Orthinox hip replacements.

The adverse effects of nickel ions on the human body have prompted the development of high-nitrogen, nickel-free austenitic stainless steels for medical applications. Nitrogen replaces nickel for austenitic FCC structure stability, as well as improving the overall steel structural properties. By combining the benefits of stable austenitic structure, high strength and good plasticity, better corrosion and wear resistances, and superior biocompatibility compared to the currently used 316L stainless steel, the high-nitrogen, nickel-free stainless steels (e.g., F2229) could be a better substitute. However, toughening of these alloys remains to be explored, as high nitrogen content tends to make the alloys brittle.

Finally, another major concern over the long-term performance of total hip replacements is associated with the *stress-shielding effect*, which refers to the reduction in bone density as a result of removal of normal stress from the bone by an implant. Stainless steel, as well as cobalt-based alloys and titanium-based alloys, have much higher Young's modulus (more than 200 GPa) than that of bone, which is only 10–30 GPa. The high elastic modulus of the implant may result in its carrying nearly all loads. The issue associated with the stress-shielding effect is not just that further revision surgery is required, but that failures are often complicated such that revision is impossible, due to insufficient bone support. Hence, it is desirable to have an implant with similar Young's modulus to that of bone. This forms the driving force behind active research in the development of new implant biomaterials that can minimize, if impossible to eliminate, the stress-shielding effect.

4.3   COBALT-BASED ALLOYS

The cobalt-based *superalloy* (high performance alloy) was originally developed by Haynes for use in aircraft engines, and called stellite. It exhibited higher strength at elevated temperatures and better corrosion resistance when compared to other superalloys. Cobalt-based alloys were first used in medical implants in the 1930s. The CoCrMo alloy vitallium was used as a cast dental alloy and then adapted to orthopedic applications in the 1940s. By modifying vitallium, a range of alloys have been developed, with compositions listed in Table 4.6.

4.3.1   Corrosion Resistance of Cobalt–Chromium Alloys

Like iron, pure cobalt is not resistant to corrosion according to its Pourbaix diagram (Figure 4.11). However, cobalt–chromium-based alloys are superior to stainless steels in corrosion resistance, demonstrating excellent performance in a chloride-rich environment, which is related to its chemical composition. The high chromium content

Table 4.6
CoCr-Based Alloys Used in Surgical Implants

ASTM Standard	Nominal Compositions	Cast/Wrought Status	Medical Application
F75-98	Co-28Cr-6Mo	Cast	Permanent implant
F90-97	Co-20Cr-15W-10Ni	Wrought	Short-term implant
F562-95	Co-35Ni-20Cr-10Mo	Wrought	Permanent implant
F563-95	Co-Ni-Cr-Mo-W-Fe	Wrought	Short-term implant
F799-99	Co-28Cr-6Mo	Forged	Permanent implant
F961-96	Co-35Ni-20Cr-10Mo	Forged	Permanent implant
F1058-97	Co-Cr-Ni-Mo-Fe	Wrought	Permanent implant
F1537-94	Co-28Cr-6Mo	Wrought	Permanent implant

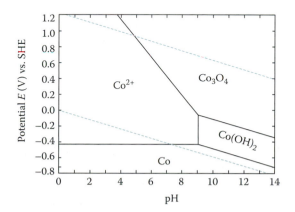

Figure 4.11
In seawater, E_{corr} of Co-Cr alloy is $-0.25V$ (SCE) $= -0.008V$ (SHE). When pH = 3.5, or 7.4, Co^{2+} ion is stable, and thus corrosion is possible. When pH = 9.0, Co_3O_4 is stable and thus passivity is possible.

Table 4.7
The Roles of Alloying Elements

Elements	On Corrosion Resistance	On Microstructure	On Mechanical Properties
Cr	Cr_2O_3 to corrosion resistance	Forms $Cr_{23}C_6$	• Enhances wear resistance
Mo	Increases corrosion resistance	Refines grain size	• Enhances solid–solution strengthening
Ni	Increases corrosion resistance		• Enhances solid–solution strengthening • Increases castability
C		Forms $Cr_{23}C_6$	• Enhances wear resistance • Increases castability
W	Decreases corrosion resistance	Reduces shrinkage cavity, gas blow hole, and grain boundary segregation	• Enhances solid–solution strengthening • Decreases corrosion fatigue strength

leads to spontaneous formation of a passive oxide (Cr_2O_3) layer within the human body fluid environment. The roles of Cr and other alloying elements are summarized in Table 4.7. In brief, Cr, Mo, and Ni are responsible for the corrosion resistance, very much like their roles in stainless steels. Tungsten, which is added to increase solid-solution strengthening and to control the distribution and size of carbides, can however impair the corrosion resistance and corrosion fatigue strength of Co-based alloys. As such, Co-20Cr-15W-10Ni and Co-Ni-Cr-Mo-W-Fe alloys are restricted to short-term implants, such as bone plates and wire, due to both unsatisfactory corrosion resistance and a high amount of toxic nickel release.

Cobalt alloys were initially used as cast (Figure 4.6a) components, with wrought (Figure 4.6b) alloys coming into use later. The casting and forging conditions of these alloys have significant influences on their corrosion resistance and mechanical properties. In general, casting gives rise to coarse grains, grain boundary segregations, gas blow holes, and shrinkage cavities in the CoCrMo alloys. Although the cast alloys are superior to noncast alloys in wear resistance, pitting resistance, and crevice corrosion resistance, they are inferior to wrought alloys in terms of fatigue strength and fracture toughness.

4.3.2 Biocompatibility of Cobalt Alloys

The first application of cobalt alloy in hip implants was in 1939, slightly later than stainless steels. In vitro evaluation showed that the CoCrMo alloy is much less toxic than pure cobalt or nickel due to its excellent corrosion resistance. The huge clinical success of CoCrMo stems in total hip replacements in the 1960s demonstrated that CoCrMo alloys are well-tolerated in the body. However, patients with CoCrMo metal-on-metal bearing systems are still exposed to wearing debris over a long period. The debris liberates cobalt and chromium into the blood via the synovial fluid, before being excreted in the urine. There have been increasing concerns over elevated serum metal ion levels, potential teratogenic effects, and potent adverse local tissue reactions; however, the specific pathogenesis of these incidents remains unclear. The toxicities of major metallic biomaterials are ranked as follows:

$$\underset{\text{Poor} \qquad \text{Biocompatibility} \qquad \text{Good}}{3.16\text{L} < \text{Orthinox} < \text{CoCrMo} < \text{Ti-6A1-4v}} \longrightarrow$$

4.3.3 Mechanical Properties of Medical-Grade Cobalt Alloys

While the excellent corrosion resistance of CoCr-based alloys is primarily imparted by alloying chromium, their superior mechanical properties over stainless steels are due to the crystallographic nature of the base element cobalt. With an atomic number of 27, cobalt falls between iron and nickel on the periodic table. The physical properties of cobalt are very similar to those of iron and nickel (Table 4.8). The elastic modulus of pure cobalt is about 210 GPa in tension and about 180 GPa in compression, which do not stand out of those of iron and nickel. The superior wear and fatigue resistances of cobalt alloys over iron alloys primarily arise from their two closely packed structures: HCP and FCC (Figure 1.4). The strengthening mechanism is the solid-state phase transformation of part of the matrix from an FCC crystal structure to an HCP structure in response to stress during cold working. The presence of two equally closely packed but distinct crystal structures poses a barrier to the motion of dislocations and leads to pronounced strengthening. In addition, the solid-solution-strengthening effects of chromium, tungsten, and molybdenum, and the formation of metal carbides all contribute to the superb fatigue resistance of this alloy system. While 316 stainless steels are wrought alloys, CoCr alloys can be used as either cast or wrought forms.

For the purpose of comparison, it should be mentioned that the presence of the second BCC-structured phase also strengthens and hardens the FCC-structured austenitic steels. However, BCC structure is relatively loosely packed, and makes the alloy susceptible to SCC and fatigue. For this reason, duplex stainless steels (FCC matrix with the second BCC structured phase) are not used in the biomedical field.

The data listed in Table 4.9 show that the wrought (cold-worked) and forged cobalt alloys have UTS in excess of 1200 MPa and fatigue strength close to or in excess of 600 MPa, well above the maximal loading stress value (300 MPa) in the stem of total hip replacements. Hence, wrought CoCr alloys are regarded to be safe for orthopedic

Table 4.8
Some Physical Properties of Fe, Co, and Ni Elements

Elements	Density (g/cm³)	Structure	Young's Modulus (GPa)		Shear Modulus (GPa)	Melting Point
			Tensile	Compressive		
Fe	7.9	BCC below 912°C FCC between 912°C and 1394°C BCC above 1394°C	210	170	82	1538°C
Co	8.8	HCP below 417°C FCC above 417°C	210	180	75	1493°C
Ni	8.9	FCC	200	180	76	1455°C
Ti	4.5	HCP below 885°C BCC above 885°C	116	110	44	1668°C

Table 4.9

Mechanical Properties of Cast and Wrought Cobalt-Based Alloys

Alloys	Young's Modulus (GPa)	UTS (MPa)	0.2% Yield Strength (MPa)	Elongation (%)	Fatigue Strength
F75/cast, annealed	210	650–890	450–520	15	200–310
F75/P/M HIP	250	1280	840		725–950
F799/forged	210	1400–1590	900–1030	28	600–900
F90/annealed	210	950–1220	450–650		NA
F90/44% cold-worked	210	1900	1610		590
F562/forged	230	1210	960–1000		500
F562/cold worked, aged	230	1800	1500	8	690–790
F563/annealed	230	600	280	50	
F563/cold-worked	230	1000–1310	830–1170	12–18	
F563/cold-worked, aged	230	1590	1310		
F1058 wire	230	1860–2280	1240–1450		

Source: Davies, J.R. (ed.), Mettalic materials, in Handbook of Materials for Medical Devices, Materials Park, OH, ASM International, 2003, pp. 21–50.

implant applications in the leg. ASTM F75, F799, and F562 alloys are the most widely used cobalt alloys for implant applications.

ASTM F75 is a cast Co-Cr-Mo alloy, and has a long history in the aerospace and biomedical implant industries. In addition to its excellent corrosion resistance, the main attribute of this alloy is wear resistance. Distribution of Cr-rich carbides $M_{23}C_6$ and the work-hardening ability of this alloy greatly enhance wear resistance. Total artificial hip joints (head and cup) made from this alloy are even more viable, due to its excellent tribological properties against plastic sockets, that is, in a metal-on-plastic joint. A further feature of F75 is the extremely large grain size observed in the original castings. A finer grain size in general results in superior mechanical properties. Hence, wrought Co alloy came into use.

ASTM F799 is a wrought version of F75 alloy, which is mechanically processed by hot forging rough billets to make the final shape. To have a good ability to be forged, the carbon content of a wrought alloy must be sufficiently low. Although the low carbon content compromises wear resistance of wrought alloys, they are superior in fatigue strength imparted by the wrought microstructure. As mentioned earlier, the primary strengthening mechanism in wrought cobalt alloys is the solid-state phase transformation of part of the matrix from an FCC crystal structure to an HCP structure by cold working. The presence of two distinct crystal structures poses a barrier to the motion of dislocations and leads to pronounced strengthening. The strength (fatigue strength, yield strength, and UTS) of F799 alloy are approximately twice those of as-cast F75 (Table 4.9). Modern metal-on-metal joint prostheses are almost exclusively made from the F799 alloy (Figure 4.12).

ASTM F562 is a wrought Co-Ni-Cr-Mo alloy. The microstructure of worked F562 is the HCP solid-state phase formed from the FCC matrix by cold working. Subsequent

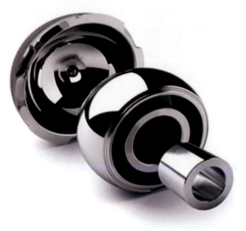

Figure 4.12
Femoral bearing head and cups made from the F799 CoCrMo alloy. (From http://www.zimmer. co.uk/z/ctl/op/global/action/1/id/9226/template/MP.)

age hardening in the 425°C–650°C range acts to further strengthen these two phases through the precipitation of carbides, primarily $Cr_{23}C_6$. Cold-worked and aged F562 can reach tensile strength levels in excess of 1795 MPa, which is the highest strength of any of the surgical implant alloys (Table 4.9).

4.3.4 Medical Applications of Cobalt Alloys

The superior fatigue resistance of CoCrMo alloys makes them a major choice of materials for total joint replacements. The medical implant application of CoCrMo alloys started as a stem material in total hip replacement in the 1950s. Currently, ~20% of total hip replacements have stems and/or the hard-on-hard joint system (Figure 4.13) made out of wrought CoCrMo alloys. As for total knee and ankle replacements, the prostheses are almost exclusively made out of CoCrMo alloys with hard polymer

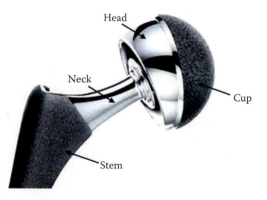

Head

Neck

Cup

Stem

Figure 4.13
CoCrMo alloys can be used as the stem, head, and cup in total hip replacements.

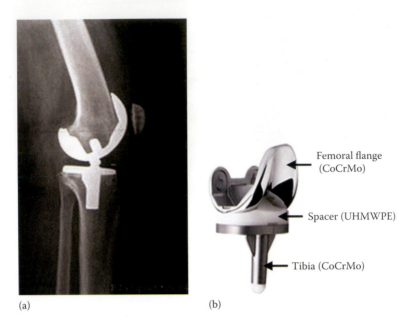

(a)   (b)

Figure 4.14

Total knee prostheses usually have a metallic femoral component (replacing the femoral condyle) fabricated from wrought CoCrMo alloys and a spacer made from ultrahigh-molecular-weight polyethylene (UHMWPE). The tibia backup (attached to tibial bone) is made of the same CoCrMo alloy. (a) An x-ray image of a total knee replacement in the body (the polymer spacer is invisible). (From the WikimediaCommons @ http://en.wikipedia.org/wiki/File:PTG_P.jpeg.) (b) Components of total knee replacement.

(ultrahigh-molecular-weight polyethylene, UHMWPE) as a lining (Figures 4.14 and 4.15). The use of wrought cobalt-based alloy for fracture-fixation purposes is not as common as stainless steels, as a result of its increased cost compared with that of stainless steel. In short, wrought CoCrMo alloys are used in permanent implants at highly stressed regions of the body.

4.3.5 Current Issues and Challenges

Wrought CoCrMo alloys are expensive, which has limited their demand in the medical market, compared with stainless steels. Other issues associated with cobalt-based alloys include stress-shielding effects and metal toxicity. Cobalt alloys have a high Young's modulus (220–230 GPa), which is much higher than that of cortical bone (10–30 GPa). The interface between a stress-shielded bone and an implant deteriorates as the bone is weakened. Loosening and fracture of the bone, the interface, or the implant itself may occur. The combination of stress shielding, wear debris, and motion at an interface is especially damaging and often leads to failure. There are also concerns about the elements released from cobalt-based alloys, as Ni, Cr, and Co each has toxic effects. They may cause systemic allergic reactions in the host body, which can increase inflammation.

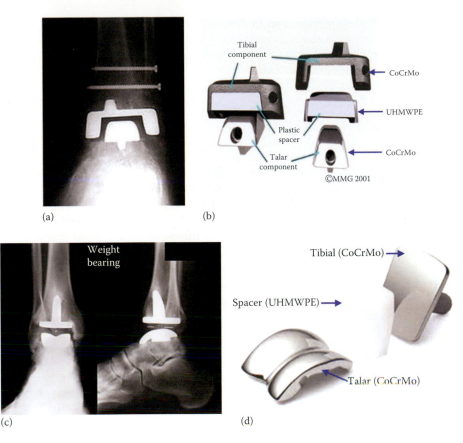

Figure 4.15
Two types of total ankle prostheses usually have metallic tibial and talar components fabricated from wrought CoCrMo alloys, and a spacer component made from ultrahigh-molecular-weight polyethylene (UHMWPE): (a) X-ray image of an Agility™ total ankle replacement in the body (the polymer spacer is invisible); (b) components of total ankle replacements; (c) X-ray image of a Zenith™ total ankle replacement; and (d) components of Zenith total ankle replacement.

4.3.6 Summary

Cobalt, as the matrix element, forms the foundation of high-strength properties of this alloy system, thus ensuring superior fatigue resistance. Cr, Mo, and Ni provide excellent corrosion resistance. As a result, CoCrNiMo alloys are superior to stainless steels in terms of resistance to corrosion, SCC, fatigue, and wear. The range of properties available for cobalt alloys make them suitable for a wide range of orthopedic applications, including all metallic components of all joint replacements. Wrought CoCrMo alloys are currently the choice of structural materials in permanent implants at high load-bearing sites (i.e., the joint systems rather than the stem), providing a more than 20 years service longevity. Long-term clinical use has proved that these alloys have good biocompatibility in bulk form. However, a number of issues remain with these alloy systems, including failures due to fretting fatigue and corrosion fatigue, aseptic loosening due to wearing, stress-shielding effects, and biological reactions due to released Co, Cr, and Ni ion or particle toxicity. Although imperfect, wrought CoCrMo alloys remain the most popular metallic implant materials of joint (bearing) systems, improving the quality of life for thousands of people worldwide.

4.4 TITANIUM ALLOYS

Titanium is a low-density element (approximately 60% of the density of iron and nearly half of the density of cobalt). Pure titanium undergoes an allotropic transformation at approximately 885°C, changing from an HCP crystal structure (α phase) to a BCC crystal structure (β phase) (Figure 1.4). Based on their microstructure after processing, titanium alloys are categorized into four classes: α alloys, near-α alloys, α–β alloys, and β alloys. The α–β alloy Ti-6Al-4V is the most widely used titanium alloy, accounting for approximately 45% of total titanium production. In terms of biomedical applications, Ti-6Al-4V and commercial pure Ti grades are the most widely used, although the past decade has seen increased use of β-titanium alloys for surgical implant applications. Table 4.10 lists ASTM standards for titanium and its alloys used for medical implants.

4.4.1 Corrosion Resistance of Titanium and Its Alloys

Titanium and its alloys provide excellent resistance to general localized attack under most oxidizing, neutral, and inhibited reducing conditions. They remain passive under mildly reducing conditions. The corrosion resistance of titanium metal is due to a stable, protective, strongly adherent oxide film, as discussed in Chapter 2, with the Pourbaix diagram of titanium shown in Figure 2.8c. The oxide film on titanium is very stable and attacked by only a few substances, most notably, hydrofluoric

Table 4.10
Titanium and Titanium Alloys Used for Medical Implants

Category	ASTM	UNs No.	Materials
α microstructure (HCP)	F67	R50250	CP-Ti grade 1
		R50400	CP-Ti grade 2
		R50550	CP-Ti grade 3
		R50700	CP-Ti grade 4
α–β microstructure (HCP + BCC)	F136	R56401	Ti-6Al-4V ELI (currently standardized)
	F1472	R56400	Ti-6Al-4V (currently standardized)
	F1295	R56700	Ti-6Al-7Nb (standardized)
	F2146	R56320	Ti-3Al-2.5V (not currently standardized)
β microstructure (BCC)	F1713		Ti-13Nb-13Zr
	F1813	R58120	Ti-12Mo-6Zr-2Fe
	F2066	R58150	Ti-15Mo

Source: Davies, J.R. (ed.), Mettalic materials, in Handbook of Materials for Medical Devices, Materials Park, OH, ASM International, 2003, pp. 21–50.

acid. Titanium is capable of healing this film almost instantly when a fresh surface is exposed to air or moisture (such as at body temperatures and in physiological fluids) because of its strong affinity for oxygen.

The use of titanium alloys as biomaterials has been increasing primarily due to their better corrosion resistance and superior biocompatibility compared to stainless steels and cobalt-based alloys, as well as relatively low Young's moduli. These attractive properties drove the early commercial introduction of pure titanium (CP-Ti) and α–β Ti-6Al-4V alloys, as well as the more recent development of β alloys.

4.4.2 Biocompatibility of Titanium Alloys

Among the long list of alloying elements of Ti alloys, V, Al, Nb, Zr, Mo, Fe, and Ta are the most important for medical implantable Ti alloys, as shown in Table 4.10. Compared with stainless steel and cobalt alloys, titanium alloys have proven to be superior in terms of biocompatibility, not only because of their excellent corrosion resistance but because of the nonreactivity of elemental titanium. Titanium implants are not rejected by the body, and generally make good physical connections with the host bone. Mutagenicity is not significant, as determined by in vitro mutation assays, indicating that the titanium alloys are safe for animals and humans.

However, the first-generation titanium alloys, represented by Ti-6Al-4V (Ti64), have been reported in clinical reports to cause toxicity and allergic reactions in the human body due to vanadium. Vanadium is added to the alloys to stabilize the β (BCC) phase, which is tougher than the α (HCP) phase. However, vanadium compounds such as oxides are all toxic. Because of this, Ti-6Al-4V has been replaced by Ti-6Al-4Nb. Titanium and its alloys designed for use in implant devices have little or no reaction with surrounding tissues.

The second-generation titanium alloys (β-titanium alloys) have been developed, driven by their low Young's modulus that can potentially address the stress-shielding effect. Some β structure stabilizing elements, such as Mo, Ta, Nb, and Zr, are used as alloying elements. These elements are considered to be relatively safe for the living body, compared with vanadium and aluminum (Figure 2.2). So far, there is a lack of long-term follow-up data on the biocompatibility of β-titanium alloys.

4.4.3 Bone-Bonding Ability of Ti and Ti Alloys

The family of titanium-based biomaterials are favored by most clinicians, surgeons, materials scientists, and medical device designers, not only because they are more inert and more biocompatible in implant applications than stainless steels and cobalt alloys, but due to a unique feature of titanium. Among all metallic biomaterials, titanium alloys are the only material system with the ability to fuse with host bone. In general, once a virtually bioinert device (such as those made of cobalt alloys) is implanted into the bone, the body naturally forms a capsule around that material in recognition of it as a foreign body (Figure 4.16a). Although this is a perfectly natural defense mechanism, the formation of capsule tissue also contributes to the loosening of permanent implants. To the surprise of surgeons, titanium implants demonstrate intimate integration with host bone tissue (Figure 4.16b).

The detailed mechanism of bone-bonding ability will be discussed in Chapter 5 with bioactive ceramics. Briefly, titanate (e.g., Na_2TiO_3) can form on the surface of Ti alloys via ion exchange. Further exchange of ions between titanate and the surrounding

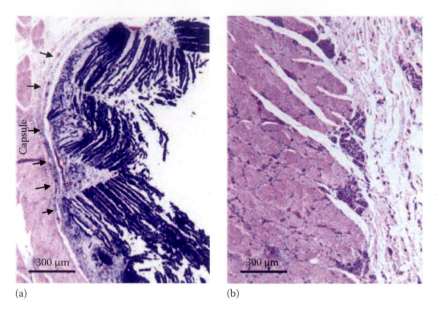

(a)   (b)

Figure 4.16
(a) The capsule tissue formed at the interface between cobalt alloy implant and bone. (b) The fused interface between a Ti alloy implant and host bone.

solution results in the formation of bone minerals (calcium and phosphorus) on the surface of titanium implants, which encourage the host bone to attach. Coating of TiO_2 on Ti alloys has been reported to enhance bone-bonding as early as 8 weeks after implantation. In the absence of any surface modification, direct bone contact was only observed after implantation for 6 months.

While the ability to bond with host bone is generally desired from the fixation point of view, this could be a problem for temporary implants or those that need to be retrieved due to rupture. As such, titanium and its alloys are primarily used in permanent implants or short-term temporary devices that are removed before bone-bonding occurs, rather than in long-term temporary implants, such as spinal corrective devices, which remain in the body for several years before removal (Figure 4.1a).

4.4.4 Mechanical Properties of Titanium Alloys

4.4.4.1 Commercial Pure Titanium The elastic modulus of titanium and its alloys is about half compared to those of stainless steels and cobalt–molybdenum alloys (Table 4.11). Except for Young's modulus, the mechanical properties of titanium alloys are sensitively affected by their alloying compositions, as shown in Table 4.11.

In commercial pure titanium (98.9%–99.6% Ti), which is essentially all α titanium with relatively low strength and high ductility, UTS and yield strengths vary from 240 to 550 MPa, and from 170 to 480 MPa, respectively, as a result of variations in the interstitial and impurity levels. Oxygen and iron are the primary variants in the CP-Ti grades, with strength increasing as their content increases. Similarly, fatigue strengths are also increased with higher levels of oxygen (Table 4.12). At 0.085% O

Table 4.11

Basic Mechanical Properties of Titanium and Titanium Alloys Developed for Orthopedic Implants

Materials	Young's Modulus (GPa)	0.2% Yield Strength (MPa)	Ultimate Tensile Strength (MPa)	Elongation (%)
α *microstructure*				
ASTM grade 1	115	170	240	24
ASTM grade 2	115	280	340	20
ASTM grade 3	115	380	450	18
ASTM grade 4	115	480	550	15
α–β *microstructure*				
Ti-6Al-4V	110	860	930	10–15
Ti-6Al-7Nb	105	795	860	10
Ti-5Al-2.5Fe	110	820	900	6
Ti-3Al-2.5V	100	585	690	15
β *microstructure*				
Ti-13Nb-13Zr	79–84	840–910	970–1040	10–16
Ti-12Mo-6Zr-2Fe (TMZF)	74–85	1000–1060	1060–1100	18–22
Ti-15Mo	78	655	800	22
Ti-15Mo-5Zr-3Al	75–88	870–970	880–980	17–20
Ti-15Mo-2.8Nb-0.2Si-0.26O(21SRx)	83	950–990	980–1000	16–18
Ti-16Nb-10Hf	81	730–740	850	10
Ti-(10–80)Nb	65–93	760–930	900–1030	
Ti-35.5Nb-7.3Zr-5.7Ta (TNZT)	55–66	800	830	20
Ti-(70–80)Ta	80–100	350–600	600–650	10–25
Ti-Ta-Nb/Nb/Sn	40–100	400–900	700–1000	17–26
Ti-Zr-Nb-Ta	46–58	—	650–1000	5–15
Stainless steels and co alloys				
316L	200	200–700	500–900	10–40
Orthinox	200	400–1550	700–1700	10–50
Co alloys	240	500–1500	900–1800	10–50

(within grade 1 oxygen level), the fatigue limit (10^7 cycles) is approximately 88 MPa, while at 0.27% O (close to grade 2 oxygen level), the fatigue limit is approximately 215 MPa.

Alpha alloys that contain small additions of β stabilizers have further been classed as super-α or near-α alloys. Although they contain some β phase, these alloys behave more like CP-Ti alloys than α–β alloys. A major mechanical limitation of α titanium alloys is their poor bending ductility due to HCP structure. The HCP structure has only three slip systems, while FCC and BCC structures have 12 slip systems. To date, α and near-α alloys have not found applications in medical implants. Their utility for medical devices has been limited by their low strength and bending ductility at ambient conditions when compared to α–β or β alloys (Table 4.13). For nonload-bearing, corrosion-resistant applications (such as the pacemaker case, Figure 1.8c), CP-Ti grades are preferred. Therefore, the rest of this section is devoted to α–β and β titanium alloys.

Table 4.12

Fatigue Strength of Orthopedic Implant Alloys in Comparison with Stainless Steels and Cobalt Alloys

Alloy	Test Condition[a]	Fatigue Limit at 10^7 Cycles (MPa)	Fatigue Strength/Yield Strength
α *microstructure*			
CP-Ti (Grade 1)	RBF($R = -1$, 100 Hz)	88	0.5
CP-Ti (Grade 2)	RBF($R = -1$, 100 Hz)	215	0.8
CP-Ti (Grade 3 and 4)	RBF($R = -1$, 100 Hz)	430	0.6
α–β *microstructure*			
Ti-6Al-4V	Axial ($R = -1$, 292 Hz)	500	0.6
	Axial ($R = -1$, 292 Hz)	330	0.4
	RBF($R = -1$, 60 Hz)	610	0.7
Ti-6Al-7Nb	RBF($R = -1$)	500–600	0.7
Ti-5Al-2.5Fe	RBF($R = -1$)	580	0.8
Ti-15Mo-5Zr-3Al	RBF($R = -1$, 100 Hz)	560–640	0.5
(aged α + β microstructure)			
β *microstructure*			
Ti-13Nb-13Zr	RBF($R = 0.1$, 60 Hz)	500	0.6
Ti-12Mo-6Zr-2Fe (TMZF)	RBF($R = -1$, 67 Hz)	525	0.5
Ti-15Mo-3Nb-0.3O (21SRx)	RBF($R = -1$, 60 Hz)	490	0.5
TNZT	RBF($R = -1$, 60 Hz)	265	0.5
TNZT-0.4O	RBF($R = -1$, 60 Hz)	450	0.5
Stainless steels and co alloys			
316L	Axial ($R = -1$, 120 Hz)	300	0.5
Orthinox	Axial ($R = -1$, 120 Hz)	500	0.5
CoCrMo (cast)	Axial ($R = -1$, 100 Hz)	200–300	0.5–0.6
CoCrMo (wrought)	Axial ($R = -1$, 20–100 Hz)	400–600	0.5–0.6

Source: Davies, J.R. (ed.), *Mettalic materials*, in *Handbook of Materials for Medical Devices, Materials Park, OH, ASM International*, 2003, pp. 21–50.

[a] RBF, rotating bending fatigue.

4.4.4.2 α–β Titanium Alloys The fatigue strengths of α–β alloys are higher than those of 316L stainless steels and comparable with those of Orthinox steel and cobalt alloys (Table 4.12). Among the four ASTM standardized α–β alloys used in medical devices, Ti-6Al-4V and Ti-6Al-4V ELI are the most widely applied titanium alloys. Ti-6Al-7Nb and Ti-5Al-2.5Fe are metallurgically similar to Ti6Al-4V, except for the absence of vanadium, which has been reported to be toxic and to show adverse tissue effects [1], as discussed earlier.

4.4.4.3 β Titanium Alloys β titanium alloys are often described as second-generation titanium biomaterials. The rapid development of β alloys for orthopedic implant applications took place in the 1990s. One of the rationales behind their development has been to address the stress-shielding effect associated with the high Young's moduli of

Table 4.13

Comparison of α, Near-α, α–β, and β Ti Alloys

Ti Alloys	Advantages	Disadvantages	Medical Applications
CP-Ti	1. Excellent corrosion resistance 2. Excellent biocompatibility 3. Good weldability	1. Cannot be significantly strengthened by heat treatment 2. Poor forgeability, especially below β transus due to HCP structure 3. Having a narrow forging temperature range 4. Low strength at ambient temperature	For nonload-bearing, corrosion-resistant applications: 1. Pacemaker case 2. Housings for ventricular assist devices 3. Implantable fusion drug pump 4. Dental implants 5. Maxillofacial and craniofacial implants 6. Screws and staple for spinal surgery
α or near α microstructure	As above	As above	Not yet
α–β microstructure	1. Can be strengthened by heat treatment		Ti-6Al-4V and Ti-6Al-4V ELI 1. Total joint replacement arthroplasty (hips and knees) Ti-6Al-7Nb 2. Femoral hip stems 3. Fracture fixation plates 4. Spinal components 5. Fasteners, nails, rods, screws, and wires Ti-3Al-2.5V 6. Tubing and intramedullary nails
β microstructure	1. High hardenability 2. Good ductility and toughness, excellent forgeability and good cold rolling capability (formability) at the solution-treated condition 3. Good fractural toughness	1. High density 2. Low creep strength 3. Low tensile ductility in the aged state 4. Low resistance to wearing	

metallic implant materials. The major advantage of β alloys is their low elastic moduli closer to that of bone. The Ti-Nb-Zr-Ta system (TNZT alloys) possesses the lowest elastic moduli (~45 MPa) of any metallic implant alloy developed to date (Table 4.11). Moreover, these alloys are vanadium-free, with the principal alloying elements being niobium, zirconium, molybdenum, tantalum, and iron, all of which exhibit suitable biocompatibility (Figure 2.4).

In β alloys, after aging (heat treatment for precipitation) at 450°C–550°C, fine α phase particles can precipitate and distribute throughout the β matrix, which is a desired microstructure in terms of precipitate-strengthening. Compared with α–β alloys, precipitate-strengthened β alloys generally have enhanced strength (including UTS, yield strength, and fatigue strength) and fracture toughness, but compromised tensile ductility [1].

It is useful to compare α–β and β alloys with stainless steels and cobalt alloys. The UTS values of α–β and β titanium alloys are comparable with those of 316L stainless steels, but lower than those of cobalt alloys. The yield strength values of α–β and β titanium alloys are also comparable with those of 316 type stainless steels and on the lower side of the yield strength range of cobalt alloys (Table 4.11). A comparison of fatigue strength of these alloys (Table 4.12) indicates that α–β titanium alloys collectively have higher fatigue strength values than 316L stainless steels, and quite similar fatigue strength to cobalt alloys. However, fatigue strength values of β alloys are lower than cobalt alloys, and this forms one of the major drawbacks of β titanium alloys. Another significant drawback of β alloys is their poor resistance to wear.

There are two approaches to enhance fatigue strength of β alloys, while retaining low Young's modulus. One method is to add Y_2O_3 particles, which cause dispersion strengthening effects that prevent dislocation sliding. In addition to refinement of the microstructure and improvement of mechanical properties, the addition of Y_2O_3 also enhances the corrosion resistance and thus the biocompatibility of β alloys. Another method is to precipitate a small amount of ω phase. This can be achieved by ageing alloys at low temperature for a short time. However, caution must be taken, as too much ω phase will cause alloy embrittlement and increased Young's modulus.

4.4.5 Wear Resistance

Hip simulation testing has shown that the wear rates of UHMWPE against Ti-6Al-4V are 35% greater than that against CoCrMo alloy. The high UHMWPE wear rates against Ti alloys have been related to the mechanical instability of the metal oxide layer [7]. It has been proposed that the surface passivated oxide layer of Ti alloys can be broken down by externally applied stresses much more easily than Co oxides. The damaged surface layer may not be able to heal immediately, leading to further loss of alloy material locally. This localized loss of metal material increases the roughness of the metal surface, which further increases UHMWPE wear rates. Moreover, the breakdown of the oxide layer produces hard oxide debris, which acts as a third abrasive body, resulting in further surface damage. Hence, titanium is not used to articulate against any materials, but is used for components of modular constraints, for example, where a titanium femoral stem is used with a cobalt–chromium or a ceramic ball to articulate against a UHMWPE line.

Wear of joint prosthetic materials is a key factor affecting the longevity of total joint replacements in the body. The incidence of nonspecific pain and prosthesis loosening has been attributed to the accumulation of UHMWPE and, to a lesser extent, metal or ceramic wear debris. Nonspecific pain is a result of adverse tissue reactions, such as chronic joint inflammation. Prosthesis loosening is a result of body's adverse reaction to implant materials' wear debris. In fact, aseptic loosening accounts for approximately 80% of all surgical revisions. The revision surgery at the same site is not only expensive, but its success rate is usually lower compared to the first implantation.

Some surface modifications are applied to increase wear resistance of titanium alloys, such as nitriding or plasma surface treatment. Methods such as physical vapor deposition coating (TiN, TiC), ion implantation (N⁺), thermal treatments (nitriding and oxygen diffusion hardening), and laser alloying with TiC have been examined for improving wear. Of these, ion implantation has been the most common treatment employed so far [7].

4.4.6 Clinical Applications of Titanium Alloys

Due to the ability of titanium to fuse with bone, titanium alloys are recommended to be used in either permanent devices such as hip replacements, or relative short-term (<6 months) temporary devices such as screws. The poor bending performance of titanium alloys excludes them as fracture plates, which are subjected to severe bending stress (Figure 4.17a). Because of both bone-bonding ability and poor bending ductility, titanium-based alloys are never used in spinal corrective devices (Figure 4.17b), which are subject to bending stresses and are typically expected to service in the body for

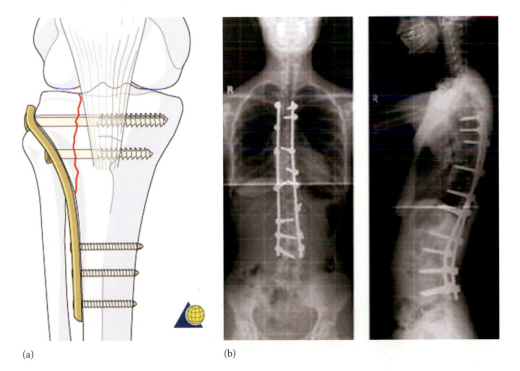

(a)   (b)

Figure 4.17
Two medical devices for which Ti alloys are not recommended to be used. (a) A fracture plate is subject to bending stresses, and α–β Ti alloys are not recommended for this application. (With permission of AO foundation) (b) A spinal corrective device is subject to bending stresses and is expected to be in the body for a number of months or even years. Hence, Ti alloys are never used in this application. (Courtesy of Retro Robot Geekery.)

several months or even years, long enough to develop bone bonding. For patients who suffer from severe metal allergy, titanium metals are the only option in procedures that require a metal implant which will be permanent.

More specifically, titanium CP-Ti and Ti-6Al-4V ELI are the most commonly used titanium materials for implant applications. Examples of biomedical applications for CP-Ti grades include pacemaker cases (Figure 1.8c), housings for ventricular assist devices and implantable infusion drug pumps, dental implants, maxillofacial and craniofacial implants, and screws or staples for spinal surgery.

The applications of Ti-6Al-4V include dental implants (e.g., tooth root) and parts for orthodontic surgery; joint replacement parts for hip, knee, shoulder, spine, elbow, and wrist; bone fixation materials like nails, screws, nuts, housing device for the pacemakers, and artificial heart valves; surgical instruments; and components in high-speed blood centrifuges. However, both Al and V released from Ti-6Al-4V alloy are found to be linked to long-term health problems, such as Alzheimer's disease, other neuropathies, and osteomalacia. Vanadium-free Ti-6Al-7Nb and Ti-5Al-2.5Fe (not currently standardized by ASTM) have therefore been developed. Both are metallurgically quite similar to Ti-6Al-4V. Ti-6Al-7Nb has been used for femoral hip stems, fracture fixation plates, spinal components, fasteners, nails, rods, screws, and wire.

4.4.7 Current Issues and Challenges

In general, titanium alloys produce adverse tissue reaction from fretting of the prostheses, and these alloys show relatively poor wear resistance in an articulating situation, compared with cobalt alloys. While α–β Ti alloys are superior in UTS and fatigue strength, they have relatively poor bending ductility due to the HCP structure of the α phase. Although BCC structured β-Ti alloys have enhanced shearing deformation ability, their UTS and fatigue strength are compromised, compared with α–β alloys. A most recent clinical failure case revealed the unreliability of current titanium hip joint implants (Figure 4.18). Premature fracture in the neck of total hip replacements more often occurred with stems made of Ti64 alloys than stainless steels and cobalt alloys. According to Figure 3.9, the maximal bending stress at the neck of hip prostheses is ~300 MPa, so the poor bending performance of α–β alloys is primarily responsible for the premature neck fractures of total hip prostheses made from these titanium alloys.

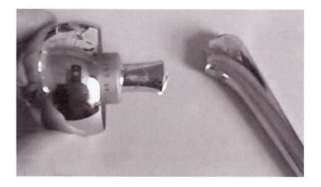

Figure 4.18
A broken stem of titanium total hip replacement in a patient. (From Briant-Evans, T.W. et al., J. Bone Joint Surg. [Br.], 89(8), 393–395, 2007. Reproduced with permission from The Bone & Joint Journal, London, U.K.)

To address the drawback of poor bending behavior of α–β titanium alloys, Ti-Mo-Zr-Fe (TMZF), a β-titanium alloy, was introduced by Stryker as a stem material in total hip replacement, trade name Accolade, in the early 2000s.* However, Accolade TMZF Plus Hip Stems were recalled in 2011 due to grit blast media, which was observed in the drive hole. Apparently, *grit blast media*, a term referring to any fine powder used as an abrasive, was found as the wearing debris due to the compromised wearing resistance of this soft β (BCC structure) titanium alloy. A satisfactory titanium alloy that has excellent bending fatigue strength and wearing resistance has yet to be developed. The wear resistance of Ti alloys could be improved by the incorporation of refractory hard metal elements (e.g., Ta, Zr, W, and Nb), and/or by surface modification of the final product.

4.4.8 Summary of Titanium Alloys

The use of titanium alloys as implant biomaterials has increased over the past two decades because of their higher corrosion resistance, better biocompatibility, and lower modulus than both stainless steels and cobalt-based alloys. Titanium and its alloys are the only metallic material system that has the ability to fuse with bone. Compared with stainless steels and cobalt–chromium alloys, however, titanium alloys are inferior in tribological properties. Hence, titanium alloys are not recommended to be used to articulate against any materials, but can be used as a femoral stem in total hip replacements. Comparing with CP-Ti and α–β (Ti-6Al-4V/Nb) alloys, the second-generation β-Ti alloys have reduced elastic modulus. However, the compromised wear resistance of β titanium alloys has hampered their applications as stem in total hip replacements. A mechanically reliable titanium implant alloy has yet to become a reality.

4.5 COMPARISON OF STAINLESS STEELS, COBALT, AND TITANIUM ALLOYS

Although these three metals are not perfect implant materials, they predominate in current orthopedics. Each alloy has its own advantages and disadvantages, as summarized in Table 4.14. A common issue is the stress-shielding effect, associated with their high Young's modulus. In a physiological solution, the fatigue life of CoCrMo constructs tends to be greater than Ti constructs. Titanium alloys are desirable for their light weight and superb biocompatibility, with low metal-related toxicity. However, they have low resistance to wear and friction, suffering from fretting fatigue associated with friction, which remains the main reason for failure in orthopedic implants, especially in stems of hip-joint prostheses.

In short, the ideal bone repair alloy should have the modulus of bone, the strength of cobalt–chromium alloys, the corrosion resistance and biocompatibility of titanium, and the fabrication cost of stainless steels (Table 4.14) [1]. However, no available materials can simultaneously have the Young's modulus of bone and the mechanical strengths of CoCr-based alloys due to the intrinsic relationship between these properties (Equation 3.3). To understand the challenges of achieving such an ideal material, it is useful to compare the mechanical properties of metallic materials with

---

* *http://www.accessdata.fda.gov/scripts/cdrh/cfdocs/cfres/res.cfm?id=99392.*

Table 4.14

Advantages and Disadvantages of Stainless Steels, Co Alloys, and Titanium Alloys

Alloys	Advantages	Disadvantages	Typical Applications
Fe-based	• Good corrosion and fatigue resistance in short-term applications • Low cost • Easy to be machined	• Tend to corrode in long-term applications • High modulus (stress-shielding effect) • Ni and Cr allergy	• Instruments • Temporary devices (316L) • Permanent implants (Orthinox stem)
Co-based	• Long-term corrosion resistance • Best fatigue and wear resistance • Biocompatibility	• Difficult to machine and thus expensive to process • High modulus (stress-shielding effect) • Co, Ni, and Cr allergy	• Permanent joint implants
Ti-based	• Light • Greatest corrosion resistance • Best biocompatibility, free of metal-related allergy • Low Young's modulus	• Lower shear strength • Low wear resistance • Still have, though to a lesser degree, stress-shielding effect	• Permanent implant • Stem of hip prostheses • Dental screws • Temporary device

bone (Figure 4.19). The data in Figure 4.19 indicate that the three orthopedic metallic implant materials are much stronger and tougher than bone, in terms of their general mechanical properties and fatigue strength. Why, then, do these metallic materials not have the longevity of healthy bone? It is certain that corrosion and wearing associated with the aggressive environment and harsh mechanical working conditions in joints contribute in many clinical failures. However, these conditions could also theoretically cause subclinical microdamage to bone as well. The difference lies in the critical feature of bone, unlike inert artificial materials, in that bone responds to mechanical impacts and heals while being subjected to them. Cancellous bone has a complex microstructure, comprising directional fibers, multiple layers, and porosity, which collectively dissipate the energy from impacts through the bone itself, while remaining light and strong compared to synthetic materials. Healing bone also undergoes gradual increases in modulus as it heals, from cartilaginous to osseous. Without this biological structure and self-healing ability, the ideal metallic biomaterial that imposes no stress-shielding effect on host bone, while having a satisfactory working longevity longer than 30 years is unlikely to be realized. Researchers have to face this reality and seek for alternative strategies, such as tissue engineering and regeneration using degradable materials (Chapter 5), as well as smarter materials with more complex micro- and nanostructure.

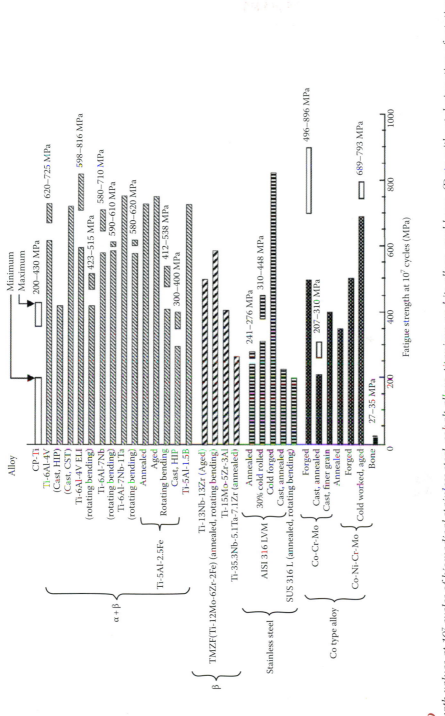

Figure 4.19

Fatigue strength values at 10^7 cycles of biomedical stainless steel, cobalt alloys, titanium and its alloys, and bone. (Data without designation of rotating bending are those obtained from uniaxial fatigue tests in the air. (From Niinomi, M., Int. J. Fatigue, 29, 992, 2007.)

4.6   SUMMARY AND REMARKS

While imperfect, stainless steels, cobalt-based, and titanium-based implant materials remain dominant in orthopedic surgery. Although these alloys are much stronger and tougher than bone in laboratory, their service longevity is limited to 20–25 years, much shorter than the life span of humans (except elderly patients), and the incidence of failure after 15 years' service is unsatisfactorily high. Until now, major attempts to reduce stress-shielding effects have involved reducing the Young's modulus of bulk materials (e.g., the development of β-Ti alloys), which inevitably compromises the fatigue resistance. While it is possible to achieve metallic materials that would have the Young's modulus of bone while maintaining a fatigue resistance of longer than 20 years, this remains unlikely. This is because biological tissues like bone have the ability to heal and remodel their mechanical properties in vivo while subjected to cyclic wearing, whereas synthetic materials do not. Hence, any bulk material that has a Young's modulus similar to that of bone would be at a high risk of premature failure. Hence, it is believed that the most promising strategy to achieve a synthetic permanent substitute that has Young's modulus of bone would be porous metallic implant. Such a porous networks could be tailored to mechanically match the host bone, and the porous structure can also encourage host bone to grow into it.

4.7   CHAPTER HIGHLIGHTS

1. Stainless steels remain popular for implant applications because of their lower cost, accepted biocompatibility, and toughness. The 316L stainless steel is predominant in a large number of temporary devices. Orthinox, a high-nitrogen stainless steel, plays the leading role as a stem material in permanent total hip prostheses.

2. Cobalt-based alloys are superior to other alloys in terms of fatigue strength and wear resistance. Wrought CoCrMo alloys are the most popular metallic implant materials of bearing systems, providing a more than 20 years' service longevity.

3. The use of titanium alloys as implant biomaterials has increased over the past two decades because of their higher corrosion resistance, better biocompatibility, and lower modulus, than both stainless steels and cobalt-based alloys. Titanium and its alloys are the only metallic materials that have the ability to fuse with bone.

4. Titanium alloys are inferior in tribological properties and have a poor bending performance. Titanium alloys are not recommended to be used to articulate against any materials. Commercially pure Ti is used in nonload-bearing sites (e.g., pacemaker case). α–β (Ti-6Al-4V/Nb) alloys can be used in permanent devices (e.g., stem of total hip replacements) or short-term temporary devices (<6 months). α–β (Ti-6Al-4V/Nb) alloys are not recommended for long-term temporary devices or devices subjected to bending stresses.

5. Compared with CP-Ti and α–β (Ti-6Al-4V/Nb) alloys, the second-generation β-Ti alloys have reduced elastic modulus. The compromised wear resistance of

β titanium alloys has hampered their applications as implant materials in joint replacement. A mechanically reliable titanium implant alloy has yet to become a reality.

6. A number of common issues associated with long-term performance remain with the three predominant metallic materials. They are failures due to fretting fatigue and corrosion fatigue, aseptic loosening due to wearing, stress-shielding effect, and biological toxicity due to release of Co, Cr, and Ni ions or particles.

7. The ideal alloy, which has a satisfactory working longevity longer than 30 years, should have the modulus of bone, the strength of cobalt–chromium alloys, the corrosion resistance and biocompatibility of titanium, and the fabrication cost of stainless steels. Due to lack of self-healing ability, such an ideal alloy is unlikely to be realistic. Researchers have to face this reality and seek for alternative strategies, such as tissue engineering and regeneration using degradable materials, and innovative prosthesis design.

ACTIVITIES

1. Watch video (SBS TV program): Hip replacement warning: http://video.au.msn.com/watch/video/hip-replacement-warning/xyru2u1orhttp://video.au.msn.com/watch/video/hip-replacement-warning/xyru2u1?cpkey=4f682b25-a7bd-4737-aa8a-60c2b42a2d92%257c%257c%257c%257c.

2. Become familiar with the Medical Devices and Database pages of US Food and Drug Administration (FDA) and read "Class 2 Recall Accolade TMZF Plus Hip Stem" on the website of FDA: http://www.accessdata.fda.gov/scripts/cdrh/cfdocs/cfres/res.cfm?id=99392.

SIMPLE QUESTIONS IN CLASS

1. What is the corrosion-resistant mechanism of Cr in stainless steels?
   a. Chemically inert
   b. Trapping carbon
   c. Passivation (protected by oxide film formation on its surface)
   d. Closely packed crystalline structure, that is, FCC structure
2. What is the corrosion-resistant mechanism of Mo in stainless steels?
   a. Chemically inert
   b. Trapping carbon
   c. Passivation (protected by oxide film formation on its surface)
   d. Closely packed crystalline structure, that is, FCC structure
3. What are the corrosion-resistant mechanisms of Ni in stainless steels?
   a. Chemically inert
   b. Trapping carbon
   c. Passivation (protected by oxide film formation on its surface)
   d. Closely packed crystalline structure, that is, FCC structure

4. 316L Which of the following stainless steels are recommended to be used in?
    a. Total shoulder replacements
    b. Fixation plates and screws of load-bearing bone
    c. Total hip replacements
    d. Total elbow replacements
5. Which of the following alloys is the best in terms of mechanical strength?
    a. Stainless steels
    b. Ti alloys
    c. CoCr-based alloys
    d. High-nitrogen stainless steels (Orthinox)
6. Which of the following alloys is the best in terms of biocompatibility?
    a. Stainless steels
    b. Ti alloys
    c. CoCr-based alloys
    d. High-nitrogen stainless steels (Orthinox)
7. Which of the following alloys is the best in terms of low cost?
    a. Stainless steels
    b. Ti alloys
    c. CoCr-based alloys
    d. High-nitrogen stainless steels (Orthinox)
8. Which part of a total hip replacement implant cannot be made from Ti-based alloys?
    a. Stem
    b. Head
    c. Lining
    d. Cup

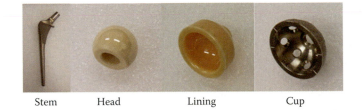

| Stem | Head | Lining | Cup |

PROBLEMS AND EXERCISES

1. What are the three dominant orthopedic implant biometallics? What is their common major drawback that has driven people to search for mechanically compatible metal implants, such as Mg alloys?
2. Describe the mechanisms of corrosion resistance of Cr, Mo, and Ni alloying elements in stainless steel.
3. Describe the application principles of stainless steels, CoCr-based, and Ti-based alloys, and explain the rationale behind their applications.

4. In the artificial knee given in the following

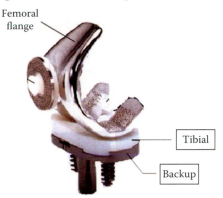

Femoral flange

Tibial

Backup

   a. Which parts are made from Co-based alloys?
   b. Which parts are NOT made from Co-based alloys?
   c. Explain its design principles from the materials science point of view.
   d. Can Ti be used in this implant? Explain your answer.

5. In the artificial ankle given in the following

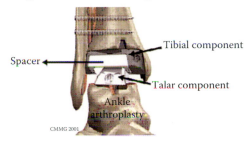

Tibial component

Spacer

Talar component

Ankle arthroplasty

CMMG 2001

   a. Which parts are made from Co-based alloys?
   b. Which parts are NOT made from Co-based alloys?
   c. Explain its design principles from the materials science point of view.
   d. Can Ti be used in this implant? Explain your answer.

6. In addition to its excellent biocompatibility, what is the major reason for the employment of Ti in short-term temporary or permanent implants, rather than long-term temporary devices?

7. Among Co-based alloys, stainless steels, and Ti alloys, which are not recommended for application in the fracture fixation plate given in the following? Which are ideal? Explain your reasons.

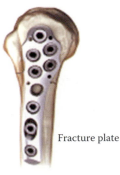

Fracture plate

8. What are the advantages and disadvantages of stainless steels, CoCr-based, and Ti-based alloys?
9. What is the stress-shielding effect? What strategies could potentially address the issue?
10. The mechanical strength of stainless steels, CoCr-based, and Ti-based alloys are all much higher than that of bone. Explain why none of them could survive as long as bone in the body.
11. What is the best feature of the following metallic implant materials? Briefly describe their main applications as orthopedic implants
    a. 316L stainless steel
    b. Cobalt alloys
    c. Titanium alloys
    d. Magnesium alloys

BIBLIOGRAPHY

References

1. Metallic materials. In *Handbook of Materials for Medical Devices*, J.R. Davies, ed. Materials Park, OH: ASM International, 2003, pp. 21–50.
2. Walczak, J., F. Shahgaldi, and F. Heatley, In vivo corrosion of 316L stainless-steel hip implants: Morphology and elemental compositions of corrosion products. *Biomaterials*, 1998;**19**(1–3):229–237.
3. Kamath, A.F. et al., Impaction bone grafting with proximal and distal femoral arthroplasty. *Journal of Arthroplasty*, 2011;**26**(8):1520–1526.
4. Tavares, S.S.M. et al., Characterization of prematurely failed stainless steel orthopedic implants. *Engineering Failure Analysis*, 2010;**17**(5):1246–1253.
5. Reigstad, O. et al., Excellent long-term survival of an uncemented press-fit stem and screw cup in young patients—Follow-up of 75 hips for 15–18 years. *Acta Orthopaedica*, 2008;**79**(2):194–202.
6. van Doorn, W.J. et al., Fracture of an Exeter stem 3 years after impaction allografting—A case report. *Acta Orthopaedica Scandinavica*, 2002;**73**(1):111–113.
7. Long, M. and H.J. Rack, Titanium alloys in total joint replacement—A materials science perspective. *Biomaterials*, 1998;**19**(18):1621–1639.
8. Niinomi, M., Fatigue characteristics of metallic biomaterials. *International Journal of Fatigue*, 2007;**29**(6):992–1000.
9. Røkkum, M. et al., *Acta Orthopaedica*, 1995;**66**(5):435–439.
10. Briant-Evans, T.W., M.R. Norton, and E.D. Fern, Fractures of Corin 'Taper-Fit' CDH stems used in 'cement-in-cement' revision total hip replacement, *The Journal of Bone & Joint Surgery [British volume]*, 2007;**89**(8):393–395.

Websites

https://www.aofoundation.org/Structure/Pages/default.aspx.
(Arbeitsgemeinschaft für Osteosynthesefragen (German for "Association for the Study of Internal Fixation", or **AO**).
https://www2.aofoundation.org/wps/portal/!ut/p/c1/04_SB8K8xLLM9MSSzPy8xBz9 CP0os3hng7BARydDRwN3QwMDA08zTzdvvxBjIwN_I6B8JJK8haEFUD7U09nP2MkPqNSEg G4_j_zcVP2C3IhyADJvFMw!/dl2/d1/L2dJQSEvUUt3QS9ZQnB3LzZfQzBWUUFCMUEwRzE wMDBJNklGS05UMzIwTzI!/?showPage=startpage.
http://www.fda.gov/default.htm.

http://www.fda.gov/MedicalDevices/default.htm.
http://www.njrcentre.org.uk/njrcentre/default.aspx.
http://orthoinfo.aaos.org/.
http://teamwork.aaos.org/ajrr/default.aspx.

Further Readings

American Joint Replacement Registry (AJRR). Annual report. Fall 2013 update. http://teamwork.
    aaos.org/ajrr/AJRR%20Documents/AJRR%20Fall%202013_F11062013.pdf.

Chapter 4: Principles of internal fixation, Chapter 5: Locking plates: Development, biomechanics, and clinical application. In *Skeletal Trauma*, B.D. Browner et al., eds. Saunders Co, Philadelphia PA, an imprint of Elsevier, 2009.

Davis, J.R. (ed.), Chapter 3: Metallic materials; Chapter 5: Failure analysis of metallic orthopedic implants. In *Handbook of Materials for Medical Devices*. Materials Park, OH: ASM International, 2003.

Lütjering, G. and J.C. Williams, Chapter 5: Alpha + beta alloys; Chapter 7: Beta alloys. *Titanium*, 2nd edn. Springer-Verlag, Berlin, 2007.

National Joint Registry for England, Wales and Northern Ireland, 10th Annual Report, Surgical data to 31 December 2012. http://www.njrcentre.org.uk/njrcentre/
    Reports,PublicationsandMinutes/Annualreports/tabid/86/Default.aspx.

Park, J. and R.S. Lakes, Chapter 5: Metallic implant materials. In *Biomaterials: An Introduction*, 3rd edn. New York: Springer, 2007.

METALLIC BIOMATERIALS
Miscellaneous Others

LEARNING OBJECTIVES

After a careful study of this chapter, you should be able to do the following:

1. Describe the special requirements of tooth filling materials, in addition to biocompatibility.
2. Describe major applications of biomaterials in restorative dentistry.
3. Describe the mechanism of the shape-memory effect of metals.
4. Describe the medical applications of NiTi alloys and related issues.
5. Describe the three generations of metallic biomaterials in terms of clinical outcomes.
6. Describe the rationale of the development of Mg alloys and related issues and challenges.

5.1 DENTAL MATERIALS

The most common oral diseases are dental caries (tooth decay) and periodontal disease (gum disease). Standard treatments for these conditions include (1) tooth restoration for dental caries (tooth fillings), (2) scaling of teeth to treat periodontal problems, (3) endodontic root canal treatment to treat abscessed teeth, (4) surgical removal of teeth which cannot be restored (extraction), and (5) surgical implantation of tooth protheses. *Restorative dentistry* encompasses all these dental treatments, except for surgical extraction.

Dental biomaterials for restorative dentistry involve all the different types of materials described in Chapter 1: Metallic, ceramic, polymeric, and composite materials, specifically including the following [1]:

- Amalgam alloys for direct fillings
- Noble metals and alloys for direct fillings, crowns, bridges, and porcelain fused to metal restorations

- Base metals and alloys for partial-denture framework, porcelain–metal restorations, crowns and bridges, orthodontic wires and brackets, and implants
- Ceramics for implants, porcelain–metal restorations, crowns, inlays, veneers, cements, and denture teeth
- Composites for replacing missing tooth structure and modifying tooth color and contour
- Polymers for denture bases, plastic teeth, cements, and other applications

Metallic biomaterials have long been applied in dentistry for dental restoration (e.g., fillings) (Figure 1.8a), endodontic implantations (e.g., tooth roots) (Figure 5.1a), and orthodontics (e.g., corrective arch wires) (Figure 5.1b), as listed in Tables 5.1 and 5.2. Specifically, cobalt-based alloys and Ti–6Al–4V/Nb are used to replace tooth roots; stainless steels and NiTi alloys are applied as corrective archwires; HgAgSn amalgam is used for tooth filling, and noble metals are used for tooth crowns or total tooth replacements. A tooth root is subject to compressive loading with little bending stress. Hence, σ-β Ti alloys, which are strong under compressive loading conditions and have an ability to bond with bone, are ideal for use in permanent tooth root implants.

Dental alloys are grouped into three broad categories:

1. Amalgam alloys
2. Noble metals
3. Base metals

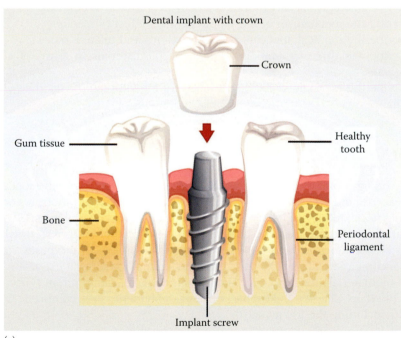

(a)

Figure 5.1
Some applications of metallic materials in dentistry. (a) Tooth roots made of Ti–6Al–4Nb alloy.
(Continued)

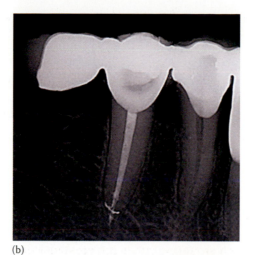

(b)

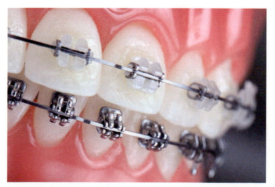

(c)

(d)

Figure 5.1 (Continued)
Some applications of metallic materials in dentistry. (b) an endodontic implant made of Ti–6Al–4Nb alloy; (c) gold crown, gold inlays, and amalgam fillings; (d) archwires made of stainless steels, CoCrNiMo alloys, or NiTi shape-memory alloys.

Table 5.1

Metallic Materials Currently Used in Dentistry

Alloys	Compositions (wt.%)
HgAgSn amalgam	45–55Hg, 25–35Ag, 15Sn, 8Cu
Noble metals	
Au alloys	58–75Au, 10–26Ag, 7–18Cu, 1–10Pd, 5–25Pt, 0–19Ir, 1–2Ni
Platinum	
Palladium	
Iridium	
Rhodium	
Base alloys	
Stainless steels	45–84Fe, 8–30Cr, 8–25Ni, 0.1–0.2C
CoCrNiMo alloys	40Co, 20Cr, 16Fe, 15Ni, 7Mo, 2Mn, 0.15C, 0.04Be
CP-Ti	99Ti, <0.10C, <0.50Fe, <0.06H, <0.40N, <0.40O
α-β Ti alloys	88–91Ti, 5–7Al, 3–5V
β-Ti alloys	
TMZS	76–82Ti, 10–12Mo, 5–7Zr, 3–5Sn
Ti–Nb	50–60Ti, 40–50Nb
Ti–Ta–Nb/Zr/Sn	50–60Ti, 25–35Ta, 5–25Nb
Ti–Zr	Ti–10Zr–5Nb–5Ta
NiTi-martensitic	44–52Ni, 45–51Ti, 5–6Cu, 0.2–0.5Cr, 0–3Co
NiTi-austenitic	44–52Ni, 45–51Ti, 5–6Cu, 0.2–0.5Cr, 0–3Co
Ni–Ta	50–70Ni, 30–50Ta

Source: Kusy, R.P., Angle Orthod., 72(6), 501, 2002.

Table 5.2

Mechanical Properties of Dental Metallic Implant Materials

Alloys	Young's Modulus (GPa)	Yield Strength (MPa)	UTS/MPa
HgAgSnCu	Varying with time	Varying with time	150–160 (compressive)
Au alloys	85–110	170–570	320–1120
Stainless steel	180–220	790–2450	930–2860
CoCrNiMo alloys	180–230	960–2140	1210–2540
CP–Ti	100–110	170–1000	240–1100
α-βTi	100–120	740–1130	860–1220
β-Ti	65–70	520–1380	690–1500
Ti–Nb	65–93	760–930	900–1030
Ti–Ta	65–110	300–600	500–700
Ti–Zr	45–60	NA	650–1000
NiTi-martensite	28–44	70–1240	900–1930
NiTi-austenite	80–110	180–690	800–1670
Ni–Ta	173–220	65–500	300–850

Source: Kusy, R.P., Angle Orthod., 72(6), 501, 2002.

Base metals include stainless steels, cobalt-based and titanium-based alloys. They are not different from those used in the orthopedics. Readers can refer to Chapter 4 for these three metal systems. In this section, we focus on amalgam alloys and noble metals. NiTi alloys represent a relatively new system, which has found applications not just in dentistry but in other important clinical areas. Hence, the NiTi system will be described in a separate section (Section 5.2).

5.1.1 HgAgSn Amalgam as Tooth Fillings

5.1.1.1 Corrosion Resistance of Amalgam

The standard electrode potentials of silver (Ag) and mercury (Hg) are +0.800 and +0.851 V, respectively, which place them on the noble side of the standard electrode potential series (Figure 2.7).

$$Hg^{2+} + 2e^- \rightleftarrows Hg\ (l) + 0.851\ V$$

$$Ag^+ + e^- \rightleftarrows Ag + 0.800\ V$$

$$Sn^{2+} + 2e^- \rightleftarrows Sn - 0.140\ V$$

In seawater, the corrosion potentials E_{corr} of silver and tin (Sn) are around −0.12 and −0.32 V (SCE) (Figure 2.5) or 0.122 and −0.078 V (SHE) according to Equation 2.1. Using these values as the first approximation, the Pourbaix diagrams of silver (Figure 2.8a) and tin (Figure 5.2) indicate that immunity and passivity are possible, respectively, for

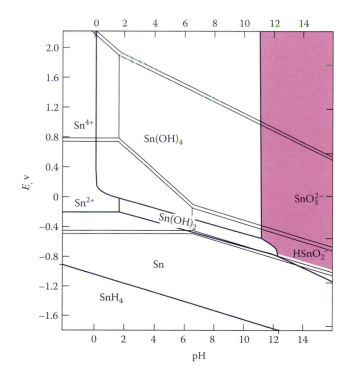

Figure 5.2
Pourbaix diagram of tin (Sn). E_{corr} = −0.32 (SCE) = −0.078 (SHE). When pH = 3.5, 7.4 or 9.0, Sn (OH)$_4$ is stable. Hence, passivity is possible.

these two metals to resist corrosion under oral conditions (pH = 6.5–6.9). Indeed, during their long application history as tooth fillings, HgAgSn amalgam alloys have proven to possess a reasonably good corrosion resistance.

5.1.1.2 Special Requirements of Tooth Fillings

Besides a satisfactory corrosion resistance and thus biocompatibility, there are additional special requirements of tooth fillings:

1. In situ solidification at a temperature reasonably close to body temperature: this is because the tooth fillings have to be liquid when implanted so as to fill the irregular shape of tooth defects. The solidification rate should be such that it allows a dentist to manipulate the filling easily within a reasonable time.
2. Low shrinkage: the change in the volume of tooth fillings during solidification causes problem of detachment, which has been a major challenge in the field of dental biomaterials. Amalgam expands with time, introducing stresses as well. In the field of dental restorative materials, minimization of volume change (typically shrinkage) is an active research area.
3. These materials are required to have good compressive strength and especially superb resistance to friction and wear due to the major function of teeth, chewing food.

5.1.1.3 Properties of HgAgSn Amalgam

HgAgSnCu (50% Hg, 22%–32% Ag, 14% Sn, and 8% Cu) amalgam has been used in dentistry as a restorative material for a number of reasons. First, its melting point is around 300°C, which can be well tolerated by the human teeth in a short time. Second, its solidification rate is such that it is easy to manipulate during placement. It remains soft for a short time so it can be packed to fill any irregular volume, and then forms a hard compound. Typically, the amalgam attains one quarter of its final strength after 1 h, and almost all of its final strength after 1 day. Third, it has satisfactory longevity, and lastly, it is inexpensive. Nonetheless, HgAgSn amalgam has been increasingly replaced by white tooth fillings (composite resins) (Figure 5.3), primarily driven by cosmetic reasons as well as due to the toxicity of Hg ions.

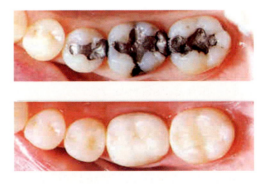

Figure 5.3
Comparison of traditional amalgam with white tooth fillings.

5.1.2   Noble Metals

5.1.2.1   Corrosion Resistance   Metals located near the positive end of the standard electrode potential series are referred to as *noble* metals. These metals have a good resistance to oxidation, tarnish and corrosion during heating, casting and soldering, with a bright surface and ability to retain surface integrity in dry or humid air, such as in the mouth. The list of noble metals typically includes gold (Au), platinum (Pt), palladium (Pd), iridium (Ir), rhodium (Rh), osmium (Os), ruthenium (Ru), and silver (Ag). However, silver is not considered a noble metal in dentistry because it corrodes considerably in the oral cavity. Gold has been the most commonly used noble metal for dental restorations, being inert and nonallergenic to the body, despite rising prices and development of cheaper substitutes.

5.1.2.2   Alloying Composition and Properties   Gold alloys used for cast restorations (e.g., crowns and bridges) are classified by the American Dental Association (ADA) into three broad groups, as listed in Table 5.3. High-noble and noble alloys are further categorized into three and four subclasses, respectively (Table 5.4). Important properties of the high noble and noble alloys are summarized in Table 5.5 [3].

5.1.2.3   Dental Applications of Noble Alloys   According to the first book on dentistry, *Operator for the Teeth*, published in 1539 by Artzney Buchlein, gold leaves were used to fill out cavities over 3000 years ago. The earliest found records of gold being used in dentistry stretches back to 700 BC, with Estrucan dentists using gold wires for positioning of replacement teeth. The modern use of gold in dentistry is usually in the form of wrought or cast gold and gold alloys, included in components

Table 5.3
Classification of Cast Gold Alloys by American Dental Association (ADA)

High-noble alloys	With a noble metal content ≥60 wt.% and a gold content of ≥40%
Noble alloys	With a noble metal content of ≥25%
Predominantly base metal alloys	With a noble metal content of <25%

Table 5.4
Seven Subclasses of High-Noble and Noble Alloys

Three classes of high-noble alloys:
  Gold–silver–platinum (>70% Au + Pt)
  Gold–copper–silver–palladium-I (>70% Au)
  Gold–copper–silver–palladium-II (50%–65% Au)

Four classes of noble alloys:
  Gold–copper–silver–palladium-III (40% Au)
  Gold–silver–palladium–indium (20% Au)
  Palladium–copper–gallium (77% Pd and 2% Au)
  Silver–palladium (25% Pd and 0% Au)

Table 5.5
Physical and Mechanical Properties of Noble Dental Casting Alloys

Alloys	Solidus–Liquidus (°C)	Color	Density (g/cm^3)	Yield Strength $\sigma_{0.2}$ (MPa)	Elongation at Break	Vickers Hardness (kg/mm^2)
High noble						
78.1Au–10.5Ag–9.9Pt (Ir trace)	1045–1140	Yellow	18.4	420–470	9–15	175–195
76.0Au–10.5Cu–10.0Ag–2.4Pd–1.0Zn–0.1Pt (Ru trace)	910–965	Yellow	15.6	270–400	12–30	135–195
56.0Au–11.8Cu–25.0Ag–5.0Pd–1.7Zn–0.4Pt (Ir trace)	870–920	Yellow	13.8	350–600	10–30	175–260
Noble						
47.0Ag–40.0Au–7.5Cu–4.0Pd–1.5Zn (Ir trace)	865–925	Yellow	12.4	325–520	10–27.5	125–215
38.7Ag–21.0Pd–20.0Au–16.5In–3.8Zn	875–1035	Light yellow	11.4	300–370	8–12	135–190
77.0Pd–7.0Ga–2.0Cu	1100–1190	White	10.6	1145	8	425
70.0Ag–25.0Pd–3.0In–2.0Zn	1020–1100	White	10.6	260–320	8–10	140–155

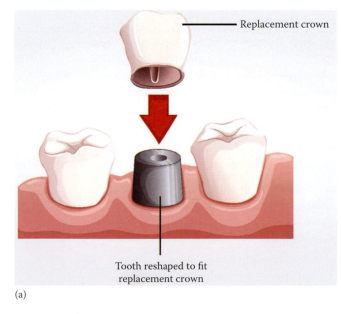

(a)

Figure 5.4
Dental applications of noble metals. (a) Application of a dental crown. *(Continued)*

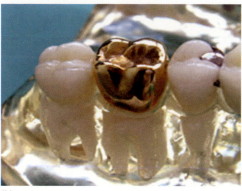

(b)

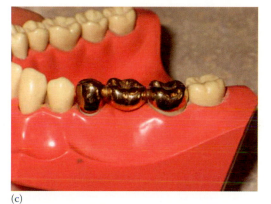

(c)

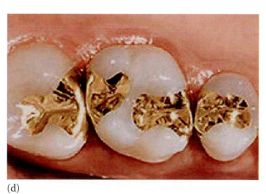

(d)

Figure 5.4 (Continued)
Dental applications of noble metals. (b) gold dental crown and ceramic metal restoration; (c) gold dental bridge; (d) wrought gold fillings.

such as bridges, fillings, crowns and orthodontic appliances. Cast gold alloys are typically used for crowns (Figure 5.4a and b), bridgework (Figure 5.4c), and ceramic metal restorations. Pure gold is used in wrought form for fillings (Figure 5.4d) or as a cast material for bridges and crowns. Some palladium-based alloys are also used for similar applications.

5.2 NiTi SHAPE-MEMORY ALLOYS

The shape-memory effect refers to the ability of materials to return to their predefined dimensions upon heating, induced by deformation training. Subjected to a proper entrainment, shape-memory alloys can undergo reversible deformation via a phase transformation mechanism, also referred to as *pseudoelasticity*. The shape-memory effect exists in a number of alloy systems: Au–Cd alloys discovered by Ölander in 1932, Cu–Zn alloys by Greninger and Mooradian (1938), and NiTi alloys (also known as Nitinol) by Buehler and his coworkers in the 1960s. In addition to these alloys, the shape-memory effect has also been discovered in InTl, NiAl, FePt, FePd, MnCu, and FeMnSi. Among these alloys, NiTi is the most attractive one in terms of large superelasticity, relatively stable cyclic performance (stable memory), good workability, and good resistance to corrosion and fatigue. Today, most shape-memory devices are produced from NiTi.

In the medical field, research to exploit the potential of NiTi as an implant material was triggered in 1968 by the finding that NiTi showed excellent corrosion resistance in seawater. The use of NiTi for medical applications was first reported in 1973, leading to clinical trials orthopedics in the early 1980s. It was only in the mid-1990s, however, that the first widespread commercial in vascular stent applications made their medical breakthrough (Figure 5.5).

5.2.1 Mechanism of the Shape-Memory Effect

The special character that allows shape-memory alloys to revert to their original shape after temperature change is that their crystal transformation (called *phase transformation* in the field of materials science) is *thermodynamically reversible*. Thermodynamics is a theory about how (heat) energy causes motion of substances. Thermodynamics in materials science is more specifically about how (heat) energy causes atomic/molecular movement and thus causes a phase (structural and/or compositional) change in a material when it is heated up. In thermodynamics, a *reversible process* is defined as

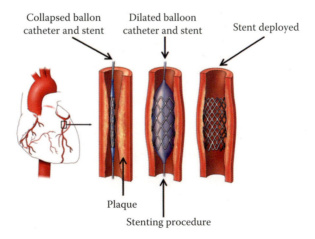

Collapsed balloon catheter and stent   Dilated balloon catheter and stent   Stent deployed

Plaque

Stenting procedure

Figure 5.5
Use of NiTi in stents is based on its superelasticity and shape-memory effect.

one that, after it has taken place, can be reversed and causes no change in either the material (also called the *thermodynamic system*) or its surroundings. In a reversible cycle, the thermodynamic system and its surroundings will be exactly the same after each cycle.

Most phase transformations involve not only a change in structure but a change in composition. In the case of a compositional change, atoms will need to travel through the material via thermal motion, called *diffusion*. Since diffusion is of random nature, it is impossible for any atoms to retrace their diffusion route so as to go back to their original position. Hence, *a diffusive transition process is irreversible*.

However, certain phase transformations do not involve the thermal diffusion of atoms. Instead, an entire network of atoms shifts at the same time to form a new structure (Figure 5.6). This type of transformation is referred to as *martensitic trans-formation*, which is also called *displacive* or *diffusionless* transformation. The phase formed at low temperature is called *martensite*, named after the German metallur-gist Adolf Martens (1850–1914), and the one stable at higher temperature is named *austenite* after Sir William Chandler Roberts-Austen (1843–1902). Unlike a diffusive transition, which is a time-dependent process, the martensitic transition from one structure to another is only dependent on temperature and stress, not time. More precisely, the amounts of the two phases are temperature-dependent (Figure 5.7). In Figure 5.7, M_f is the temperature at which the alloy is completely in the martensite phase. A_s and A_f are the temperatures at which the transformation from martensite to austenite starts and finishes. M_s and M_f are the temperatures at which the trans-formation from austenite to martensite starts and finishes. Repeated operation of the shape-memory effect will typically lead to a shift of these four characteristic trans-formation temperatures, an effect known as *functional fatigue*, which is caused by changes in microstructure.

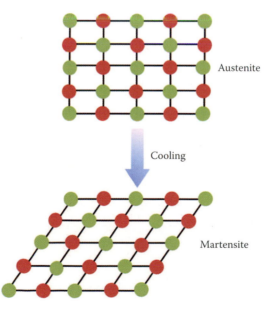

Austenite

Cooling

Martensite

Figure 5.6
Martensitic (displacive or diffusionless) phase transformation.

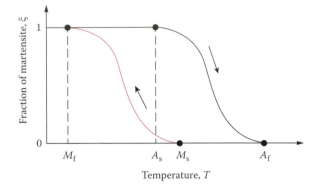

Figure 5.7
Typical heating–cooling curves of a shape-memory alloy.

A reversible transformation must be diffusionless, but a diffusionless transformation is not necessarily reversible. The martensitic transformation from FCC austenite to BCC ferrite in a Fe–C alloy during cooling, for example, is nonreversible. This is because the backward transition from ferrite BCC to austenite FCC encounters a high energy barrier (called *activation energy* in the theory of phase transformation) such that the transition can only take place at a high temperature, at which the energy barrier can be overcome and thermal diffusion of atoms has started. Eventually, in Fe–C alloys ferrite BCC reverts to austenite FCC via diffusion rather than lattice displacement, though the martensitic transition from FCC to BCC is displacive.

5.2.1.1   One-Way Shape-Memory Effect

As indicated in Figure 5.6, martensite transformation involves a shape change, thus resulting in large strains in the parent (austenitic) phase around the martensite plate. To reduce the strain energy, martensitic transformation opts for a mechanism called lattice invariant shear (LIS). There are two possible LIS mechanisms, slipping and twinning (Figure 5.8), which are necessary processes in martensite transformation. Which of these two mechanisms takes place depends on the alloy compositions. In low carbon steels, for example, slipping is the typical accommodation mechanism, while in high carbon steels, both slipping and twinning are involved. Twinning is usually the mechanism of a LIS in shape-memory alloys.

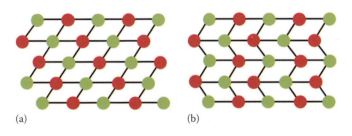

(a)   (b)

Figure 5.8
Slipping and twinning mechanisms involved in martensite transformation. (a) Slipping accommodation mechanism of martensite in low carbon steels, for example; and (b) twinning mechanism in martensite transformation of shape-memory alloys.

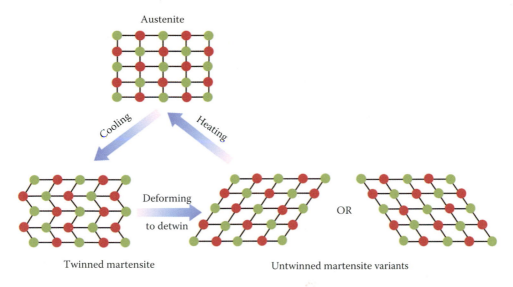

Austenite

Cooling   Heating

Twinned martensite   Deforming to detwin   OR   Untwinned martensite variants

Figure 5.9
One-way shape-memory effect. Note: the shape change at the lower temperature M_f is the result of mechanical deformation done by a user. Different users could introduce different shape change. Hence, the shape at M_f is not remembered by the alloy.

The important difference between slipping and twinning is that the former involves breaking of atomic bonds, while all bonds remain intact in the latter process. In fact, if a stress is applied to the twinned structure, the twin boundaries can move during this deformation to produce a shape that better accommodates the applied stress. This results in a transition from poly-twin variants to a single variant. This process is called *detwinning*, as shown in Figure 5.9. Twinning and detwinning processes are the mechanisms behind the shape memory in alloys.

Upon cooling to M_f from austenite, the self-accommodating (i.e., twinned) variants of martensite are formed (Figure 5.9). In the subsequent deformation process, twin boundaries move and, as a result, most twinned variants, if all is impossible, are detwinned. The metal will then hold those shapes until heated above the transition temperature. It is important to note that the shape changes of all grains collectively produce a shape change to the polycrystalline alloy during deformation at M_f, and that the shape change of each single grain is not exclusive (Figure 5.9). Different users could introduce different variants and thus different shape change at M_f. Hence, the shape at M_f is not remembered by the alloy. However, no matter what the distribution of martensite variants is, it is the austenitic structure and original orientation that each variant can displacively revert to. Therefore, heating to A_f (the heating step of Figure 5.9), the martensitic variants can collectively return back to their original shape after transforming back to austenite structure; that is, the metal remembers its original shape at A_f. When the metal cools to M_f again, it will remain in the original shape (the rectangular shape in this case), until deformed again; that is, the metal does not remember the parallelogram shape obtained at M_f by cooling and deformation. One-way shape-memory effect is the property used in self-expandable stents (Figure 5.5). This is one of the most innovative concepts introduced in the field of metallic biomaterials.

5.2.1.2 Two-Way Shape-Memory Effect   The two-way shape-memory effect is the effect that the material remembers two different shapes: one at low and one at high temperature. A material that shows a shape-memory effect during both heating and cooling is called *two-way shape-memory*. This can be obtained without the application of an external force. The two-way shape memory of an alloy lies in its memory of preferential starting sites (called nucleation sites) of forward and backward phase transformations. If the alloy could remember the nucleation site of the transformation, it will remember the shape of the alloy in the resultant structure. Displacive phase transformations sensitively prefer to initiate from structural defects, especially dislocations. Hence, one method to make an alloy remember a shape is to seed structural defects into it by repeated deformation, a process called *training*. It is these structural defects that remember the transformation routes, which lead to the shapes of the alloys at targeted temperatures. A trained alloy heated beyond a certain point will lose the *permanent* defects and thus lose the two-way memory effect, which is known as *amnesia*. The two-way shape-memory property has not yet found medical applications.

5.2.2   Corrosion of NiTi Alloys

As discussed in Chapter 2, the human body provides a surprisingly aggressive environment for long-term implants. Table 5A.16 in Appendix 5.A lists the major results on the corrosion behaviors of NiTi alloys. In general, NiTi has a better corrosion resistance than 316L stainless steel or CoCrMo but is more sensitive to corrosion than titanium. The corrosion resistances of these metallic biomaterials are ranked as follows:

$$\text{Stainless steels} < \text{CoCrMo} < \text{TiNi} < \text{Ti–6Al–4V}$$

Poor ————————— Corrosion resistance ————————— Good →

5.2.3   Biocompatibility of NiTi Alloys

5.2.3.1 In Vitro Evaluation   The biocompatibility of NiTi remains controversial. Although we do not know the exact concentrations of metallic compounds released from implanted material due to the complicated local conditions (pH, fretting, etc.), the high nickel content of NiTi (50 at.%) is of concern as it may cause biocompatibility problems if deleterious amounts of it are released [4]. Up to now, there are only a small number of reported in vitro studies on cytocompatibility of NiTi (Table 5A.17). In general, the cytocompatibility of NiTi is comparable with CoCrMo alloys, 316 stainless steel, and Ti alloys. However, it must be mentioned that the releasing kinetics of metal ions from alloys designed to be anticorrosive, such as NiTi, is slow, and thus the toxicity of released metal ions from such materials could only be diagnosed after years of implantation. Hence, the short-term in vitro evolution data on the toxicity associated with metal ion release from bulk specimens should not be regarded as a reliable indicator of long-term in vivo effects of the implants.

5.2.3.2 In Vivo Evaluation in Animals   Comprehensive evaluation of NiTi biocompatibility was first made by Castleman and coworkers in 1976 [5] in a canine implant model. In their work, neutron analyses were carried out on a number of tissues including liver, spleen, brain, and kidney, showing no metallic contamination of these organs due to atom or ion release from the implants. The majority of the data summarized in Table 5A.18 suggest that NiTi is quite well accepted into bone; however, there are conflicting studies, in which NiTi has been found to have inferior properties compared to the other implant materials tested, including stainless steel, Co-, and Ti alloys.

5.2.3.3 In Vivo Trials of NiTi Implants in Humans

NiTi has been used as an implant material in humans for both hard and soft tissue. The overall inflammatory response and the capsule membrane thickness around NiTi in recent studies have been found to be similar to those of stainless steel and Ti alloys (Tables 5A.19 through 5A.21).

Based on published studies, NiTi appears to have good potential for clinical use as its biocompatibility in vivo is also good. A commercially produced bone anchor (Mitec G2®) includes a small piece of NiTi wire, and this device has been approved by the FDA, although this and other NiTi long-term implant devices remain to have been proven in long term follow-up of biocompatibility. There are reports that NiTi material has been successfully used in bone-related human applications in Russia and China in a large number of patients (Table 5A.19). Although the studies summarized in Table 5A.19 apparently indicate that the NiTi material in itself has no deleterious effects in human use, the number and quality of clinical trial studies are such that no clear conclusion can be made so far. Because of this, worldwide medical applications of NiTi have been hindered for a long time.

5.2.3.4 Biocompatibility of NiTi Wires as Stents (Filters)

The most exciting clinical application of NiTi is as an alloy for cardiovascular stents (also called filters), which provides a minimally invasive treatment instead of major surgery. The first stent implant experiments were conducted by Cragg and coworkers in 1983 [6]. Based on the studies summarized in Table 5A.20, the biocompatibility of NiTi stents seems to be equal or better compared to stainless steel stents.

To minimize ion release from NiTi implants, especially in stents that have high surface area and are in a dynamic flow, polymer coatings have been applied. However, severe inflammation associated with polyester- or polyurethane coatings has been consistently reported with coated NiTi stents (Table 5A.21).

5.2.4 Mechanical Properties of NiTi Alloys

5.2.4.1 General Mechanical Properties

The mechanical properties of NiTi alloys are unique. First, the mechanical properties of NiTi alloys sensitively depend on the deformation temperatures, whether in austenite or martensite phase (Table 5.6).

Table 5.6

Mechanical Properties of NiTi Alloys in Comparison with 316L Stainless Steel and Cortical Bone

Alloys	Young's Modulus (GPa)	Yield Stress (MPa)	Maximal (Pseudo-) Elastic Strain/%	UTS/MPa	Elongation at Rupture (%)	Fracture Toughness (MPa m$^{1/2}$)
316L	200	200–700	0.1–0.3	500–850	10–40	100–150
NiTi (austenite)	50–110	200–700	8–15	800–1500	<20	30–60
NiTi (martensite)	30–70	70–140	8–15	100–1100	<60	30–35
Cortical bone	10–30	100–120	0.5–1	50–150	3	2–12

Second, the Young's modulus of NiTi alloys is in the range of 30–80 GPa, most close to that of the cortical bone of humans, compared with stainless steel, Co-based alloys, and β Ti alloys (Table 3.3). The lower Young's modulus in NiTi alloys does affect their yield strength and UTS, which are comparable with those of stainless steels (Table 5.6). Third and most attractively, austenitic NiTi alloys have a large elastic strain, ~10%, which is one to two orders of magnitude higher than that of any traditional alloys.

5.2.4.2 Fatigue Properties of NiTi Alloys

The fatigue properties of NiTi alloys sensitively depend on the deformation temperature, whether in austenite or martensite phase. The fatigue strength of austenitic NiTi alloys is in general higher than that of martensitic alloys, and the fatigue strength of austenitic NiTi alloys is higher at elevated temperatures. At both room and body temperatures, the fatigue strength of austenitic NiTi alloys is typically around 400 MPa.

A comparison of fatigue properties of NiTi alloys with those of stainless steel, and Co- and Ti-based alloys (Table 5.7) reveals that nitinol alloys are not advantageous over other alloys in terms of fatigue properties, which explains why these alloys are not the choice for joint replacements.

5.2.5 Medical Applications of NiTi Alloys

Since the early 1970s, NiTi wires have found a variety of applications, including orthodontic archwires, vascular stents, and orthopedic devices for closure or fixation. Among these applications, the most successful ones have been self-expandable stents in gastroenterology and cardiovascular applications (Figure 5.5). Using stents, major surgical operations can be avoided. For critically ill patients, a stent may be the only choice.

5.2.5.1 Cardiovascular Applications of Self-Expandable Stents

The first commercial vascular NiTi device was the Simon Nitinol Filter (SNF, Figure 5.9a) used to treat pulmonary embolism. The filter is inserted as a straight, thin wire via a small bore catheter inserted into a distant vein, and carefully moved within the vessel using live angiography. Upon reaching the lumen of the inferior vena cava and sensing body temperature, it reverts to its preset complex filter shape and locks into place permanently, trapping any further emboli from the pelvis or the lower limbs.

Table 5.7

Fatigue Strength of NiTi Alloys in Comparison with Stainless Steel, Cobalt, and Titanium-Based Alloys

Alloys	Fatigue Strength (MPa) in the Air at 10^7 cycles	Fatigue Strength (MPa) in Solution at 10^7 Cycles
NiTi alloys	100–400 (strain control)	NA
Wrought 316L	300–350 (unnotched stress control)	100–200 (stress control)
Wrought CoCrMo alloys	600–900 (unnotched stress control)	200–300 (stress control)
Ti alloys	500–600 (unnotched stress control)	400–600 (stress control)

Source: Niinomi, M., Int. J. Fatigue, 29(6), 992, 2007.

The SNF was approved by the FDA in 1990. Self-expandable NiTi-based stents have since become the general trend in stent production, whereby a thin stent is placed in the narrowed artery to then expand and dilate the vessel. Today, there are a number of self-expandable stents/filters approved by the FDA, commercially available in medical markets and applied widely in clinics (Figures 5.10 and 5.11).

5.2.5.2 Gastrointestinal Applications of Self-Expandable Stents Self-expanding stents have been applied for esophageal strictures (Figure 5.12). NiTi stents are routinely implantable, providing effective palliation of obstructions due to esophageal adenocarcinoma, and have a low risk of severe complications. The only disadvantage has been incomplete initial stent expansion, as well as tumor ingrowth/overgrowth occurring in nearly one third of the patients tested. Biliary stents (Figure 5.10g) are also effective in achieving long-term palliation in patients with cholangiocarcinomas (bile duct tumor)

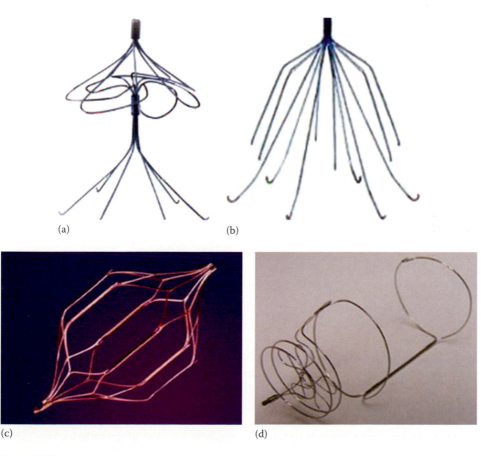

(a)

(b)

(c)

(d)

Figure 5.10
Various nitinol (NiTi) stents/filters. (a) Simon Nitinol Filter, FDA approved in 1990. (b) G2 (Bard Peripheral Vascular), FDA approved for permanent use in 2005 and for retrievable use in 2008. (c) OptEase, FDA approved for permanent use in 2002 and retrievable use in 2004. (d) SafeFlo, FDA approved for permanent use in 2009. (Continued)

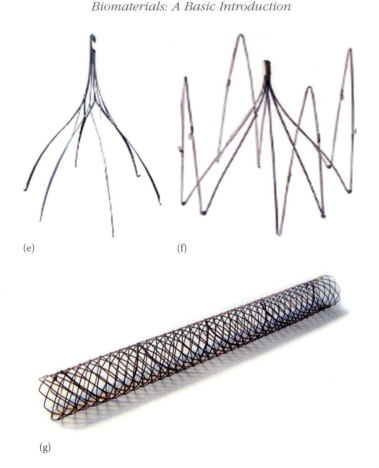

(e) (f)

(g)

Figure 5.10 (Continued)
Various nitinol (NiTi) stents/filters. (e) Option. (f) Vena Tech LP, FDA approved in 2001. (g) Biliary stent, FDA approved in 1999. (From http://www.whichmedicaldevice.com/editorial/article/104/a-brief-history-of-inferior-vena-cava-filters-and-analysis-of-current-devices.)

and in 1999, the FDA released a stent for this purpose. For benign biliary strictures, metallic stent placement is associated with a low long-term patency rate.

5.2.5.3 Urological and Other Applications of Self-Expandable Stents The use of NiTi stents has also been extended to the treatment of prostatic obstruction. For patients with a high operative risk, the insertion of a permanent metal stent system offers a useful alternative to treat urethral obstruction caused by prostatic carcinoma and benign prostatic hyperplasia. NiTi stents have also been used to prevent major airway occlusion, such as in inoperable tracheal or bronchial stenosis due to intraluminal tumor protrusion and invasion. NiTi alloys are also used as detachable clamps for gastrointestinal tract surgery and stapes prosthesis for ossicular fixation after stapedectomy, in the middle ear.

5.2.5.4 Orthopedic and Orthodontic Applications of NiTi Implants Since the 1960s, studies have been carried out on the application of NiTi for orthopedic procedures, including correction rods for scoliosis of the spine and fixation staples for long

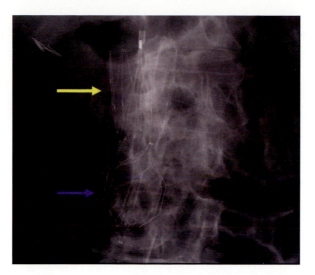

Figure 5.11
Radiograph of the inferior vena cava implanted with Vena Tech LP (yellow arrow) and OptEase (blue arrow) stents. (From http://www.ceessentials.net/article12.html.)

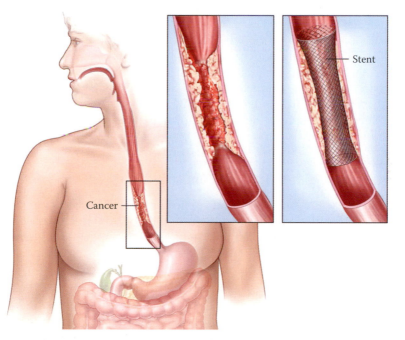

Figure 5.12
Esophageal stent. (From Terese Winslow LLC, U.S. Govt. has certain rights, Alexandria, VA. Copyright 2005, reproduced with permission.)

bones (Table 5A.22). Early trials have indicated that NiTi may not provide any improvements compared to the traditional implant systems. However, a follow-up study from China in 1986 [8] reported satisfactory performance of NiTi rods in 26 scoliosis patients. Successful applications of NiTi in spinal correction of 38 scoliosis patients were reported in another more recent follow up report in 2011 [9].

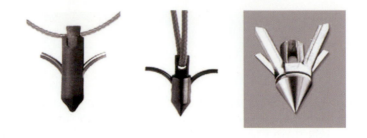

Figure 5.13
Nonscrew anchors Mitek G2, Mitek Rotator Cuff Anchor, and Linvatec Ultrafix RC from left to right. (From Ritchie, P.K. and McCarty, E.C., Oper. Techn. Sport. Med., 12(4), 215, 2004.)

NiTi compression staples were first introduced in China in 1981. After that, NiTi staples and clamps were used in fractures of short tubular bone, for fixation of mandibular fractures, metatarsal osteotomies, anterior cervical decompression and fusion, fixation of small bone fragments, and for several other cursory applications. The only NiTi-containing orthopedic implant widely used in western countries is the Mitek G2 suture anchor (Figure 5.13). It has NiTi wings that prevent the anchor from pulling out of the bone after insertion and securing of tendons or ligaments back onto the bone. Another potential application of NiTi is a hook used to restore the dislocated acromioclavicular joint of the shoulder.

Most published studies in orthopedics have not satisfied the basic quality criteria of scientific study. The data are not convincing enough to say that a certain NiTi implant can be used without harm. To be considered fully successful, it must be proved to be better than the existing competitors. At present, there are no comparative clinical studies and the sample groups have generally been small. Randomized prospective studies are needed for applying new NiTi implant devices for long-term clinical use in humans [4].

5.2.6 Issues and Challenges of NiTi Implants

Despite the most exciting and successful applications of NiTi as stents in the treatment of the occlusion of various vessels and ducts in the body, there are concerns over the systemic toxicity associated with the release of Ni element over a long-term implantation, especially in applications of NiTi as a bone implant material in humans. New nickel-free shape-memory alloys are under development.

5.2.7 Summary

The shape-memory property of NiTi (Nitinol) alloy has put it in a special place for minimally invasive surgical applications. Today, self-expandable stents, clamps, and clips made out of NiTi alloys have been applied in various types of surgery. Despite extensive investigation on the biocompatibility of NiTi alloys, reports have been controversial, especially those of orthopedic implant trials. So far, many researchers believe that NiTi alloy has excellent corrosion resistance and biocompatibility, while on the other hand there are serious concerns over its long-term systemic toxicity due to nickel ion release. The development of new nickel-free shape-memory alloys may offer new opportunities to obviate these concerns.

5.3 OTHER CLINICALLY APPLIED METALLIC MATERIALS

5.3.1 Tantalum

Tantalum is one of the refractory metals, among others, including niobium, molybdenum, tungsten, and rhenium. Except for two of the platinum-group metals (osmium and iridium), the refractory metals have the highest melting temperatures (>2000°C) and the lowest vapor pressures of all metals. The use of niobium, molybdenum, and tungsten for biomedical applications is confined to alloying in stainless steels, cobalt alloys, and titanium alloys. Radioactive rhenium is occasionally used in stents to prevent restenosis. Tantalum has found a number of clinical applications, due to its excellent biocompatibility, flexibility, and corrosion resistance.

5.3.1.1 Corrosion and Biocompatibility of Tantalum   Pure tantalum has excellent resistance to corrosion in a large number of acids, most aqueous solutions of salts, organic chemicals, and various combinations and mixtures of these agents. The corrosion resistance of tantalum is approximately the same as that of glass. Tantalum has no known biological role and is nontoxic. Compounds containing tantalum are rarely encountered in the natural environment. Tantalum is among the most biocompatible metals used for implantable devices (Figure 2.2). The compositional requirements for medical-grade tantalum are given in Table 5.8. Requirements for the mechanical properties of annealed and cold-worked unalloyed tantalum are listed in Table 5.9.

5.3.1.2 Clinical Applications of Tantalum   Since the 1950s, tantalum has been used in closure in the form of suture wires for skin closure, tendon, and nerve repair; foils and sheets for nerve anastomoses; clips for the ligation of vessels; staples for abdominal procedures; and in the form of pliable sheets and plates for cranioplasty and reconstructive surgery. Sintered tantalum capacitor electrodes are also used in electrical stimulation devices.

Tantalum has also been used to coat other metals, such as titanium implants, and carbon foam skeletons used as a biocompatible replacement for vertebral bodies of the spinal column. Tantalum coatings, which are 70%–80% porous, have a macroporous structure similar to that of cancellous bone. Besides spinal implants, carbon–tantalum cellular materials have potential applications for hip and knee re-construction and bone scaffold void filling applications. Porous scaffolds have also been made from tantalum, including Trabecular Metal™, which contains pores, the size of which makes this material very good for bone ingrowth. It is believed that Trabecular Metal™ has an elastic nature that aids bone remodeling.

5.3.2 Zirconium Alloys

5.3.2.1 Corrosion and Biocompatibility of Zirconium   Zirconium is mainly used as an alloying element for its strong resistance to corrosion. Similar to titanium in that it is refractory, zirconium has a high affinity for oxygen, forming an adherent, protective oxide film spontaneously on its surface, in both dry and wet oxygen-rich conditions. Moreover, this film is self-healing and protects the base metal from chemical attack at temperatures up to 300°C. As a result, zirconium is very resistant to corrosive attack in most mineral and organic acids, strong alkalis, and saline solutions. Zirconium metal exhibits the highest biocompatibility of all metals in the body (Figure 2.2), and zirconium compounds are of low toxicity.

Table 5.8

Compositions, Maximum Weight Percent Allowed for Unalloyed Tantalum in Accordance with ASTM F 560

	Ta	Carbon	Oxygen	Nitrogen	Hydrogen	Niobium	Iron	Titanium	Tungsten	Molybdenum	Silicon	Nickel
UNS R05200[a]	Bal	0.010	0.0150	0.010	0.0015	0.100	0.010	0.010	0.05	0.020	0.0050	0.010
UNS R05400[b]	Bal	0.010	0.030	0.010	0.0015	0.100	0.010	0.010	0.05	0.020	0.0050	0.010

[a] *Electron beam or vacuum arc cast tantalum.*
[b] *Sintered tantalum.*

Table 5.9

Mechanical Properties for Unalloyed Tantalum

Processing Condition	Hardness, HV	Young's Modulus (GPa)	Yield Strength (MPa)	UTS (MPa)	Elongation (%)
Annealed	80–110	186–191(±27–28)	140 ± 20	205 ± 30	20–30
Cold-worked	120–300	186–191(±27–28)	345 ± 50	480 ± 70	1–25

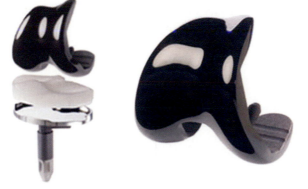

Figure 5.14
OXINIUM™ oxidized zirconium has been introduced to reduce the wear rate over CoCrMo alloy total knee implants. (From http://www.oxinium.co.uk/surgeons/knee_implants.php)

5.3.2.2 Clinical Application of Zirconium Alloy   A zirconium alloy, Zr-2.5Nb, is used in a new ceramic knee implant (Figure 5.14). The Zr-2.5Nb alloy has a relatively low modulus of 100 GPa, strengthened with small additions of oxygen and coated with a hard ceramic surface. The ceramic coating is developed through heating at 500°C, at which the zirconium reacts with oxygen to produce zirconium oxide (zirconia). It is believed that this new knee could last for 20–25 years, substantially longer than the 15–20 years over which existing cobalt chromium alloy and polyethylene implants last. Another important characteristic of this material is that it is systemically more biocompatible, meaning that sufferers of nickel allergies who may not tolerate knee implants made of cobalt chromium alloy may well tolerate a zirconium alloy alternative.

5.3.3 Silver

5.3.3.1 Biocompatibility of Silver   Silver has no known biological roles. Although silver itself is nontoxic, most silver salts are, and some maybe, carcinogenic.

5.3.3.2 Medical Application of Ag   Silver ions and silver compounds show moderate toxicity to humans, although they also have potent, broad-spectrum antimicrobial effects. The antimicrobial properties of silver are mainly used in the form of silver salts and nanoparticles that break down to release silver ions (Ag^+). These forms of silver compounds are impregnated into wound dressings, topical antiseptics, and antimicrobial surface treatments for devices such as catheters. Metallic silver is also used in surgical applications for structural devices (e.g., cranial support plates, suture wire, aneurysm clips, and tracheostomy tubes). Silver tubing is also used in the urinary tract, for urethral catheters, and penile prosthetic implants.

5.3.4   Metals Used as Medical Electrodes

An important and challenging medical use of implanted electrodes is in prosthetic devices for neural or muscle stimulation. These devices employ metal electrodes to transmit the current required for electrical stimulation of appropriate areas of the nervous system. Neural prostheses for direct control of peripheral organs include the cardiac pacemaker, the phrenic stimulator for respiratory control, and spinal cord stimulators for bladder control. More complex neural control devices include auditory prostheses for deafness, experimental visual prostheses for blindness, and neuromuscular prostheses for muscular entrainment to restore limb function in paralyzed individuals. Some external devices also require metal electrodes, such as those used for polygraph detection of transdermal electrical activity from internal organs, including the heart (e.g., electrocardiography, ECG), brain (electroencephalography, EEG), and muscle (electromyography, EMG).

The most frequently considered metals for electrical stimulation are the noble or precious metals: platinum, iridium, rhodium, gold, and palladium. This is because of their resistance to chemical and electrochemical corrosion. However, all of these metals show corrosion effects during both in vitro and in vivo electrical stimulation. Corrosion effects include weight loss, formation of unstable surface films that tend to spall from the surface, and dissolution of metal. Of the noble metals, platinum and platinum–iridium alloys containing 10%–30% irridium are the most widely used for electrical stimulation.

Metal oxides such as iridium oxide have also shown promise. Some non-noble metals are candidates for electrode applications requiring high mechanical strength and fatigue resistance such as that demanded of intramuscular electrodes. These include vacuum melted type 316L stainless steel, cobalt alloys Elgiloy and MP35N, pure forms of zirconium, tantalum, titanium, tungsten, and tungsten bronzes made by powder metallurgy processing.

5.4   NEW METALLIC MATERIALS: MAGNESIUM ALLOYS

5.4.1   Three Generations of Biomaterials in Terms of Degradability

The development of biomaterials has witnessed three distinct generations, which meet three levels of clinical requirements. In the early stages, biomaterials were expected to meet the most essential clinical requirement, that is, no harm to the tissue being repaired. To meet this criterion, virtually inert biomaterials were designed and tested as implant materials. Examples include Co-alloys and Orthinox, which are typical first-generation biomaterials. Loosening of implants made from these biomaterials drove researchers to seek materials with surface bioactivity that could allow them to bond to the host tissue. These surface bioactive materials formed the so-called second-generation of biomaterials, represented by titanium alloys. However, the limited longevity of both first- and second-generation biomaterials, as well as the low probability of overcoming this limitation, has driven scientists to adopt a new strategy of tissue engineering and regeneration. Biomaterials are now sought to act as a temporary structure, which requires them to be able to degrade and allow native tissue to integrate with the implant and eventually replace it. Degradable biomaterials therefore form the so-called third generation of biomaterials. The essential requirements of the third generation

Table 5.10
Three Generations of Metallic Biomaterials

Generation	Biodegradability	Clinical Requirements	Examples
First	Biologically inert	No harm to tissues	CoCr alloys
Second	Surface erosion	Tissue-bonding	Titanium alloys
Third	Biodegradation	Tissue regeneration	Magnesium alloys

of metallic implant materials include that they be nontoxic, mechanically compatible (with a minimal stress-shielding effect), and degradable. Table 5.10 summarizes the three generations of biomaterials.

5.4.2 Rationale of Developing Mg Alloys as Medical Implants

Magnesium alloys fall into the third category of implant biomaterials. The potential application of this alloy system for orthopedic implant materials is based on the following potential benefits of these alloys. First, magnesium is a benign macro-element in the body (Table 2.1). As early as the 1930s, feasibility studies showed good resorbability and high biocompatibility of magnesium bone-fixation implants [11]. Second, magnesium has a density (1.74 g/cm^3) close to that of bone ($1.8–2.1$ g/cm^3) and a Young's modulus also similar to that of bone (Table 5.11). Third, magnesium alloys have controllable corrosion rates (and thus resorbability) in physiological media. In short, magnesium and alloys are likely to meet all three essential requirements for third generation metallic implant biomaterials: biologically not harmful, mechanically matched to bone, and degradable. Table 5.12 provides a list of the compositions of major magnesium alloys.

5.4.3 Corrosion of Mg Alloys

The basic electrochemical characteristic of magnesium, with standard electrode potential of -2.375 V, leads to a low corrosion resistance. The surface of magnesium passivates and builds up a thin layer of magnesium oxide, when exposed to air, which prevents further chemical reactions. However, magnesium is severely attacked in the saline environments of the human tissues, the characteristics that actually enable Mg alloys, particularly Mg–Ca varieties, to be effectively used as absorbable implant materials. Magnesium can be entirely absorbed in the human body.

Table 5.11
Mechanical Properties of Metallic Materials and Cortical Bone

Materials	Density (g/cm^3)	Young's Modulus E (GPa)	Yield Strength σ_y (MPa)	Ultimate Tensile Strength (MPa)
316L stainless steel	7.8	200	200–700	500–900
CoCr alloys	8.8	240	450–1500	600–1600
Ti alloys	4.5	105–125	350–1050	600–1100
Magnesium	1.74	45	20	120
Cortical bone	1.8–2.1	10–30	100–120	130–150

Table 5.12

Composition (wt.%) of Magnesium Alloys

Type	Group (Example)	Al	Mn	Si	Zn	Ag	Cu	Zr	Nd	Ni	Y
Cast	AM series (AM20)	2	0.5	—	—	—	—	—	—	—	—
	AS series (AS21)	2	0.4	1	—	—	—	—	—	—	—
	AZ series (AZ61)	6	0.2	—	0.7	—	—	—	—	—	—
	EQ series (EQ21)	—	—	—	—	1.5–2	0.075	0.7	2.25	—	—
	EZ series (EZ33)	—	—	—	2–3.1	—	0–0.1	0.5–1	3	0–0.01	—
	QE series	—	—	—	—	2–2.5	—	0.6	2	—	—
	WE series (WE43)	—	—	—	—	—	—	0.5	3.25	—	4
	ZC series (ZC63)	—	0.5	—	6	—	2.7	—	—	—	—
	ZE series (ZE41)	—	0–0.15	—	3.5–5	—	0–0.1	0.4–1	1.3	0–0.01	—
Wrought	AZ series (AZ31)	3	0.3	—	1	—	—	—	—	—	—
	EA series (EA55RS)	5	—	—	5	—	—	—	4.9	—	—
	WE series (WE54)	—	—	—	—	—	—	0.5	3.15	—	5.1
	Z series (Z6)	—	—	—	6	—	—	—	—	—	—
	ZC series (ZC71)	—	0.75	—	6.5	—	1.25	—	—	—	—
	ZK series (ZK60A-F)	—	—	—	6	—	—	0.45	—	—	—
	ZM series (ZM21)	—	1	—	2	—	—	—	—	—	—
	ZW series (ZW3)	—	—	—	3.25	—	—	0.6	—	—	—

Magnesium alloys corrode/degrade in aqueous conditions via several different oxidation–reduction reactions, which are influenced by the alloying elements. Generally, the corrosion of magnesium in water will yield magnesium hydroxide and hydrogen gas evolution. The net reaction is given as follows:

$$Mg + H_2O \rightarrow Mg\ (OH)_2 + H_2. \tag{5.1}$$

Typically, zinc is used as an alloying element, as it also possesses the ability to displace hydrogen ions from solution. If zinc is used in magnesium–zinc alloys, then the following reactions would also occur:

$$Zn + H_2O \rightarrow Zn\ (OH)_2 + H_2. \tag{5.2}$$

Magnesium metal can also remove zinc ions from solution:

$$Mg + Zn^{2+} \rightarrow Mg^{2+} + Zn. \tag{5.3}$$

The hydrogen evolution due to fast corrosion rates is a significant problem in the application of magnesium alloys as implants. Because of this drawback, a slow corrosion rate in magnesium alloys is more desirable.

There have been a number of alloying elements used in magnesium-based materials in an attempt to tune down their corrosion properties to make them more feasible as implants. Elements like Mn, Cu, Al, Ca, Zr, Gd, and Zn have all been explored (Table 5.13). A minor addition of calcium (Ca) to Mg-based alloys in general has been shown to enhance their corrosion resistance significantly, with similar effects following addition of manganese. The use of copper increases the strength of magnesium casts, but at the same time can accelerate the corrosion rates of magnesium alloys in NaCl solutions. Magnesium alloys containing aluminum generally possess a good combination of mechanical properties and corrosion resistance. Aluminum is a passivative element, and thus enhances corrosion resistance of alloys. The important benefit of adding zinc to magnesium is that Zn-rich alloys form less hydrogen gas. Zinc is actually the most commonly used alloying element in magnesium alloys. It can effectively improve the yield strength of magnesium, while retaining its Young's modulus of $\sim$40 GPa.

However, the solubility of alloying elements in crystalline Mg is limited, and thus corrosion rates can only be altered within a limited range. Hydrogen evolution thus remains a problem during the degradation of crystalline Mg alloys. In contrast, there is a much greater range for elements to be alloyed in an amorphous structure, which allows the production of metallic glasses with significantly improved corrosion characteristics. It has been shown that the hydrogen evolution during degradation can be significantly reduced or even prevented completely in glassy MgZnCa alloys [12].

5.4.4 Biocompatibility/Toxicity of Mg Alloys

As described earlier, the chemical toxicity of these metals inside the body depends not only on the toxicity of the elements and their compounds but also on the concentration of released ions or wear particles. Even a poisonous substance may be less toxic in sufficiently low concentrations, while micronutrients can cause adverse responses when present in excessive amounts. Hence, to design biologically safe, degradable magnesium alloys, it is important to know the release kinetics (corrosion rates) of the implanted material (Table 5.13) and the biological safe limit of relevant elements in the body (Table 5.14). It is also important to understand the tissue-specific accumulation of

Table 5.13

In Vitro and In Vivo Corrosion Rates of Magnesium Alloys

| Alloys | In Vitro Electrochemical Corrosion Rate ($\mu A/cm^2$) | | | | In Vitro Immersion Corrosion Rate ($mg/cm^2/h$) | | | | In Vivo Corrosion Rate ($mg/cm^2/Year$) |
	0.9 wt.% NaCl	Hank's Solution	SBF	m-SBF	0.9 wt.% NaCl	Hank's Solution	SBF	m-SBF	
Pure Mg (99.85%)		15.98	80.06			0.011	0.038		1.17
AZ31	34	31.60				0.0065			1.38
AZ91	10			65.70		0.0028			1.56
WE43	22.56	30.60	16.03				0.085		
ZE41	27					0.0626			0.39
LAE442	30			17.80					
AZ91Ca				36.50					
AZ61Ca									
Cast Mg–Mn–Zn		1.45–1.60				0.003–0.010			0.92
Extruded Mg–Mn–Zn			79.17				0.05		
Extruded Mg–Zn–Y		1.88–4.47					0.015–0.04		1.28
Cast Mg–1Ca			546.09				0.136		
Extruded Mg–1Ca			75.65				0.040		

Source: Gu, X.N. and Zheng, Y.F., Front. Mater. Sci. Chin., 4(2), 111, 2010.

Table 5.14
Biological Safe Limit of Mg and Its Alloying Elements

Elements	Blood Serum Level	Daily Allowance
Mg	0.9 mmol/L	0.7 g
Ca	1.3 mmol/L	0.8 g
Cu	1.1–1.5 μg/mL	2–3 mg
Zn	46 μmol/L	15 mg
Mn	1 μmol/L	4 mg
Li	2–4 ng/g	0.2–0.6 mg
Al	2.1–4.8 μg	Total amount in humans <300 mg
Zr	Total <250 mg	3.5 mg
R and RE	<47 μg	

elemental metals. Extra magnesium ions in the body, for example, are mainly filtered and removed by the kidney. Hence, excessive magnesium could place patients at the risk of renal dysfunction, and magnesium implants should not be recommended for patients with renal diseases.

As mentioned earlier, the hydrogen evolution could be a problem with Mg-based implants. The hydrogen evolution in implants with a filigree structure, such as cardiovascular stents, seems to be of minor importance, where gas can freely diffuse away from the material surface. However, in bone biosynthesis applications, where vascularization and nutrient transport is minimal, hydrogen evolution remains problematic. Poor transport mechanisms can result in gas pockets occurring around Mg alloy implants. In animal studies, subcutaneous gas bubbles have had to be removed by means of puncture procedures.

5.4.5 Mechanical Properties of Mg Alloys

Magnesium alloys have UTS and rupture elongation in the range of 90–280 MPa and 3%–20%, respectively (Table 5.15). In principle, the rapid reduction in strength due to degradation is not an issue-to-tissue engineering application, as the degradable implant is expected to provide temporary support rather than permanent substitution of bone.

Table 5.15
Mechanical Properties of Mg–Zn- and Mg–Ca-Based Alloys

Alloys	Young's Modulus (GPa)	0.2% Yield Strength (MPa)	UTS (MPa)	Rupture Elongation (%)
Mg-cast	41	21	87	13
AZ91D-die cast	45	150	230	3
AZ31-extruded	45	125	235	7
LAE442		148	247	18
AE43-extruded T5	44	195	280	10
AM60B-die cast	45		220	6–8
Mg–Zn–Mn extruded		246	180	22
Mg–1Ca extruded		140	220	14

The mechanical properties of magnesium alloys can be tuned by the alloying composition and processing history. The addition of Al, Ag, In, Si, Sn, Zn, and Zr can improve both the strength and elongation of magnesium alloys, with further strength imparted by processes such as hot rolling and hot extrusion.

5.4.5.1 Mg–Zn-Based Alloys In general, the addition of Zn up to 3 wt.% reduces the grain size and enhances the mechanical properties of the alloy matrix, with Young's modulus, UTS, and yield strength increasing from 41 to 45 GPa, 90 to 230, 20 to 130 MPa, respectively (Table 5.15). Beyond 3 wt.% Zn, grain size and strength remain the same, while elongation decreases significantly (Table 5.15). The fracture behavior of Mg alloy also changes from nearly complete cleavage fracture to quasi-cleavage fracture with the addition of Zn. When Zn content exceeds 3 wt.%, (Mg, Zn)-rich particles act as the crack initiation sites.

5.4.5.2 Mg–Ca-Based Alloys The addition of calcium up to 1.0 wt.% leads to an increase in tensile strength up to approximately 220 MPa. The 0.2% yield strength also increases to ~140 MPa with increasing concentration of calcium. No significant further increase in the tensile strength can be achieved above 2.0 wt.% calcium. Calcium content dramatically affects the elongation at rupture, which reaches a maximum value of 14% at the composition of 1 wt.% Ca (Table 5.15).

5.4.6 Potential Applications of Magnesium Alloys and Challenges

The development of magnesium alloys as third-generation degradable biomaterials has been primarily driven by applications in tissue engineering. A number of issues must be addressed prior to any clinical applications, among which hydrogen generation and related infection are the most challenging. Caution is advised also for the toxicity of any alloying elements used in new alloy compositions.

5.4.7 Summary

The hope of metallic implants with long-term success will probably lie in the development of degradable metallic materials. Using this strategy, researchers must take great caution in the choice of metal to prevent metal-related toxicity, because biological safety levels of most metal elements are lower than 0.01%. The corrosion rate of a degradable implant must be lower than the tolerable level of the individual alloying elements in the body. In this regard, careful design must be conducted based on the biological profile of each alloying element (toxicity, storage versus excreting mechanism and rate, etc.) and the corrosion profile of the implant in an appropriately simulated physiological environment combined with appropriate nonhuman implant models.

Magnesium alloys attract much attention from the field of orthopedic implant materials and tissue engineering because the major alloying elements (Mg and Ca) can be tolerated by the body at a relatively high level. Magnesium alloys are also mechanically compatible to bone and biodegradable. However, several issues must be addressed prior to clinical applications, including the alleviation of hydrogen bubble generation and implant related infection. Glassy magnesium alloys seem to offer a highly suitable alternative to crystalline alloys as an opportunity to address the issue associated with the hydrogen bubble effect.

5.5   CHAPTER HIGHLIGHTS

1. Dental restorative biomaterials involve all types of materials described in Chapter 1: Metallic, ceramic, polymeric, and composite materials. Dental alloys are grouped into three broad categories: amalgam alloys, noble metals, and base metals. Base (non-noble metals) metals are included in stainless steels, cobalt-based, and titanium-based alloys.

2. Besides nontoxicity, special requirements of tooth fillings are as follows:
   • In situ solidification at a temperature close to body temperature
   • Minimal shrinkage
   • Good compressive strength and superb resistance to friction and wear

3. The shape-memory effect is the result of reversible crystal transition, which does not involve any thermal diffusion of atoms.

4. One-way shape-memory effect: When a shape-memory alloy is in its cold state, the metal can be bent or stretched and will hold those shapes until heated above the transition temperature. Upon heating, the shape changes to its original state. When the metal cools again it will remain in the shape achieved during its heated state, until deformed again. One-way shape-memory effect is the property used in self-expandable stents.

5. Two-way shape-memory effect: The material remembers two different shapes: one at low and one at high-temperature. The ability of a material that shows a shape-memory effect during both heating and cooling is called two-way shape memory. The two-way shape-memory property has not yet found medical applications.

6. The one-way shape-memory property of NiTi (nitinol) alloy has been used in self-expandable stents, clamps, and clips in various types of surgery. Despite these successes, the biocompatibility of NiTi alloys remains controversial, especially in orthopedic implants. There are serious concerns over the long-term systemic toxicity of the alloys from nickel ion release.

7. Three generations of biomaterials: The first generation of materials are bio-inert, a character aimed to ensure that materials are not harmful to tissues. The second generation of materials are surface bioactive, a character aimed to achieve effective tissue bonding. The third generation of biomaterials are biodegradable, a character which allows them to be replaced by regenerating tissues.

8. In the development of biodegradable metallic biomaterials, researchers must take great caution in the choice of metal to prevent metallic element–related toxicity. The corrosion rate of a degradable implant must be lower than the tolerable level of each individual alloying element in the body.

9. Mg alloys are the choice of materials as a third-generation material system since the major alloying elements (Mg and Ca) can be tolerated by the body at relatively high levels. The alloys are also mechanically compatible to bone and biodegradable. One of the major issues is hydrogen bubble due to fast corrosion rates.

LABORATORY PRACTICE 2

Introduce one-way shape-memory effect in NiTi alloys.

5.A APPENDIX DATA ON CORROSION RESISTANCE AND BIOCOMPATIBILITY OF NiTi ALLOYS

Table 5A.16
Corrosion Behaviors of NiTi Alloys

Testing Conditions	Major Results	Refs.
37°C, Hank's solution	NiTi has better corrosion resistance than Co–Cr–Mo or 316L stainless steel.	[14]
37°C, 0.9 wt.% NaCl solution	NiTi is more sensitive to corrosion than titanium. Pitting of the NiTi surface was observed.	[15]
37°C, Hanks' solution	NiTi has a better resistance to the chemical breakdown of passivity, compared to 316L.	[16]
37°C, 0.9 wt.% NaCl solution	When stainless steel (316L) was coupled with NiTi, 316L was found to suffer from crevice corrosion	[17]
Retrieved implants	NiTi wires are no more subject to corrosion than stainless steel.	[18]
Tested in artificial saliva	The release rates of nickel from stainless steel and nickel–titanium arch wires were not significantly different.	[19]
Evaluated in physiological simulating fluids	The Ni ion release was three times higher for NiTi than for austenitic stainless steels. The characteristics of the passive film formed on NiTi are not so good as those on Ti6–Al–4V but are comparable or inferior to those on austenitic stainless steels.	[20]
Ringer's solution	Annealed NiTi to be more corrosion-resistant than cold-worked material. Thus, the heat treatment and mechanical working had a significant influence on corrosion behavior. The same study also indicated that straining of NiTi led to significant improvements in corrosion resistance. This may be due to the development of a single martensite variant during deformation.	[21]
In vivo: NiTi plates, 17 months after implantation in dogs	No generalized or localized corrosion on NiTi. Neutron activation analysis of distant organs in the same study showed no accumulation of trace metals from NiTi.	[5]
Implanted 44 NiTi intraluminal stents in the iliac arteries of 22 sheep	Only minimal corrosion was seen at 6 months. Pitting was the predominant type of corrosion. The pit penetration rate was estimated to be approximately 0.0046 cm/year. Corrosion product analysis around the pit sites indicated that the main product of pitting was a titanium-bearing compound, probably an oxide.	[22]

Source: Ryhanen, J., Biocompatibilty evaluation of nickel-titanium shape memory metal alloy, Phd thesis, Oulu University Library, Oulu, Finland, 1999.

Table 5A.17

In Vitro Studies on Biocompatibility of NiTi Alloys

Cells	Control Materials	Major Results	Refs.
Human fetal lung fibroblasts	316L stainless steel and CoCr alloy	316L stainless steel and CoCr alloy did not differ in cell growth from the negative control cultures, but NiTi and titanium significantly reduced cell growth. The morphological changes of cells with NiTi and titanium were also more pronounced.	[23]
Human fibroblasts	No	Nickel induces a significant inhibition of mitosis in human fibroblasts, whereas no significant effects of this kind were found for titanium or NiTi. NiTi was considered biocompatible and comparable to titanium.	[24]
L-929 fibroblasts	316L stainless steel and CoCr alloy	All metals induced a mild biological reaction. The cytotoxicity of NiTi was found to be approximately equal to that of Co–Cr–Mo, both being more than that of pure titanium, Ti–6A1–4V or 316L stainless steel.	[25]
Human gingival fibroblast spreading	No	Human plasma fibronectin (pFN), an adhesive protein, can be covalently immobilized onto NiTi substrate and human gingival fibroblast spreading significantly improved, suggesting that this chemical modification enables the controlling of metal/cell interactions.	[26,27]
Rat splenocytes	No	Cells exposed to NiTi are critically affected by the surface preparation. The hydrogen peroxide surface treatment of NiTi caused a toxic effect comparable to that of pure nickel. However, the situation changed tremendously when NiTi was treated by autoclaving in water or steam. The reaction with these NiTi specimens was clearly nontoxic.	[28]
Human peripheral blood lymphocytes	316L stainless steel	The NiTi alloy showed no cytotoxic, allergic, or genotoxic activity. The findings were similar to those on 316L stainless steel. Conclusion: The NiTi alloy can be regarded as a biologically safe implant material.	[29]

(Continued)

Table 5A.17 (Continued)
In Vitro Studies on Biocompatibility of NiTi Alloys

Cells	Control Materials	Major Results	Refs.
Human peripheral blood lymphocytes	CP-titanium and 316L stainless steel	These three alloys induced similar DNA strand breaks of interphase chromatin, but stainless steel induction of metaphase chromatin damage was more intense than with NiTi or pure titanium. Conclusion: NiTi genocompatibility is promising in view of its biocompatibility approval.	[30]
Fibroblasts	316L stainless steel, CoCr alloy, β-titanium alloy wires	NiTi, stainless steel, and β-titanium alloy wires had no effect on the rate of cell proliferation. The most severe growth inhibition was induced by the CoCrNi alloy.	[31]
Murine fibroblasts and osteoblasts	No	No cytotoxicity was detected in the direct-contact evolution testing.	[32]
Human osteoblast-like osteosarcoma cells (SAOS-2, MG-63), primary human osteoblasts (HOB), and murine fibroblasts (3T3)	No	The results indicate a good biocompatibility for a nickel content up to about 50%.	[33]
Rat osteosarcoma cell line ROS-17	Stainless steel, pure titanium and pure nickel	In the NiTi and Ti groups, the number of dead cells was significantly lower than in the Ni group. Conclusion: NiTi is well tolerated by the osteoblastic type ROS-17 cells.	[34]
Osteoblasts	Stainless steel	The plasma-treated surfaces are cytologically compatible, allowing the attachment and proliferation of osteoblasts. The sample with surface titanium nitride exhibits the largest degree of cell proliferation whereas stainless steel fares the worst.	[35–37]
MG63 cells	No	Oxidized NiTi surfaces enhance differentiation of osteoblast-like cells.	[38]
Osteoblasts	No	The adhesion, spreading, and proliferation of osteoblasts on the implanted NiTi surface were assessed by cell culture tests. Our results indicate that the nanoscale surface morphology that is altered by the implantation frequencies impacts the surface free energy and wettability of the NiTi surfaces, and in turn affects the osteoblast adhesion behavior.	[39]

Table 5A.18

In Vivo Studies on Biocompatibility of NiTi Alloys with Animals

Animal Model/ Maximal Duration of Implantation	Control Materials	Major Results	Refs.
45 rats subcutaneously/9 weeks	316 stainless steel	The tissue reaction was minimal. A dense, relatively avascular fibrous connective tissue capsule formed around implants. Conclusion: NiTi compares favorably with stainless steel and could be used in deep tissues.	[40]
5 dogs, 12 beagles/17 months	316L stainless steel and CoCr alloy	The muscle tissue in dogs exposed to NiTi implants for 17 months showed some variability.	[5]
		There was no evidence of either localized or general corrosion on the surfaces of the bone plates and screws. No signs of adverse tissue reactions (e.g., bone resorption) resulting from the NiTi implants were seen. In the NiTi group, some high nickel concentrations were observed in bone due to contamination.	
		Overall, the gross clinical, radiological, and morphological observations of tissue at the implantation sites at autopsy revealed no signs of adverse tissue reactions resulting from the NiTi implants. The authors concluded that NiTi alloy is sufficiently compatible with dog tissue to warrant further investigation of its potential as a biomaterial.	
NA/3 months	No	After 3 months' implantation, no corrosion was observed on the plate surfaces. Conclusion: Ti50Ni50–xCux (x = 2, 6, 8) shape-memory alloys also have good biocompatibility.	[41]
Femoral shafts of 15 dogs/12 weeks	316L stainless steel	Since the elastic modulus of the NiTi shape-memory alloy was lower, the stress-shielding effect in the bone underneath the NiTi device is less than 316 stainless steel. The axial compression stress of the fracture line was kept greater and the contact of that NiTi device with the bone was not so close. This might be beneficial for the recovery of blood supply and bone remodeling.	[42]

(Continued)

Table 5A.18 (Continued)
In Vivo Studies on Biocompatibility of NiTi Alloys with Animals

Animal Model/ Maximal Duration of Implantation	Control Materials	Major Results	Refs.
Frontal bone of 7 rabbits/12 weeks	Hydroxyapatite	Porous NiTi No adjacent macrophage cells were seen for either implant type. Both materials made bone contact with the surrounding cranial hard tissue, and the percentage of ingrowth increased with the surgical recovery time. The bone in contact with the implants was similar in quality to the surrounding cranial bone. Porous NiTi implants appear to allow for significant cranial bone ingrowth after as few as 12 weeks. Conclusion: Porous NiTi appears to be suitable for craniofacial applications.	[43]
Long crus of the incus and the incus of 24 ears of 12 cats/355 days	No	With the exception of pressure-induced bone erosions, there was no progressive bone resorption which was prosthesis-induced. The authors concluded that the biocompatibility of the nickel–titanium alloy stapes prosthesis with the long crus of the incus was satisfactory.	[44]
Paravertebral implantation in 4 rabbits/4 weeks		The blood Ni concentration after implantation reached twice the normal level in 6–9 h (28 ± 11 vs. 13 ± 5 ppb). After 4 weeks, the Ni concentration was 4-fold in the kidneys (140 ± 43 ppb), 2-fold in the liver (40 ± 18 ppb), and 10-fold in urine (90 ± 35 ppb). The authors concluded that Ni elution readily occurred, and suggested this may be prevented by surface coatings.	[45]
Six rabbit tibias/12 weeks	Vitallium, CP–Ti, Duplex austenitic-ferritic stainless steel (SAF), and 316 stainless steel	The biocompatibility results of NiTi screws compared with screws made of control metals showed a slower osteogenesis process characterized by **no close contacts between the implant and bone**, disorganized migration of osteoblasts around the implant, and a lower activity of osteonectin synthesis.	[46]

(Continued)

Table 5A.18 (Continued)
In Vivo Studies on Biocompatibility of NiTi Alloys with Animals

Animal Model/ Maximal Duration of Implantation	Control Materials	Major Results	Refs.
Medullary canal of 15 rat tibiae/168 days	Pure titanium, anodic oxidized titanium (AO-Ti), Ti–6Al–4V alloy and pure nickel	While NiTi and the other materials were progressively encapsulated with bone tissues, Ni was encapsulated with connective tissues and showed no bone contact through the 168-day experimental period. No significant differences between the tissue reactions to Ti, AO-Ti, and Ti–6Al–4V, but **NiTi implants showed a significantly lower percentage of bone contact and bone contact area than any of the other titanium or titanium alloy materials**. In terms of bone contact thickness, there were no significant differences between NiTi and the other three materials (Ti, AO-Ti, and Ti–6Al–4V).	[47]
12 adult white rabbits/2 years	No	The bioactivity and biocompatibility of NiTi alloy were significantly improved by coating the alloy with HA through chemical treatment. However, the untreated NiTi showed good biocompatibility after long term implantation.	[48]
6 rabbits/3 weeks	No	All six rabbits successfully completed the surgical distraction procedure. A continuity in the newly formed bone with similar transversal and horizontal dimensions as the original bone were observed in the gap between bone surfaces. Conclusion: the application of a constant force on distraction osteogenesis, using NiTi, may be a successful alternative to conventional gradual distraction.	[49]
Femur/tibia of New Zealand rabbits/15 weeks	No	New bone tissues adhere and grow well on the external surfaces as well as exposed areas on the inner pores of the NiTi scaffold.	[50]
Rabbits/20 weeks	No	The cell adherence and bone tissue inducing capability were respectively enhanced over 1.1–1.2 and 9–10 times by sputtering a uniform TiO_2 film on the surfaces of porous NiTi, compared with untreated NiTi.	[51]

Table 5A.19
In Vivo Trials of NiTi Implants in Humans

Applications	Number of Patients/ Implant Duration	Major Outcomes	Refs.
Clamps for the fixation of mandibular fractures	77 patients, 93 fractures using 124 clamps/6 weeks	In 72 patients the treatment progressed satisfactorily, while in five cases infections occurred. After removal of the clamps from 58 patients, there were no pathologic or atypical tissue reactions or signs of disturbed cell maturation. Conclusion: the application of NiTi for the surgical treatment of mandibular fractures facilitates treatment while ensuring stable fixation of the bone fragments.	[52]
Maxillofacial fractures		The surgical treatment of these fractures by NiTi devices ensured a good stability of the fracture surfaces, reduced the time needed for operative procedures and rehabilitation, and allowed rapid bone healing.	[53, 54]
Ventral intercorporeal lumbar spondylodesis	51 patients/9 months	In view of the easier operative technique, the earlier mobilization of the patients and the good fusion rate, the NiTi spondylodesis seems to have important advantages over the transplantation of bone chips.	[55]
Staple to lock a tricortical iliac bone graft in cervical anterior fusion was used	50 patients/7 weeks	Very good clinical results were reported in 80% of the cases, with rapid bone fusion rates.	[56]
The diseased cervical and lumbal spine were treated with anterior fusion and porous NiTi implant grafts	84 patients	Porous NiTi implants can be successfully used, probably because their mechanical properties were similar to those of the vertebral bodies, and the material itself showed a high degree of biocompatibility.	[57]

(Continued)

Table 5A.19 (Continued)
In Vivo Trials of NiTi Implants in Humans

Applications	Number of Patients/ Implant Duration	Major Outcomes	Refs.
Internal fixation of compression staple for hallux valgus	36 patients	The recovery period preceding return to light work averaged 19 days, and normal work and normal walking were resumed an average of 41 days postoperatively. All the osteotomies united, and the average angle of hallux valgus and the intermetatarsal angle improved. The distal fragment during the healing of the osteotomy was stable. No external fixation by plaster splintage was needed. The benefits of this internal fixator were that the period of bone healing was shortened and the patients were allowed to bear weight earlier than usual.	[58]
Fixation of small bone fragments with NiTi clamps	64 patients	Nonunion occurred in four patients treated with only one fixative. Two clamps implanted in nonparallel planes seem to be advisable to exclude the need for longer immobilization. Neither toxic manifestation nor episodes of allergic reaction occurred. The study suggests that by using NiTi clamps in an appropriate way, satisfactory outcomes could be achieved with respect to both biological functionality and biocompatibility.	[59]

Summary: So far, there have been no reports of tissue necrosis, granulomas, or signs of tissue dystrophy of calcification in vivo. The general immune response to nitinol has been found to remain low also during long term implantation. For muscular tissue, NiTi implants are nearly inert, with porous NiTi found to exhibit a thin, tightly adherent fibrous capsule with fibers penetrating into implant pores. In neural and perineural tissue, NiTi implants were also reported to be nontoxic and nonirritating after NiTi implantation. In relation to bone and related connective tissues, nitinol wire might be a very promising new tendon suture material because of high mechanical strength compared to the conventional materials. The biocompatibility of NiTi in tendon tissue is excellent. NiTi has no negative effect on new bone formation and bone contact to NiTi has been found to be very close, indicating good tissue tolerance. Osteotomy healing with porous NiTi has also been found to be good, with normal osteoclastic and osteoblastic activity. After long term implantation, no difference in nickel concentration between the NiTi and stainless steel groups has been found in any distant organs. The surface corrosion changes of retrieved NiTi implants were minimal.

Table 5A.20
Biocompatibility of Bare NiTi Wires as Stents and Closures (without Coating)

Number of Patients/Implant Duration	Major Outcomes	Refs.
Intravascular stents		
66 endovascular NiTi prostheses implanted in 36 dogs/14 months	Good and prolonged permeability of the NiTi prostheses.	[60]
	The endovascular prosthesis was wrapped by a thin layer of connective tissue, while inside it was lined with a layer of endothelial cells.	
12 intravascular NiTi stents implanted in the iliac and femoral arteries of 6 normal dogs/2 years	No migration, erosion, inflammation, surface thrombus, or stenosis of the side branches was seen. Nor were any histopathologic effects detected.	[61]
	Conclusion: The good biocompatibility manifested as a completely endothelialized, thin and stable neointima, satisfactory delivery and long-term patency at 2 years.	
44 NiTi intraluminal stents implanted in the iliac arteries of 22 sheep/6 months.	All but one stent remained widely patent during the follow-up period. Minimal corrosion was seen at 6 months, and the stent appeared to be biocompatible.	[6,22]
	Conclusion: A stent can be reliably and safely deployed in the vascular system.	
14 vascular stents in 14 dogs/9 months	No incompletely occluded aneurysms were visible after the implantation of NiTi stents. After 9 months, significantly more abundant intimal fibrocellular tissue growth surrounded the tantalum filaments than the NiTi filaments, which were covered with a smooth, thin neointimal layer.	[62]
	Conclusion: NiTi stents may become the treatment of choice for broad-based and fusiform aneurysms of the internal carotid artery.	
Iliac artery of 6 pigs	The early proliferative reaction of smooth muscle cells in the media of the iliac artery following percutaneous transluminal angioplasty [63] was compared with the reaction on the insertion of NiTi stents. The cell reaction appeared to be more pronounced after PTA than after the insertion of a self-expanding stent.	[64,65]

(Continued)

170

Table 5A.20 (Continued)
Biocompatibility of Bare NiTi Wires as Stents and Closures (without Coating)

Number of Patients/Implant Duration	Major Outcomes	Refs.
NiTi stents implanted in low flow velocity, vertebral arteries in 6 dogs/9 months	Five arteries remained patent without significant narrowing. The total mean thickness of the intima covering the stents showed no significant differences over time. The histologic findings on the stented vessels showed atrophic compression of the media, but intact endothelial cell linings without necrosis or perforation were observed. Conclusion: No significant risk of thromboembolic events exists after the implantation of NiTi stents in the vertebral arteries in dogs.	[66]
Eleven NiTi and 11 stainless steel stents implanted in 11 mature pigs	At 3 days, the stainless steel stents had more inflammatory cells adjacent to the stent wires than their NiTi counterparts. After 28 days, the vessel response was similar for the NiTi and stainless steel designs. The mean neointimal area and the percentage of stenosis were significantly lower in the NiTi than in the stainless steel group. Conclusion: A NiTi stent exerts a more favorable effect on vascular remodeling with less neointimal formation, than a balloon-expandable design. Progressive intrinsic stent expansion after the implantation does not appear to stimulate neointimal formation and may therefore prevent in-stent restenosis.	[67–69]
Nitinol stents implanted in carotid artery for up to 14 days in 8 rabbits	Nitinol stents showed less extensive vascular damage than stainess steel stents; stainless steel stents showed extensive thrombogenicity at histological level	[70]
22 self-expandable NiTi coil stents implanted in 16 dogs/1–2 weeks, 1–12 months	Angiographic artery dimensions measured immediately after stent implantation did not differ from those noted at follow-up. Outward stent pressure compressed the internal elastic membrane and the media in most cases. Intimal hyperplasia started at 2 weeks and was most apparent at 3 and 6 months. Conclusion: The NiTi self-expandable stent provoked a moderate cellular proliferative response that reached its maximum in 3–6 months without further progression.	[71]

(Continued)

Table 5A.20 (Continued)
Biocompatibility of Bare NiTi Wires as Stents and Closures (without Coating)

Number of Patients/Implant Duration	Major Outcomes	Refs.
27 NiTi wire devices implanted into the venae cavae of 16 dogs and 1 sheep/1 week to 4 years	All cleaned NiTi wire filters remained patent, but some showed venographic filling defects caused by adherent organized thrombi. The filters in larger veins tended to have less thrombus formation. Surface polishing and filter shape had no observable effect on thrombogenicity. Observation of patchy chronic inflammation on the surface of uncleaned filters, but only a benign fibrous tissue reaction on cleaned filters. Neointimal tissue overgrowth was observed in the contact area of the vena cava. Platelet adhesion and plasma coagulation effects of NiTi wire were tested in vitro in human blood and found to be similar to those of stainless steel. Conclusion: NiTi may be a promising material for human intravascular prosthetic applications.	[72]
Urethral stents		
18 urethral NiTi stents implanted in 18 dogs/1 week and 1, 3, 6, 12, and 18 months	Conclusion: Despite the excellent biocompatibility of the material with no evidence of foreign body reactions or corrosion, there were no complete incorporations of the stent by epithelialization. Clinical application therefore appears to be problematic.	[73]
Urethral stents implanted in 39 patients (human)/26 months	39 patients with benign prostatic hyperplasia had NiTi urethral stents implanted with a clinical success rate of 89%. Follow-up for 26 months showed no incrustation or migration of the spiral.	[74,75]
Closures		
Atrial septal defect closure device in 20 adult dogs/8 weeks	Percutaneous transcatheter closures were attempted using the new device. The closures were successful in 19 studies and unsuccessful in one. At 8 weeks, 3 dogs showed the devices to be covered by smooth endocardium enmeshed in mature collagen tissue, with minimal mononuclear cell infiltration. Conclusion: This new device permits effective and safe atrial septal defect closure in a canine model.	[76]
50 patients operated on with NiTi	No problems related to early migration and expulsion were observed, and no anastomotic leakage and bleeding occurred. Conclusions: Intestinal anastomosis with the NiTi was safe and feasible without anastomotic leakage and reoperation compared with the stapling technique.	[77]

Table 5A.21

Biocompatibility of Coated NiTi Stents Compared with Bare NiTi Stents

Number of Patients/Implant Duration	Major Outcomes	Refs.
Intravascular stents		
14 patients	Perivascular inflammation was seen in 79% of patients with polyester-covered NiTi stents. Clinical symptoms were seen in 57% of these patients. No reaction was evident among the controls with uncovered NiTi stents and the subjects who underwent peripheral percutaneous transluminal angioplasty. Conclusion: The polyester-covered NiTi stent may induce systemic and severe local reactions.	[78]
10 PTFE[a] (Dacron)-coated NiTi stents implanted in 10 patients/1 month	Clinical signs of acute inflammation manifested as fever and local tenderness. No inflammation was found in the control groups with bare NiTi stents.	[79]
Heparin-coated Dacron-covered NiTi stent-grafts in 4 sheep/6 months	Severe inflammatory perigraft responses, marked vascular wall thickening and adhesions around the Dacron fabric, and a pronounced inflammatory foreign-body response. There was almost no response to bare NiTi stents. Conclusion: The use of noncovered stents should thus be preferred to the use of Dacron-covered stent-grafts.	[80]
6 polyurethane-coated and 6 bare NiTi stents implanted in rabbit carotid arteries/4 weeks	At 4 weeks, all stent struts were endothelialized. Mild proliferative responses with some neovascularization around both stent types were seen. No differences in the degree of neointimal proliferation between the stents were found, but the polyurethane coating was associated with an inflammatory tissue response consisting of lymphocytic infiltration and foreign-body reaction and the appearance of multinucleated giant cells. Conclusion: A low biocompatibility of polyurethane, which may thus not be an ideal material for coating intravascular devices.	[81]

[a] *PET = polyethylene terephthalate.*

Table 5A.22

Outcomes of Orthopedic and Orthodontic Applications of NiTi Alloys

Animal Models	Major Outcomes	Refs.
Correction rods of scoliosis The functional principle of the NiTi memory wire was demonstrated in an experiment carried out on *a plastic model*.	NiTi wire prestretched by 7% was led through eyelets on the convex side and fixed at the ends. On being heated, the wire shortened, righting the model so that it assumed a straight shape.	[82]
26 patients	Correction was reported to be good and there were no complications.	[8]
1 scoliosis monkey/4 weeks	The blood Ni concentration after implantation of the NiTi alloy rod reached twice the normal level after 6–9 h. After 4 weeks, the Ni concentration increased 4-fold in the kidneys, 2-fold in the liver, and 10-fold in the urine. Scoliosis with a Cobb angle of 43° was completely corrected.	[45]
6 goats with experimental scoliosis were implanted with 6-mm nitinol rods	The rods were transformed, and the scoliosis corrected, in the awakened goats by 450 kHz radio frequency induction heating. The curves averaged 41° before instrumentation, 33° after instrumentation, and 11° after rod transformation. The animals tolerated the heating without discomfort, neurologic injury, or evidence of thermal injury to the tissues or the spinal cord. The use of shape-memory alloys allows continuous true rotational correction by rod torsion.	[83]
6 pigs/3 and 6 months	The induced curve of about 40° Cobb angle remained constant during the follow-up. The postoperative serum nickel measurements were around the detection limit, and were not significantly higher compared to the preoperative nickel concentration. The device was almost overgrown with newly formed bone. Corrosion and fretting processes were not observed. No evidence of a foreign body response in the lungs, liver, spleen, and kidneys.	[84]

(Continued)

Table 5A.22 (Continued)

Outcomes of Orthopedic and Orthodontic Applications of NiTi Alloys

Animal Models	Major Outcomes	Refs.
38 scoliosis patients (ranging from 50° to 120°; 22 cases over 70°) who underwent NiTi-assisted correction/4 months	The major Cobb angle improved from an average 78.4° preoperatively to 24.3° postoperatively (total percent correction 71.4%). In 16 patients with a major curve <70° and flexibility of 52.7%, the deformity improved from 58.4° preoperatively to 12.3° postoperatively (percent correction, 78.9%). In 22 patients with a major curve >70° and flexibility of 25.6%, the deformity improved from 94.1° preoperatively to 30.1° postoperatively (percent correction, 68.1%). Only one case had a deep infection. There were no neurologic, vascular, or correction-related complications such as screw pullout or metal fracture. The study showed that the intraoperative use of a NiTi rod was a safe and effective method to correct scoliosis.	[9]
Compressive staples, clamps, or clips 133 NiTi clips were applied in 119 patients/2–8 years	No procedural complication or adverse reaction to the clip was noted. There was no movement at the operated level in the dynamic lateral view x-ray of the cervical spine at the first postoperative day as well as on follow-up. Graft extrusion was seen in one patient on the second day after surgery and was reoperated. Bony fusion occurred in all patients after 9–12 months of surgery. There was no incidence of breakage or dislodgement of the clip from the site where it was inserted. Conclusion: NiTi clips proved a simple alternative for cervical spine stabilization after discoidectomy. Their insertion was simple, minimally invasive, did not require any special set of instruments and they were much more economical than other established methods of treatment. These clips were accepted well by human tissue and did not interfere with MRI.	[63,85]

SIMPLE QUESTIONS IN CLASS

1. Which of following properties is a persisting issue in tooth filling material?
   a. Poor wear resistance
   b. High toxicity
   c. Unsatisfactory shrinkage
   d. Brittleness

2. Which of following mechanisms is responsible for the shape memory of TiNi alloys?
   a. Diffusive phase transformation
   b. Any diffusionless phase transformation
   c. Reversible diffusive phase transformation
   d. Reversible diffusionless phase transformation
3. Which of following mechanisms is the working principle of self-expandable stents?
   a. Reversible elastic deformation
   b. One-way memory
   c. Two-way memory
   d. Reversible superstretchability
4. NiTi is NOT applied to which of following applications?
   a. Vascular stent
   b. Orthopedic implants
   c. Tooth archwires
   d. Surgical clips
5. Which of following materials is used for tooth fillings?
   a. Gold
   b. Amalgam
   c. Ti alloys
   d. Pure silver
6. Which of following materials is used for tooth prosthesis?
   a. Amalgam
   b. Stainless steels
   c. Gold
   d. Mg alloys
7. Which of following materials is used for tooth root implants?
   a. Gold
   b. Amalgam
   c. Ti alloys
   d. Silver
8. Which of the following statements about Mg and its alloys is incorrect?
   a. Magnesium is a micro (trace) element of the body.
   b. Magnesium is a macroelement of the body and can thus be used at a high amount.
   c. Magnesium is a macroelement of the body and can be used at a relatively high amount with caution.
   d. Mg alloys are not recommended for patients with renal dysfunction.

PROBLEMS AND EXERCISES

1. What is restorative dentistry? List five vastly different dental materials (not slightly different in composition) used as dental implants.
2. In addition to biocompatibility, what are the other important requirements of tooth filling biomaterials? Explain your answers. What is the common issue of tooth fillings?
3. Among all metallic biomaterials, which alloy system is the best choice for the implantation of a tooth root? Explain your answer.

4. Hg is used in amalgam primarily because of its low melting point. The toxicity of liquid Hg is well documented. Based on the Pourbaix diagram of Hg, discuss the safety to use Hg alloys in the body.

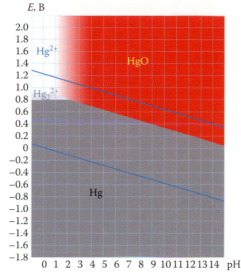

5. How is *thermodynamically reversible* defined? Ice melts to water, and the water is then frozen into ice again. Is this cycle a thermodynamic reversing process?

6. If an austenite iron (γ-Fe) alloy is cooled rapidly to room temperature, it can transform to the α-Fe structure without involving diffusion; that is, the transformation from γ to α phase can be displacive. Explain, using the following phase diagram, why this displacive phase transformation is irreversible.

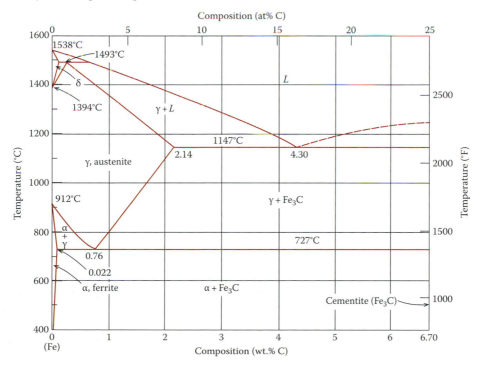

7. In NiTi alloy, the phase transformation that is responsible for its shape-memory alloys is between B2 (CsCl structure) and B19′ phases, which occurs around room temperature, as shown in the following phase diagram. Explain, using the following phase diagram, why the displacive phase transformation (B2→ B19′) is reversible.

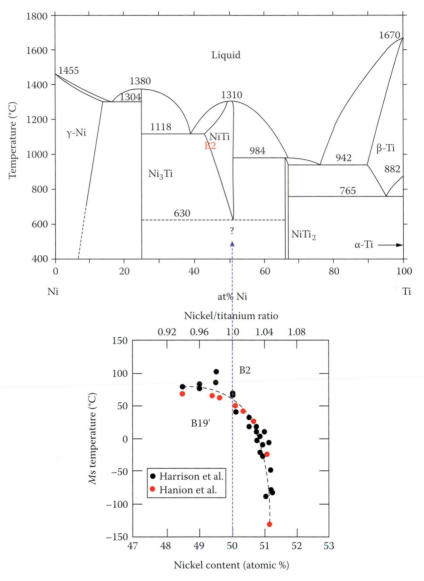

8. Explain why one-way shape-memory alloys cannot remember the shape at a low temperature, and how two-way shape-memory alloys remember the shapes at both low and high temperatures.

9. Using the data provided in Table 5.11, rationalize why magnesium and its alloys have a potential to be used in orthopedic implants. Discuss the advantages of Mg and its alloys and the issues and challenges associated with potential medical implants made from Mg and its alloys.

10. Assume a rod-shaped implant (2 cm in diameter and 10 cm in length) made from AZ31 magnesium alloy is placed in the body. Estimate, based on the corrosion rates provided in Table 5.13, the amount of materials released into the body each day. Compared with the data in Table 5.14, is the implant safe to use? Explain your answer.

BIBLIOGRAPHY

References for Text

1. Davies, J.R. (ed.), Chapter 10 Biomaterials for dental applications. In *Handbook of Materials for Medical Devices*, Materials Park, OH: ASM International, 2003.
2. Kusy, R.P., Orthodontic biomaterials: From the past to the present. *Angle Orthodontist*, 2002;**72**(6):501–512.
3. Craig, R.G. and J.M. Powers, *Restorative Dental Materials*, 11th edn. St. Louis, MO: Mosby Inc. (an affiliate of Elsevier Science), 2002.
4. Ryhanen, J., Biocompatibilty evaluation of nickel-titanium shape memory metal alloy, PhD thesis, Oulu, Finland: Oulu University Library, 1999.
5. Castleman, L.S. et al., Biocompatibility of nitinol alloy as an implant material. *Journal of Biomedical Materials Research*, 1976;**10**(5):695–731.
6. Cragg, A. et al., Non-surgical placement of arterial endoprostheses—A new technique using nitinol wire. *Radiology*, 1983;**147**(1):261–263.
7. Niinomi, M., Fatigue characteristics of metallic biomaterials. *International Journal of Fatigue*, 2007;**29**(6):992–1000.
8. Lu, S.B., J.F. Wang, and J.F. Guo, Treatment of scoliosis with a shape-memory alloy rod. *Chinese Journal of Surgery*, 1986;**24**(3):129–187.
9. Wang, Y. et al., Temporary use of shape memory spinal rod in the treatment of scoliosis. *European Spine Journal*, 2011;**20**(1):118–122.
10. Ritchie, P.K. and E.C. McCarty, Metal and plastic suture anchors for rotator cuff repair. *Operative Techniques in Sports Medicine*, 2004;**12**(4):215–220.
11. Salahshoor, M. and Y.B. Guo, Biodegradable orthopedic magnesium-calcium (MgCa) alloys, processing, and corrosion performance. *Materials & Design*, 2012;**5**:135–155.
12. Zberg, B., P.J. Uggowitzer, and J.F. Loeffler, MgZnCa glasses without clinically observable hydrogen evolution for biodegradable implants. *Nature Materials*, 2009;**8**(11):887–891.
13. Gu, X.N. and Y.F. Zheng, A review on magnesium alloys as biodegradable materials. *Frontiers of Materials Science in China*, 2010;**4**(2):111–115.

Websites

http://global.smithnephew.com/us/patients/OXINIUM.htm.
http://www.ada.org/(American Dental Association).
http://www.ceessentials.net/article12.html.
http://www.whichmedicaldevice.com/editorial/article/104/a-brief-history-of-inferior-vena-cava-filters-and-analysis-of-current-devices.

References for Appendix

1. Davies, J.R. (ed.), Biomaterials for dental applications. In *Handbook of Materials for Medical Devices*. Materials Park, OH: ASM International, 2003.
2. Kusy, R.P., Orthodontic biomaterials: From the past to the present. *Angle Orthodontist*, 2002;**72**(6):501–512.

3. Craig, R.G. and J.M. Powers, *Restorative Dental Materials*, 11th edn. St. Louis, MO: Mosby Inc. (an affiliate of Elsevier Science), 2002.

4. Ryhänen, J., Biocompatibilty evaluation of nickel-titanium shape memory metal alloy, PhD thesis, Oulu, Finland: Oulu University Library, 1999.

5. Castleman, L.S. et al., Biocompatibility of nitinol alloy as an implant material. *Journal of Biomedical Materials Research*, 1976;**10**(5):695–731.

6. Cragg, A. et al., Non-surgical placement of arterial endoprostheses - a new technique using nitinol wire. *Radiology*, 1983;**147**(1):261–263.

7. Niinomi, M., Fatigue characteristics of metallic biomaterials. *International Journal of Fatigue*, 2007;**29**(6):992–1000.

8. Lu, S.B., J.F. Wang, and J.F. Guo, Treatment of scoliosis with a shape-memory alloy rod. *Zhonghua wai ke za zhi [Chinese Journal of Surgery]*, 1986;**24**(3):129–187.

9. Wang, Y. et al., Temporary use of shape memory spinal rod in the treatment of scoliosis. *European Spine Journal*, 2011;**20**(1):118–122.

10. Ritchie, P.K. and E.C. McCarty, Metal and plastic suture anchors for rotator cuff repair. *Operative Techniques in Sports Medicine*, 2004;**12**(4):215–220.

11. Salahshoor, M. and Y.B. Guo, Biodegradable orthopedic magnesium-calcium (MgCa) alloys, processing, and corrosion performance. *Materials & Design*, 2012;**5**:135–155.

12. Zberg, B., P.J. Uggowitzer, and J.F. Loeffler, MgZnCa glasses without clinically observable hydrogen evolution for biodegradable implants. *Nature Materials*, 2009;**8**(11):887–891.

13. Gu, X.N. and Y.F. Zheng, A review on magnesium alloys as biodegradable materials. *Frontiers of Materials Science in China*, 2010;**4**(2):111–115.

14. Speck, K.M. and A.C. Fraker, Anodic polarization behavior of Ti-Ni and Ti-6A1-4V in simulated physiological solutions. *Journal of Dental Research*, 1980;**59**(10):1590–1595.

15. Sarkar, N.K. et al., The chloride corrosion behavior of 4 orthodontic wires. *Journal of Oral Rehabilitation*, 1983;**10**(2):121–128.

16. Wever, D.J. et al., Electrochemical and surface characterization of a nickel-titanium alloy. *Biomaterials*, 1998;**19**(7–9):761–769.

17. Platt, J.A. et al., Corrosion behavior of 2205 duplex stainless steel. *American Journal of Orthodontics and Dentofacial Orthopedics*, 1997;**112**(1):69–79.

18. Edie, J.W., G.F. Andreasen, and M.P. Zaytoun, Surface corrosion of nitinol and stainless-steel under clinical conditions. *Angle Orthodontist*, 1981;**51**(4):319–324.

19. Barrett, R.D., S.E. Bishara, and J.K. Quinn, Biodegradation of orthodontic appliances.1. Biodegradation of nickel and chromium in vitro. *American Journal of Orthodontics and Dentofacial Orthopedics*, 1993;**103**(1):8–14.

20. Rondelli, G., Corrosion resistance tests on NiTi shape memory alloy. *Biomaterials*, 1996;**17**(20):2003–2008.

21. MonteroOcampo, C., H. Lopez, and A.S. Rodriguez, Effect of compressive straining on corrosion resistance of a shape memory Ni-Ti alloy in ringer's solution. *Journal of Biomedical Materials Research*, 1996;**32**(4):583–591.

22. Cragg, A.H. et al., Nitinol intravascular stent - results of preclinical evaluation. *Radiology*, 1993;**189**(3):775–778.

23. Castleman, L.S. and S.M. Motzkin, The biocompatibility of Nitinol. In *Biocompatibility of Clinical Implant Materials*, D.F. Williams, ed. Boca Raton, FL: CRC Press, Inc., 1981, pp. 129–154.

24. Putters, J.L.M. et al., Comparative cell-culture effects of shape memory metal (nitinol(r)), nickel and titanium—A biocompatibility estimation. *European Surgical Research*, 1992;**24**(6):378–382.

25. Assad, M. et al., Cytotoxity testing of the nickel-titanium shape-memory alloy. *Annales De Chirurgie*, 1994;**48**(8):731–736.

26. Endo, K., Chemical modification of metallic implant surfaces with biofunctional proteins (Part 1). Molecular structure and biological activity of a modified NiTi alloy surface. *Dental Materials Journal*, 1995;**14**(2):185–198.

27. Endo, K., Chemical modification of metallic implant surfaces with biofunctional proteins (Part 2). Corrosion resistance of a chemically modified NiTi alloy. *Dental Materials Journal*, 1995;**14**(2):199–210.

28. Shabalovskaya, S.A., On the nature of the biocompatibility and on medical applications of NiTi shape memory and superelastic alloys. *Bio-Medical Materials and Engineering*, 1996;**6**(4):267–289.

29. Wever, D.J. et al., Cytotoxic, allergic and genotoxic activity of a nickel-titanium alloy. *Biomaterials*, 1997;**18**(16):1115–1120.

30. Assad, M. et al., In vitro biocompatibility assessment of a nickel-titanium alloy using electron microscopy in situ end-labeling (EM-ISEL). *Journal of Biomedical Materials Research*, 1998;**41**(1):154–161.

31. Rose, E.C., I.E. Jonas, and H.F. Kappert, In vitro investigation into the biological assessment of orthodontic wires. *Journal of Orofacial Orthopedics = Fortschritte der Kieferorthopadie: Organ/Official Journal Deutsche Gesellschaft fur Kieferorthopadie*, 1998;**59**(5):253–264.

32. Nie, F.L. et al., In vitro corrosion and cytotoxicity on microcrystalline, nanocrystalline and amorphous NiTi alloy fabricated by high pressure torsion. *Materials Letters*, 2010;**64**(8):983–986.

33. Bogdanski, D. et al., Rapid analysis of biocompatibility with graded test samples exemplified by Ni-NiTi-Ti. Biomedizinische Technik. *Biomedical Engineering*, 2002;**47**(Suppl 1 Pt 1):500–502.

34. Kapanen, A. et al., Behaviour of Nitinol in osteoblast-like ROS-17 cell cultures. *Biomaterials*, 2002;**23**(3):645–650.

35. Yeung, K.W.K. et al., Corrosion resistance, surface mechanical properties, and cytocompatibility of plasma immersion ion implantation-treated nickel-titanium shape memory alloys. *Journal of Biomedical Materials Research Part A*, 2005;**75A**(2):256–267.

36. Yeung, K.W.K. et al., Investigation of nickel suppression and cytocompatibility of surface-treated nickel-titanium shape memory alloys by using plasma immersion ion implantation. *Journal of Biomedical Materials Research Part A*, 2005;**72A**(3):238–245.

37. Yeung, K.W.K. et al., Nitrogen plasma-implanted nickel titanium alloys for orthopedic use. *Surface & Coatings Technology*, 2007;**201**(9–11):5607–5612.

38. Michiardi, A. et al., Oxidized NiTi surfaces enhance differentiation of osteoblast-like cells. *Journal of Biomedical Materials Research Part A*, 2008;**85A**(1):108–114.

39. Liu, X.M. et al., Nano-scale surface morphology, wettability and osteoblast adhesion on nitrogen plasma-implanted NiTi shape memory alloy. *Journal of Nanoscience and Nanotechnology*, 2009;**9**(6):3449–3454.

40. Cutright, D.E. et al., Tissue reaction to nitinol wire alloy. *Oral Surgery Oral Medicine Oral Pathology Oral Radiology and Endodontics*, 1973;**35**(4):578–584.

41. Wen, X.J. et al., Electrochemical and histomorphometric evaluation of the TiNiCu shape memory alloy. *Bio-Medical Materials and Engineering*, 1997;**7**(1):1–11.

42. Yang, P.J. et al., Ni-Ti memory alloy clamp plate for fracture of short tubular bone. *Chinese Medical Journal*, 1992;**105**(4):312–315.

43. Simske, S.J. and R. Sachdeva, Cranial bone apposition and ingrowth in a porous nickel-titanium implant. *Journal of Biomedical Materials Research*, 1995;**29**(4):527–533.

44. Kasano, F. and T. Morimitsu, Utilization of nickel-titanium shape memory alloy for stapes prosthesis. *Auris, Nasus, Larynx*, 1997;**24**(2):137–142.

45. Matsumoto, K., N. Tajima, and S. Kuwahara, Correction of scoliosis with shape-memory alloy. *Nihon Seikeigeka Gakkai zasshi*, 1993;**67**(4):267–274.

46. BergerGorbet, M. et al., Biocompatibility testing of NiTi screws using immunohistochemistry on sections containing metallic implants. *Journal of Biomedical Materials Research*, 1996;**32**(2):243–248.

47. Takeshita, F. et al., Histomorphometric analysis of the response of rat tibiae to shape memory alloy (nitinol). *Biomaterials*, 1997;**18**(1):21–25.

48. Li, C.Y. et al., In vivo histological evaluation of bioactive NiTi alloy after two years implantation. *Materials Science and Engineering C-Biomimetic and Supramolecular Systems*, 2007;**27**(1):122–126.

49. Idelsohn, S. et al., Continuous mandibular distraction osteogenesis using superelastic shape memory alloy (SMA). *Journal of Materials Science—Materials in Medicine*, 2004;**15**(4):541–546.

50. Liu, X. et al., Relationship between osseointegration and superelastic biomechanics in porous NiTi scaffolds. *Biomaterials*, 2011;**32**(2):330–338.

51. Yuan, B. et al., In vitro and in vivo evaluation of porous NiTi alloy modified by sputtering a surface TiO$_2$ film. *Science China-Technological Sciences*, 2012;**55**(2):437–444.

52. Drugacz, J. et al., Use of tinico shape-memory clamps in the surgical-treatment of mandibular fractures. *Journal of Oral and Maxillofacial Surgery*, 1995;**53**(6):665–671.

53. Sysolyatin, P.G. et al. The use of Ni-Ti implants in maxillofacial surgery. In *Shape Memory and Superelastic Technologies, Proceedings of SMST-94, SMST*, Pacific Grove, CA, 1994.

54. Itro, A. et al., Experience with a rigid fixation device in maxillofacial surgery using shape-memory clips. *Minerva Stomatologica*, 1997;**46**(7–8):381–389.

55. Vonsalissoglio, G.F., Memory-spondylodesis in the lumbar spine - results after 76 operations. *Zeitschrift Fur Orthopadie Und Ihre Grenzgebiete*, 1989;**127**(2):191–196.

56. Ricart, O. The use of memory shape staple in cervical anterior fusion. In *Shape Memory and Superelastic Technologies, Proceedings of SMST -97, SMST*, Pacific Grove, CA, 1997.

57. Silberstein, B. Subtotal and total vertebral body replacement and interbody fusion with porous Ti-Ni implants. In *Shape Memory and Superelastic Technologies, Proceedings of SMST-97, SMST*, Pacific Grove, CA, 1997.

58. Tang, R.G., K.R. Dai, and Y.Q. Chen, Application of a NiTi staple in the metatarsal osteotomy. *Bio-Medical Materials and Engineering*, 1996;**6**(4):307–312.

59. Musialek, J., P. Filip, and J. Nieslanik, Titanium-nickel shape memory clamps in small bone surgery. *Archives of Orthopaedic and Trauma Surgery*, 1998;**117**(6–7):341–344.

60. Rabkin, D.I. et al., Experimental-morphological study of the Roentgeno-endovascular prosthesis. *Meditsinskaia Radiologiia*, 1986;**31**(10):55–63.

61. Sutton, C.S. et al., Titanium-nickel intravascular endoprosthesis—A 2-year study in dogs. *American Journal of Roentgenology*, 1988;**151**(3):597–601.

62. Wakhloo, A.K. et al., Self-expanding and balloon-expandable stents in the treatment of carotid aneurysms—An experimental-study in a canine model. *American Journal of Neuroradiology*, 1994;**15**(3):493–502.

63. Singh, D. et al., Use of nitinol shape memory alloy staples (NiTi clips) after cervical discoidectomy: Minimally invasive instrumentation and long-term results. *Minimally Invasive Neurosurgery*, 2011;**54**(4):172–178.

64. Cwikiel, W. et al., Self-expanding stent in the treatment of benign esophageal strictures—Experimental-study in pigs and presentation of clinical cases. *Radiology*, 1993;**187**(3):667–671.

65. Cwikiel, W. et al., Proliferative response in smooth muscle cells after angioplasty or insertion of self-expanding stents—An experimental study in pigs. *Acta Radiologica*, 1997;**38**(1):124–128.

66. Wakhloo, A.K. et al., Self-expanding nitinol stents in canine vertebral arteries—Hemodynamics and tissue-response. *American Journal of Neuroradiology*, 1995;**16**(5):1043–1051.

67. Carter, A.J. and T.A. Fischell, Current status of radioactive stents for the prevention of in-stent restenosis. *International Journal of Radiation Oncology Biology Physics*, 1998;**41**(1):127–133.

68. Carter, A.J. et al., Vascular remodeling and neointimal formation depend on stent design and strut geometry in small diameter coronary arteries. *Circulation*, 1998;**98**(17):189–189.

69. Carter, A.J. et al., Progressive vascular remodeling and reduced neointimal formation after placement of a thermoelastic self-expanding nitinol stent in an experimental model. *Catheterization and Cardiovascular Diagnosis*, 1998;**44**(2):193–201.

70. Sheth, S. et al., Subacute thrombosis and vascular injury resulting from slotted-tube nitinol and stainless steel stents in a rabbit carotid artery model. *Circulation*, 1996;**94**(7):1733–1740.
71. Grenadier, E. et al., Self-expandable and highly flexible nitinol stent—Immediate and long-term results in dogs. *American Heart Journal*, 1994;**128**(5):870–878.
72. Prince, M.R. et al., Local intravascular effects of the nitinol wire blood-clot filter. *Investigative Radiology*, 1988;**23**(4):294–300.
73. Latal, D. et al., Nitinol urethral stents - long-term results in dogs. *Urological Research*, 1994;**22**(5):295–300.
74. Qiu, C.Y., Shape memory alloy spiral for urethrostenosis caused by benign prostatic hyperplasia. *Zhonghua wai ke za zhi [Chinese journal of surgery]*, 1993;**31**(5):272–274.
75. Qiu, C.Y. et al., Stent of shape-memory alloy for urethral obstruction caused by benign prostatic hyperplasia. *Journal of Endourology*, 1994;**8**(1):65–67.
76. Das, G.S. et al., Experimental atrial septal-defect closure with a new, transcatheter, self-centering device. *Circulation*, 1993;**88**(4):1754–1764.
77. Kim, H.R. et al., Early surgical outcomes of NiTi endoluminal compression anastomotic clip (NiTi CAC 30) use in patients with gastrointestinal malignancy. *Journal of Laparoendoscopic & Advanced Surgical Techniques*, 2012;**22**(5):472–478.
78. Kellner, W. et al., MR imaging of soft-tissue changes after percutaneous transluminal angioplasty and stent placement. *Radiology*, 1997;**202**(2):327–331.
79. Hayoz, D. et al., Acute inflammatory reaction associated with endoluminal bypass grafts. *Journal of Endovascular Surgery*, 1997;**4**(4):354–360.
80. Schurmann, K. et al., Perigraft inflammation due to Dacron-covered stent-grafts in sheep iliac arteries: Correlation of MR imaging and histopathologic findings. *Radiology*, 1997;**204**(3):757–763.
81. Rechavia, E. et al., Biocompatibility of polyurethane-coated stents: Tissue and vascular aspects. *Catheterization and Cardiovascular Diagnosis*, 1998;**45**(2):202–207.
82. Baumgart, F. et al., Dwyers scoliosis operation using memory alloy wire. *Archives of Orthopaedic and Trauma Surgery*, 1978;**91**(1):67–75.
83. Sanders, J.O. et al., A preliminary investigation of shape-memory alloys in the surgical-correction of scoliosis. *Spine*, 1993;**18**(12):1640–1646.
84. Wever, D.J. et al., Scoliosis correction with shape-memory metal: Results of an experimental study. *European Spine Journal*, 2002;**11**(2):100–106.
85. Dai, K.R., Orthopedic application of a Ni-Ti shape-memory alloy compression staple. *Zhonghua wai ke za zhi [Chinese Journal of Surgery]*, 1983;**21**(6):343–345.

Further Readings

Avedesian, M.M. (ed). Section: Properties of unalloyed magnesium. In *Magnesium and Magnesium Alloys*. Materials Park, OH: ASM International, 1999.
Craig, R.G. and J.M. Powers (eds.), *Restorative Dental Materials*, 11th edn. St. Louis, MO: Mosby Inc (an affiliate of Elsevier Science), 2002.
Davies, J.R. (ed.), *Handbook of Materials for Medical Devices*. Materials Park, OH: ASM International, 2003.
Otsuka, K. and C.M. Waymen (eds.), Chapter 2 Mechanism of shape memory effect and super-elasticity, Chapter 3 Ti-Ni shape memory alloys, and Chapter 12 Medical and dental applications of shape memory alloys. In *Shape Memory Materials*. Cambridge, U.K.: Cambridge University Press, 1998.

CHAPTER 6

BIOINERT CERAMICS

LEARNING OBJECTIVES

After a careful study of this chapter, you should be able to do the following:

1. Describe three generations of biomaterials.
2. Discuss the sensitivity of ceramics to stress concentration.
3. Describe two types of joints.
4. Select proper materials for various artificial joints.
5. Describe the application principles of bioceramics of the first generation.

6.1 OVERVIEW OF BIOCERAMICS

6.1.1 Classification of Bioceramics

Ceramics encompass any inorganic, nonmetallic solids. This category of materials can be further divided in a number of ways. Based on the level of crystallinity, for example, the three subgroups include ceramics (crystalline inorganic, nonmetal materials), glasses (amorphous inorganic, nonmetal materials), and glass-ceramics (partially crystalline inorganic, nonmetal materials). In industry, ceramics are often classified according to their applications, as listed here:

- Structural clay products, including bricks, pipes, and floor and roof tiles.
- Refractories, such as furnace linings, crucibles to contain steel and glass melts, and gas fire radiants.
- Whitewares, including tableware, cookware, wall tiles, pottery products, and sanitary ware.
- Abrasives, such as SiC powders.
- Cements and plaster.
- Porcelain enamel.
- Technical ceramics, such as semiconductors, structural ceramics, and biomedical implant ceramics. The raw materials of technical ceramics do not include clays, and thus this type of ceramics is often called fine ceramics.

Bioceramics are also classified as technical ceramics. The successful use of bioceramics inside the human body as implants is relatively new, compared with metal materials. Bioceramics are frequently classified according to their biological reactivity in the body, according to the following groups:

- *Biological near-inert ceramics* (e.g., Al_2O_3 and ZrO_2). The formation of a nonadherent fibrous capsule is the most common response of tissue to an implant made from these materials. The tissue attempts to reject the implant by essentially creating a barrier around it.
- *Surface bioactive ceramics* (e.g., crystalline hydroxyapatite and calcium phosphate). A bond forms across the interface between implant and the tissue. The interfacial bond prevents motion between the two surfaces and mimics the type of interface that forms when tissues undergo self-repair.
- *Biodegradable ceramics* (e.g., glasses SiO_2-CaO-P_2O_5-Na_2O). The implant material is dissolved and absorbed by the surrounding tissues (i.e. is resorbable).

In general, the aforementioned bioceramics have low toxicity. Inert and near-inert ceramics (e.g., Al_2O_3) have excellent corrosion resistance due to almost no ion release. Bioactive hydroxyapatite and related calcium phosphates closely resemble bone minerals in terms of chemical composition. Bioresorbable glasses (e.g., SiO_2-CaO-P_2O_3-Na_2O) are biocompatible because they are composed of ions commonly found in the physiological environment (Ca^{2+}, K^+, Na^+, etc.). Except for silicon, which is a trace element, these elements are macroelements of the body, rather than trace elements. For detailed description on the toxicity of bioactive ceramics, the reader can refer to Chapter 7.

6.1.2 Three Generations of Bioceramics

The concept of three generations of biomaterials actually emerged from the development of bioceramics, which were later found to represent a process of development common to all biomaterial types. Table 6.1 summarizes the three generations of all biomaterials.

Table 6.1
Three Generations of Biomaterials

Generation	Biodegradability	Clinical Requirements	Examples
First	Biologically inert	No harm to tissues	Al_2O_3 CoCr alloys UHMWPE
Second	Surface erosion	Tissue-bonding	Hydroxylapatite Calcium phosphate Titanium alloys Surface bioactive glasses
Third	Biodegradation	Tissue regeneration	Magnesium alloys Degradable Bioglass® Degradable polymers

6.1.3 Mechanical Sensitivity of Ceramics to Stress Concentration

In day-to-day life, we often apply the stress concentration effect to open a food bag (Figure 6.1a), almost without an awareness of the mechanical principle behind the application. A small V-shaped crack on the edge of a plastic bag allows us to open it easily, which otherwise we might not be strong enough to open manually. Workers of glass manufacturers also use the stress concentration effect to cut glass (Figure 6.1b). The working principle behind these applications is that the *opening* (i.e., tensile) stress we apply is amplified tens or hundreds of times at the tip of a tiny crack.

However, the useful stress concentration effect in the food packaging industry is undesirable in the applications of structural materials, especially ceramics. A force that is not damaging when it is applied homogenously on a glass window could break the same window when it is focused on a point (Figure 6.2).

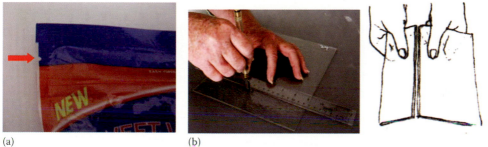

(a) (b)

Figure 6.1
Applications of the stress concentration effect. (a) V-shaped cracks of food bags. (b) Cutting of glass.

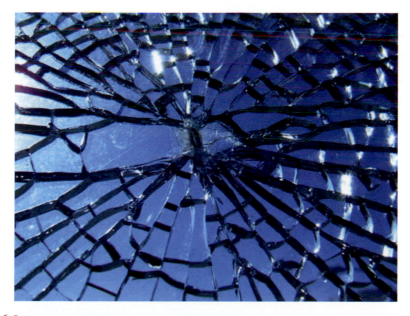

Figure 6.2
A piece of glass cracked by a concentrated force shock.

As depicted in Chapter 1, the brittleness of ceramics is due to the fact that their covalent or ionic bonds lack tolerance of deformation in their lattice structures. Structural imperfections are the preferential sites of deformation due to the stress concentration effect. Hence, the mechanical performance of ceramics is highly sensitive to defects. As a matter of fact, the fracture of ceramics is always initiated by the unavoidable microscopic flaws (microcracks and micropores) that result during cooling after the melt, with particular sensitivity to surface defects. The concentrated stresses (i.e., deformation) around these flaws lead to the breakage of chemical bonds, which propagate as linear cracks, usually along crystal planes. Unfortunately, the microscopic flaws cannot be eliminated in manufacturing, and their location, either within the material or on its surface, is of random nature; this leads to a large variability (scatter) in the fracture strength of ceramic materials. The compressive strength is typically 10 times the tensile strength. This makes ceramics good structural materials under compressive loads (e.g., bricks in houses, stone blocks in the pyramids), but not in conditions of tensile stress, such as under flexure.

In summary, the mechanical performance of ceramics is highly sensitive to the stress concentration effect, and thus to the presence of material imperfections. As a general rule, ceramics cannot be used where tensile, bending, or concentrated stresses occur. They are typically used at compressive load-bearing sites where the stresses are homogenously distributed across the bulk material.

6.2   INERT BIOCERAMICS: Al_2O_3

6.2.1   Corrosion Resistance and Biocompatibility

It is widely known that the good corrosion resistance of aluminum is due to the formation of a thin film of aluminum oxide or alumina (Al_2O_3), which is dense and chemically stable. In fact, Al_2O_3 as a material has excellent corrosion resistance. The inertness of Al_2O_3 makes it very biocompatible, having almost no chemical impact on the body.

The human body has a useful defense system that can recognize and remove both macro- and microscopic foreign bodies. In the case of microscopic particles, specialized cells will engulf and digest them. For larger materials, such as a splinter, the surrounding tissue will form a fibrous tissue barrier around the object. This isolates the material, preventing surface release from the material, or reaction with the tissue. It also prevents further biological reactions such as immune reactions, allergic responses, or sepsis. Ultimately, the splinter is removed, assisted by the growth of new tissue. Using the same mechanisms, the formation of a nonadherent fibrous capsule (Figure 6.3) is the most common response of tissue to an inert implant material like Al_2O_3.

6.2.2   Mechanical Properties

Highly dense, highly pure Al_2O_3 bulk materials also have high wear resistance and high strength. The International Organisation for Standards (ISO) describes the required physical properties for alumina. Alumina implants that meet or exceed ISO standards have excellent resistance to fatigue, and resist subcritical crack growth and implant failure. It is essential that Al_2O_3 implants be produced with the highest standards of quality assurance.

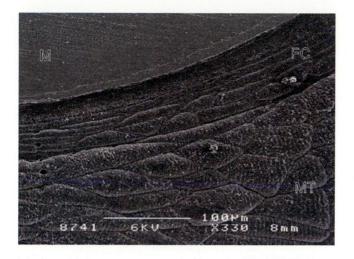

Figure 6.3
Electron micrograph of a nonadhesive fibrous capsule (FC) formed between muscular tissue (MT) and a bioinert material (M). (Reprinted from Biomaterials, 20, Ryhänen, J. et al., 1309–1317, 2014, Copyright 1999, with permission from Elsevier.)

6.2.3   Medical Applications of Al_2O_3

The main problem with the total hip replacement system is loosening of the acetabular component (Figure 6.4), which is caused by wearing between the two load-bearing surfaces. The major application of alumina is as the head, with the stem made from stainless steel (Orthinox), Ti alloy or CoCr alloys, the line is made from ultrahigh-molecular-weight polyethylene (UHMWPE) and the cup is made from a Ti alloy (Figure 6.5). The Ti cup protects, through bone bonding, the host bone from wearing damage. The line, which is fixed with the cup, protects the cup from wearing damage. Overall, the head-on-line is designed to have good wearing resistance and reduced pain.

Back in the 1960s, the head and stem were predominately made from stainless steels in one piece (Figure 4.5a). With the development of ceramics Al_2O_3 and hard wrought CoCrMo alloys, the heads of many total hip replacement products are now also made of Al_2O_3 or Co-based alloys (Section 4.3.4). In Charnley's designs between 1958 and 1962 (see Advanced Topics: Total Joint Replacement), the acetabular cup was made from polytetrafluoroethylene (PTFE). Although the PTFE cup effectively released patients from their debilitating pain, the short-term benefit was counteracted by the risks associated with revision surgery and loss of bone stock caused by PTFE debris. Figure 6.6 shows that the retrieved PTFE cup is severely worn. Since 1962, UHMWPE has been used as the line of Charnley's *double-cup* design.

Al_2O_3-on-UHMWPE and metal-on-UHMWPE are collectively called hard-on-soft joints. The wearing of the polymer component and associated aseptic loosening remains to be the major problems of a hard-on-UHMWPE system (Section 3.7.2). This drawback has triggered the development of hard-on-hard bearings. The improved mechanical properties of Al_2O_3 ceramics and CoCrMo alloy together with significantly advanced surface polishing technique have made the hard-on-hard joint system feasible, including both Al_2O_3-on-Al_2O_3 and CoCrMo-on-CoCrMo (Figure 6.7). Table 6.2 gives a ranking of various ball head-on-cup socket joint systems in terms of wear resistance.

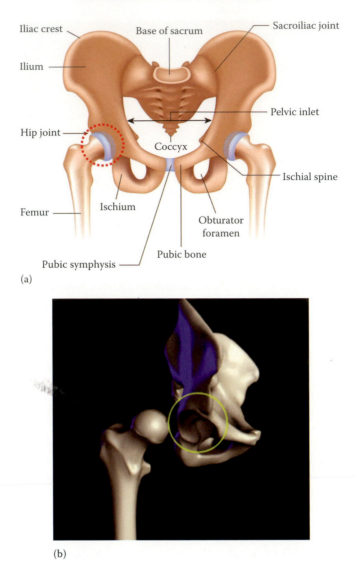

Figure 6.4
The structure of the natural hip joint. (a) Structure of pelvic girdle, the circled area is hip joint. (b) Acetabular component (circled area) of the hip joint.

However, the hard-on-hard systems have their own problems. The Al_2O_3-on-Al_2O_3 system has a high incidence of fracture due to the brittle nature of the ceramics. The CoCrMo-on-CoCrMo system releases more metal debris than any other joint system, placing patients at a high risk of systemic toxicity. Table 6.3 summarizes the advantages and disadvantages of various ball head-on-cup socket bearing systems. Currently, hard-on-soft systems are still playing the leading role in the clinical application of total hip replacement, with CrCoMo-on-UHMWPE being ~60% and Al_2O_3-on-UHMWPE being ~20% (Figure 6.8). The hard-on-hard system is dominated by CoCrMo-on-CoCrMo, which occupies almost the remaining 20%, with few Al_2O_3-on-Al_2O_3 applications.

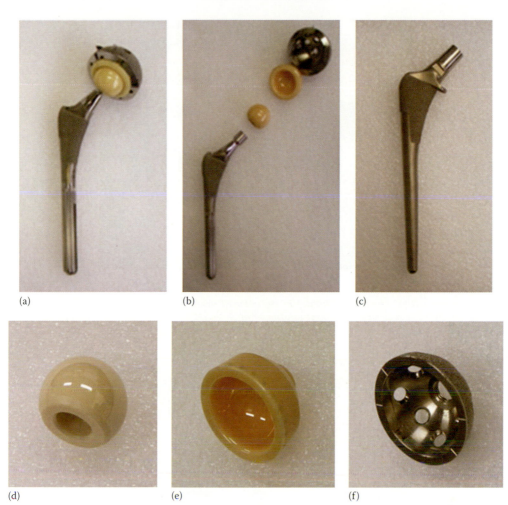

(a)   (b)   (c)

(d)   (e)   (f)

Figure 6.5
The structure of a modern total hip replacement. (a) Total hip replacement. (b) Structure of the hip replacement. (c) Stem made from Ti alloy or CoCr alloy. (d) Head made from Al_2O_3 or wrought CoCrMo alloy. (e) Line made from UHMWPE. (f) Cup made from Ti alloys.

6.2.4 Strategies to Minimize the Wear of Bearing Surfaces

The wear of joints can be minimized by the following strategies:

- In selection of a joint system: to choose good joint systems.
- In fabrication: to achieve extremely low surface roughness.
- It is very important that the alumina ball and socket have an extremely smooth surface, polished with a roundness deviation between 0.1 and 1 μm.
- In surgery: immediately applying lubricant.
- The high surface energy of alumina results in the fast and strong adsorption of biological molecules. This layer of adsorbed molecules provides a liquid-like covering which limits the direct contact of the articulating solid surfaces, acting like a lubricant.

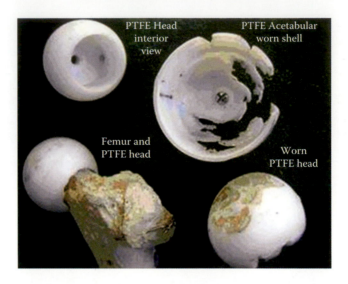

Figure 6.6
Worn cup of a total hip replacement. (From www.uhmwpe.org, reproduced with permission, Prof Steve Kurtz, School of Biomedical Engineering, Science & Health Systems, Drexel University, Philadelphia, PA.)

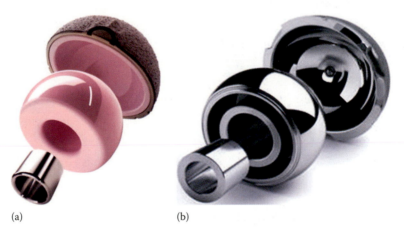

(a)   (b)

Figure 6.7
Hard-on-hard joint systems. (a) Al_2O_3-on-Al_2O_3. (b) CoCrMo-on-CoCrMo.

Table 6.2
Joint Articular Surfaces

Ball and Socket	Wearing Resistance
Ceramic-on-ceramic (Al_2O_3 or ZrO_2)	Superior
CoCrMo-on-CoCrMo	Excellent
Al_2O_3-on-CoCrMo	Excellent
Al_2O_3-on–UHMWPE	Excellent
CoCrMo-on–UHMWPE	Good
Ti6Al4V-on–UHMWPE	Unsatisfactory
Metal-on-metal (Metal = stainless steels or titanium alloys)	Poor

Table 6.3
Comparison of Bearing Systems in Total Hip Replacement

Ball on Socket	Advantages	Disadvantages
Al_2O_3-on-Al_2O_3	Superior resistance to wear	High incidence of fracture
CoCrMo-on-CoCrMo	No fracture	Metal debris related toxicity
Al_2O_3-on-CoCrMo	Low incidence of fracture	Metal debris related toxicity
Al_2O_3-on-UHMWPE	No fracture, less pain	Wear quickly, aseptic loosening
CoCrMo-on-UHMWPE	No fracture, less pain	Wear quickly, aseptic loosening

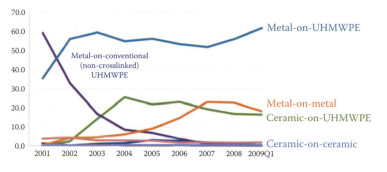

Figure 6.8
Percentage of bearing systems currently used in total hip replacements. (From Paxton, E.W. et al., Pharmacoepidemiol. Drug Saf., 21, 53, 2012.)

6.2.5 Other Applications of Al_2O_3 as an Implant Material

- Elbow prostheses
- Shoulder prostheses
- Wrist prostheses
- Finger prostheses
- Alveolar ridge and maxillofacial reconstruction
- Ossicular bone substitutes
- Keratoprostheses (corneal replacements)
- Segmental bone replacements
- Dental implants

6.3 INERT BIOCERAMICS: ZrO_2

Bioceramics made from zirconium oxide or zirconia (ZrO_2) have advantages over Al_2O_3 ceramics, which include higher fracture toughness, higher flexural strength, and lower Young's modulus. However, there are three major problems with ZrO_2 applications:

1. Strength reduction with time in physiological fluids
2. Unfavorable wear and friction properties
3. Potential radioactivity of the material

ZrO_2 is often accompanied by radioactive elements with a very long half-life such as Th and U. These elements are difficult and expensive to separate from ZrO_2. The level of gamma radiation in commercially available ZrO_2 bioceramics is not a major concern, however, the alpha emission from femoral head prostheses made from zirconium is potentially dangerous due to short range absorption and mutagenesis in the tissue.

6.4 TWO TYPES OF JOINTS

In addition to the hip, the skeletal system contains several other types of mobile joints between long bones (e.g., knee, ankle, shoulder, elbow, and inter-digital joints) (Figure 6.9) and static but slightly flexible joints (e.g., skull, wrist, and tooth). There are also other low-motility joints, representing combinations of these two main types, including rib-cage joints (congruent, slightly curved articulation, mostly fibrous) and intervertebral joints (congruent but not articulated, mostly fibrous, absorption of compressive loads). Wear is a primary concern in any artificial joints no matter what materials are used, and this together with the type of mobile joint determines the choice of prosthetic material.

Mobile joints can be categorized as two major types, congruent or incongruent, depending on how closely the opposed bone surfaces fit together. In *congruent* joints such as hip and shoulder, a ball-shaped head fits snugly into a cup-like socket, and the stress is distributed evenly (Figure 6.10). Such mechanical loads can be sustained

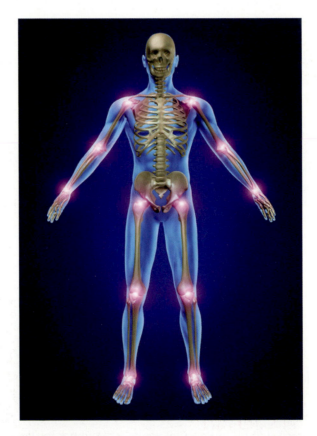

Figure 6.9
Mobile joints between long bones in the human body.

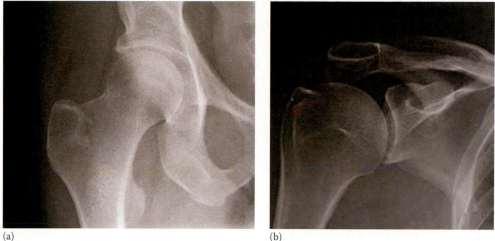

(a) (b)

Figure 6.10
X-ray images of two congruent joints in human bodies: (a) hip and (b) shoulder.

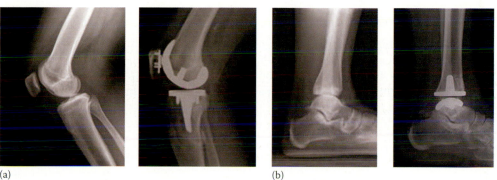

(a) (b)

Figure 6.11
Four healthy and artificial incongruent joints: (a) knee and (b) ankle.

by any strong materials, including brittle ceramic materials, as listed in Table 6.2. In *incongruent* joints, such as the knee and ankle joints, contact of the two opposed hard surfaces is more or less like a ball on a flat plate (Figure 6.11). At the contact point, there are highly concentrated (heterogeneous) stresses. Brittle ceramic materials cannot sustain such stress impacts, so metallic and hard polymeric materials are preferred in these joints, as discussed in Chapter 4 (Figures 4.14 and 4.15).

6.5 SUMMARY AND REMARKS ON Al$_2$O$_3$ AND ZrO$_2$

The low fracture toughness, deterioration of toughness with time, and high sensitivity to tensile stresses are all serious concerns for the applications of these two ceramics in high load-bearing sites. Al$_2$O$_3$ and ZrO$_2$ bioceramics should be restricted to applications involving compressive loading or very limited tensile loads.

Table 6.4
Young's Modulus of Ceramics (GPa)

Cortical Bone	Cancellous Bone	Al_2O_3 (Alumina)	ZrO_2 (Zirconia)
10–30	0.05–0.5	380–420	150–200

The high elastic modulus of these vertically inert bioceramics is also a limitation on their use in the body. There is significant modulus mismatch between bone and Al_2O_3 implants. One approach to address this issue is by compositing materials. The high modulus of elasticity of Al_2O_3 does not limit its ability to serve as an articulating surface (Table 6.4).

6.6   DENTAL CERAMICS

Dental ceramic materials fall into two broad categories: implant ceramics and dental porcelains that have the general composition of vitrified feldspar with metallic oxide pigments added to simulate natural tooth enamel color [3].

6.6.1   Dental Implant Ceramics

Although dental implants are conventionally made from titanium alloys (Section 5.1), there has been interest in the use of alumina ceramics (Figure 6.12). Bioceramic dental implants may be shaped as tapered cylinders, with a series of circumferential stops providing the taper. This design is aimed at achieving optimal load transfer to the implant. Other ceramic materials that have been used for dental implants include zirconia and bioinert glasses. Alumina, however, is used much more than these other ceramics.

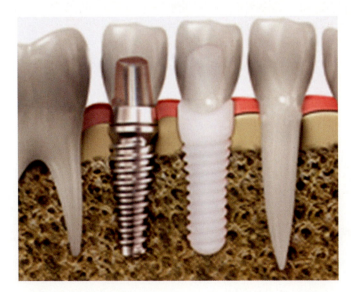

Figure 6.12
Dental implants made of Ti alloy or alumina ceramics.

6.6.2 Dental Porcelains

Generally, dental porcelains must fulfill the following three requirements:

1. Not excessively abrade opposing host teeth
2. Simulate the appearance of natural teeth
3. Withstand the oral environment

Figure 6.13 illustrates popular applications of dental porcelains. All-ceramic crowns, inlays, onlays, and veneers are used for cosmetic purposes (Figure 6.13a,b). All-ceramic materials contain up to 90 vol.% of the crystalline phases (Table 6.5) to reinforce the glass matrix.

Denture porcelains (Figure 6.13c) are melted in metal molds to form the shape of the denture teeth, with raw materials based on feldspar, with additions of ~15% quartz, ~4% kaolin, and pigment oxides (Table 6.5). Kaolin ($Al_2Si_2O_5(OH)_4$) improves the molding qualities of the mixture. Denture teeth are used as full dentures for replacement of all teeth, or just the upper or lower arch. Porcelain denture teeth show a natural translucency that simulates that of natural teeth. A cosmetic problem with denture teeth is their geometric appearance without the defects and asymmetries of

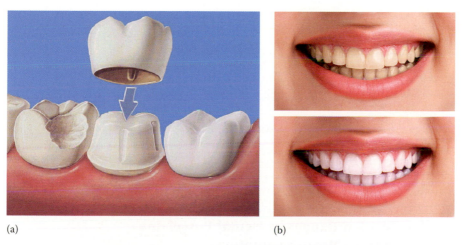

(a) (b)

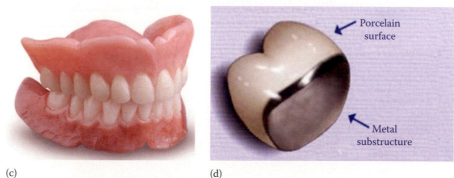

(c) (d)

Figure 6.13

Application of ceramics in dentistry. (a) All ceramic dental crown. (b) Veneers for cosmetic purposes (all ceramics). (c) Ceramic denture made from feldspar. (d) porcelain fused metal crown.

Table 6.5
Classification of Dental Ceramics for Fixed Restorations and Denture Teeth

Type	Fabrication	Crystalline Phase/Percentage Present
All-ceramic	Machined	Alumina (Al_2O_3)
		Feldspar ($KAlSi_3O_8$)
		Mica ($KMg_{2.5}Si_4O_{10}F_2$)/50%–70%
	Slip cast	Alumina (Al_2O_3)/>90%
		Spinel ($MgAl_2O_4$)/NR
	Heat pressed	Leucite ($KAlSi_2O_6$)/35%–55%
		Lithium disilicate ($Li_2Si_2O_5$)/60%
	Sintered	Alumina (Al_2O_3)/40–50 wt.%
		Leucite ($KAlSi_2O_6$)/45 vol.%
Ceramic–metal	Sintered	Leucite ($KAlSi_2O_6$)/10%–20%
Denture teeth	Manufactured	Feldspar

Source: Chapter 10: Biomaterials for dental applications, in Handbook of Materials for Medical Devices, J.R. Davies, ed., ASM International, Materials Park, OH, 2003.

natural teeth, which make them look artificial. Denture teeth are also brittle, making a characteristic clicking sound during biting.

The glass-ceramics used in porcelain fused metal (PFM) restorations (Figure 6.13d) must fulfill another two requirements in addition to the three criteria stated earlier, that is,

1. Simulate the appearance of natural teeth.
2. Withstand the oral environment.
3. Not excessively abrade opposing host teeth.

Table 6.6
Composition Ranges of Dental Porcelains for Ceramic–Metal Restorations

Component	Opaque Powder, %	Dentin (Body) Powder, %
SiO_2	50–59	57–62
Al_2O_3	9–15	11–16
Na_2O	5–7	4–9
K_2O	9–11	10–14
TiO_2	0–3	0–0.6
ZnO_2	0–5	0.1–1.5
SnO_2	5–15	0–0.5
Rb_2O	0–0.1	0–0.1
CeO_2	…	0–3
Pigments	…	Trace

Source: Chapter 10: Biomaterials for dental applications, in Handbook of Materials for Medical Devices, J.R. Davies, ed., ASM International, Materials Park, OH, 2003.

4. Fuse at relatively low temperature.
5. Have thermal expansion coefficients compatible with the metals used for ceramic–metal bonding. Most porcelains have coefficients of thermal expansion between 13.0 and $14.0 \times 10^{-6}/°C$ and metals between 13.5 and $14.5 \times 10^{-6}/°C$.

PFM materials are comprised primarily of SiO_2, Al_2O_3, Na_2O, and K_2O (Table 6.6), mostly as glass matrix embedded with crystalline phases, with TiO_2, ZrO_2, SnO_2 used as opacifiers. To match the appearance of tooth structures, small amounts of fluorescent pigments (e.g., CeO_2) are added. Pigments and opacifiers together produce the color and translucency of natural teeth.

6.7   CHAPTER HIGHLIGHTS

1. There are three generations of biomaterials:
   The first generation of materials are bioinert, a characteristic aimed to ensure they are not harmful to human tissue. The second generation of materials are surface bioactive, a characteristic aimed at achieving tissue bonding. The third generation of biomaterials are biodegradable, a requirement of tissue regeneration.
2. Because the chemical bonds of ceramic materials lack tolerance of structural deformation, their mechanical performance can be sensitively compromised by stress concentration around defects. As a general rule, ceramics cannot be used when tensile, bending, or concentrated stressing occurs. They are typically used at compressive load-bearing sites where the stresses are homogeneously distributed.
3. There are two types of motile joints: congruent and incongruent.
   In *congruent* joints such as hip and shoulder, a ball-shaped head is on a cup-like socket, and the stress is distributed evenly. In *incongruent* joints such as the knee and ankle joints, contact of two incongruent hard surfaces is like a ball on a flat plate. At the contact point, there are highly concentrated (heterogeneous) stresses.
4. Selection of materials for joint replacements:
   For congruent joints:
   a.   CoCrMo-on-UHMWPE
   b. Al_2O_3-on-UHMWPE
   c.   CoCrMo-on-CoCrMo
   d. Al_2O_3-on-Al_2O_3
   For incongruent joints:
   a.   CoCrMo-on-UHMWPE
   Ceramics are completely excluded from incongruent joints.
5. Dental porcelains must fulfill three requirements:
   a.   Have the appearance of natural teeth
   b.   Withstand the oral environment
   c.   Not excessively abrade opposing host teeth

ACTIVITIES

1. Watch videos from http://morphopedics.wikidot.com/total-hip-arthroplasty and Youtube on total hip, knee, or ankle joint replacements.

2. Visit E-leaning on http://dental-materials.blogspot.com.au/ and you can learn about most recent dental materials.
3. Visit http://www.rightdiagnosis.com/h/hip_replacement/stats-country.htm and calculate how many surgical joint replacements are performed annually worldwide.

SIMPLE QUESTIONS IN CLASS

1. Which of the following materials are first-generation biomaterials, which primarily address the most essential concern associated with biocompatibility of implants in vivo?
   a. Co-based alloys
   b. Al_2O_3
   c. Ti alloys
   d. ZrO_2
2. Which of the following materials are second-generation biomaterials, which aim to achieve tissue integration (e.g., bone-bonding) in vivo?
   a. Co-based alloys
   b. Al_2O_3
   c. Ti alloys
   d. Hydroxylapatite
3. Which of following materials are third-generation biomaterials, which are bioresorbable and aim to achieve tissue regeneration in vivo?
   a. Co-based alloys
   b. Mg alloys
   c. Crystalline hydroxylapatite
   d. Bioactive glasses
4. Which part of a total hip replacement implant is widely made of Al_2O_3?
   a. Stem
   b. Head
   c. Lining
   d. Cup
5. Which of the following artificial articulate systems is the best in terms of wear resistance?
   a. Co alloy/Co alloy
   b. Al_2O_3/UHMWPE
   c. Co alloy/UHMWPE
   d. Al_2O_3/Al_2O_3
6. Rank the following artificial articulate systems, from the best (1) to the worst (4) in terms of wear resistance.
   a. Co alloy/ceramic ____
   b. Al_2O_3/UHMWPE ____
   c. Co alloy/UHMWPE ____
   d. Al_2O_3/Al_2O_3 ____
7. In the following artificial joints, which are incongruent?
   a. Knee prostheses
   b. Ankle prostheses
   c. Shoulder prostheses
   d. Hip prostheses

8. Give the name of each part of a total hip replacement in the following:

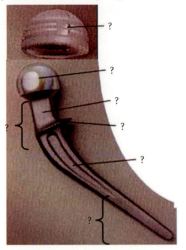

PROBLEMS AND EXERCISES

1. Describe the three generations of bioceramics, including their bioactivities and the main clinical concerns addressed.
2. What is the common response of host tissues to inert implants? Explain your answer.
3. How can wear problems at joints be alleviated in terms of material selection, implant manufacture, and clinical applications?
4. Describe the two types of joints: congruent and incongruent. Discuss the selection principles of biomaterials for these two types of joints.
5. In the artificial knee given in the following, what materials can be used to make the joint? What type of materials cannot be used? Explain your answer.

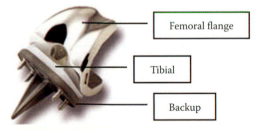

6. In the artificial ankle given in the following, what materials can be used to make the joint? What type of materials cannot be used? Explain the reasons.

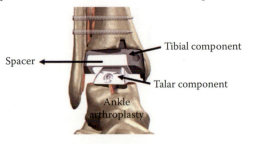

7. Rank, based on Figure 6.8, bearing systems currently used in total hip replacements in terms of their clinical application fractions. Compare your rank with the rank of various joints in terms of wearing resistance (Table 6.2). What do you find? Discuss your discovery.
8. What is the major concern with metal-on-metal joints? What consequences are anticipated?
9. What is the major concern with ceramic-on-ceramic joints?
10. What is the major issue with hard-on-soft joints? What is the adverse clinical result that has been reported associated with the issue? Describe the pathological mechanism.

ADVANCED TOPIC: TOTAL JOINT REPLACEMENT

Historical Retrospect of the Development of Total Joint Replacement

Developments in metallic implant materials have centered around repairing long bones and joints. It is interesting to consider the evolution of total joint replacement [1–4], which is one of the most successful operations of modern times, generally considered a development of the twentieth century [5,6]. The innovative German surgeon Themistocles Glück (1853–1942) led the way in the development of joint implant fixation. In May 1890, Glück produced an ivory ball and socket joint, which he inserted into the knee of a 17-year-old girl and fixed the materials to bone with nickel-plated screws (Figure 6.14) [7,8]. Later versions of early constrained total knee arthroplasty prosthesis introduced in the second half of the twentieth century were not dissimilar to the original design of Glück. He reported performing 14 arthroplasties in that year, including a hip, but only provided details of five cases: three knee, a wrist, and an elbow [6,9]. The procedures appeared successful over the short term; however, all of the five patients in the report suffered from tuberculosis, and all developed complications of chronic infection. Three of the five prostheses were removed (the wrist and

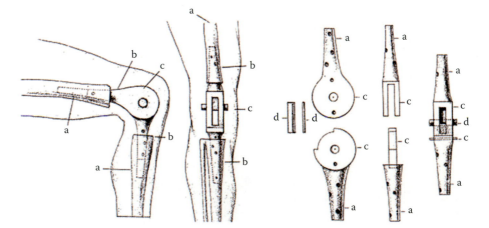

Figure 6.14
Illustrations of joints suggested by Gluck. (From Brand, R.A. et al., Clin. Orthop. Relat. Res., 469, 1525, 2011; Gluck, T., Arch. Klin. Chir., 41, 187, 1891.)

one of the knees were left in situ). He later realized that prior joint infection was a contraindication to joint arthroplasty [6].

In 1893, Jules Pean, one of the great French surgeons of the nineteenth century, attempted total joint arthroplasty with a prosthesis made of a platinum tube and a rubber ball. It had to be removed 2 years later due to infection. It was not until 1919 that French surgeon Pierre Delbet used a rubber femoral prosthesis to replace a one-half hip joint [10]. A subsequent trial with a more advanced prosthesis was performed in 1925 by Marius Nygaard Smith-Petersen from Boston. The glass and bakelite design that he used could not withstand the mechanical demands and inevitably failed [11]. Smith-Petersen modified it over a period of time with celluloid, Bakelite, and finally Pyrex [7,12], which had been introduced to the dentistry market.

Since the late 1930s, several passionate and well-known surgeons had sought to improve the clinical performance of hip replacement surgeries with unique design changes and revolutionary surgical procedures, using standard and innovative materials [3]. In 1938, Philip Wiles at the Middlesex Hospital, London, undertook six operations with the first metal-on-metal THR made of stainless steel, which were fixed to the bone with screws and bolts, but all failed due to loosening (Figure 6.15a) [13]. In 1939, surgeons Frederick R. Thompson of New York and Austin T. Moors of South Carolina separately developed the entire ball of the hip joint. This hemiarthroplasty

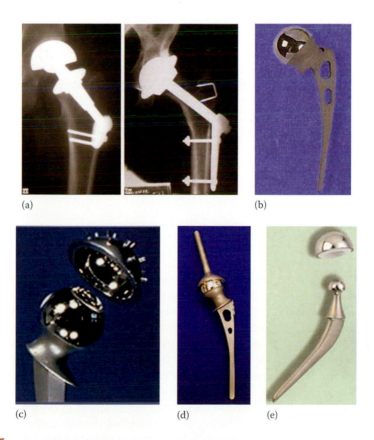

(a) (b)

(c) (d) (e)

Figure 6.15
(a) Philip Wiles's metal-on-metal prosthesis made out of stainless steel. (b) Austin Moors prosthesis made out of CoCr alloys. (c) McKee–Farrar prosthesis. (d) Ring prosthesis. (e) Charnley's prosthesis.

addressed the diseased femoral head only, but the acetabulum (hip socket) was not replaced. In the same year, Austin Moors designed the now popular long-stemmed prosthesis (Figure 6.15b). The original prosthesis they designed was a proximal femoral replacement, with a large fixed head made of Vitallium, a CoCr alloy [3,14,15]. Moore performed the metallic hip replacement surgery. This prosthesis functioned well and influenced the development of subsequent long-stem femoral head prostheses [16].

In 1948, much attention was generated by the Judet brothers from Paris, who developed an acrylic prosthesis. The Judet prostheses turned out to be exceptionally susceptible to wear, and ultimately failed [10]. Edward Haboush of the Hospital for Special Surgery and Kenneth McKee of Norwich, England, also developed acrylic prostheses in the late 1940s, experimenting with acrylic cement for fixation. Their high incidence of failure also resulted from loosening of the components [17].

In the 1950s, McKee designed the first metal-on-metal joint, which had been modified throughout 1950s and 1960s. Later versions of McKee's design, referred to as the McKee–Farrar prosthesis (Figure 6.15c) were widely accepted and successfully applied clinically in the 1960s [18–20]. His early arthroplasties provided surprisingly good results with up to 97% of implants surviving for as long as 17 years [21]. During the same period, another Briton, Peter Ring of Redhill in Surrey, started his clinical experience with cementless components as part of a metal-on-metal articulation in 1964 (Figure 6.15d) [22,23]. However, McKee's metal-on-metal joints were challenged by Professor Sir John Charnley of Wrightington Hospital in the United Kingdom. Charnley's work on tribology resulted in a design (Figure 6.15e) that almost completely replaced the other designs by the 1970s, resulting in perhaps the most successful total hip arthroplasty yet devised. By the late 1970s, usage of metal-on-metal hip devices was replaced by metal-on-polyethylene; however, McKee–Farrar's metal-on-metal implants continued to function well in many patients [24–26].

During the 1980s, the hard-on-hard joint model was reevaluated because of wearing of the UHMWPE in metal-on-polymer implants. Today, another wave of metal-on-metal bearings is on the rise [10]. It is likely that the use of hard-on-hard bearings will remain or even continue to increase, especially in young and active patients [26]. The chronology of total hip replacement is summarily provided in Table 6.7.

Materials Used in Total Joint Replacements

As reviewed earlier, hip replacement has gone through many early stages of failures with the use of inappropriate materials (e.g., ivory and acrylic resin), which later improved tremendously with the use of appropriate materials. Charnley's modern total hip replacements comprise primarily two components: a stem with attached head (ball) in one piece, and a socket (cup) as a second piece (Figure 6.16), replacing the femoral stem and head, and pelvic acetabulum (Figure 6.4), respectively.

Table 6.8 summarizes the materials used in hip replacement prostheses. Stainless steels were first used in total hip replacements by Philip Wiles in 1938, and a CoCr alloy was wisely chosen by Austin Moore in the 1950s. The issues associated with the poor corrosion, fatigue, and wear resistances of stainless steels and the consequent issue of heavy metal toxicity have since barred them from applications in permanent implants, and stainless steels are rarely used in permanent implant devices anymore.

Today, the stem portions of most hip implants are made of high-nitrogen containing Orthinox stainless steel, CoCr- or Ti-based alloys. Cobalt–chromium-based alloys

Table 6.7
Historical Evolution of Total Joint Replacement

Year(s)	Inventor(s)	Joints	Materials	Clinical Outcomes
1890	Themistocles Glück/ Berlin, Germany	Knee Hip Wrist Elbow	Ivory ball and socket joint	Failed due to chronic infection
1893	Jules Pean/Paris, France	Shoulder	Platinum tube and a rubber ball	Removed 2 years later due to infection
1919	Pierre Delbet/La Ferte Gaucher, France	Hip	Rubber femoral	Failed due to wearing
1925– 1939	Smith-Petersen/Boston, USA	Hip	Glass, celluloid, pyrex, bakelite, and Vitallium	Failed due to mechanical fracture
1938	Philip Wiles/London, UK	Hip	Metal-on-metal stainless steel	Poor clinical results
1948	Robert and Jean Judet brothers/Paris, France	Hip	Acrylic resin	Removed due to loosening
1950	Austin Moore/South Carolina, USA	Hip	Metal-on-metal CoCr alloy (Vitallium)	Removed due to loosening
1950– 1970	Kenneth McKee/ Norwich, UK	Hip	Metal-on-metal stainless steels or Co alloys	Successful with surviving for up to 17 years
1960– 1970	Peter Ring/Redhill, UK	Hip	Metal-on-metal stainless steel, Co alloy)	Successful with surviving for up to 17 years
1962– present	John Charnley/UK	Hip	Metal-on-UHMWPE (stainless steel, Co alloy, or Ti alloys)	Successful with surviving for about 25 years

Source: Pramanik, S. et al., *Trends Biomater. Artif. Organs, 19, 15, 2005.*

or ceramic materials (aluminum oxide or zirconium oxide) are used in making the ball portions, which are polished smooth to allow easy rotation within the prosthetic socket. Sockets can be made of metal, UHMWPE, or a combination of polyethylene backed by metal. Table 6.9 lists current major manufacturers of hip replacement prostheses and the materials used.

Recent market data (Figure 6.8) show that Charnley's model metal-on-UHMWPE bearing surfaces still accounts for the largest proportion (approximately 60%) of all total hip arthroplasty devices. Ceramic-on-UHMWPE joints account for ~20%, with the remainder metal-on-metal, which has recently risen to ~20% [2].

With the huge success of application in total hip replacements, cobalt alloys were soon used in other total joint replacements [4] for load-bearing sites, including knee and ankle joints, and less stressed sites, such as shoulder joints. Figures 4.14 and 4.15 demonstrate the structures of knee and ankle prostheses. As discussed in Section 5.3, knee and ankle joints are incongruent, which involves stress concentration at their dynamic working conditions. Hence, brittle ceramic is forbidden. Cobalt–chromium

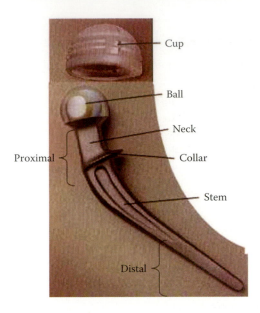

Figure 6.16
Terminologies of components of a modern total hip replacement.

alloys are suitably tough and almost exclusively used in knee and ankle implants. Cobalt-based alloys are used to make the femoral and tibial components of total knee replacements, and tibial and talar components in total ankle replacements, between which UHMWPE is used. Ta and Zr have also been explored for use in knee prostheses (Figure 5.13).

The glenohumeral joint (shoulder joint) is a ball-and-socket joint, similar to the hip joint. The shoulder joint is made up of three bones (Figure 6.17):

1. The scapula, or the shoulder blade
2. The humerus, or the upper arm bone
3. The clavicle, or the collarbone

In modern total shoulder prostheses, humeral stems are widely made from Ti alloys and CoCr alloys are used to make the head, which rotates against the UHMWPE glenoid (Figure 6.17).

Total joint replacement represents one of the greatest achievements in surgery of the twentieth century. Nowadays, approximately two and half million hip replacements are performed each year globally. Recent years have also seen continuous increases in the number of total knee and ankle replacements. Shoulder replacements are relatively less common, although from 1996 to 2002 approximately 7000 total shoulder replacements were performed annually in the United States.

Current Issues and Challenges

The cumulative survival rate of joint replacements has been improving over the past half century, with the revision rate at 15 years survival decreasing from 50% in the middle of the 1990s [27] to around 10% in the late 2010s [1,25,28,29]. Despite the huge

Table 6.8
Biomaterials Used in Modern Total Joint Replacements

Products	Stem	Head	Line	Cup	Year(s)
Metal-on-metal before the 1960s					
Philip Wiles	Stainless steels	Stainless steels	No line	Stainless steels	1938
Austin Moore	CoCr alloy (Vitallium)	CoCr alloy (Vitallium)	No line	No cup	1950s
McKee–Farrar	Stainless steels CoCrMo alloys	Stainless steels CoCrMo alloys	No line	Stainless steels Co alloys	1950s
Peter Ring	Stainless steels CoCrMo alloys	Stainless steels CoCrMo alloys	No line	Stainless steels CoCrMo alloys	1950s
Metal-on-UHMEPE					
Charnley	Stainless steels[a] CoCrMo alloys Ti alloys	Stainless steels[a] CoCrMo alloys Ceramics (Al_2O_3 or ZrO_2)	UHMWPE	Stainless steels[a] CoCrMo alloys Ti alloys	1960s
Metal-on-metal since the 1960s					
	CoCrMo alloys Ti alloys	CoCrMo alloys	No line	CoCrMo alloys	1960s
Ceramic-on-ceramic					
	CoCrMo alloys Ti alloys	Ceramics (Al_2O_3 or ZrO_2)	No line	Ceramics (Al_2O_3 or ZrO_2)	1980s
Ceramic-on-metal					
	CoCrMo alloys Ti alloys	Ceramics (Al_2O_3 or ZrO_2)	No line	CoCrMo alloys	2000s

Source: Zywiel, M.G. et al., Expert Rev. Med. Devices, 8, 187, 2011.

[a] *Today, stainless steels are rarely used in the joint couplings of total hip replacements, though some previously implanted stainless steel prostheses are still in service. Stainless steel 316L/CoCr couplings should be avoided.*

success, failure of the femoral stem and loosening caused by wearing of acetabular components remain the most serious postimplantation complications of all total joint replacements (Figure 6.18) [30,31]. The failure incidence is especially high after 20 years implantation, being 30%–40% [28]. Failure analysis has consistently revealed that fretting corrosion fatigue is the major cause of stem fracture, with *wearing between bearing surfaces being responsible for the aseptic loosening* [30–32]. The corrosion fatigue strength value of wrought CoCrMo alloys in simulated body fluid is around 200 MPa after 10 years of service, a similar level to the working stress of 200 MPa for a stem of hip prosthesis under normal walking conditions. Hence, fatigue or corrosion fatigue is likely to cause the fracture of the stem. It is also important to bear in mind that the difference between estimates of material parameters under in vitro versus in vivo conditions is such that the corrosion fatigue and fretting corrosion fatigue strengths of metallic material implants may be overestimated by in vitro testing. The in vivo

Table 6.9

Major Orthopedic Implant Manufacturers and Materials of Some Hip Replacements

Company	Products	Materials
Zimmer Holdings (ZMH)	Zimmer®ML Taper Hip Prosthesis with Kinectiv® Technology	Metal-on-UHMWPE Wrought Co-based alloy
	Metasul® Metal-on-Metal articulation	Forged Co-based alloy
Depuy (Johnson and Johnson) (JNJ)	AML® Total Hip System	CoCrMo alloy
	Austin Moore Hemi-Arthroplasty	CoCrMo alloy
	Prodigy® Total Hip System	CoCrMo alloy
Stryker Corp.	Accolade TMZF (recalled)	TMZF alloy (recalled)
	Accolade C Femoral Component	Forged cobalt-chrome alloy
Biomet (BMET)	Echo™ Hip System	Forged cobalt-chrome alloy
	Taperloc® Complete Hip Stem	Titanium alloy Ti-6Al-4V
Smith & Nephew (SNN)	SMF Short Modular Femoral Hip	Cobalt-chrome alloy
Wright Medical	Perfecta® RS Stem	Titanium alloy
	Perfacta Plasma Spray Stems	Titanium alloy
Exactech	AcuMatch® L-Series (Cemented Stems)	Forged cobalt-chrome alloy
	AcuMatch L-Series (Press-Fit Stems)	Forged titanium alloy

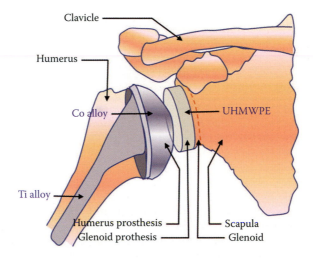

Figure 6.17
Total shoulder replacements.

working conditions are mechanically and biologically complicated. Normal physiological loading provokes a combination of various deformation strains in bone, including compression, tension, shear, torsion, and vibration. Complex biological conditions include the changes in pH, low-level infection, inflammation, tissue remodeling, and the presence of macrophages and debris. Hence, the in vivo working environment may be far more aggressive than we estimate.

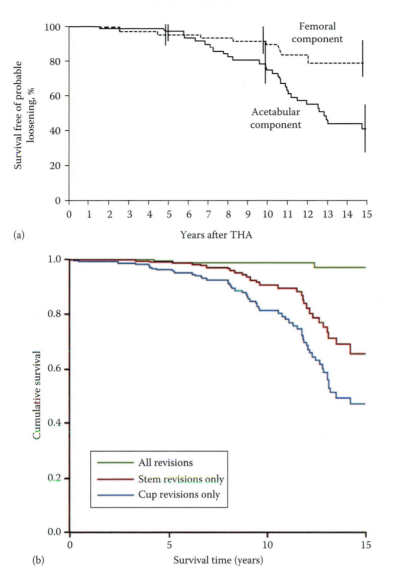

Figure 6.18
Cumulative improvements in survival rate reported in (a) 1996 [27] and (b) 2007 [28]. (a) (Reprinted with permission from Torchia, M.E. et al., J. Bone Joint Surg. [Am.],78A(7), 995, 1996. Copyright 1996, Rockwater Inc., Lexington, SC.) (b) (Reprinted from Lancet, 370(9597), Learmonth, I.D., C. Young, and C. Rorabeck, The operation of the century: Total hip replacement, 1508–1519, 2007, Copyright 2007, with permission from Elsevier.)

BIBLIOGRAPHY

References for Text

1. Ryhanen, J. et al., Bone modeling and cell-material interface responses induced by nickel-titanium shape memory alloy after periosteal implantation. *Biomaterials 1999*, 2014;**20**:1309–1317.

2. Paxton, E.W. et al., Evaluation of total hip arthroplasty devices using a total joint replacement registry. *Pharmacoepidemiology and Drug Safety*, 2012;**21**:53–59.
3. Chapter 10: Biomaterials for dental applications. In *Handbook of Materials for Medical Devices*, J.R. Davies, ed. Materials Park, OH: ASM International, 2003.

Websites

http://ceramics.org/about-us/international-ceramic-societies.
http://morphopedics.wikidot.com/total-hip-arthroplasty.
http://www.ada.org/.
http://www.fpnotebook.com/ortho/Anatomy/HpAntmy.htm (family practice notebook, an excellent website, with a medical book list and other websites).
http://www.journals.elsevier.com/dental-materials/.
http://www.njrcentre.org.uk/njrcentre/default.aspx.
https://academydentalmaterials.org/scripts/default.asp.

References for Advanced Topics

1. Paxton, E.W. et al., Evaluation of total hip arthroplasty devices using a total joint replacement registry. *Pharmacoepidemiology and Drug Safety*, 2012;**21**:53–59.
2. Biomaterials for dental applications. In *Handbook of Materials for Medical Devices*, J.R. Davies, ed. Materials Park, OH: ASM International, 2003.
3. Pramanik, S., A.K. Agarwal, and K.N. Rai, Chronology of total hip joint replacement and materials development. *Trends in Biomaterials and Artificial Organs*, 2005;**19**(1):15–26.
4. Luetjring, G. et al., The influence of soft, precipitate-free zones at grain boundaries in Ti and Al alloys on their fatigue and fracture behavior. *Materials Science and Engineering A-Structural Materials Properties Microstructure and Processing*, 2007;**468**:201–209.
5. Eynonlewis, N.J., D. Ferry, and M.F. Pearse, Gluck, Themistocles—An unrecognized genius. *British Medical Journal*, 1992;**305**(6868):1534–1536.
6. Brand, R.A., M.A. Mont, and M.M. Manring, Biographical sketch: Themistocles Gluck (1853–1942). *Clinical Orthopaedics and Related Research*, 2011;**469**(6):1525–1527.
7. Hughes, S. and I. McCarthy, *Science Basic to Orthopaedics*. Philadelphia, PA: WB Saunders Company Ltd, 1998.
8. Rang, M., *Anthology of Orthopaedics*. London, U.K.: Churchill Livingstone, 1966.
9. Gluck, T., Referat über die durch das moderne chirurgische Experiment gewonnenen positiven Resultate, betreffend die Naht und den Ersatz von Defecten höherer Gewebe, sowie über die Verwethung resorbirbarer und lebendiger Tampons in der Chirurgie. *Arch Klin Chir*, 1891;**41**:187–239.
10. Gomez, P.F. and J.A. Morcuende, Early attempts at hip arthroplasty—1700s to 1950s. *The Iowa Orthopaedic Journal*, 2005;**25**:25–29.
11. Pospula, W., Total hip replacement: Past, present and future. *Kumait Medical Journal*, 2004;**36**(4):250–255.
12. Smith-Petersen, M.N., Arthroplasty of the hip, a new method. *The Journal of Bone and Joint Surgery. British Volume*, 1939;**21B**:269–288.
13. Wiles, P., The surgery of the osteo-arthritic hip. *British Journal of Surgery*, 1958;**45**(193):488–497.
14. Moore, A.T. and H.R. Bohlman, Metal hip joint—A case report (Reprinted from *J Bone Joint Surg*, 25, 688, 1943). *Clinical Orthopaedics and Related Research*, 2006;**453**:22–24.
15. Moore, A.T. and H.R. Bohlman, Metal hip joint: A case report. *Journal of Bone and Joint Surgery*, 1943;**25**:688–692.
16. Welch, R.B. and J. Charnley, Low friction arthroplasty of hip in rheumatoid arthritis and ankylosing spondylitis. *Arthritis and Rheumatism*, 1970;**13**(3):358.
17. McKee, G.K., Development of total prosthetic replacement of hip. *Clinical Orthopaedics and Related Research*, 1970;**72**:85–103.

18. McKee, G.K., Artificial hip joint. *Journal of Bone and Joint Surgery. British Volume*, 1958;**40**(2):345–345.

19. McKee, G.K. and J. Watson-Farrar, Artificial hip joint. *Journal of Bone and Joint Surgery. British Volume*, 1963;**45**(3):624–624.

20. McKee, G.K., Development and use of artificial hip joints. *Journal of Bone and Joint Surgery. British Volume*, 1963;**45**(3):616–616.

21. Ring, P.A., Replacement of the hip joint. *Annals of the Royal College of Surgeons of England*, 1971;**48**(6):344–355.

22. Ring, P.A., Total hip replacement. *Proceedings of the Royal Society of Medicine-London*, 1967;**60**(3):281–284.

23. Ring, P.A., Complete replacement arthroplasty of the hip by the ring prosthesis. *The Journal of Bone and Joint Surgery. British Volume*, 1968;**50**(4):720–731.

24. Verheyen, C.C.P.M. and J.A.N. Verhaar, Failure rates of stemmed metal-on-metal hip replacements. *Lancet*, 2012;**380**(9837):106.

25. Smith, A.J. et al., Failure rates of stemmed metal-on-metal hip replacements: Analysis of data from the National Joint Registry of England and Wales. *Lancet*, 2012;**379**(9822):1199–1204.

26. Zywiel, M.G. et al., State of the art in hard-on-hard bearings: How did we get here and what have we achieved? *Expert Review of Medical Devices*, 2011;**8**(2):187–207.

27. Torchia, M.E., R.A. Klassen, and A.J. Bianco, Total hip arthroplasty with cement in patients less than twenty years old—Long-term results. *Journal of Bone and Joint Surgery. American Volume*, 1996;**78A**(7):995–1003.

28. Learmonth, I.D., C. Young, and C. Rorabeck, The operation of the century: Total hip replacement. *Lancet*, 2007;**370**(9597):1508–1519.

29. Labek, G. et al., Revision rates after total joint replacement: Cumulative results from world-wide joint register datasets (vol 93, 293, 2011). *Journal of Bone and Joint Surgery. British Volume*, 2011;**93B**(7):998–998.

30. Rostoker, W., E.Y.S. Chao, and J.O. Galante, Defects in failed stems of hip prostheses. *Journal of Biomedical Materials Research*, 1978;**12**(5):635–651.

31. Sumita, M., T. Hanawa, I. Ohnishi, and T. Yoneyama, Failure processes in biometallic materials. In *Bioengineering*. Milne, I., R.O. Ritchie, and B. Karihaloo, (Eds.) London, U.K.: Elsevier Science Ltd., 2003, pp. 131–167.

32. Antunes, R.A. and M.C. Lopes de Oliveira, Corrosion fatigue of biomedical metallic alloys: Mechanisms and mitigation. *Acta Biomaterialia*, 2012;**8**(3):937–962.

33. Ryhänen, J. et al., *Biomaterials*, 2014;**20**:1309–1317.

Further Readings

Chapter 2: The use of alumina and zirconia in surgical implants. In *Introduction to Bioceramics*, L.L. Hench and J. Wilson, eds. World Scientific Publishing Company, Incorporated, Singapore, 1993.

Chapter 6: Ceramic implant materials. In *Biomaterials: An Introduction*, J. Park and R.S. Lakes, eds., 3rd edn. New York: Springer, 2007.

Chapter 10: Biomaterials for dental applications. In *Handbook of Materials for Medical Devices*, J.R. Davies, ed. Materials Park, OH: ASM International, 2003.

Hussain, S., *Textbook of Dental Materials*. New Delhi, India: Japee Brothers Medical Publishers (P) Ltd, 2004.

The most recent National Joint Registry (NJR). Annual report http://www.njrcentre.org.uk/njrcentre/Portals/0/Documents/England/Reports/10th_annual_report/NJR%2010th%20Annual%20Report%202013%20B.pdf

The most recent The American Joint Replacement Registry (AJRR). Annual report http://teamwork.aaos.org/ajrr/AJRR%20Documents/AJRR%20Fall%202013_F11062013.pdf

CHAPTER 7

BIOACTIVE AND BIORESORBABLE CERAMICS

LEARNING OBJECTIVES

After a careful study of this chapter, you should be able to do the following:

1. Accurately define the term "bioactive" used in the field of biomaterials.
2. Describe apatite formulae and name them using the nomenclature.
3. Describe bone bonding mechanisms of surface bioactive ceramics.
4. Describe the biodegradation mechanism of ceramics.
5. Apply strategies to design bioactivity and tune biodegradation rates.

7.1 OVERVIEW OF SURFACE BIOACTIVE AND BULK DEGRADABLE CERAMICS

The term "bioactive" has been used with different definitions in different scientific fields. In the biochemistry field, for example, the bioactive component of an enzyme refers to its biochemically reactive part. In the field of biomaterials, *bioactive* often refers to a material, which upon being placed within the human body interacts with the surrounding tissue [1,2]. According to the aforementioned definition, *bioactive* is restricted to surface bioactive materials, as opposed to bulk bioresorbable materials. Surface bioactive ceramics are virtually nonresorbable in the body but exhibit an ability to bond with the bone. *Surface-erodible* and *surface-bioactive* are often used interchangeably. There are three types of surface bioactive ceramics:

1. Hydroxyapatite and related calcium phosphates
2. Bioactive glasses
3. Glass-ceramics

Most surface bioactive ceramics can, however, be tuned to become bulk biodegradable via the alteration of crystallinity and/or composition. In general, crystalline ceramics are more stable in aqueous environments than their amorphous counterparts of the same compositions, and many glass bioceramics (e.g., amorphous calcium phosphates) are biodegradable.

7.2   CALCIUM PHOSPHATES AND HYDROXYAPATITE

7.2.1   Calcium Phosphate

Calcium phosphate [3] refers to a family of compounds (minerals) containing calcium ions Ca^{2+} and orthophosphates $(PO_4)^{3-}$. For example,

- Tricalcium phosphate: $Ca_3(PO_4)_2$
- Dicalcium phosphate anhydrous: $Ca_2H_2(PO_4)_2$
- Dicalcium phosphate dihydrate: $Ca_2H_2(PO_4)_2 \cdot 2H_2O$

Similar salts can be formed from magnesium and other positively charged metal ions.

7.2.2   Apatite

Apatite is a group of phosphate minerals. The general formula for this group is given in Table 7.1. Figure 7.1 illustrates the crystal structure of apatite.

The four most common members of apatite include hydroxyl-apatite, fluor-apatite, chlor-apatite, and brom-apatite. Their formula is written as $\mathbf{Ca_{10}(PO_4)_6(OH/F/Cl/Br)_2}$, and the crystal unit cell formulae of the individual minerals are written as follows:

- Hydroxyl-apatite—$\mathbf{Ca_{10}(PO_4)_6(OH)_2}$
- Fluor-apatite—$\mathbf{Ca_{10}(PO_4)_6F_2}$
- Chlor-apatite—$\mathbf{Ca_{10}(PO_4)_6Cl_2}$
- Brom-apatite—$\mathbf{Ca_{10}(PO_4)_6Br_2}$

7.2.3   Bone Minerals (Biological Apatite)

Almost two-thirds of the weight of the bone is hydroxyapatite $Ca_{10}(PO_4)_6(OH)_2$. However, the biological apatite is usually Ca-deficient and always carbonate $(CO_3)^{2-}$ substituted. The composition of bone mineral can be written as follows:

$$\mathbf{(Ca/Mg/Zn/Na/K)_{10}(PO_4/CO_3)_6(OH/F/Cl/CO_3)_2}$$

For this reason, biological apatite is also referred to as *carbonate apatite*, rather than simply as hydroxyapatite.

Table 7.1
Formula of Apatite

$A_{10}(BO_4)_6(OH/F/Cl/Br)_2$
- The **A** cations can be any of several metal ions such as Ca, Mg, Br, Na, Ba, Pb, Sr, La, and/or Ce.
- The **B** cations can be either P or V.
- Carbonate anion groups **CO$_3$** and silicate anion groups **SiO$_4$** can substitute to a limited extent for the **BO$_4$** groups.

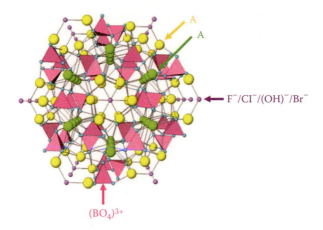

A
A

$F^-/Cl^-/(OH)^-/Br^-$

$(BO_4)^{3+}$

Figure 7.1
Crystal structure of apatite. (From Prof. Anton Chakhmouradian, Department of Geological Sciences, University of Manitoba, Winnipeg, Manitoba, Canada. Copyright, reproduced with permission.)

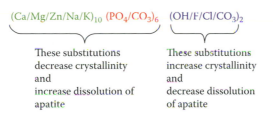

$(Ca/Mg/Zn/Na/K)_{10}$ $(PO_4/CO_3)_6$ $(OH/F/Cl/CO_3)_2$

| These substitutions decrease crystallinity and increase dissolution of apatite | These substitutions increase crystallinity and decrease dissolution of apatite |

Figure 7.2
Stability of substituted apatite.

The aforementioned ion substitutions change the stability of apatite, by modifying its solubility, which is directly related to its crystallinity. In general, a loosely packed amorphous structure is more soluble than its closely packed crystalline counterpart. The substitution of Ca with metal ions decreases the crystallinity of apatite and thus makes the apatite less stable (Figure 7.2). The substitution of phosphate with carbonate also reduces the crystallinity of apatite, and thus increases the solubility of apatite. The substitution of OH^- with F^- will give greater chemical stability due to the closer coordination of F (symmetric shape) as compared to the hydroxyl (nonsymmetric) by the nearest calcium. This is the major reason for the better caries resistance of teeth following fluoridation (e.g., in the water supply, tooth paste products) (Figure 7.3).

7.2.4 Biocompatibility of Synthetic Calcium Phosphates and Hydroxyapatite

Synthetic hydroxyapatite and related calcium phosphates have been intensively investigated. As expected, calcium phosphates have an excellent biocompatibility due to their close chemical and crystal resemblance to bone mineral. A large number of in vivo and in vitro assessments have been reported, showing that calcium phosphates, no matter which forms (bulk, coating, powder, or porous) and which phases (crystalline or amorphous) they are in, always support the attachment, differentiation, and proliferation of osseous (bone) cells (such as osteoblasts), with hydroxyapatite being the most effective.

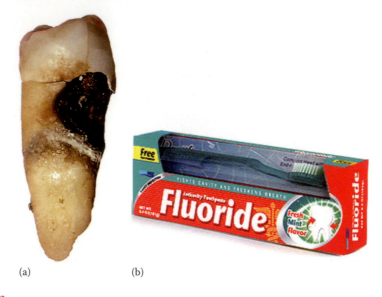

(a)   (b)

Figure 7.3
Regular exposure to fluoride anions can enhance caries resistance of teeth: (a) Dental caries; (b) fluoride toothpaste.

The ability of implant biomaterials to enhance bone healing occurs under different conditions. *Osteoinduction* is the ability to induce bone formation in osseous and nonosseous tissues. *Osteoconduction* is the ability to encourage the growth of host bone tissue into the structure of an implant, or onto the surface of the graft in situ. Although hydroxyapatite and related calcium phosphates do not show osteoinductive ability, they certainly possess osteoconductive properties, having a remarkable ability to bond directly to bone.

7.2.5   Stability of Synthetic Calcium Phosphates and Hydroxyapatites in Physiological Solutions

In laboratory studies, the dissolution rate of synthetic hydroxyapatites depends on several factors related to the solutions used (composition, pH, saturation limit) and the material itself (time in suspension, composition, crystallinity) (Figure 7.2). For fully crystalline hydroxyapatite, the degree of micro- and macroporosities, defect microstructure, amount, and type of other phases present also have a significant influence on its dissolution kinetics. Crystalline hydroxyapatite exhibits the slowest dissolution rate, compared with other calcium phosphates. This is by no means a surprise, given that nano-sized crystalline hydroxyapatite is a relatively stable component of natural bone in the body. Nature would be unlikely to select an unstable mineral to constitute 70% of bone, which provides support and protection to the body. The dissolution rate decreases in the following order:

Amorphous CaP > Amorphous HA > Crystalline CaP > Crystalline HA

While crystalline calcium phosphates typically are very stable in the body, they are surface bioactive. Clinical follow-ups have shown that implanted hydroxyapatite and tricalcium phosphates are virtually inert, remaining in the body for as long as 7 years postimplantation [4].

7.2.6 Mechanical Properties of Synthetic Calcium Phosphates and Hydroxyapatite

The properties of synthetic calcium phosphates vary significantly with their crystallinity, grain size, porosity, and composition (e.g., calcium deficiency). In general, the mechanical properties of synthetic calcium phosphates decrease significantly with increasing content of amorphous phase, microporosity, and grain size. High crystallinity, low porosity, and small grain size tend to give higher stiffness, higher compressive and tensile strength, and greater fracture toughness. The flexural strength and fracture toughness of dense hydroxyapatite are also lower in dry compared to wet conditions [5]. Table 7.2 provides the typical range of mechanical properties of hydroxyapatite and calcium phosphates.

If we compare the properties of hydroxyapatite and calcium phosphates with those of bone (Table 7.2), we find that bone has a reasonably good compressive strength, though it is lower than that of hydroxyapatite. Bone also has better tensile strength and significantly better fracture toughness than hydroxyapatite. The apatite crystals in bone tissue make it strong enough to tolerate compressive loading. The high tensile strength and fracture toughness of bone are attributed to the tough and flexible collagen fibers that make up the remaining 30% of bone mass. Hence, calcium phosphates and hydroxyapatite alone cannot be used for load-bearing implants in spite of their good biocompatibility and osteoconductivity. Elimination of the stress shielding effect is another motivation for the development of bioceramic–polymer composites.

7.2.7 Applications of Synthetic Calcium Phosphates and Hydroxyapatites as Implant Materials

While the excellent biological performance of hydroxyapatite and related calcium phosphates has been well documented, the brittleness of these ceramics restricts their application in load-free regions as bone fillers, or in composite bone cements and pastes as reinforcements, as illustrated in Figure 7.4a and b. Hydroxyapatite, a relatively nonresorbable form of calcium phosphate, has also been used with some success as a coating material for metallic implants (Figure 7.4c) and as a ridge augmentation material. Studies indicate that the hydroxyapatite increases the rate of bone growth toward the implant. Bone tissue engineering scaffolds made from calcium phosphates (Figure 7.4d) have been intensively explored.

Table 7.2
Mechanical Properties of Calcium Phosphates, Hydroxyapatite, and Human Bone

Ceramics	Compressive Strength (MPa)	Tensile Strength (MPa)	Elastic Modulus (GPa)	Fracture Toughness (MPa) $\sqrt{m}$
CaP	~900	~200	~100	<1.0
HA	>400	~40	~100	~1.0
Cortical bone	130–180	130–150	10–30	6–12

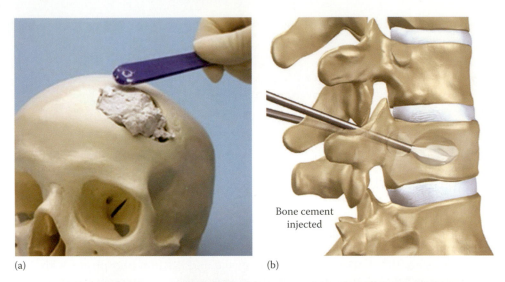

(a)   (b)

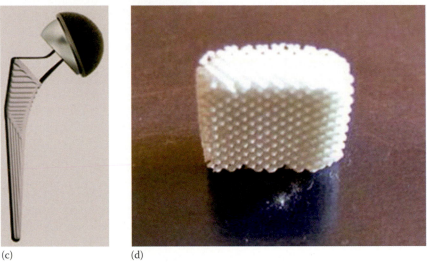

(c)   (d)

Figure 7.4
Medical applications of hydroxyapatite and calcium phosphates: (a) bone filler to heal a critical-sized defect in skull; (b) bone cement to heal a critical-sized defect in spine; (c) coating on a total hip replacement; (d) tissue engineering scaffold made from β-tricalcium phosphate.

7.3 BIOACTIVE GLASSES

7.3.1 Bioactive Silicate Glasses

7.3.1.1 Composition and Biodegradability of Bioactive Silicate Glasses
Before we look into bioactive glasses, let us first look at the most familiar type of glass, soda-lime glass, which has been used for centuries in windows and drinking vessels. Silica (SiO_2) is a common fundamental constituent of glass. Pure silica glass, however, has a high melting point (1723°C), which increases the manufacture cost in the glass industry. To reduce the melting point of glass, Na_2O is added, whereas other components such as CaO and MgO are also added to stabilize this glass, which would otherwise

be rendered water soluble. Soda-lime glass is typically composed of about 75% silica (SiO_2) plus sodium oxide (Na_2O), lime (CaO), and other minor additives.

The constituent of bioactive glasses is similar to that of soda-lime glass. The most bioactive glasses are composed of SiO_2, Na_2O, CaO, and P_2O_5. The well-known 45S5 Bioglass® (first bioactive composition) contains 45% SiO_2, 24.5% Na_2O, 24.4% CaO, and 6% P_2O_5, in wt.%. The bioreactivity of these materials is composition-dependent. In the 1960s, Larry Hench [1,2] systematically studied a series of glasses in the four-component systems with a constant 6 wt.% P_2O_5 content. This work is graphically summarized in the ternary SiO_2-Na_2O-CaO diagram shown in Figure 7.5. The major features are listed as follows:

- In region A, the glasses are bioactive and bond to bone.
- In region B, glasses are nearly inert when implanted.
- In region C, the compositions are resorbed within 10–30 days in tissue.
- In region D, the compositions are not technically practical.

The key advantage that makes bioactive glasses attractive bioceramics is the possibility of controlling the bone-bonding ability and biodegradation kinetics by modification of their chemical properties. The structure and chemistry of glasses can thus be tailored at the molecular level by varying either composition or thermal processing parameters. It is possible to design glasses with properties specific to a particular clinical application.

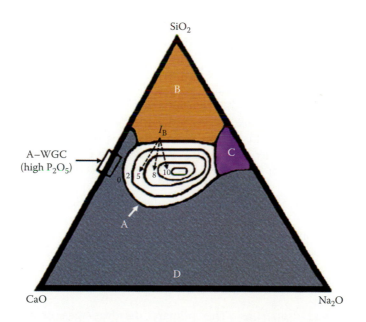

Figure 7.5

Compositional dependence (in wt.%) of bone bonding and soft tissue bonding for bioactive glasses and glass ceramics. Bioactivity index I_B is defined as $I_B = 100/t_{0.5}$, where $t_{0.5}$ is the time taken for 50% of the interface to bond to bone. All compositions have a constant 6 wt.% of P_2O_5. In region A, the glasses are bioactive and bond to bone. In region B, glasses are nearly inert when implanted. Compositions in region C are resorbed within 10–30 days in tissue. In region D, the compositions are not technically practical. In the region where $I_B > 8$ (called region E), soft tissue bonding occurs. Apatite–wollastonite glass ceramic (A–WGC) has higher P_2O_5 content. (From Hench, L.L. and Wilson, J., Science, 226, 630, 1984.)

Crystallization of certain bioactive glasses decreases the level of bioactivity and can even turn a bioactive glass into an inert material (see Section 7.4). This is one of the disadvantages that limit the application of these glasses as bioactive implants, as full crystallization happens prior to significant densification upon heat-treatment (i.e., sintering). Extensive sintering is necessary to densify the material, which would otherwise be made up of loosely packed particles, and thus be too fragile to be used as implants. There is one exception, sintered (crystallized) 45S5 Bioglass, which has been found to retain bioactivity and even degradability while its mechanical properties are improved by the sintering [7].

7.3.1.2 Biocompatibility of Bioactive Silicate Glasses

As briefly mentioned in Chapter 5, bioactive glasses SiO_2-Na_2O-CaO-P_2O_3 are generally biocompatible because they are composed of ions commonly found in the physiological environment (Ca^{2+}, K^+, and Na^+). These elements are macroelements of the body, rather than trace elements.

Silicon, an element below carbon in the periodic table, has been proposed to be an ultra trace nutrient, and is considered to be necessary for synthesis of elastin and collagen in connective tissue, such as in the aorta, which contains the highest quantity of silicon. Awareness of the role of silicon in improving bone density and strength is also increasing, such as improvements seen after the treatment of women of 50 years or older (the age susceptible to osteoporosis) with bioavailable forms such as silicic acid. Furthermore, it has been found that higher levels of silica in water appear to decrease the risk of dementia. The study found an association between an increase of 10 mg/day of the intake of silica in drinking water with a decreased risk of dementia of 11%.

In contrast, as for all trace elements, an excessive level of silicon or silica is toxic. In the body, crystalline silica particles do not dissolve over clinically relevant periods of time. However, the condition of silicosis occurs due to the inhalation of finely divided crystalline silica dust in very small quantities over time, similar to asbestosis. There is also an increased risk bronchitis and cancer, as the dust becomes lodged in the lungs and continuously irritates them and causes reduced lung capacity. Amorphous silica, such as fumed silica, is not associated with development of silicosis, but may cause irreversible lung damage.

In general, the biocompatibility of bioactive glasses can be compromised by their composition and crystallinity. For instance, a faster release of Na_2O from amorphous Na_2O-containing glass can be toxic, due to over alkalinization of the physiological microenvironment. This explains why sintered 45S5 Bioglass-ceramics have improved biocompatibility compared with the original unsintered form of 45S5 Bioglass.

7.3.1.3 Mechanical Properties

The primary disadvantages of bioactive glasses are their mechanical weakness and low fracture toughness (Table 7.3) due to their amorphous structure. Hence, bioactive glasses alone have limited application in load-bearing situations owing to poor mechanical reliability. However, they can be used in combination with polymers to form composite materials having bone repair potential. Alternatively, certain Na_2O-containing glasses, such as 45S5 Bioglass, can be sintered to improve their mechanical properties, while remaining bioactive and even biodegradable for the application of bone tissue engineering.

Table 7.3

Mechanical Properties of Hydroxyapatite, 45S5 Bioglass®, Glass-Ceramics, and Human Cortical Bone

Ceramics	Compression Strength (MPa)	Tensile Strength (MPa)	Elastic Modulus (GPa)	Fracture Toughness (MPa) $\sqrt{m}$
Hydroxyapatite	>400	~40	~100	~1.0
45S5 Bioglass®	~500	42	35	0.5–1
Cortical bone	130–180	130–150	10–30	6–12

Sources: Hench, L.L. and J. Wilson, An Introduction to Bioceramics, 2nd edn., Word Scientific, London, U.K., 1999; Yamamuro, T. et al., eds., Handbook of Bioactive Ceramics, CRC Press, Boca Raton, FL, 1990.)

7.3.1.4   Medical Applications of Bioactive Glasses   The advantages of 45S5 Bioglass (Figure 7.6) described earlier have allowed its successful clinical application as a treatment for periodontal disease (PerioGlas®) and as a bone filler material (NovaBone®). Bioglass implants have also been used to replace damaged middle ear bones, restoring hearing in patients. Bioactive glasses overall have gained much attention as promising tissue engineering scaffold materials.

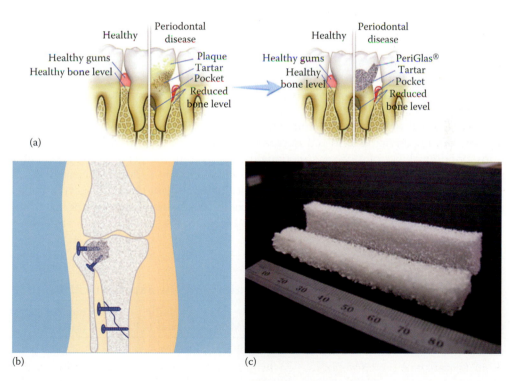

Figure 7.6
Medical applications of 45S5 Bioglass®: (a) treatment of periodontal disease with PerioGlas®, (b) filling a bone void with bone cement after tumor removal, and (c) bone tissue engineering scaffolds.

7.4 BIOACTIVE GLASS-CERAMICS

Glass-ceramics are fine-grained polycrystalline materials formed when glasses of suitable compositions are heat treated and thus undergo controlled crystallization to the lower energy crystalline state. Only specific glass compositions are suitable precursors for glass-ceramics, such as some bioactive glasses. Some glasses are too stable and difficult to crystallize (e.g., window glass), whereas others crystallize too readily in an uncontrollable manner, resulting in undesirable microstructures.

Usually a glass-ceramic is not fully crystalline; typically, the microstructure is 50–95 vol.% crystalline, with the remainder being residual glass. The mechanical properties of glass-ceramics are superior to those of the parent glass. Almost all bioactive glasses can be strengthened by the formation of crystalline particles upon heat-treatment into a glass-crystal region of its phase diagram. The resultant glass-ceramics can exhibit better mechanical properties than both the parent glass and sintered crystalline ceramics (Table 7.4). There are many biomedical glass-ceramics available for the repair of damaged bone. Among them, apatite–wollastonite (A–W), Ceravital®, and Bioverity® glass-ceramics have been intensively investigated in clinical applications [1,2].

7.4.1 A–W Glass-Ceramic

In A–W glass-ceramic, the glass matrix is reinforced by β-wollastonite ($CaSiO_3$) and a small amount of apatite phase, which precipitate successively at 870°C, and again at 900°C. Some mechanical properties of this glass-ceramic are listed in Table 7.4. The high bending strength (215 MPa) of A–W glass-ceramic is due to the precipitation of both the wollastonite and the apatite. These precipitates also give the glass-ceramic a higher fracture toughness than both the glass or ceramic phases separately. It is believed that the wollastonite effectively prevents straight propagation of cracks, causing them to turn or branch out.

A–W glass-ceramics are also capable of binding tightly to living bone in a few weeks after implantation, and the implants do not deteriorate in vivo. The excellent bone-bonding ability of A–W glass-ceramic is attributed to the glass matrix and apatite precipitates, whereas the in vivo stability as a whole implant is due to the inertness of β-wollastonite. Although the long-term integrity of A–W glass-ceramics in vivo makes them suitable for the application of nonresorbable prostheses, this does not match the goal of tissue engineering which demands a biodegradable scaffold.

Table 7.4

Mechanical Properties of Glass-Ceramics and Human Cortical Bone

Ceramics	Compression Strength (MPa)	Tensile Strength (MPa)	Elastic Modulus (GPa)	Fracture Toughness (MPa) $\sqrt{m}$
A–W	1080	215 (bend)	118	2.0
Parent Glass of A–W	NA	72 (bend)	NA	0.8
Bioverit® I	500	140–180 (bend)	70–90	1.2–2.1
Cortical bone	130–180	130–150	10–30	6–12

Sources: Hench, L.L. and J. Wilson, An Introduction to Bioceramics, 2nd edn., Word Scientific, London, U.K., 1999; Yamamuro, T. et al., eds., Handbook of Bioactive Ceramics, CRC Press, Boca Raton, FL, 1990.

7.4.2 Ceravital® Glass-Ceramics

Ceravital was coined in reference to a product made from a number of different compositions of *ceramic* and glasses (i.e., *vitreous*) materials. The basic network components of these materials include SiO_2, $Ca(PO_2)_2$, CaO, Na_2O, MgO and K_2O, with a range of ceramic additions including Al_2O_3, Ta_2O_5, TiO_2, B_2O_3, $Al(PO_3)_3$, SrO, La_2O_3 or Gd_2O_3. This material system was developed for use as solid fillers in load-bearing conditions for the replacement of bone and teeth. It turned out, however, that their mechanical properties did not serve this purpose. The surface bioactivity of Ceravital products is such that the long-term stability of the materials is eventually compromised, however this degradability is a useful property in many other tissue engineering applications.

7.4.3 Bioverit® Glass-Ceramics

Bioverit products are mica-apatite glass-ceramics. Mica crystals (aluminum silicate minerals) give these materials good machinability, and apatite crystals ensure the bioactivity of the implants. The mechanical properties of Bioverit materials (Table 7.4) allow them to be used effectively as fillers in dental application, and implants are resistant to hydrolytic degradation in vivo.

7.5 BONE-BONDING MECHANISMS

As early as in 1969, Larry Hench discovered that certain silicate glass compositions had not only excellent biocompatibility but also the ability to bond with bone. The same researchers subsequently conducted systematic studies on the bonding between bone and solid implants of Bioglass. The bone-bonding mechanisms of synthetic bioceramics (e.g., hydroxyapatites/related calcium phosphates; bioactive glasses) have since been intensively studied. The bonding strength between the host bone and the described implant materials is such that fracture of bone/implant samples often occurred in either the bone or the implant material, rather than at the interfaces, when examined after surgical retrieval (Figure 7.7). This unexpected bonding strength fascinated researchers for nearly half a century until 2004 when direct TEM observations revealed a bonding mechanism [8].

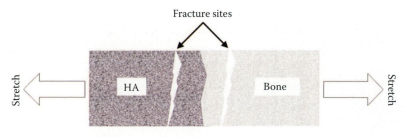

Figure 7.7
Fracture frequently occurs in either the implant or the bone examined after surgical retrieval, rather than at the interface between the two.

Historically, three fundamentally distinct mechanisms were proposed to explain bone bonding of implants:

1. Mechanical interlocking (physical bonding)
2. Chemical bonding
   - Ionic
   - Covalent
3. Biological bonding

Mechanical interlocking takes place when the implant is porous at its surface (Figure 7.8). This mechanism has been used in the surface design of metallic implants. However, unexpected bone-bonding strength has also been observed with the solid (nonporous) bioceramics. Hence, chemical bonding and biological bonding were proposed as alternative forms.

The first question is which chemical bonding could be possible in these bone-bonding phenomena. To find the answer, let us first look at all chemical bonds in

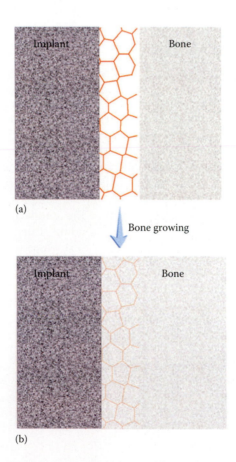

Figure 7.8
Mechanical interlocking on the porous surface of an implant. (a) Immediatly after implantation. (b) Host bone grows into the porous surface of the implant after several weeks.

Table 7.5

Strength of Chemical Bonds

Bond Type		Length (nm)	Typical Strength (kcal/mol)	
			In Vacuum	In Water
Covalent		0.15	90	90
Noncovalent	Ionic	0.25	80	1–3
	Hydrogen	0.30	4	1
	van der Waals	0.35	0.1	0.1

the body. Covalent bonds bind atoms to form molecules; however, there are three main types of noncovalent bonding between macromolecules in cells and tissue:

1. Ionic bonds
2. Hydrogen bonds
3. van der Waals attractions

The strength of these chemical bonds is summarized in Table 7.5.

Larry Hench proposed that all three noncovalent bonds were responsible for bonding between bone and bioceramics. However, Table 7.5 tells us that hydrogen and van der Walls bonds are far too weak. Ionic bonds, which are compressively strong in a dry condition, become as weak as hydrogen bonds once in an aqueous environment. Hence, only covalent bonding could provide the high level of strength revealed in these experiments. However, it is hard to envisage how hydroxyapatite and collagen proteins in the host bone could covalently bond with a bioceramic or Ti alloy (Figure 4.16).

In the 1970s, researchers from the field of medical science proposed a biological bonding theory, in which collagen fibers inserted into the bioactive material, and thus strengthened and toughened the interface [9]. The biological bonding via the insertion of collagen into biomaterials can well account for the range of bond strength observed experimentally. One may argue that this represents covalent bonding, since the collagen fiber molecular chains (polymer chains) are involved in the strengthening mechanism. However, the mechanisms of chemical bonding and biological bonding of bone to material are different (Figure 7.9). In the chemical bonding mechanisms proposed by Hench, the interface is strengthened by the chemical bonds built between the biological tissues and the implanted material (Figure 7.9a). In the biological bonding mechanism, the interface is strengthened by the covalent bonds within the collagen fibers that grow into the material (Figure 7.9b). In 2004, Chen and coworkers carried out a thorough investigation on the bone-bonding mechanism using transmission electron microscopy (Figure 7.10) [8]. A comparison of Figures 7.9 and 7.10 immediately reveals that a complex form of biological bonding is the primary mechanism.

A further question is whether pure chemical or biological bonding alone can provide strong and tough mechanical performance in bone-ceramic systems. The chemical bonding between an apatite layer (e.g., by epitaxial growth) and an implanted HA crystal should in theory be ionic in nature, like the chemical bonding within the HA crystal itself, and thus should be just as brittle. Hence, chemical bonding alone cannot toughen the interface. On the other hand, flexible collagen fibers alone cannot harden the interface without the resistance of strong HA crystallites. It is very likely that the biological interdigitation of collagen fibers with HA and chemical bonding between an

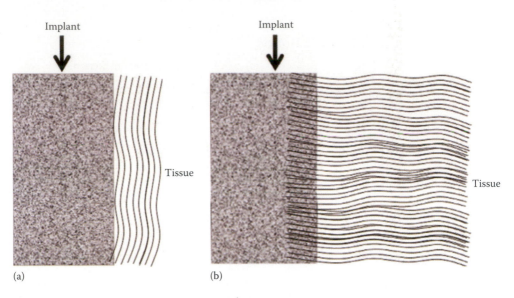

Figure 7.9
(a) Covalent bonding between implant and tissues. (b) Biological bonding.

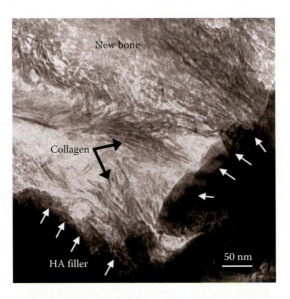

Figure 7.10
In biological bonding, collagen fibers insert into the surface layer of the hydroxyapatite implant at 3-month follow-up, delineated by the arrows. (From Chen, Q.Z. et al., Biomaterials, 25, 4243, 2004.)

apatite layer and the implant surface are both necessary in strengthening and toughening an HA/bone interface. In addition, osteoblast processes might invade into and degrade the surface layer of the implant, laying down collagen and new HA, which eventually ossifies to create a fibrous crystalline lattice.

To understand this complex bone-bonding mechanism, it is necessary to reiterate the chemistry and microstructure of bone matrix first. Hydroxyapatite $Ca_{10}(PO_4)_6(OH)_2$ accounts for nearly two-thirds of the weight of bone. These inorganic components

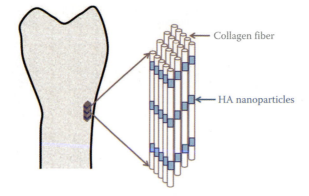

Figure 7.11
The microstructure of natural bone: collagen fibers reinforced with nano-sized CHA.

provide compression strength to bone. The remaining roughly one third of the weight of bone is from collagen fibers. These fibers are tough and flexible, and thus tolerate stretching, twisting, and bending. In natural bone, hydroxyapatite is always carbonated, with a significant amount of PO_4^{3-} being substituted by CO_3^{2-}. Natural bone is actually a polymer-matrix ceramic reinforced composite, with the collagen fiber network being strengthened by nano-sized carbonated hydroxyapatite (CHA) (Figure 7.11).

Now let us look at again what has been discovered at the interface of bone-ceramics. Although the chemical bonding mechanisms proposed in the studies of Hench and coworkers on Bioglass were less likely to occur in reality, their work revealed a number of important discoveries, among which the foremost is the formation of CHA on the surface of an implant as a critical step in the establishment of bone bonding [1,2]. Although the chemical bonding mechanism has proved to be incorrect, Hench's work supports the biological bonding mechanism. It has been revealed that through interfacial and cell-mediated reactions, bioactive glass develops a calcium-deficient, carbonated calcium phosphate surface layer that allows it to chemically bond to host bone. This bone-bonding behavior is referred to as material bioactivity, and has been associated with the formation of similar films on the surfaces of glass materials in contact with biological fluids. The stages that are involved in forming the bone bond of bioactive glasses and bioactive glass-ceramics were later summarized by Hench as shown in Figure 7.12. Although many chemical details of this complex process remain unknown, it is clearly recognized that for a bond with bone tissue to occur, a layer of biologically active CHA must form at the bone–material interface (stages 4 and 5). This conclusion is based on the finding that *CHA is the only common characteristic of all the known bioactive implant materials.* It is now widely recognized that the formation of CHA on the surface of an implant is the critical step prior to bone bonding.

The chemistry and microstructure of natural bone tell us that there is natural, intrinsic intimacy between collagen and CHA, and they would readily accept each other whenever they meet. The discovery of Hench regarding the critical step of CHA indicates that for collagen to grow in, synthetic HA and other biomaterials must first become carbonated, and that only CHA can be recognized and accepted by collagen and other biological macromolecules as appropriate minerals.

Although biological bonding involves more complexity than the chemical mechanisms proposed originally, the following two aspects represent key mechanisms. First, naturally

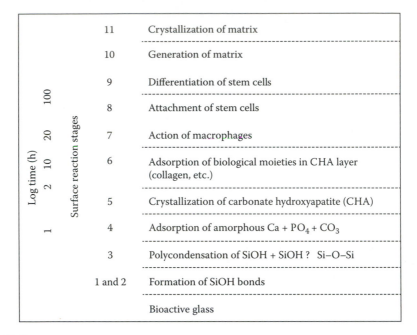

Log time (h)	Surface reaction stages	Stage	Reaction
		11	Crystallization of matrix
		10	Generation of matrix
		9	Differentiation of stem cells
100		8	Attachment of stem cells
20		7	Action of macrophages
10		6	Adsorption of biological moieties in CHA layer (collagen, etc.)
2		5	Crystallization of carbonate hydroxyapatite (CHA)
		4	Adsorption of amorphous $Ca + PO_4 + CO_3$
1		3	Polycondensation of SiOH + SiOH ? Si–O–Si
		1 and 2	Formation of SiOH bonds
			Bioactive glass

Figure 7.12

Sequence of interfacial reactions involved in forming a bond between bone and bioactive ceramics and glasses. (From Hench, L.L. and J. Wilson, An Introduction to Bioceramics, 2nd edn., Word Scientific, London, U.K., 1999; Yamamuro, T. et al., eds., Handbook of Bioactive Ceramics, CRC Press, Boca Raton, FL, 1990.)

occurring collagen proteins and CHAs have a strong tendency to mingle with each other. Second, it is apparent that once a CHA is formed on the surface of an implant, the collagen fibers of the host tissue tend to infiltrate, thus forming a biological bonding between the implant and host tissue, depending on the orientation and thickness of the bone–material interface. Also, natural movement between the two surfaces further induces collagen because healing osteoblasts are responsive to directional stress and strain. In brief, the bone-bonding mechanism involves two major steps described as follows:

- *First step*: Formation of a CHA layer on the surface of bioactive ceramics. This occurs through a time-dependent kinetic modification of the surface, triggered by their implantation within the living bone. An ion-exchange reaction between the bioactive implant and surrounding body fluids results in the formation of a biologically active carbonate apatite layer on the implant that is chemically and crystallographically equivalent to the mineral phase in bone.
- *Second step*: The collagen fibers of host bone insert into the above carbonated apatite layer.

In the case of bioactive glasses, the composition of glass material is rapidly modified toward that of CHA upon contact with a physiological solution (Figure 7.13a), apparently via ion exchange. Concurrently, CHA crystallizes from nano-sized fibers on the surface of bioactive glasses (Figure 7.13b). In vivo, collagen fibers of the host bone grow into this carbonated apatite fibrous layer.

In the case of Ti alloy (refer to Section 4.4.3) the key question is how a CHA could form on these metallic materials, and what is the nature of the interaction. Although the

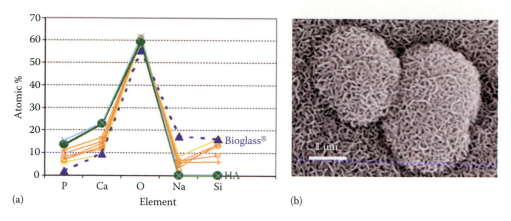

(a)   Element   (b)

Figure 7.13

Changes in chemical composition on the surface of Bioglass® during soaking in a simulated body fluid. (a) The blue line represents the original composition of the bioactive glass. The green line represents the composition of hydroxyapatite. The orange lines are the experimental data measured during the soaking. (b) Carbonated crystalline hydroxyapatite formed on the surface of Bioglass.

aforementioned process is still not fully understood, a widely accepted mechanism has been proposed by Kokubo and coworkers [10]. In their work, after being treated with 10 M NaOH aqueous solution and subsequently heat-treated at 600°C, Ti alloys had a thin sodium titanate (Na_2TiO_3) layer formed on its surfaces. Amorphous sodium titanate exchanges Na^+ for H_3O^+ and forms hydrated titania on the implant surface. The Ti–OH groups in this hydrated titania then induce the formation of carbonated apatite. Hence, a similar mechanism has been proposed for the bonding between bone and Ti alloys. That is,

- *First step*: Titanate (e.g., Na_2TiO_3) forms on the surface of Ti alloy via ion exchange, and further exchanges ions with the surrounding solution, resulting in the formation of carbonated apatite.
- *Second step*: The collagen fibers of the host bone insert into the carbonated apatite layer.

7.6   BIODEGRADABLE CERAMICS

The third generation of biomaterials aims to assist tissue regeneration, by ultimately being completely replaced by host tissue. Hence, biocompatibility and degradability are two essential properties. The following types of biomaterials represent degradable bioceramics:

- Amorphous hydroxyapatite
- Amorphous calcium phosphates
- Silicate glasses and glass-ceramics

One aspect that makes bioactive glasses different from hydroxyapatites and calcium phosphates is the possibility of controlling a range of chemical properties, rates of bonding to tissue and degradation kinetics. It is possible to design glasses with properties specific to a particular clinical application.

7.6.1   Biodegradation Mechanisms of Amorphous Structures

Ion exchange between implants and dissolved moieties in aqueous biological environ-ments is slow but inevitable, similar to erosion. Ion diffusion breaks down materials into fine pieces (Figure 7.14), which continues until sufficiently small-sized particles can be cleared by cells, a process called phagocytosis, or until ions are dissolved into body fluids solution and drained by the vascular systems. The chemical bonds of silica (O=Si=O) (Figure 7.14a) are difficult to be broken by body fluid. However, Na^+ ions can be easily displaced from the chemical network of Na−O−Na, leading to structural weakening. Hence the addition of Na_2O into the silicate network can significantly enhance the biodegradation kinetics (Figure 7.14b).

7.6.2   Biodegradation Mechanisms of Crystalline Structures

These mechanisms are very much similar to those of amorphous glass networks, that is, via ion exchange between the implant material and the fluid environment. Ion dif-fusion distorts the periodic, regular shape of the crystal network to such an extent that an amorphous structure eventually forms (Figure 7.15). This has been observed in sintered 45S5 Bioglass-ceramics (Figure 7.16) [7]. The amorphous structure then breaks down into fine pieces or even ions, which can be cleared by the physiological system of the body.

7.6.3   Design of Degradation Kinetics of Degradable Biomaterials

In principle, the degradation of degradable biomaterials should occur in a timed/timely fashion that matches the healing kinetics of host tissue. In Figure 7.17, the mechanical strength of a healthy bone is represented by the green line. If the healing kinetics of an injured bone in terms of mechanical strength is represented by the red curve, the degradation kinetics of the implant material should ideally follow the profile of the blue curve, that is:

Strength of plate + Strength of healing bone = Strength of healthy bone

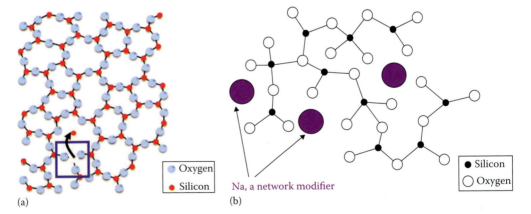

(a)

(b)

Oxygen
Silicon
Na, a network modifier

Silicon
Oxygen

Figure 7.14
Ion diffusion breaks down amorphous networks into fine pieces: (a) hard to break Si−O bonds; (b) easy to break Na−O bonds.

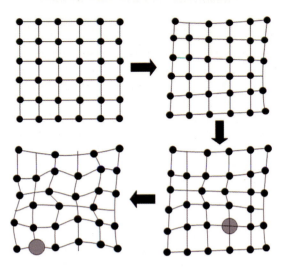
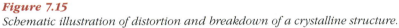

Figure 7.15
Schematic illustration of distortion and breakdown of a crystalline structure.

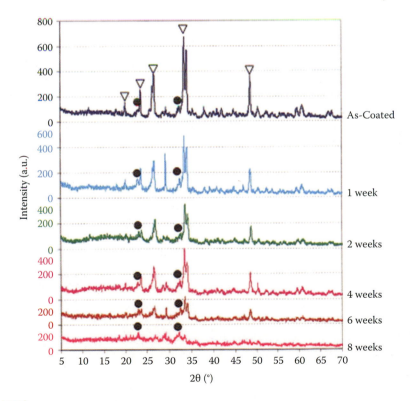

Figure 7.16
X-ray spectra of sintered Bioglass®-ceramics soaked in a simulated body fluid. The crystalline diffraction peaks continuously reduced with soaking time, and eventually an amorphous spectrum was obtained from samples soaked for 8 weeks.

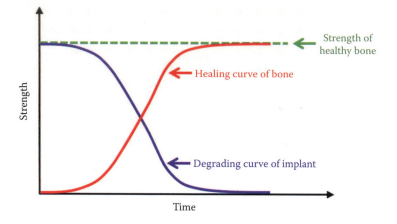

Figure 7.17
The design of blue curve depends on the knowledge about the red curve, which however remains to be elucidated.

The healing rate of injured or diseased tissue changes from one patient to another, and from one anatomical location to another within the body of the same patient. The design of a degradation profile of biomaterials therefore relies on the knowledge of healing kinetics of bone. Unfortunately, the latter largely remains unexplored.

7.6.4 How to Tune Bioactivity and Degradation Kinetics of Bioceramics

As mentioned previously, the biological reactivity of ceramics depends on their composition and crystallinity. Diffusion, a key step in the degradation mechanism, is much faster in amorphous (loosely packed) than crystalline (closely packed) structures. Hence there are various methods available to engineer either parameter:

- Crystallinity can be changed via composition (Figure 7.2).
- Cooling rate is another effective method to change crystallinity. Figure 7.18 is a typical T-t-t diagram of solidification kinetics. Crystallization solidification involves thermal motion of atoms, which needs time to start (t_{start}) and end (t_{end}). The starting and ending times both vary with the temperature at which the material is solidified, typically exhibiting C-shape (blue and green curves in Figure 7.18). If the cooling rate is high such that there is not sufficient time for crystallization to start (e.g., the yellow cooling curve 1), the liquid structure will be frozen down at room temperature. This is how fully glassy materials are produced. The cooling rate 2 (yellow line 2) will lead to a fully crystalline material, and the cooling rate 3 will result in a partially glass and partially crystalline material.
- Change of chemical composition can systematically tune bioactivity and degradation kinetics of any biomaterial type, as illustrated in Figure 7.5.

7.7 CHAPTER HIGHLIGHTS

1. In the field of biomaterials, *bioactive* often refers to a material that, upon being placed within the human body, interacts with the surrounding tissue.

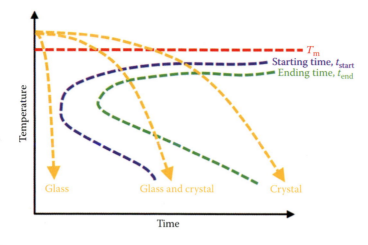

Figure 7.18
A T-T-T diagram of solidification.

2. Three types of bioactive/biodegradable ceramics:
   a. Hydroxyapatite and related calcium phosphates
   b. Bioactive glasses
   c. Glass-ceramics
3. The biological apatite (bone mineral) is substituted, usually calcium deficient and always carbonate $(CO_3)^{2-}$ substituted. The composition of bone mineral can be written as follows:

$$(Ca/Mg/Zn/Na/K)_{10}(PO_4/CO_3)_6(OH/F/Cl/CO_3)_2$$

4. *Osteoinduction* is the ability to induce bone formation. *Osteoconduction* is the ability to encourage the growth of host bone tissue into the structure of the implant or onto the surface of the graft.
5. The dissolution rate decreases in the following order:

   Amorphous CaP > Amorphous HA > Crystalline CaP > Crystalline HA.

6. Biological bonding is the primary bone-bonding mechanism, which involves two major steps:
   • *First step:* Formation of a CHA layer on the surface of bioactive ceramics. This occurs through a time dependent modification of the surface, triggered by their implantation within the living bone. An ion-exchange reaction between the bioactive implant and surrounding body fluid, results in the formation of a biologically active carbonate apatite layer on the implant that is chemically and crystallographically equivalent to the mineral phase in bone.
   • *Second step:* The collagen fibers of host bone insert into the CHA layer.
7. The biological interdigitation of collagen fibers with HA and chemical bonding of an apatite layer on the surface of HA implant are both necessary in strengthening and toughening an HA/bone interface.

8. Ion exchange between bioceramics and the surrounding physiological fluid is the main biodegradation mechanism of bioceramics.
9. The biological reactivity of ceramics can be tuned through their composition and crystallinity.

LABORATORY PRACTICE 3

The effect of surface defects (scratches) on the mechanical properties of glass materials.

SIMPLE QUESTIONS IN CLASS

1. A main component of bone is substituted with hydroxyapatite $Ca_{10}(PO_4)_6(OH)_2$. What is the phosphate usually substituted by?
   a. F–
   b. CO_3^{2-}
   c. Cl⁻
   d. OH⁻
2. A main component of bone is substituted with hydroxyapatite $Ca_{10}(PO_4)_6(OH)_2$. What is the hydroxyl ion usually substituted by?
   a. F⁻
   b. CO_3^{2-}
   c. Cl⁻
   d. Mg
3. Why does fluoridation make teeth more resistant to decay?
   a. Fluorine coating
   b. The closer coordination of element F, as compared to hydroxyl, to the nearest calcium
   c. Corrosion resistance of fluorine
   d. Decreased dissolubility of apatite
4. What would you do to develop a bioactive glass that degrades faster than the existing one?
   a. Increase the CaO component.
   b. Reduce the Na_2O component.
   c. Increase the Na_2O component.
   d. Increase the MgO component.
5. What would you do to develop a bioactive glass that degrades slower than the existing one?
   a. Increase the CaO component.
   b. Reduce the Na_2O component.
   c. Increase the Na_2O component.
   d. Increase the MgO component.
6. Which one of the following compounds most resembles the inorganic minerals in bone?
   a. Calcium phosphate
   b. Hydroxyapatite
   c. Magnesium hydroxyapatite
   d. Carbonated apatite

7. Which of following materials is virtually bioinert?
   a. Crystalline HA
   b. Amorphous calcium phosphate
   c. Amorphous HA
   d. Crystallized Na_2O-containing bioactive glasses
8. Which of following materials is biodegradable?
   a. Crystalline HA
   b. Crystalline calcium phosphate
   c. Crystallized Na_2O-free, silica bioactive glasses $-Ca(SiO_3)_2$
   d. Crystallized Na_2O-containing bioactive glasses

PROBLEMS AND EXERCISES

1. Describe the essential clinical requirements of the three generations of bioceramics, and their main features in terms of biostability.
2. Does HA and Bioglass bond to bone via chemical or biological bonds? Describe the mechanism by which synthetic HA and Bioglass bonds to bone. What is the difference between chemical boning and biological bonding?
3. Do amorphous or crystalline materials biodegrade faster? Explain your answer.
4. Describe the strategies to change biodegradability of bioceramics.
5. If the healing kinetics of a damaged bone is as follows (the red line):

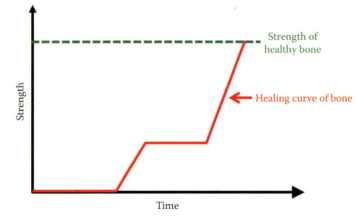

draw the ideal degradation kinetics of the bone implant.
6. What is the major reason for the enhanced cavity resistance of teeth following fluoridation?
7. What are the typical components in bioactive glasses? Explain why bioactive glasses are generally biocompatible?
8. The density of bioactive glasses is typically 2.7 g/cm^3. A porous sample of the material is 1.5 cm^3 and weighs 0.9 g. Calculate the porosity of the scaffold, using Equation 7.1.
9. The tensile strength of a sintered (crystalized) bioactive glass is 45 MPa. Calculate the mechanical strength of a fully open ($p = 78\%$) or fully closed scaffold ($p = 78\%$, $\phi = 0.5$) made from this material, using Equation 7.2 or 7.3.
10. Is it possible that the mechanical strength of a real scaffold is higher than the theoretical value? Explain your answer.

ADVANCED TOPIC: BIOCERAMIC SCAFFOLDS FOR BONE TISSUE ENGINEERING

Principles of Tissue Engineering

Tissue engineering, a term formally coined in 1987, has emerged as a distinct scientific field from the historical evolution of medicine. In this evolutionary development, the fundamental of health care in the conventional practice of medicine remains with us in tissue engineering; that is, the body heals itself [1]. This principle is based on the fact that the organs of the body have an ability to regenerate and recover when they are diseased or injured. Regeneration of serious tissue damage, however, can only occur within limits such that recovery is usually not without some form of medical or surgical intervention.

In conventional medical treatment, practitioners support a patient's vital functions by optimizing the environment most conductive to healing. Basically, physicians attempt to neutralize hostile factors and at the same time enhance the supply of oxygen and nutrients that the body needs for the healing process. Surgeons eliminate hostile factors through excising the necrotic or malign tissue that is the source of unfavorable chemical agents, reconstructing tissue through the suture of the remaining tissue, auto-/allo-/xeno-transplantation, or implantation of prosthesis, and manipulating the local environment to help the body heal itself by, for example, medication and blood supply [2].

In tissue engineering, we strive to achieve exactly the same goal. Surgeons remove the dead or malign tissue. But rather than the remaining tissues being sutured, organs being transplanted or prosthesis being implanted, living cells can now be harvested and expanded in vitro, and a designed scaffold is used to dictate the regeneration of the shape and function of the desired tissue by providing structural cues. Then the scaffold which is cultured with sufficient cells is implanted, and the tissue engineers and surgeons manipulate the local environment in precisely the same manner as the physician. Under ideal conditions, this will then enable the body to heal itself. It is when the attention of medical treatment was focused on the regeneration of living tissues in the laboratory (i.e., ex vivo) that aspects of reconstructive surgery came to be called tissue engineering [2]. In summary, tissue engineering induces the regeneration ability of the host body through a designed scaffold that is populated with cells and/or signaling molecules, aiming at regenerating functional tissue as an alternative to conventional organ transplantation and tissue reconstruction.

The aforementioned definition of tissue engineering is a specific concept. Tissue engineering has been generally defined as "the application of principles and methods of engineering and life sciences to obtain a fundamental understanding of structure–function relationships in normal and pathological mammalian tissue and the development of biological substitutes to restore, maintain, or improve tissue function" [3]. Other similar definitions exist. In 1993 Langer and Vacanti [4] defined tissue engineering as "an interdisciplinary field that applies the principles of engineering and life sciences toward the development of biological substitutes that restore, maintain or improve tissue function." In 1995, Galletti, Hellman and Nerem [5] defined tissue engineering as "the basic science and development of biological substitutes for implantation into the body or the fostering of tissue remodeling for the purpose of replacing, repeating, regenerating, reconstructing, or enhancing biological function."

Rationale for Bone Tissue Engineering

There are several clinical reasons to develop bone tissue engineering processes and practices. Although transplantation and implantation are standard methods in conventional treatment of tissue damage, shortcomings are encountered with their usage [6]. First, the application of bone grafts is limited by the size of the defect and the viability of the host body. There can be significant donor site morbidity in autografting and donor tissue scarcity for allografting. Allografting also introduces the risk of disease due to transmission of infection. Second, the revolution of material implantation, which has led to a remarkable increase in the quality of life for millions of patients in the last 30 years, has run its course. Orthopedic prostheses have an excellent 15 year survivability of 75%–85%. However, there is a requirement of longer than 30 year survivability of implants, now that the population is aging [7–9].

Tissue engineering will ultimately have a more profound impact on our life than we can now appreciate. Its technical significance lies in that this treatment will address the transplantation crisis caused by donor scarcity, immune rejection, and pathogen transfer [10]. This revolution will also reach a goal of more than 30-year implant survivability.

Tissue Engineering Approaches

The approaches of tissue engineering are established on the fact that living bodies have the potential of regeneration, and on the supposition that the employment of natural biology (e.g., cells and biomolecules) of the living body will maximize the capacity for regeneration. This will allow for greater success in developing therapeutic strategies aimed at the replacement, repair, maintenance, and enhancement of tissue function [11].

In essence, tissue engineering is a methodology that imitates nature. Natural tissues consist of three components: cells, extracellular matrix (ECM), and signaling systems. The ECM is made up of a complex of cell secretions and structural macromolecules immobilized in spaces and thus forming a scaffold for its cells, allowing cell collectives to form and communicate with each other. Hence, in a similar way, an engineered tissue construct is a triad [2], the three constituents of which correspond to the aforementioned three basic components of natural tissues. Figure 7.19 illustrates this tissue engineering triad, that is, living cells, scaffolds, and the signal molecules that mediate function.

New functional living tissue is generated by living cells in the triad system, like in a natural biological system. But the regeneration in the engineered system is achieved with the guide of a scaffold. Such scaffolds can be natural, man-made, or a composite of both. The use of signaling molecules has the potential to markedly increase scaffold effectiveness. Living cells can migrate into the implant after implantation (acellular approach) or can be associated with the matrix in cell culture before implantation (cellular approach). Such cells can be isolated as fully differentiated cells of the tissue they are hoped to be involved in repairing, or they can be manipulated to produce the desired function when isolated from other tissues or stem cell sources. These two types of approaches in tissue engineering are summarized in Table 7.6 [6,12]. In both approaches, the tissue-like matrix (scaffold, template) to which specific cell types are attached either in vivo or in vitro is one of the most important components in the engineering of new functional tissues.

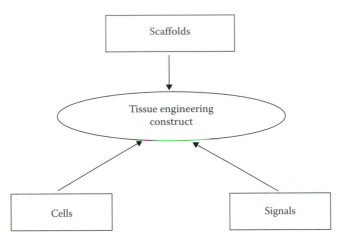

Figure 7.19

The tissue engineering triad. (From Bell, E., Tissue engineering in perspective, in Principles of Tissue Engineering, R.P. Lanza, R. Langer, and J.P. Vacanti, eds., Academic Press, San Diego, CA, 2000, pp. xxxv–xli.)

Table 7.6

Two Approaches of Tissue Engineering

1. Acellular approach

   This approach relies on guided regeneration of tissue materials that serve as templates for ingrowth of host cells and tissue in vivo.

2. Cellular approach

   This approach relies on cells that have been cultured with scaffold in vitro and then implanted as part of an engineered device. The success of such a cell-based approach for tissue engineering of bone repair is critically dependent on the developments of an ECM-like scaffold for cell delivery.

Sources: Burg, K.J.L. et al., Biomaterials, 21, 2347, 2000; Vacanti, J.P. and Vacanti, C.A., The history and scope of tissue engineering, in Principles of Tissue Engineering, R.P. Lanza, R. Langer, and J.P. Vacanti, eds., Academic Press, San Diego, CA, 2000, pp. 3–7.

Challenges in Tissue Engineering and Ideal Scaffolds

Tissue engineering involves many disciplines, including anatomy; cell, molecular, and developmental biology; immunology; materials science, and branches of engineering. Hence, the advancement of tissue engineering depends on the progress and integration of science and technology gained in each of these fields. Being a very much fledgling discipline compared to medicine, tissue engineering encounters a variety of challenges, which can be grouped into three categories associated with the science and technology of cells, materials, and interaction between them, as summarized in Table 7.7 [11]. The challenges that the material scientists encounter are linked with the required properties of ideal scaffolds. An ideal scaffold should mimic the ECM of the tissue that is to be engineered, depending on the tissue type. For bone regeneration, the biggest challenge is a scaffold suitable to replace large cortical bone defects and capable of mechanical load transmission. The specific criteria for an ideal scaffold for bone regeneration are listed in Table 7.8.

Table 7.7
Three Categories of Challenges in Tissue Engineering

1. Challenges associated with cells

   The understanding of cells and cell technology, including cell sourcing, the manipulation of cell function, and the future use of stem cell technology. The discovery that embryonic stem cells can be recovered from human fetal tissue and propagated for long periods without losing their toti- or pluripotency has a huge impact on tissue engineering, for example, bone marrow stem cells. Stem cells, together with signaling molecules, play an important role in tissue and organ development. How to direct their differentiation is a subject of high current interest.

2. Challenges associated with biomaterials and scaffolds

   The design and fabrication of tissue-like materials to provide a scaffold or template. It has been documented that there are certain biocompatible materials that enable cells to be seeded onto a synthetic scaffold, and that some types of cells are capable of undergoing subsequent differentiation to generate new functional tissue after being cultivated in vitro and implanted with scaffold into living bodies. Bone cells are in this category. One of the challenges in bone tissue engineering is to develop ECM-like scaffolds that can deliver cells, provide proper mechanical stability, and be degradable at the desired rate until replaced by newly formed bone.

3. Challenges associated with interaction between cells and scaffolds

   Integration into living systems. The interface between the cells and the scaffold must be clearly understood so that the interface can be optimized. Their design characteristics are major challenges for the field of bone tissue engineering, and should be considered at a molecular and chemical level.

Source: Nerem, R.M., The challenge of imitating nature, in Principles of Tissue Engineering, R.P. Lanza, R. Langer, and J.P. Vacanti, eds., Academic Press, San Diego, CA, 2000, pp. 9–15.

Design Considerations of Bioceramic Scaffolds

Ideal Porous Structure for Tissue Engineering Applications   A void in foam is a called *pore* or *cell*. If the material contains only pore edges (struts), the foam is termed open-pore, or reticulate foam. If the substance also exists in the form of pore faces, the foam is termed a closed-pore product and the individual pores are isolated from one another. There is clearly the possibility that porous materials can be partly open and partly closed [16,17]. Porous materials with very high porosities (above ~70%) are usually called foams or cellular solids. Below ~70%, there is a transition from a cellular structure to one which is better thought of as a solid that contains isolated pores [18].

The structure of an organ and tissue varies with its location in the body. Hence, the selection of porous configurations, as well as appropriate biomaterials, will depend on the anatomic site for regeneration, the mechanical loads present at the site, and the desired rate of incorporation. Ideally, the scaffold should be porous to support cell penetration, ingrowth, vascularization and nutrient delivery. Also, its degradation kinetics should be a match of the temporal profile of the healing process of injured tissues [19,20]. It should be mentioned that although the degradability of a scaffold is generally desirable for applications in tissue engineering, there are clinical scenarios when nondegradable biomaterials find applications, such as biostable polymers (polyurethane and polytetrafluoroethylene) used in the treatment of congenial heart defects [21]. For bone tissue engineering, there are few degradable bioceramics (e.g., 45S5 Bioglass®). However, the excellent biocompatibilities of nondegradable

Table 7.8
Criteria of an Ideal Scaffold for Bone Engineering

1. Ability to deliver cells

   The material should not only be biocompatible (i.e., harmless), but also foster cell attachment, differentiation, and proliferation.

2. Osteoconductivity

   It would be best if the material encourages osteoconduction with host bone. Osteoconductivity not only eliminates the formation of encapsulating tissue but also brings about a strong bond between the scaffold and host bone.

3. Biodegradability

   The composition of the material, combined with the porous structure of the scaffold, should lead to biodegradation in vivo at rates appropriate to tissue regeneration.

4. Mechanical properties

   The mechanical strength of the scaffold, which is determined by both the properties of the biomaterial and the porous structure, should be sufficient to provide mechanical stability to construct in load-bearing sites prior to synthesis of new ECM by cells.

5. Porous structure

   The scaffold should have an interconnected porous structure with porosity >90% and diameters between 300 and 500 μm for cell penetration, tissue ingrowth and vascularization, and nutrient delivery.

6. Fabrication

   The material should possess desired fabrication capability, for example, being readily produced into irregular shapes of scaffolds that match the defects in bone of individual patients.

7. Commercialization

   The synthesis of the material and fabrication of the scaffold should be suitable for commercialization.

Sources: Bruder, S.P. and Caplan, A.I., Bone regeneration through cellular engineering, in Principles of Tissue Engineering, R.P. Lanza, R. Langer, and J.P. Vacanti, eds., Academic Press, San Diego, CA, 2000, pp. 683–696; Jones, J.R. and Hench, L.L., Curr. Opin. Solid State Mater. Sci., 7, 301, 2003; Jones, J.R. and Boccaccini, A.R., Cellular ceramics in biomedical applications: Tissue engineering, in Cellular Ceramics: Structure, Manufacturing, Processing and Applications, M. Scheffler and P. Colombo, eds., Wiley-VCH Verlag GmbH & Co. KGaA, Weinheim, Germany, 2005, pp. 550–573.

bioceramics, such as hydroxyapatite and related calcium phosphates [22], have minimized the detrimental effects of persisting foreign bodies.

The ideal porous structure that promotes vasculature and tissue ingrowth has not been determined, and there is significant controversy regarding the optimal porosity and pore size (i.e., the diameter of the void space). It was initially thought that a pore size in the range of 100 μm was sufficient to allow for a scaffold's vascularization and tissue growth following transplantation, based on estimates of oxygen diffusion limits in tissues. Subsequent research work indicated that a pore size of ~300 μm or more might be necessary for the cell seeding efficiency and the homogeneity of the tissue engineered [19,20,23–26]. Indeed, the major disadvantage of most scaffolds reported to date is that cells tend to adhere only to the outer layer of the scaffolds [26]. This may partially explain why most scaffolds failed to vascularize, independent of their material properties [23].

Mechanical Properties of Porous Scaffolds   The requirement of the mechanical properties of scaffolds depends on the anatomic site for regeneration and the mechanical loads present at the site. To engineer bone, for example, which is strong and functions to support the body, the initial mechanical strength of the scaffold must be such that it can temporarily replace the mechanical function of the damaged bone until sufficient new bone tissue has formed. The mechanical strength of a highly porous network can be predicted by Gibson and Ashby's theory [27]. The relative density of a scaffold is defined as

$$p = 1 - \frac{\rho_{foam}}{\rho_{solid}} = 1 - \rho_{relative} \qquad (7.1)$$

where ρ_{foam} and ρ_{solid} represent the density of the foam and the solid material forming the scaffold respectively. The theoretical compressive collapse stress (σ_{theo}) of the foam with open or closed cells can be expressed as a function of the relative density of a cellular structure by Equation 7.2 and 7.3, respectively:

$$\frac{\sigma_{theo}}{\sigma_{fs}} = 0.2 \left(\frac{\rho_{foam}}{\rho_{solid}} \right)^{3/2} \qquad \text{(open cells)}, \qquad (7.2)$$

$$\frac{\sigma_{theo}}{\sigma_{fs}} = 0.2 \left(\phi \frac{\rho_{foam}}{\rho_{solid}} \right)^{3/2} + \left(1 - \phi\right) \left(\frac{\rho_{foam}}{\rho_{solid}} \right) \qquad \text{(closed cells)}, \qquad (7.3)$$

where
  ϕ is the fraction of material contained in the cell edges (thus $1 - \phi$ is the fraction of material distributed in the cell faces)
  σ_{fs} is the modulus of rupture of the strut

The modulus of rupture is typically about 1.1 times larger than the tensile strength in brittle materials [27].

These two equations are derived assuming that the cell walls (including cell edges and faces) are fully dense and perfectly uniform throughout the network. In reality there is no such a perfect network. The struts of a real porous scaffold vary in thickness and always contain cracks and holes [28,29]. Hence a scaffold will always prematurely rupture at these weak sites. A theoretical strength calculated from Gibson and Ashby's model (Equation 7.2 or 7.3) sets an upper boundary of compressive strength that could be achieved from a real scaffold.

Fabrication of Porous Ceramics

Porous ceramics can be produced by a variety of different processes [30], which may be classified into two categories: (1) manual-based processing techniques and (2) computer-controlled fabrication processes: rapid prototyping (RP) [31]. Manual-based processing techniques can further be divided into conventional powder-forming processes and sol–gel techniques [32]. A flowchart common to all powder forming processes is shown in Figure 7.20.

A slurry is a suspension of ceramic particles in a suitable liquid (e.g., water or ethanol) that will be used to prepare green bodies. Agglomeration of particles is caused by attractive forces which consist of hydrogen bonds, van der Waals forces, Coulomb's forces, and physical friction between particles. Porosity can be increased by adding

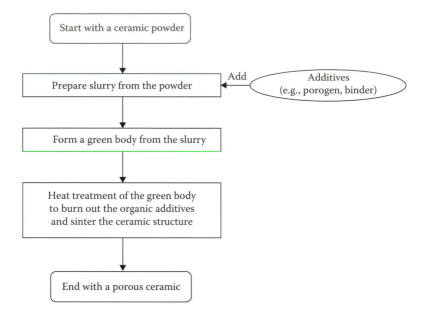

Figure 7.20
Flowchart of the powder-sintering method to produce a porous ceramic scaffold. (From Chen, Q.Z., Development of bioglass(R)-ceramic scaffolds for bone tissue engineering, in Materials Department, Imperial College London, London, U.K., 2006.)

fillers to the slurry, such as sucrose, gelatin, and PMMA micro beads and a wetting agent (i.e., a surfactant). These chemicals, which are called porogens, are evaporated or burned out during sintering, and as a result pores are formed [14,30]. One successful formulation has been the use of hydroxyapatite powder slurries (dispersed with vegetable oil) added with gelatin solution [34]. Porous scaffolds were formed with interconnected interparticle pore diameters of ~100 µm. A similar process has been used to prepare melt-derived Bioglass scaffolds using camphor ($C_{10}H_{16}O$) as the porogen [35].

Binders are also added to slurries. The most important function of the binder is to improve the strength of the green body in order to provide structural integrity for handling (green strength) before the product is sintered [32]. Frequently added binders in bioceramic slurries are polysaccharides [36], polyvinyl alcohol (PVA) [37], and polyvinyl butyl (PVB) [38].

Conventional Process: Formation of Porous Green Bodies   In porous ceramic production, a green body is porous, and its structure largely determines that of the sintered product. Table 7.9 lists different methods of obtaining porous green bodies. These methods can be classified into two categories: dry and wet processes [30]. They lead to different porous structures within green bodies. Some techniques, such as tape-casting, extrusion, slurry-dipping, and spraying, are not included here because they aim at, instead of achieving porous structure in ceramics, a geometric shape (such as rods, tubes, sheets, and coating films) of ceramic products. Except for injection-molding, all these conventional processes have been applied to synthesize ceramic scaffolds for tissue engineering.

Compaction   The simplest way to prepare green bodies is the dry process, in which the powder is directly compressed by pressing into molds or dies, thereby forming green bodies. Pore diameters decrease and mechanical properties increase as the

Table 7.9

List of Methods of Obtaining Green Bodies for 3D Porous Ceramics

Dry process
  Loose-packing
  Compaction
Uniaxial-pressing
Cold-isostatic-pressing (CIPing)
Wet process
  Slip-casting
  Injection-molding
  Phase separation/freeze-drying
  Polymer-replication
  Gel-casting

Source: Ishizaki, K. et al., Porous Materials: Processing Technology and Applications, Kluwer Academic Publisher, Dordrecht, the Netherlands, 1998, pp. 12–66.

packing density of the spheres in the green bodies increases. Mechanical properties can be altered further by hot-isostatic-pressing (HIPing), which decreases the pore diameter as well. The addition of porogens, such as sucrose and camphor, can enhance the formation of pores [30].

Slip-Casting   A slip is a creamy (relatively thick) slurry that contains solid particles. In this method, the slurry is cast into a porous mold. The liquid of the slurry is absorbed into the porous mold and as a result, the particles in the slurry are filtered and adhered on the mold surface. After this process, a porous green body is obtained through drying [17,32].

Phase Separation/Freeze-Drying   Porous structure can also be achieved through phase separation and evaporation. One approach to induce phase separation is to lower the temperature of the suspension of materials. The solvent is solidified first, forcing the polymer and ceramic mixture into the interstitial spaces. The frozen mixture is then lyophilized using a freeze-dryer, in which the ice solvent evaporates [39–42]. In a typical process with ceramics, the ceramic slurry is poured into a container which is immersed in a freezing bath. Thus, ice is stimulated to grow and ceramic particles pile up between columns of growing ice. After the slurry is completely frozen, the container is dried in a drying vessel [43].

Replication Technique   This method, which is also called the polymer-sponge method, was patented for the manufacture of ceramic foams in 1963 [44], and has been widely used to produce foams of various ceramics [45–50]. It is similar to the slip-casting technique in which ceramic particles are adhered on the mold surface. In the polymer-replication process, the green bodies of ceramic foams are prepared by coating a polymer (e.g., polyurethane) foam with a ceramic slurry. The polymer foam, having already the desired macrostructure, simply serves as a sacrificial template for the ceramic coating. The polymer template is immersed in the slurry, which subsequently infiltrates the structure and coats the ceramic particles to the surface of the polymer substrate. Excess slurry is squeezed out, leaving a ceramic coating on the foam struts. After drying, the polymer is slowly burned out in order to minimize damage to the porous coating. Once the polymer has been removed, the ceramic is sintered to

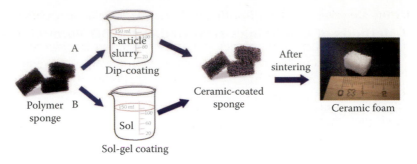

Figure 7.21
Replication technique to fabricate bioactive glass-derived scaffolds (A) using a ceramic powder; (B) combined with the sol–gel process.

the desired density. The process replicates the macroporous structure of the polymer foam, and results in a rather distinctive microstructure within the struts. A scheme of the process is given in Figure 7.21. This method has been applied for the preparation of porous calcium phosphates [51], Bioglass [52–54], and other inert bioceramics [55].

Apart from the slurry-immersion and sol–gel coating, electrospray coating techniques have also been applied together with the polymer-sponge process to produce hydroxyapatite [56], Al_2O_3 [57], and ZrO_2 [58] foams. Unlike the foams produced by the slurry-immersion method, the struts of the ceramic foams produced by electrospraying did not contain numerous holes and large cracks. This microstructure led to improved mechanical properties of the foams [57].

Gel-Casting A full term for this method should be direct-foarming/gel-casting. This method adopts mechanical stirring (one of the direct-foaming techniques listed in Table 7.10) to achieve highly porous green bodies. The foamed suspension is set through a direct-consolidation technique (Table 7.10), that is, polymerization of organic monomers (i.e., gelation) [59], in which the particles of the slurry are consolidated through polymerization reaction. A green body is formed after the gel is cast in a mold [60–62].

Table 7.10
Techniques of Direct-Foaming and Direct-Consolidation

Direct-foaming
    Injection of gasses through the fluid medium
    Mechanically agitating particulate suspension
    Blowing agents
    Evaporation of compounds
    Evaporation of gas by in situ chemical reaction
Direct-consolidation
    Gel casting
    Direct coagulation consolidation (DCC)
    Hydrolysis-assisted solidification (HAS)
    Freezing (Quick Set®)

Source: *Chen, Q.Z., Development of bioglass(R)-ceramic scaffolds for bone tissue engineering, in Materials Department, Imperial College London, London, U.K., 2006.*

Two factors are critical in the gel-casting process: (1) the gelation speed must be fast enough to prevent foam collapse; and (2) the gel rheology is important because the process involves casting. Systems of high fluidity are required in order to enable easy filling of small details in molds to allow production of high complexity shapes. Direct-foarming/gel-casting techniques have been applied to produce hydroxyapatite foams [63–65]. Gel-casting has also been combined with the replication process to produce hydroxyapatite scaffolds with interconnected pores [66].

The final step in the production of a ceramic foam is the densification of the green bodies, which are normally dried at room temperature for at least 24 h prior to sintering. In this step, controlled heating is important to prevent collapse of the ceramic network. The heating rate is 0.5°C–2°C/min for hydroxyapatite foams [51,63,65,67]. The sintering temperatures and holding time, which depend on the ceramic starting materials, are in the range of 1200°C–1350°C for 2–5 h in the case of porous hydroxyapatite [51,63,65,67].

Sol-Gel Process of Ceramic Scaffolds　The sol–gel process is defined as the chemical synthesis of ceramic materials by preparation of a sol, gelation of the sol (gel), and the removal of the solvent. That is, the sol–gel process involves the transition of a system from a liquid *sol* into a solid *gel* phase. The chemical involved in the process is based on inorganic polymerization reactions of metal alkoxide [68].

The sol–gel technique is a versatile solution process for making ceramic and glass materials. Applying the sol–gel process, it is possible to fabricate ceramic or glass materials in a wide variety of forms: ultrafine or spherical-shaped powders, thin film coatings, ceramic fibers, microporous inorganic membranes, monolithic ceramics and glasses, or extremely porous aerogel materials.

Alkoxide precursors, such as tetraethyl orthosilicate (TEOS and triethoxyl ortho-phosphate [TEP]), undergo hydrolysis and condensation reactions to form a sol. Polymerization of −Si−OH groups continued after hydrolysis is complete, beginning the formation of the silicate (−Si−O−Si−) network. The network connectivity increases until it spans throughout the solvent medium. Eventually a wet gel forms. The wet gel is then subjected to controlled thermal processes of aging to strengthen the gel, drying to remove the liquid by-product of the polycondensation reaction, and thermal stabilization (or sintering) to remove organic species from the surface of the material; and as a result, a porous aerogel or xerogel forms [14,69–71].

Highly macroporous glasses (or glass foams) have been developed by directly foaming the sol with the use of a surfactant and catalysts [72–74]. The precursors of the glass foams are $Ca(NO_3)_2$ and two alkoxides: TEOS and TEP. A flowchart of the process is given in Figure 7.22. Sol–gel derived bioactive glass foams [75,76] and gel-cast HA scaffolds [63,65] showed favorable results in both in vitro and in vivo tests for bone regeneration.

Solid Free-Form of Ceramic Scaffolds　As mentioned earlier, solid free-form (SFF) techniques are computer-controlled fabrication processes. The process chain for all SFF techniques is presented in Figure 7.23. Calcium phosphate scaffolds have been produced using the fused deposition modeling (FDM) process [77–80], selective laser sintering (SLS), 3D printing processes [31], extrusion free-forming [81] and stereo lithography [82], as well as RP combined with the replication technique [83,84]. Up to now, only a small number of SFF techniques, such as three-dimensional printing (3D-P),

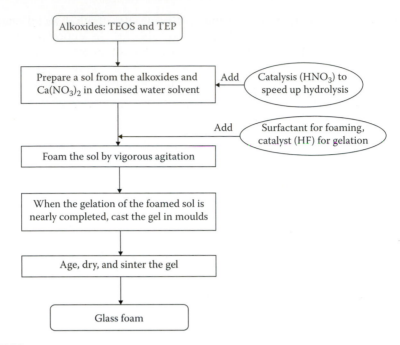

Figure 7.22

Flowchart of the production of bioactive glass foams using sol–gel technology. (From Chen, Q.Z., Development of bioglass(R)-ceramic scaffolds for bone tissue engineering, in Materials Department, Imperial College London, London, U.K., 2006; Chen, Q.Z. et al., Acta Biomater., 6, 4143, 2010.)

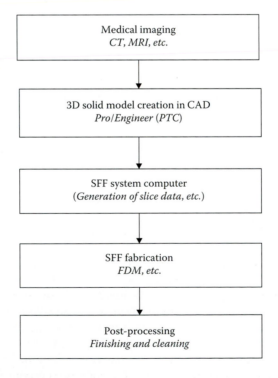

Figure 7.23

Flowchart of a typical RP process. (From Leong, K.F. et al., Biomaterials, 24, 2363, 2003.)

FDM, and SLS, have been adapted for tissue engineering scaffolds. The following paragraphs give brief introductions to the principles of these three techniques. Their technical details can be found in previous reviews available [31,85–87].

Three-Dimensional Printing   3D-p employs ink-jet printing technology for processing powder materials. Therefore, this technique is a combination of SFF and power-sintering. During fabrication, a printer head is used to print a liquid binder onto thin layers of powder following the object's profile being generated by the system computer. The subsequent stacking and printing layer recreates the full structure of the desired object.

Fused Deposition Modeling   FDM employs the concept of melt extrusion to deposit a parallel series of material roads that forms a material layer. In FDM, filament material stock (generally thermoplastic) is fed and melted inside a heated liquefier head before being extruded through a nozzle with a small orifice. An indirect fabrication method involving FDM has been applied to produce porous bioceramic implants. FDM was employed to fabricate wax molds containing the negative profiles of the desired scaffold microstructure. Ceramic scaffolds were then cast from the mold via a lost mold technique [77–80].

Selective Laser Sintering   This technique employs a CO_2 laser beam to selectively sinter polymer or polymer–ceramic composite powders to form material layers. The laser beam is directed onto the powder bed by a high-precision laser scanning system. The fusion of material layers that are stacked on top of one another replicates the object height [88,89].

Table 7.11 collects the porosity, pore size, and mechanical properties of porous ceramics produced by different techniques. Generally, they are very brittle. Eventually they become too fragile to handle when the porosity increases up to 90% [67]. An approach to improve the mechanical properties of ceramic scaffolds is to coat the scaffold network with polymeric materials [51]. However, few studies have been reported with respect to this approach.

Comparison of Fabrication Techniques for Ceramic Foams   Figure 7.24 shows typical structures of porous ceramics produced by different techniques. A comparison of the porous structures of ceramic scaffolds with that of trabecular bone reveals that the porous structure produced by the replication technique is the most similar one to that of cancellous bone, containing completely interconnective pores and solid materials forming only the struts. The ceramic foams synthesized by gel-casting and sol–gel techniques come next in terms of structural similarity to cancellous bone, but sol–gel derived foams exhibit only limited pore connectivity. Other advantages of the replication technique include (1) high commercialization potential: This technique is the simplest method, and thus most suitable for commercialization, compared with SFF. SFF rapid-prototyping is an expensive process, which may be a method for producing specific and complex scaffold architectures. (2) Safety: It does not involve any toxic chemicals, compared with sol–gel and gel-casting techniques which use HF to accelerate polymerization. (3) Irregular or complex shape production ability: It can produce a scaffold in irregular or complex shapes, compared with standard dry powder processing.

247

Table 7.11

Porous Structures and Mechanical Properties of Porous Ceramics Produced by Different Techniques

Technique	Material	Porosity (%)	Pore Size/μm	Closed (C) or Open (O)	Compressive or Flexural Strength[a]/MPa	Refs.
1. Powder-forming-sintering						
Dry process with porogens	Hydroxyapatite	NA	Predominately 0.4, but varying between 0.4–100	C	NA	[37]
	Hydroxyapatite	67	250–400	O		[90]
	45S5 Bioglass®	21	200–300	C		[35]
		42	80	C		[91]
Phase separation/freeze-drying	Al_2O_3	30–60	~50 in width, 300–500 in length	O	NA	[43]
Replication technique/coated by slurry-immersion	Al_2O_3	87	Up to 800	O	NA	[17]
	TiO_2	74	385–700	O		[36]
	Glass-reinforced HA	85–97.5	Ave: 420–560	O	0.01–0.175	[67]
	Hydroxyapatite	69–86	490–1130	O	0.03–0.29	[51]
	HA coated by PLGA	69–86	490–1130	O	0.31–4.03	[51]
Electrospray	Al_2O_3	96	~800	O		[57]
	ZrO_2	95	500–700	O	1–3	[58]
Gel-casting/foamed by						
Starch	Al_2O_3	23–70	10–80	C	NA	[60]
Vigorous stirring	Al_2O_3	70–92	Ave size:260–700 Range in 50–2000	Partly O/C	2–26[a]	[61]
	Al_2O_3	NA	NA	NA	3–20	[62]

				O/C		Ref
Replication technique	Hydroxyapatite	76.7–80.2	20–1000	Partly O/C	4.4–7.4	[63]
	Hydroxyapatite	48	50–300	Partly O/C	8[a]	[65]
	Hydroxyapatite	NA	Cell: 100–500 Window: 30–120	Partly O/C	1.6–5.8	[64]
	Hydroxyapatite	70–77	200–400	O	0.55–5	[66]
	β-TCP + HA	73	NA	O	9.8	[92]
	Bioglass	85–95	300–700	O	0.1–0.4	[52]
2. *Sol-gel/foamed by*						
a. Burning PMMA beads	$CaO–SiO_2$ glass		~0.5	Partially O/C		[93]
b. Decomposition of H_2O_2	$(CH_3O)_4Si$		< 0.7	Partially O/C		[94]
c. Burning EO–PO–EO blocks	SiO_2 glass		1–10	Partially O/C		[95]
d. Vigorous stirring	Bioactive glasses	70–95	Up to 600, size of cell windows mostly in 80–120	Partially O/C		[73]
3. *SFF*						
a. FDM	Al_2O_3	29–44	305–480	O	62–128	[96]
	β-TCP	29–44	305–480	O	0.25–1.45	[96]
	$CaO–Al_2O_3$	29–44	300	O	2–24	[97]
	PP–TCP composite	36–52	160	O	12.7–10	[78]
b. SLS	Calcium phosphates	30	200	O	13.8	[98]

Source: Chen, Q.Z., Development of bioglass(R)–ceramic scaffolds for bone tissue engineering, in Materials Department, Imperial College London, London, U.K., 2006.

[a] Flexural strength in beading of Table 7.11.

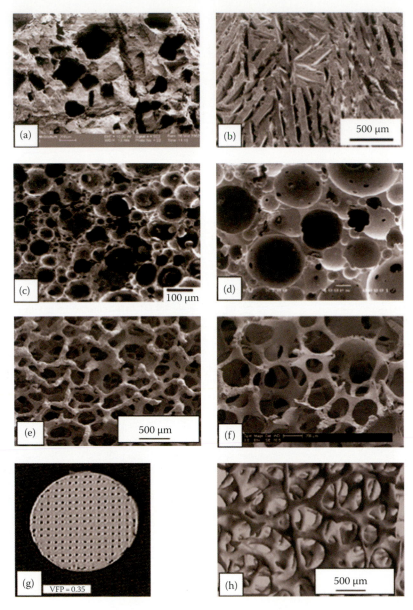

Figure 7.24

Typical structures of porous ceramics produced by different techniques. (a) Porous HA produced by the powder combined with PVA as a porogen additive. (From Tadic, D. et al., Biomaterials, 25, 3335, 2004.) (b) Porous alumina by the freeze-drying method. (From Fukasawa, T. et al., J. Mater. Sci., 36, 2523, 2001.) (c) Porous HA by the gel-casting method. (From Sepulveda, P. et al., J. Biomed. Mater. Res., 50, 27, 2000.) (d) 70S30C bioactive glass foams by the sol–gel technique. (From Sepulveda, P. et al., J. Biomed. Mater. Res., 59, 340, 2002.) (e) Porous Bioglass®-ceramic by the replication technique. (From Callcut, S. and Knowles, J.C., J. Mater. Sci. Mater. Med., 13, 485, 2002.) (f) β-TCP + HA foam produced by the gel-casting method combined with the replication technique. (From Ramay, H.R.R. and Zhang, M., Biomaterials, 25, 5171, 2004.) (g) Porous β-TCP by the SFF technique. (From Bose, S. et al., Mater. Sci. Eng. C Biomim. Supramol Syst., 23, 479, 2003.) (h) Porous structure of cancellous bone. (From Gibson, L.J., J. Biomech., 18, 317, 1985.)

Summary

A number of foaming techniques have been established to process biomaterials into porous scaffolds with large void volumes for cell seeding and sufficient surface area for cell attachment. Each technique has its advantages and disadvantages, such as ease of fabrication, unique macroporous structure, mechanical strength, or the cell seeding efficiency, but none can be considered as an ideal method of scaffold fabrication to be employed for all tissue engineering applications. Future challenges in foaming biomaterials for tissue engineering applications include the fabrication of highly porous, degradable, and yet high-strength scaffolds for tissue replacement at load-bearing sites and the ability to incorporate and deliver proteins and growth factors without being denatured. The methods reviewed in this chapter are promising ways to produce porous biomaterials for tissue regeneration and repair.

BIBLIOGRAPHY

References for Text

1. Hench, L.L. and J. Wilson, *An Introduction to Bioceramics*, 2nd edn. London, U.K.: Word Scientific, 1999.
2. Yamamuro, T., L.L. Hench, and J. Wilson, eds., *Handbook of Bioactive Ceramics*. Boca Raton, FL: CRC Press, 1990.
3. Bruder, S.P. and A.I. Caplan, Bone regeneration through cellular engineering. In *Principles of Tissue Engineering*, R.P. Lanza, R. Langer, and J.P. Vacanti, eds. San Diego, CA: Academic Press, 2000, pp. 683–696.
4. Marcacci, M. et al., Stem cells associated with macroporous bioceramics for long bone repair: 6- to 7-year outcome of a pilot clinical study. *Tissue Engineering*, 2007;**13**(5):947–955.
5. de Groot, K. et al., Chemistry of calcium phosphate bioceramics. In *Handbook of Bioactive Ceramics*, T. Yamamuro, L.L. Hench, and J. Wilson, eds. Boca Raton, FL: CRC Press, 1990, pp. 3–16.
6. Hench, L.L. and J. Wilson, Surface-active biomaterials. *Science*, 1984;**226**(4675):630–636.
7. Chen, Q.Z., I.D. Thompson, and A.R. Boccaccini, 45S5 Bioglass (R)-derived glass-ceramic scaffolds for bone tissue engineering. *Biomaterials*, 2006;**27**(11):2414–2425.
8. Chen, Q.Z. et al., Strengthening mechanisms of bone bonding to crystalline hydroxyapatite in vivo. *Biomaterials*, 2004;**25**(18):4243–4254.
9. Ganeles, J., M.A. Listgarten, and C.I. Evian, Ultrastructure of durapatiteperiodontal tissue interface in human intrabony defects. *Journal of Periodontology*, 1986;**57**:133–140.
10. Kitsugi, T. et al., Bone bonding behavior of titanium and its alloys when coated with titanium oxide (TiO_2) and titanium silicate (Ti_5Si_3). *Journal of Biomedical Materials Research*, 1996;**32**(2):149–156.

Websites

http://ceramics.org/about-us/international-ceramic-societies.
The International Society for Ceramics in Medicine. http://bioceramics.org/.

References for Advanced Topic

1. Vacanti, C.A., Foreword. In *Principles of Tissue Engineering*, R.P. Lanza, R. Langer, and J.P. Vacanti, eds. San Diego, CA: Academic Press, 2000, p. xxix.
2. Bell, E., Tissue engineering in perspective. In *Principles of Tissue Engineering*, R.P. Lanza, R. Langer, and J.P. Vacanti, eds. San Diego, CA: Academic Press, 2000, pp. xxxv–xli.

3. Skalak, R. and C.F. Fox, eds. *Tissue Engineering: Proceedings of a Workshop*, held at Granlibakken, Lake Tahoe, California, 1988. New York: Alan Liss.

4. Langer, R. and J.P. Vacanti, Tissue engineering. *Science*, 1993;**260**(5110):920–926.

5. Galletti, P.M., K.B. Hellman, and R.M. Nerem, Tissue engineering: From basic science to products. *Tissue Engineering*, 1995;**1**:147–149.

6. Burg, K.J.L., S. Porter, and J.F. Kellam, Biomaterial developments for bone tissue engineering. *Biomaterials*, 2000;**21**(23):2347–2359.

7. Hench, L.L., Biomaterials: A forecast for the future. *Biomaterials*, 1998;**19**(16):1419–1423.

8. Jones, J.R. and L.L. Hench, Materials perspective—Biomedical materials for new millennium: Perspective on the future. *Materials Science and Technology*, 2001;**17**(8):891–900.

9. Hench, L.L. and J.M. Polak, Third-generation biomedical materials. *Science*, 2002;**295**(5557):1014–1017.

10. Naughton, G.K., Emerging developments in tissue engineering and cell technology. *Tissue Engineering*, 1995;**1**:211–219.

11. Nerem, R.M., The challenge of imitating nature. In *Principles of Tissue Engineering*, R.P. Lanza, R. Langer, and J.P. Vacanti, eds. San Diego, CA: Academic Press, 2000, pp. 9–15.

12. Vacanti, J.P. and C.A. Vacanti, The history and scope of tissue engineering. In *Principles of Tissue Engineering*, R.P. Lanza, R. Langer, and J.P. Vacanti, eds. San Diego, CA: Academic Press, 2000, pp. 3–7.

13. Bruder, S.P. and A.I. Caplan, Bone regeneration through cellular engineering. In *Principles of Tissue Engineering*, R.P. Lanza, R. Langer, and J.P. Vacanti, eds. San Diego, CA: Academic Press, 2000, pp. 683–696.

14. Jones, J.R. and L.L. Hench, Regeneration of trabecular bone using porous ceramics. *Current Opinion in Solid State and Materials Science*, 2003;**7**(4–5):301–307.

15. Jones, J.R. and A.R. Boccaccini, Cellular ceramics in biomedical applications: Tissue engineering. In *Cellular Ceramics: Structure, Manufacturing, Processing and Applications*, M. Scheffler and P. Colombo, eds. Weinheim, Germany: Wiley-VCH Verlag GmbH & Co. KGaA, 2005, pp. 550–573.

16. Saggiowoyansky, J., C.E. Scott, and W.P. Minnear, Processing of porous ceramics. *American Ceramic Society Bulletin*, 1992;**71**(11):1674–1682.

17. Montanaro, L. et al., Ceramic foams by powder processing. *Journal of the European Ceramic Society*, 1998;**18**(9):1339–1350.

18. Gibson, L.J. and M.F. Ashby, *Cellular Solids: Structure and Properties*, 2nd edn. Cambridge, U.K.: Cambridge University Press, 1997, p. 2.

19. Hutmacher, D.W., Scaffolds in tissue engineering bone and cartilage. *Biomaterials*, 2000;**21**(24):2529–2543.

20. Karageorgiou, V. and D. Kaplan, Porosity of 3D biomaterial scaffolds and osteogenesis. *Biomaterials*, 2005;**26**(27):5474–5491.

21. Chen, Q.Z. et al., Biomaterials in cardiac tissue engineering: Ten years of research survey. *Materials Science and Engineering R-Reports*, 2008;**59**(1–6):1–37.

22. Wong, C.T. et al., Ultrastructural study of mineralization of a strontium-containing hydroxyapatite (Sr-HA) cement in vivo. *Journal of Biomedical Materials Research. Part A*, 2004;**70A**(3):428–435.

23. Laschke, M.W. et al., Angiogenesis in tissue engineering: Breathing life into constructed tissue substitutes. *Tissue Engineering*, 2006;**12**(8):2093–2104.

24. Eglin, D. et al., Farsenol-modified biodegradable polyurethanes for cartilage tissue engineering. *Journal of Biomedical Materials Research. Part A*, 2010;**92A**(1):393–408.

25. Rezwan, K. et al., Biodegradable and bioactive porous polymer/inorganic composite scaffolds for bone tissue engineering. *Biomaterials*, 2006;**27**(18):3413–3431.

26. Kannan, R.Y. et al., The roles of tissue engineering and vascularisation in the development of micro-vascular networks: A review. *Biomaterials*, 2005;**26**(14):1857–1875.

27. Gibson, L.J. and M.F. Ashby, *Cellular Solids: Structure and Properties*, 2nd edn. Oxford, U.K.: Pergamon Press, 1999, pp. 429–452.

28. Tulliani, J.M. et al., Semiclosed-cell mullite foams: Preparation and macro- and microme-chanical characterization. *Journal of the American Ceramic Society*, 1999;**82**(4):961–968.

29. Vedula, V.R., D.J. Green, and J.R. Hellman, Thermal shock resistance of ceramic foams. *Journal of the American Ceramic Society*, 1999;**82**(3):649–656.

30. Ishizaki, K., S. Komarneni, and M. Nanko, *Porous Materials: Processing Technology and Applications*. Dordrecht, the Netherlands: Kluwer Academic Publisher, 1998, pp. 12–66.

31. Leong, K.F., C.M. Cheah, and C.K. Chua, Solid freeform fabrication of three-dimensional scaf-folds for engineering replacement tissues and organs. *Biomaterials*, 2003;**24**(13):2363–2378.

32. Reed, J.S., *Principles of Ceramic Synthesis*, 2nd edn. Chichester, U.K.: Wiley & Sons, 1988, pp. 173–174.

33. Chen, Q.Z., Development of bioglass(R)-ceramic scaffolds for bone tissue engineering. In *Materials Department*. London, U.K.: Imperial College London, 2006.

34. Komlev, V.S. and S.M. Barinov, Porous hydroxyapatite ceramics of bi-modal pore size dis-tribution. *Journal of Materials Science. Materials in Medicine*, 2002;**13**(3):295–299.

35. Livingston, T., P. Ducheyne, and J. Garino, In vivo evaluation of a bioactive scaffold for bone tissue engineering. *Journal of Biomedical Materials Research*, 2002;**62**(1):1–13.

36. Haugen, H. et al., Ceramic TiO_2-foams: Characterisation of a potential scaffold. *Journal of the European Ceramic Society*, 2004;**24**(4):661–668.

37. Andrade, J.C.T. et al., Behavior of dense and porous hydroxyapatite implants and tis-sue response in rat femoral defects. *Journal of Biomedical Materials Research*, 2002;**62**(1):30–36.

38. Kim, H.W. et al., Porous ZrO_2 bone scaffold coated with hydroxyapatite with fluorapatite intermediate layer. *Biomaterials*, 2003;**24**(19):3277–3284.

39. Boccaccini, A.R. et al., Bioresorbable and bioactive composite materials based on polylac-tide foams filled with and coated by Bioglass (R) particles for tissue engineering applica-tions. *Journal of Materials Science. Materials in Medicine*, 2003;**14**(5):443–450.

40. Verrier, S. et al., PDLLA/Bioglass (R) composites for soft-tissue and hard-tissue engineering: An in vitro cell biology assessment. *Biomaterials*, 2004;**25**(15):3013–3021.

41. Yin, Y.J. et al., Preparation and characterization of macroporous chitosan-gelatin beta-tricalcium phosphate composite scaffolds for bone tissue engineering. *Journal of Biomedical Materials Research. Part A*, 2003;**67A**(3):844–855.

42. Zhang, R.Y. and P.X. Ma, Poly(alpha-hydroxyl acids) hydroxyapatite porous composites for bone-tissue engineering. I. Preparation and morphology. *Journal of Biomedical Materials Research*, 1999;**44**(4):446–455.

43. Fukasawa, T. et al., Pore structure of porous ceramics synthesized from water-based slurry by freeze-dry process. *Journal of Materials Science*, 2001;**36**(10):2523–2527.

44. Schwartzalder, K. and A.V. Somers, Method of making a porous shape of sintered refractory ceramic articles. United States Patent No. 3090094, 1963.

45. Bao, X., M.R. Nangrejo, and M.J. Edirisinghe, Preparation of silicon carbide foams using polymeric precursor solutions. *Journal of Materials Science*, 2000;**35**(17):4365–4372.

46. Bao, X., M.R. Nangrejo, and M.J. Edirisinghe, Synthesis of silicon carbide foams from poly-meric precursors and their blends. *Journal of Materials Science*, 1999;**34**(11):2495–2505.

47. Bao, X., M.R. Nangrejo, and M.J. Edirisinghe, Preparation of ceramic foams from poly-meric precursors. In *Ceramics: From Processing to Production*, J. Yeomans, ed. Institute of Materials, Minerals and Mining, London, UK, 2001, pp. 1–16.

48. Nangrejo, M.R., X. Bao, and M.J. Edirisinghe, Silicon carbide-titanium carbide composite foams produced using a polymeric precursor. *International Journal of Inorganic Materials*, 2001;**3**(1):37–45.

49. Nangrejo, M.R., X.J. Bao, and M.J. Edirisinghe, Preparation of silicon carbide-silicon nitride composite foams from pre-ceramic polymers. *Journal of the European Ceramic Society*, 2000;**20**(11):1777–1785.

50. Nangrejo, M.R. and M.J. Edirisinghe, Porosity and strength of silicon carbide foams pre-pared using preceramic polymers. *Journal of Porous Materials*, 2002;**9**(2):131–140.

51. Miao, X. et al., Preparation and characterisation of calcium phosphate bone cement. *Materials Processing and Properties Performance* (MP3), 2004;**3**:319–324.

52. Chen, Q.Z., I.D. Thompson, and A.R. Boccaccini, 45S5 Bioglass (R)-derived glass-ceramic scaffolds for bone tissue engineering. *Biomaterials*, 2006;**27**(11):2414–2425.

53. Chen, Q.Z. and A.R. Boccaccini, Coupling mechanical competence and bioresorbability in Bioglass (R)-derived tissue engineering scaffolds. *Advanced Engineering Materials*, 2006;**8**(4):285–289.

54. Chen, Q.Z. et al., Surface functionalization of Bioglass((R))-derived porous scaffolds. *Acta Biomaterialia*, 2007;**3**(4):551–562.

55. Kim, H.W., H.E. Kim, and J.C. Knowles, Hard-tissue-engineered zirconia porous scaffolds with hydroxyapatite sol-gel and slurry coatings. *Journal of Biomedical Materials Research. Part B, Applied Biomaterials*, 2004;**70B**(2):270–277.

56. Muthutantri, A.I., M.J. Edirisinghe, and A.R. Boccaccini, Improvement of the microstructure and mechanical properties of bioceramic scaffolds using electrohydrodynamic spraying with template modification. *Journal of the Mechanical Behavior of Biomedical Materials*, 2010;**3**(3):230–239.

57. Jayasinghe, S.N. and M.J. Edirisinghe, A novel method of forming open cell ceramic foam. *Journal of Porous Materials*, 2002;**9**(4):265–273.

58. Chen, Q.Z. et al., Improved mechanical reliability of bone tissue engineering (Zirconia) scaffolds by electrospraying. *Journal of the American Ceramic Society*, 2006;**89**(5):1534–1539.

59. Tuck, C. and J.R.G. Evans, Porous ceramics prepared from aqueous foams. *Journal of Materials Science Letters*, 1999;**18**(13):1003–1005.

60. Lyckfeldt, O. and J.M.F. Ferreira, Processing of porous ceramics by 'starch consolidation'. *Journal of the European Ceramic Society*, 1998;**18**(2):131–140.

61. Sepulveda, P. and J.G.P. Binner, Processing of cellular ceramics by foaming and in situ polymerisation of organic monomers. *Journal of the European Ceramic Society*, 1999;**19**(12):2059–2066.

62. Ortega, F.S., F.A.O. Valenzuela, and V.C. Pandolfelli, Gelcasting ceramic foams with alternative gelling agents. In *Advanced Powder Technology III*. Uetikon, Zurich, Switzerland: Trans Tech Publications Ltd, 2003, pp. 512–518.

63. Sepulveda, P. et al., Production of porous hydroxyapatite by the gel-casting of foams and cytotoxic evaluation. *Journal of Biomedical Materials Research*, 2000;**50**(1):27–34.

64. Sepulveda, P. et al., In vivo evaluation of hydroxyapatite foams. *Journal of Biomedical Materials Research*, 2002;**62**(4):587–592.

65. Tamai, N. et al., Novel hydroxyapatite ceramics with an interconnective porous structure exhibit superior osteoconduction in vivo. *Journal of Biomedical Materials Research*, 2002;**59**(1):110–117.

66. Ramay, H.R. and M.Q. Zhang, Preparation of porous hydroxyapatite scaffolds by combination of the gel-casting and polymer sponge methods. *Biomaterials*, 2003;**24**(19):3293–3302.

67. Callcut, S. and J.C. Knowles, Correlation between structure and compressive strength in a reticulated glass-reinforced hydroxyapatite foam. *Journal of Materials Science. Materials in Medicine*, 2002;**13**(5):485–489.

68. Brinker, C.J. and G.W. Scherer, *Sol-Gel Science: The Physics and Chemistry of Sol-Gel Processing*. Boston, MA: Harcourt Brace Jovanovich, 1990, pp. 1–10.

69. Saravanapavan, P. and L.L. Hench, Mesoporous calcium silicate glasses. I. Synthesis. *Journal of Non-Crystalline Solids*, 2003;**318**(1–2):1–13.

70. Saravanapavan, P. and L.L. Hench, Mesoporous calcium silicate glasses. II. Textural characterisation. *Journal of Non-Crystalline Solids*, 2003;**318**(1–2):14–26.

71. Chen, Q.Z. et al., A new sol-gel process for producing Na_2O-containing bioactive glass ceramics. *Acta Biomaterialia*, 2010;**6**(10):4143–4153.

72. Sepulveda, P., J.R. Jones, and L.L. Hench, Bioactive sol-gel foams for tissue repair. *Journal of Biomedical Materials Research*, 2002;**59**(2):340–348.

73. Jones, J.R. and L.L. Hench, Factors affecting the structure and properties of bioactive foam scaffolds for tissue engineering. *Journal of Biomedical Materials Research. Part B, Applied Biomaterials*, 2004;**68B**(1):36–44.

74. Jones, J.R., S. Ahir, and L.L. Hench, Large-scale production of 3D bioactive glass macroporous scaffolds for tissue engineering. *Journal of Sol-Gel Science and Technology*, 2004;**29**(3):179–188.

75. Lenza, R.F.S. et al., In vitro release kinetics of proteins from bioactive foams. *Journal of Biomedical Materials Research. Part A*, 2003;**67A**(1):121–129.

76. Gough, J.E., J.R. Jones, and L.L. Hench, Nodule formation and mineralisation of human primary osteoblasts cultured on a porous bioactive glass scaffold. *Biomaterials*, 2004;**25**(11):2039–2046.

77. Bose, S., S. Suguira, and A. Bandyopadhyay, Processing of controlled porosity ceramic structures via fused deposition. *Scripta Materialia*, 1999;**41**(9):1009–1014.

78. Kalita, S.J. et al., Development of controlled porosity polymer-ceramic composite scaffolds via fused deposition modeling. *Materials Science and Engineering C-Biomimetic and Supramolecular Systems*, 2003;**23**(5):611–620.

79. Hattiangadi, A. and A. Bandyopadhyay, Modeling of multiple pore ceramic materials fabricated via fused deposition process. *Scripta Materialia*, 2000;**42**(6):581–588.

80. Lous, G.M. et al., Fabrication of piezoelectric ceramic/polymer composite transducers using fused deposition of ceramics. *Journal of the American Ceramic Society*, 2000;**83**(1):124–128.

81. de Sousa, F.C.G. and J.R.G. Evans, Tubular hydroxyapatite scaffolds. *Advances in Applied Ceramics*, 2005;**104**(1):30–34.

82. Chu, T.M.G. et al., Mechanical and in vivo performance of hydroxyapatite implants with controlled architectures. *Biomaterials*, 2002;**23**(5):1283–1293.

83. Jun, I.K., Y.H. Koh, and H.E. Kim, Fabrication of a highly porous bioactive glass-ceramic scaffold with a high surface area and strength. *Journal of the American Ceramic Society*, 2006;**89**(1):391–394.

84. Koh, Y.H., I.K. Jun, and H.E. Kim, Fabrication of poly(epsilon-caprolactone)/hydroxyapatite scaffold using rapid direct deposition. *Materials Letters*, 2006;**60**(9–10):1184–1187.

85. Sachlos, E. and J.T. Czernuszka, Making tissue engineering scaffolds work. Review on the application of solid freeform fabrication technology to the production of tissue engineering scaffolds. *European Cells and Materials Journal*, 2003;**5**(1):29–40.

86. Yang, S.F. et al., The design of scaffolds for use in tissue engineering. Part II. Rapid prototyping techniques. *Tissue Engineering*, 2002;**8**(1):1–11.

87. Curodeau, A., E. Sachs, and S. Caldarise, Design and fabrication of cast orthopedic implants with freeform surface textures from 3-D printed ceramic shell. *Journal of Biomedical Materials Research*, 2000;**53**(5):525–535.

88. Bourell, D.L. et al., Selective laser sintering of metals and ceramics. *International Journal of Powder Metallurgy*, 1992;**28**(4):369–381.

89. Nelson, J.C. et al., Model of the selective laser sintering of bisphenol-a polycarbonate. *Industrial and Engineering Chemistry Research*, 1993;**32**(10):2305–2317.

90. Tadic, D. et al., A novel method to produce hydroxyapatite objects with interconnecting porosity that avoids sintering. *Biomaterials*, 2004;**25**(16):3335–3340.

91. Kaufmann, E., P. Ducheyne, and I.M. Shapiro, Evaluation of osteoblast response to porous bioactive glass (45S5) substrates by RT-PCR analysis. *Tissue Engineering*, 2000;**6**(1):19–28.

92. Ramay, H.R.R. and M. Zhang, Biphasic calcium phosphate nanocomposite porous scaffolds for load-bearing bone tissue engineering. *Biomaterials*, 2004;**25**(21):5171–5180.

93. Yan, H.W. et al., In vitro hydroxycarbonate apatite mineralization of CaO-SiO$_2$ sol-gel glasses with a three-dimensionally ordered macroporous structure. *Chemistry of Materials*, 2001;**13**(4):1374–1382.

94. Gun, J. et al., Sol-gel formation of reticular methyl-silicate materials by hydrogen peroxide decomposition. *Journal of Sol-Gel Science and Technology*, 1998;**13**(1–3):189–193.

95. Sato, Y. et al., Formation of ordered macropores and templated nanopores in silica sol-gel system incorporated with EO-PO-EO triblock copolymer. *Colloids and Surfaces A-Physicochemical and Engineering Aspects*, 2001;**187**:117–122.

96. Bose, S. et al., Pore size and pore volume effects on alumina and TCP ceramic scaffolds. *Materials Science and Engineering C-Biomimetic and Supramolecular Systems*, 2003;**23**(4):479–486.

97. Kalita, S.J. et al., Porous calcium aluminate ceramics for bone-graft applications. *Journal of Materials Research*, 2002;**17**(12):3042–3049.

98. Lee, G.H. et al., Biocompatibility of SLS-formed calcium phosphate implants. In *Proceedings of Solid Freeform Fabrication Symposium*, Austin, TX, 1996, pp. 15–22.

99. Gibson, L.J., The mechanical-behavior of cancellous bone. *Journal of Biomechanics*, 1985;**18**(5):317–328.

Further Readings

Chapter 6: Ceramic implant materials. In *Biomaterials: An Introduction*, J. Park and R.S. Lakes, eds., 3rd edn. New York: Springer, 2007.

Chapter 10: Biomaterials for dental applications. In *Handbook of Materials for Medical Devices*, J.R. Davies, ed. Materials Park, OH: ASM International, 2003.

Hench, L.L. and Wilson, J. *Introduction to Bioceramics*, Chapters 3–11. World Scientific Publishing Company Inc., Hackensack, NJ, 1993.

CHAPTER 8

POLYMERIC BIOMATERIALS
Fundamentals

LEARNING OBJECTIVES

After a careful study of this chapter, you should be able to do the following:

1. Describe polymers of various types, including atactic, isotactic, syndiotactic polymers; homopolymers and copolymers; block polymers and graft polymers, thermoplastics and thermosets; thermoset elastomers and thermoplastic elastomers.
2. Describe the mechanism of flexibility of carbon–carbon bonds.
3. Discuss strategies to strengthen/harden polymers.
4. Discuss strategies to adjust the ability of polymers to degrade and the degradation rate.
5. Describe the general design/selection principles of polymeric biomaterials.

8.1   BASIC CONCEPTS ON POLYMERS

The Nobel laureate Herman Staudinger first believed that polymers were composed of very large molecules containing long sequences of simple chemical units linked together by covalent bonds and introduced the word *macromolecules* to describe them. By the early 1930s, most scientists in the field were convinced of the macromolecular structure of polymers. In the next two decades, the Nobel laureate Paul Flory established the fundamental principles of polymer science, with his prominent theoretical and experimental work. Flory's magnum opus *Principles of Polymer Chemistry*, which was published in 1953, quickly became a standard text for all workers in the field of polymers and is widely used to this day.

8.1.1 What Are Polymers?

A polymer (*poly* means many, *mer* means unit) is a large molecule (macromolecule) composed of *repeating units*, also known as *monomer residues* or *building blocks*. Carbon is the most important element in polymers, starting with four valence (unpaired) electrons and sharing (pairing with) four more. Most importantly, carbon forms strong bonds with itself. Long, strong chains or nets made of thousands of carbon atoms form the backbone of most polymers [1]. Let us look at six simple polymers.

The simplest polymer is polyethylene (often abbreviated as PE)* (Figure 8.1). In addition to the carbon *backbone*, only hydrogen atoms are used to achieve four covalent bonds per carbon atom. The repeating building block of polyethylene is $-CH_2-CH_2-$ (NOT $-CH_2-$), and the molecular formula of this polymer is represented by $(-CH_2-CH_2-)_n$. The side hydrogen atoms can be replaced by other atoms, such as $-CH_2-$ or $(-CH_2-)_n$, which are often called *side chains*, and often denoted by a capital "R" (derived from the original term, *radical*). Polyethylene has been widely used to produce a range of food-grade plastic containers. As a biomaterial, polyethylene is used for the line of total hip replacements (Figure 8.2).

The carbon backbone and hydrogen side atoms can both be replaced by a variety of atoms and chains, which results in an immense variety of polymers. The backbone atoms of carbon can be replaced by silicon, divalent oxygen, or sulfur. Although silicon is in the same group as carbon, it does not form strong bonds with itself. Silicones, long chains of alternating silicon and oxygen atoms (Figure 8.3), can be synthesized to make soft polymers, such as those used in contact lenses (Figure 1.14).

Many nonmetal atoms and molecular groups can be covalently attached to a polymer backbone. Groups of atoms that contribute some properties besides C–C and C–H bonds are called *functional groups*. They affect the chemical and physical properties of a polymer. Examples of functional groups that appear in polymeric biomaterials are given in Table 8.1.

If the side hydrogen atoms are replaced by fluorine atoms, the resultant polymer $(-CF_2-CF_2-)_n$ is polytetrafluoroethene (abbreviated as PTFE), with the brand name Teflon®. This highly stable and nonwettable polymer is used as a coating in the production of the nonstick cookware. The same properties also find medical applications in artificial blood vessels (Figure 8.4).

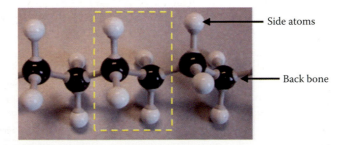

Side atoms

Back bone

Figure 8.1
The molecular structure of the simplest polymer, polyethylene. Note: each pair of hydrogen atoms is placed alternatively on the opposite side of the backbone. Hence, the repeating building block of polyethylene is $-CH_2-CH_2-$, rather than $-CH_2-$.

---

* *For nomenclature, refer to publications of The International Union of Pure and Applied Chemistry (IUPAC).*

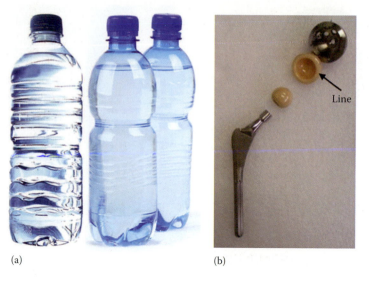

(a)   (b)

Figure 8.2
Applications of polyethylene: (a) drinking bottles; (b) the line in total hip replacement.

Figure 8.3
The molecular structure of silicone.

Table 8.1

Examples of Functional Groups Appearing in Polymeric Biomaterials

Name	Molecular Structure
Carboxylic acid group (–COOH)	(a)
Hydroxyl (also called alcohol) group (–OH)	(b)
Amino group (–NH₂)	(c)
Halide (–Cl, –F, etc.)	–F, –Cl
Styrene (–C₆H₆)	(d)

259

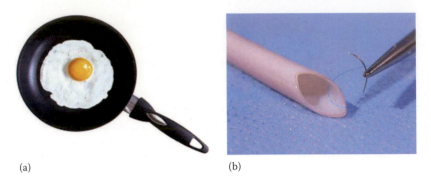

(a)   (b)

Figure 8.4
Applications of PTFE: (a) Teflon-coated nonstick saucepan; (b) artificial blood vessel made from PTFE.

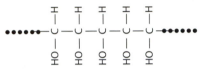

Figure 8.5
Molecular structure of polyglycerol.

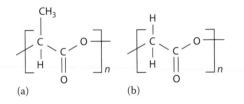

(a)   (b)

Figure 8.6
Molecular structures of two polyesters: (a) PLA; (b) PGA.

   If one of the pair of side hydrogen atoms on each carbon is replaced by a hydroxyl group −OH (Figure 8.5), the resultant polymer is called polyglycerol. The molecular formula of this polymer is $H(HC-OH)_nH$, and is often written as $H(C \cdot H_2O)_nH$. Hence, polyglycerol is a hydrogenated (referring to the hydrogen atoms at the two ends of each polymer chain) *carbohydrate* compound. This *sugar alcohol* is found in many foods, as well as in our body. Glycerol and polyglycerol have also been used as an additive in cough syrup.

   Figure 8.6 illustrates the molecular structures of two polymers which contain carboxylic groups (also called ester group), −COO−; hence, these polymers are also called polyesters. Both poly(lactic acid) (PLA) and poly(glycolic acid) (PGA) are applied in self-resorbable surgical sutures (Figure 1.14).

   It must be mentioned that most biological tissues are regarded as polymers in materials science. However, biological polymers are structurally more complicated than synthetic polymers, with vastly different properties, synthesis requirements, and working conditions. Biological materials will be described in Chapter 16, Part II, of this book. In this and the next two chapters, we focus on synthetic polymers.

8.1.2 Simplified Illustration of Molecular Structures of Polymers

Simplified or *skeleton* structures can be used to emphasize the functional groups of polymers (Figure 8.7a). Carbon–carbon bonds of the framework are represented by line segments, with each vertex representing the location of a carbon atom. Most hydrogen atoms and all lone pairs are omitted. This type of diagram de-emphasizes the hydrocarbon skeleton, since it is so strongly bonded as to be unreactive, and does not affect the chemical properties of the polymer. Polyethylene is the simplest polymer, and since it has no functional groups, the skeleton structure of a polyethylene fragment looks like it does not have any atoms (Figure 8.7a). It is possible to figure out which information is missing, as there should be a carbon atom at the end of each line segment, with six connected by five single bonds (Figure 8.7b). Since each carbon atom must have four bonds per molecule, they must be missing bonds to hydrogen atoms. For the carbon atoms on the ends of the molecule, adding three C–H bonds to each will achieve octets. Two C–H bonds should be added to each of the inner carbons (Figure 8.7c). To emphasize again, only hydrogen atoms are omitted in a *skeleton* structure, and any other atoms, such as F and Cl, should be notated clearly.

8.1.3 Why Many Polymers Are Flexible?

Polymers are generally softer and more stretchable than metals and ceramics, a mechanical property related directly to the long flexible polymer chain. The flexibility of polymer chains lies in the rotational movement of sigma bonds between carbon atoms. Carbon has four unpaired electrons ready for pairing. A simple reaction is the covalent bonding between carbon and hydrogen (Figure 8.8a), which also has an unpaired electron. Carbon atoms can also react with each other, as they both have unpaired electrons. However, unlike that of the smaller hydrogen atoms, which can easily fit into carbons, the electron clouds of two carbon atoms are more crowded, causing them to rearrange themselves in order to achieve a comfortable (low energy)

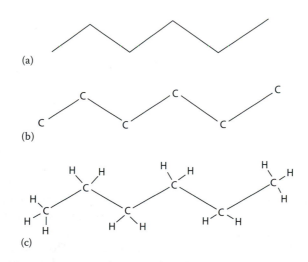

Figure 8.7
Simplified and complete Lewis structures for polyethylene fragment: (a) most simplified "skeleton" structure; (b) simplified structure showing carbons; (c) complete Lewis structure showing side groups.

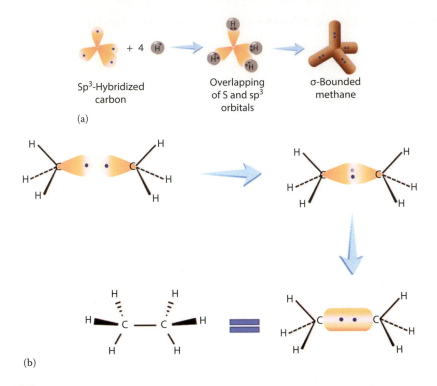

Sp³-Hybridized
carbon

Overlapping
of S and sp³
orbitals

σ-Bounded
methane

(a)

(b)

Figure 8.8
The rotational sigma bonding between two carbon atoms: (a) the unpaired four electrons of a carbon atom; (b) sigma bond (C–C) between carbon atoms.

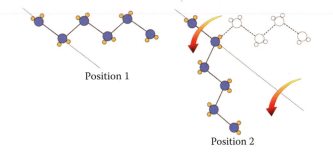

Position 1

Position 2

Figure 8.9
The rotation (the red curved arrow) of the C_1–C_2 bond about their bonding axis (the dash line) can move the rest of the chain from position 1 to position 2. A physical barrier can immobilize the chain and prevent it from moving to position 2.

state. Eventually, the shape of the electron cloud of C–C covalent bond (called a sigma bond) forms an ellipse, which is symmetric about the bonding axis (Figure 8.8b).

As described in Chapter 1, covalent bonds are typically rigid and lack tolerance to any deformation that attempts to change their bonding direction. Then how do the rigid covalent C–C bonds in the backbone allow for the flexibility of polymer chains? The answer lies in the symmetric nature of the C–C bond. The symmetry of sigma bonds gives the C–C bonds a freedom to rotate about the bonding axis without changing the bonding direction. Assume in Figure 8.9 that carbon Atom 1 is fixed and Atom 2 can rotate about the C_1–C_2

bonding axis. This rotation will move the rest of the chain from Position 1 to Position 2, while the bonding direction between C_1 and C_2 is maintained. This rotation can be easily observed using carbon back-bone models similar to the one appearing in Figure 8.1. It is the rotating ability of sigma bonds that produces the flexibility of a polymer chain. To emphasize this, *the flexibility of polymer chains is the result of the rotation of C–C sigma bonds, not due to the redirection of C–C bonds which would lead to brittle fracture.*

The flexibility of a polymer chain is directly controlled by its moving freedom, but this motion can be inhibited by several strengthening/hardening mechanisms. Specifically, the moving ability of a chain is influenced by:

- Its length: long, tangled chains are more difficult to move around than short chains.
- The existence of physical barriers (second particles in composites) (Figure 8.9).
- Restraining of other chains (physical tangling and chemical bonding between chains).

8.1.4 Classification of Homo- and Copolymers

The identity of the repeating units in a polymer is its most important attribute, with polymer nomenclature generally based upon the type of monomer residues. A *homopolymer* is a polymer whose structure can be represented by the repetition of a single type of unit (monomer) which may contain one or more species, such as silicone. The polymers described earlier are all homopolymers. PLA, for example, is composed only of lactic acid monomer residues, and is therefore classified as a homopolymer. The attachment of the side-group (one species) to the C–C backbone chain introduces a stereo-structure along the chain. The notation used to describe this distribution is *tacticity* (Figure 8.10), summarized as follows:

- *Atactic polymers*: where side groups are placed randomly along the chain
- *Isotactic polymers*: where all the side-groups are located on the same side of the chain
- *Syndiotactic polymers*: the substituents have alternating positions along the chain

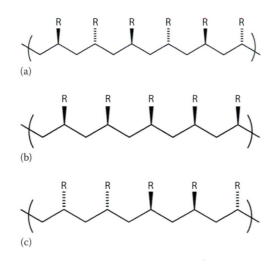

(a)

(b)

(c)

Figure 8.10
Tacticity of homopolymers: (a) atactic, (b) isotactic, and (c) syndiotactic.

Table 8.2
Homopolymers and Different Types of Copolymers

Classification	Arrangement of the Repeating Units
Homopolymer	–A–A–A–A–A–A–A–A–A–A–A–A–A–A–A–A–A–A–
Alternating copolymer	–A–B–A–B–A–B–A–B–A–B–A–B–A–B–A–B–A–B–
Periodic copolymers	–(A–B–A–B–B–B)–(A–B–A–B–B–B)–(A–B–A–B–B–B)–
Statistical (or random) copolymers	–A–B–A–A–B–B–A–B–B–A–A–A–B–A–B–A–B–B–
Block copolymers	–A–A–A–A–A–A–A–A–B–B–B–B–B–B–B–B–B–B–
Graft copolymers	–A–A–A–A–A–A–A–A–A–A–A–A–A–A–A–A–A–A–
	| |
	–B–B–B–B–B B–B–B–B–B–B–

A *copolymer* (or *heteropolymer*) is a polymer whose molecules contain two or more different types of repeating units, as opposed to a homopolymer where only one monomer is used. Poly(lactic acid-*co*-glycolic acid) (PLGA) contains two types of repeating units, lactic acid and glycolic acid, and is thus a copolymer. A *terpolymer* is a copolymer consisting of three distinct monomers, derived from *ter* (Latin) meaning *third*. Based on the arrangement of the repeating units in polymer chains, copolymers are further classified as follows (see also Table 8.2) [2]:

- *Alternating copolymers* with regular alternating A and B units.
- *Periodic copolymers* with A and B units arranged in a repeating sequence, for example, (A–B–A–B–B–B)$_n$
- *Statistical (random) copolymers* are copolymers in which the sequence of monomer residues follows a statistical rule. If the probability of finding a given type of monomer residue at a particular point in the chain is equal to the mole fraction of that monomer residue in the chain, then the polymer may be referred to as a truly random copolymer.
- *Block copolymers* comprise two or more homopolymer subunits linked by covalent bonds. The union of the homopolymer subunits may require an intermediate nonrepeating subunit, known as a *junction block*. Block copolymers with two or three distinct blocks are called *diblock copolymers* and *triblock copolymers*, respectively.
- *Stereo-block copolymers*: A special structure can be formed from one monomer where the distinguishing feature is the tacticity of each block. Hence, strictly speaking, a stereoblock copolymer is not a true copolymer.
- *Graft copolymers* are a special type of branched copolymer in which the side chains are structurally distinct from the main chain. However, the individual chains of a graft copolymer may be homopolymers or copolymers.

Finally, a polymer molecule containing ionizable subunits is known as a *polyelectrolyte* or *ionomer*.

8.1.5 Classification of Skeletal Structures

The skeletal structure of polymer chains can broadly be classified into the following four types (Figure 8.11): linear, branched, cross-linked, and networked [2].

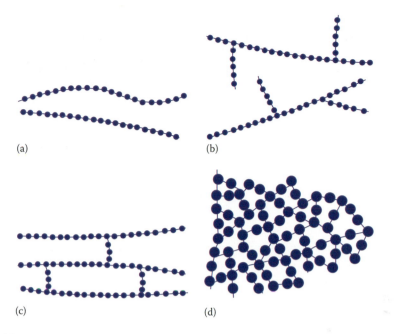

Figure 8.11
Four types of skeletal structures of polymers. (a) linear, (b) branched, (c) cross-linked, and (d) networked polymers.

8.1.5.1 Linear or Branched Chain Structures: Thermoplastic Polymers *Linear* polymers only consist of a main chain (Figure 8.11a), whereas *branched* polymers consist of a main chain with one or more polymeric side chains (Figure 8.11b). Branching occurs by the replacement of a substituent (e.g., a hydrogen atom) on a monomer by another covalently bonded chain of that polymer, or in the case of a graft copolymer, by a chain of another type (Table 8.2). Other special types of branched polymer structures include star, brush, and comb copolymers. In gradient copolymers, the monomer composition changes gradually along the chain. Polymers which are branched but not cross-linked are generally thermoplastic.

8.1.5.2 Cross-Linked (Elastomeric) or Networked (Rigid) Structures: Thermoset Polymers *Cross-linking* (i.e., *curing*, in common parlance) is a process in which polymer chains are chemically bonded together (Figure 8.11c). As with many chemical reactions, cross-linking can be initiated thermally or by ultraviolet (UV) light radiation (Figure 8.12a). In the case of polyethylene, UV light can kick off hydrogen atoms and leave unpaired electrons behind. The activated carbon atoms are ready to react with each other, resulting in chemical bonds (i.e., cross-links) between chains (Figure 8.12b).

In a chemically cross-linked polymer, the whole material is actually one giant molecule. There is no clear-cut boundary between the so-called cross-linked and networked structures, which are both cross-linked in structure. The former typically refers to sparsely linked and thus elastomeric polymers, and the latter is frequently used to describe a highly cross-linked solid. In fact, any soft elastomers can be further

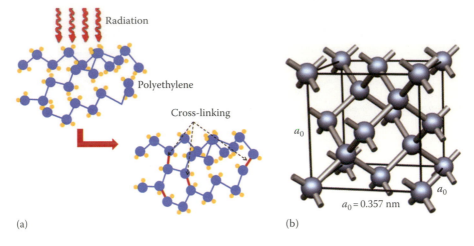

Figure 8.12
*The cross-linking process of polyethylene under UV light radiation. (a) Schematic drawing show-
ing how radiation is used to "cross-link" polyethylene chains (e.g. the cup of total hip replacement
bearings) resulting in a more durable product. (b) Diamond can be regarded as an extreme case
of cross-linked network.*

cured to become a fully cross-linked rigid solid. Diamond can be regarded as an
extreme case, where all hydrogen atoms are removed and the network is fully linked
by C–C bonds (Figure 8.12b). These polymers are collectively called *thermoset*, and
are characterized by their cross-link density, which is directly related to the number of
junction points per unit volume.

8.1.6 Phase Separation of Polymers

8.1.6.1 Crystallinity of Polymers   In general, polymers have a low degree of crystallinity, compared with metal and ceramic materials. Long chains reduce the degree of
crystallization and prevent complete crystallization. As a matter of fact, no polymers are
fully crystallized. Many polymers have a crystallinity between 50% and 90%. In semicrystalline polymers, there are two separated phases, the crystalline rigid domains and
amorphous soft segments (Figure 8.13). In an extreme case, a cross-linked polymer can
be a single giant molecule that is completely amorphous.

8.1.6.2 Segmented Copolymers   Many copolymers possess a two-phase microstructure due to incompatibility between the two different building blocks, one
separating into either crystalline or glassy rigid segments, the other into amorphous soft segments. The International Union of Pure and Applied Chemistry
(IUPAC) defines *segmented copolymers* as "containing phase domains of microscopic or smaller size, with the domains constituted principally of single types of
structural unit."

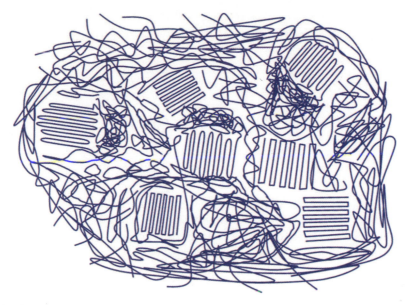

Figure 8.13
A schematic illustration of a semicrystalline polymer.

8.1.7 Molar Mass (Molecular Weight) of Polymers

The average molar mass of mixtures $\bar{M}$ can be calculated from the mole fractions x_i of the components and their molar masses $\bar{M}_i$:

$$\bar{M}_n = \sum_i x_i M_i.$$ (8.1)

It can also be calculated from the mass fractions w_i of the components:

$$\frac{1}{\bar{M}} = \sum_i \frac{w_i}{M_i}.$$ (8.2)

as summarized in Table 8.3.

8.1.8 Mechanical Properties of Polymers

8.1.8.1 Thermoplastics Thermoplastics are linear or branched (not cross-linked) polymers. These polymers become pliable or moldable above a specific temperature, and return to a solid state upon cooling. Their phase state is characterized by their melting temperature T_m or glass transition temperature T_g. Their mechanical properties depend on the temperature and applied strain rate (Figure 8.14), with their main features including [2]:

- Small elastic limits (typically <5%).
- Large plastic strains (>100%).

Table 8.3

Molar Mass of Polymers

Number Average $\bar{M}_n$	Weight Average $\bar{M}_w$	z-Average $\bar{M}_z$
$$\bar{M}_n = \sum x_i M_i$$	$$\bar{M}_w = \sum w_i M_i$$	$$\bar{M}_z = \frac{\sum w_i M_i^2}{\sum w_i M_i}$$
	$$= \frac{\sum N_i M_i^2}{\sum N_i M_i}$$	
$$x_i = \frac{N_i}{\sum N_i}$$	$$w_i = \frac{N_i M_i}{\sum N_i M_i}$$	
is the molar (or number) fraction of molecules of weight M_i.	is the weight fraction of molecules of weight M_i.	
Number average degree of polymerization	Weight average degree of polymerization	
$$\bar{x}_n = \frac{\bar{M}_n}{M_0}$$	$$\bar{x}_w = \frac{\bar{M}_w}{M_0}$$	

Polydispersity: $\dfrac{\bar{M}_w}{\bar{M}_n}$

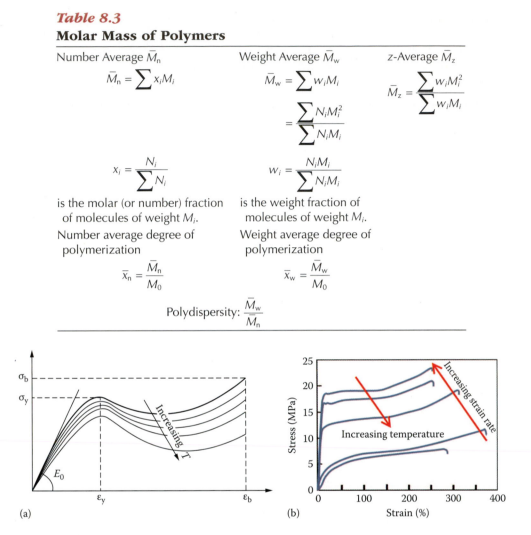

(a)   **(b)**

Figure 8.14
*(a) Typical stress–strain curves of thermoplastics and definitions of five mechanical properties.
(b) Stress–strain curves of fluoropolymer (e.g., PTFE).*

- Sensitivity to strain rate and temperature:
- The strength of polymers increases with decreasing temperature and increasing strain rate (Figure 8.14b).
- Effects of crystallinity: Crystalline polymers are stronger than their amorphous counterparts.
- Effects of molecular weight (length):
- The longer the polymer chains, the stronger/harder the polymer is.
- Effects of side chains:
- Side chains make polymers more flexible due to the increased spaces between polymer chains.
- Effects of chemical composition:
- Substituting the backbone carbon with divalent oxygen or sulfur will make chains more flexible due to the increased rotational freedom.

8.1.8.2 Thermoset Elastomers Elastomers (also called rubber materials) can undergo high deformation under stress without rupture, and recover to their original state when the stress is removed. Elastomers are sparsely cross-linked networks. The cross-linkers serve as micro-springs. Their mechanical properties have the following characteristics:

- Super-elasticity: maximal elastic strains typically >100%, even up to 1000%.
- Nonlinear elasticity—S-shaped stress–strain curve (Figure 8.15).
- Viscoelasticity: Rubber materials typically show a time-dependent elastic behavior, known as *viscoelasticity*. In response to an applied stress, they do not deform instantaneously like a perfectly elastic solid. Viscoelasticity is the property of materials that exhibit both viscous and elastic characteristics when undergoing deformation. Viscous materials, like honey, resist shear flow and strain linearly with time when a stress is applied. Elastic materials strain instantaneously when stretched and just as quickly return to their original state once the stress is removed.
- Hysteresis: (Figure 8.15)
- Although, in the elastic regime, the strain is recoverable, the stress–strain curve is not the same for loading and unloading, that is, *hysteresis*.

The stress–strain (σ vs ε) curve of an elastomer can be represented by

$$\sigma = \nu RT \left(\lambda - \frac{1}{\lambda^2} \right) \tag{8.3}$$

where
   ν is the network strand density (in units of moles of strands per unit volume of polymer)
   σ and λ are the engineering stress and extension ratio $(1 + \varepsilon)$
   R is the universal gas constant
   T is absolute temperature

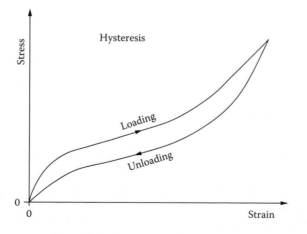

Figure 8.15
A typical full stress–strain cyclic curve of elastomers, showing hysteresis of mechanical behaviors.

For soft tissues (e.g., cardiac muscle), the maximum strain in vivo is typically 12%–15%. Hence, the mechanical properties of polymers at strains lower than 15% are relevant to those in clinical applications. Their stress–strain behavior can be described by Equation 8.3. At low strains of ≤12%, linearized Equation 8.4 only causes an error of <10%:

$$\sigma = \nu RT \left(\lambda - \frac{1}{\lambda^2} \right) \approx 3\nu RT \varepsilon. \tag{8.4}$$

For an elastic medium filled with a low percentage of rigid spherical particles, Equations 8.3 and 8.4 become

$$\sigma = \nu RT \left(\lambda - \frac{1}{\lambda^2} \right)\left(1 + 2.5\phi + 14.1\phi^2 \right) \tag{8.5}$$

or

$$E = 3\nu RT \left(1 + 2.5\phi + 14.1\phi^2 \right) \tag{8.6}$$

where ϕ is the volume percentage of the filler.

Elastomers can be divided into two categories: physically cross-linked elastomers (also called *thermoplastic rubbers*) and chemically cross-linked elastomers (frequently simply called elastomers). These two categories differ in the nature of the structure linking the chains together and imparting the elastic response. In chemically cross-linked elastomers, the flexible polymer chains or segments are linked together into a three dimensional network structure by covalent bonds, which are introduced during the vulcanization or curing process.

8.1.8.3 Thermoplastic Rubbers

Thermoplastic rubbers have the thermal properties of thermoplastics and mechanical properties of rubbers. In these rubbers, the flexible polymer chains are held together by physical linkers, either crystalline regions or glassy domains. The majority of thermoplastic elastomers have two separated phases, the glassy or crystalline rigid segments and amorphous soft segments. The rigid segments function as cross-linkers which provide mechanical strength, whereas amorphous segments provide the flexibility. Unlike chemical cross-linking which renders materials insoluble and incapable of being plastically deformed by heat and pressure, physical linkers can be melted above their melting points.

Thermoplastic rubbers are either copolymers or a physical mix of polymers (usually a plastic and a rubber) which consist of materials with both thermoplastic and elastomeric properties. A physical mix of polymers is called a *polymer blend*.

8.1.8.4 Thermoset Resins

As mentioned, chemically cross-linked elastomers and highly cross-linked rigid polymers are both thermoset in nature. In practice, the term *thermoset* is often used for the rigid cross-linked polymer materials, which are hard and brittle due to the high density of cross-linkers [2]. A comparison of mechanical properties of thermoplastics and thermoset polymers is given in Figure 8.16. Table 8.4 summarizes the structure, properties, and examples of the aforementioned three types of polymers.

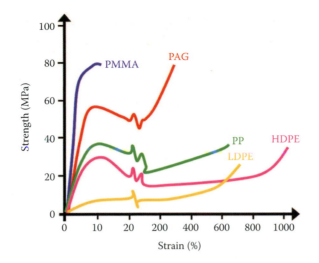

Figure 8.16

Typical stress–strain curves for various types of polymers (PMMA, polymethylmethacrylate; PA6, polyamide/nylon; ABS, acrylonitrile butadiene styrene; PP, polypropylene; HDPE, high-density polyethylene; LDPE, low density polyethylene.) (From Azom.com.)

Table 8.4

Comparison of Thermoplastics, Elastomers, and Thermosets

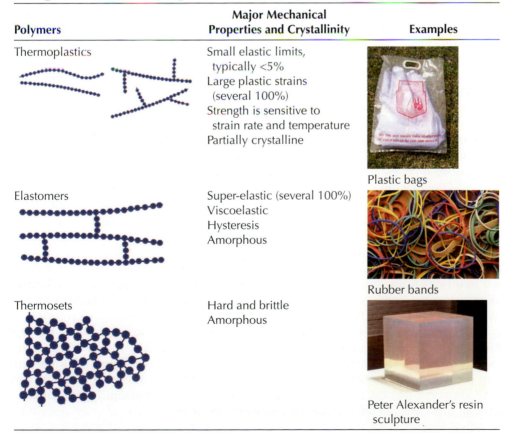

Polymers	Major Mechanical Properties and Crystallinity	Examples
Thermoplastics	Small elastic limits, typically <5% Large plastic strains (several 100%) Strength is sensitive to strain rate and temperature Partially crystalline	Plastic bags
Elastomers	Super-elastic (several 100%) Viscoelastic Hysteresis Amorphous	Rubber bands
Thermosets	Hard and brittle Amorphous	Peter Alexander's resin sculpture

8.1.9   Strategies to Strengthen/Harden Polymers

The ability of elastic and plastic materials to deform depends on the ability of polymer chains to move. Virtually all techniques for strengthening polymers rely on restricting or hindering this chain motion. These include

- Increasing the molecular weight (chain length)
- Promoting cross-linking
- Increasing crystallinity
- Introducing hard particles or fibers

8.1.10   Synthesis of Polymers

In polymer chemistry, polymerization (including cross-linking and branching) occurs via a variety of reaction mechanisms that vary in complexity due to functional groups present in reacting compounds and their inherent *steric effects*. These effects arise from the fact that each atom within a molecule occupies a certain amount of space. If atoms are brought too close together, there is an associated cost in energy due to overlapping electron clouds (Pauli or Born repulsion), and this may affect the molecule's preferred shape (conformation) and reactivity. There are a number of systems to categorize polymerization [3].

Polymer growth is defined based on the various styles of polymer chain extension. In a *step-growth polymerization* process, monomers react to first form many dimers, trimers, and even longer oligomers, which then connect with each other to eventually form long chain polymers (Figure 8.17a). In a *chain-growth polymerization* process, monomers react to form first a limited number of oligomers with active sites at any moment during the polymerization, and then unsaturated monomer molecules add onto the active site on a growing polymer chain, one at a time (Figure 8.17b).

Other forms of polymerization are classified depending on whether or not the chemical reaction results in small molecules that will be lost during the synthesis. *Addition polymerization* (Figure 8.17c) yields polymers with repeating units having molecules identical to those that make up the polymers. In addition to polymerization, the unsaturated monomers have double or triple carbon–carbon bonds (Figure 8.18), and the extra internal bonds are able to break and link up with other monomers to form a repeating chain. Addition polymerization is involved in the manufacture of polymers such as polyethylene (PE), polypropylene (PP), and polyvinyl chloride (PVC). *All chain-growth polymers are addition polymers.*

Radicals (also called *free radicals*) are atoms, molecules, or ions with unpaired electrons (Figure 8.19). Chain-growth (addition) polymerization can be further classified into free radical, anionic, cationic, and coordination polymerization. *Free radical polymerization* is a process by which a polymer forms after successive addition of free radical building blocks (Figure 8.19).

Condensation polymerization, on the other hand, involves loss of small molecules during the synthesis (e.g., the elimination of H_2O) (Figure 8.20). In another words, condensation polymerization yields polymers with repeating units having fewer atoms than present in the monomers from which they are formed. Most step-growth polymers are condensation polymers, but not all step-growth polymers release condensates; in that case, we refer to them as addition polymers.

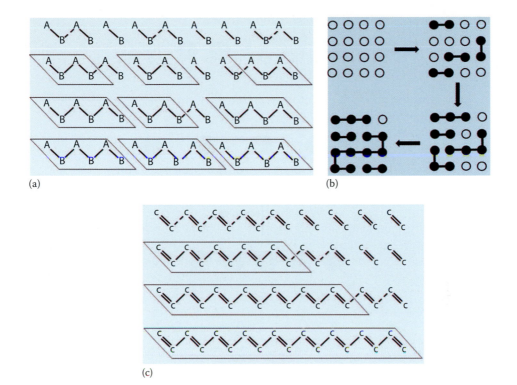

(a)

(b)

(c)

Figure 8.17
Schematic illustration of (a) step-growth polymerization, (b) chain-growth polymerization, and (c) addition polymerization.

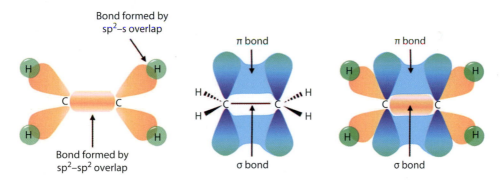

Figure 8.18
Double-bonded $CH_2=CH_2$, in which the two carbon atoms have three chemical bonds. Since they have four bonds in their saturated state, this is an unsaturated monomer.

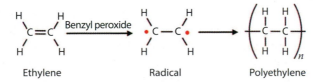

Ethylene   Radical   Polyethylene

Figure 8.19
Free radical addition polymerization of polyethylene.

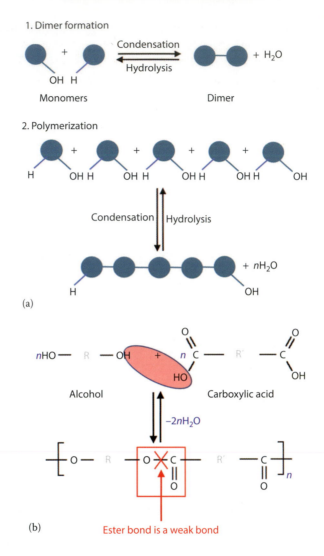

Figure 8.20
Condensation polymerization that involves loss of water molecules. (a) Condensation of one type of monomer. (b) Condensation of two types of monomers, an alcohol, and a carboxylic acid.

8.1.11 Hydrolysis and Chemical Design Principles of Medical Polymers

A typical condensation reaction is *esterification* between an alcohol group (−OH) and carboxylic group (−COOH) (Figure 8.20). The chemical bond is referred to as an *ester bond*, and the resultant polymer is called *polyester*. Ester bonds are weak, and esterification reaction has a strong tendency to be reversed. The reverse of esterification polymerization is called *hydrolysis*. Hydrolysis is the major mechanism of biodegradation in polyesters, and is always enzyme-mediated in the body. Biodegradation of polyesters breaks down polymers to their precursor monomers, that is, monomers with alcohol and carboxylic acid functional groups.

Many natural metabolic products of the body are carboxylic acids (e.g., lactic acid, glycolic acid) and alcohols (e.g., glycerol), and so on. Hence, these monomers can be used to synthesize biodegradable polymers. As a matter of fact, most medically applied degradable polymers are chosen for their metabolizable or excretable final breakdown products. To summarize, the chemical design principle of implant-grade polymers is:

- For permanent implants, choose or design inert polymers.
- For degradable polymers, priority choices of *monomers* are those metabolizable and/or excretable.

8.2 OVERVIEW OF POLYMERIC BIOMATERIALS

8.2.1 Classification

As with metallic and ceramic biomaterials, polymeric biomaterials can be classified according to their biological reactivity:

- Bioinert (thermoplastic, elastomeric, and thermoset), for example
  - Polyethylene (PE)
  - Poly(methyl methacrylate) (PMMA)
  - PTFE
  - Silicone
  - Polyurethane
- Surface bioerodible (thermoplastic and elastomeric) (Note: not aimed at tissue bonding; instead for controlled drug delivery)
  - Polyurethane
- Biodegradable (thermoplastic and elastomeric)
  - PLA
  - PGA
  - Poly(polyol sebacate) (PPS)

8.2.2 How to Adjust Degradability of Polymers

As with metals and ceramics, the ability of polymers to degrade can be changed by adjusting their chemical composition and network structure. The biostability of polymers is primarily determined by the chemical bonds on the backbone and steric interference. C–C, C–F, C–Si, and Si–O, etc. are strong bonds, giving polymers long durability, while ester bonds are weaker, making polymers degradable. *Steric hindrance*, one of the steric effects, occurs when the large size of side groups within a molecule prevents chemical reactions that are observed with smaller groups in related molecules (Figure 8.21). Although steric hindrance sometimes causes an undesired problem (e.g., decreased reaction rates), it can also be a very useful tool and is often exploited by chemists to change the reactivity pattern of a molecule by stopping unwanted side reactions (steric protection).

Cross-link density and crystallinity secondarily influence the degradation rates of a network by changing the diffusion rate. The diffusion of H_2O into a polymer network is the first step in the biodegradation mechanism. Hence, a high cross-link density and crystallinity will retard the diffusion of H_2O and thus slow down the degradation kinetics. Diffusion is much faster in an amorphous (loosening) structure than in a crystalline (more closely packed) structure. The aforementioned strategies of tuning degradation of polymers are summarily listed in Table 8.5, in comparison with those of ceramics.

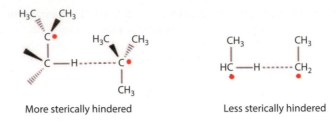

More sterically hindered   Less sterically hindered

Figure 8.21
Steric hindrance prevents the chemical reaction of unsaturated carbons.

Table 8.5

Strategies of Tuning Degradation of Polymers in Comparison with Those of Ceramics

		Polymer	Ceramic
Chemically	*Primarily*	To design chemical bonds in polymer chains, such as weak ester bond, strong C–C, C–F, Si–O bonds, etc. Steric interference	To change chemical composition, which will change chemical bonding and crystallinity, thus influencing degradation kinetics of ceramics
Structurally	*Secondarily*	To change cross-link density To change crystallinity	To change crystalline structure To change crystallinity

8.3   CHAPTER HIGHLIGHTS

1. Polymer chains have excellent flexibility due to the rotatable sigma bond between C–C. The flexibility of chains can be altered by
   a. Their length
   b. The existence of physical barriers (secondary particles)
   c. Restraint of the other polymer chains
2. A *homopolymer* is a polymer whose structure can be represented by the repetition of a single type of repeat unit (monomer)
   A *copolymer* is a polymer whose molecules contain two or more different types of repeating units.
3. Thermoplastic vs thermoset
   Linear or branched polymers are thermoplastic
   Chemically cross-linked and networked polymers are thermoset
4. Crystallinity of polymers
   Long polymer chains reduce the degree of crystallization and prevent complete crystallization, and no polymers are fully crystallized. Many polymers crystallize with crystallinity being between 50% and 90%

5. Thermoset elastomers are chemically cross-linked. Thermoplastic elastomers are copolymers or polymer blends (usually a plastic and a rubber), which are physically cross-linked

6. All strengthening techniques of polymers rely on restricting or hindering polymer chain motion. These include
   a. Increasing molecular weight (chain length)
   b. Promoting cross-link
   c. Increasing crystallinity
   d. Introducing hard particles or fibers

7. Biodegradation of polyesters breaks down polymers to their precursor monomers. Hence, the selection principles for biomaterials include using
   a. Inert polymers for permanent implants
   b. Metabolizable or excretable monomers for degradable implants

8. Degradation kinetics should match the healing rate of host tissue

9. Tuning of biodegradation kinetics
   a. Via chemical bonds
   b. Via steric interference
   c. Via crystallinity
   d. Via cross-link density

ACTIVITIES

Find nine things used in your day-to-day life that are made of thermoplastic, elastomers, and thermosets, three for each. Demonstrate sigma rotation in a plastic carbon backbone model, and note the variety of conformations from just one C–C bond rotation.

SIMPLE QUESTIONS IN CLASS

1. Which of following substances are not found in the body naturally?
   a. Sugar
   b. Alcohol
   c. Silicone
   d. Carboxylic acid

2. Complete the following molecular formula of Ethyl acrylate with C, CH, CH_2, or CH_3.

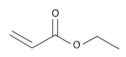

3. The flexibility of polymer chains is due to
   a. Nondirectional nature of C–C bonds
   b. Weak bonding between carbon atoms on the backbone of chains
   c. Side chains
   d. Rotational nature of C–C bonds

4. The following polymer is

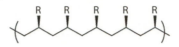

   a. Atactic
   b. Isotactic
   c. Syndiotactic

5. The following polymer is

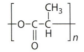

   a. An alternating copolymer
   b. A homopolymer
   c. A block copolymer
   d. Graft copolymer

6. The following scheme describes a

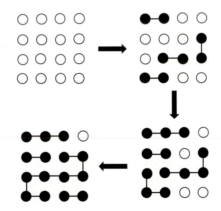

   a. Step reaction
   b. Chain reaction
   c. Addition polymerization
   d. Polycondensation

7. The nature of all strengthening/hardening methods of polymers is
   a. To strengthen C–C bonds
   b. To make polymer chain motion difficult
   c. To increase chemical cross-links
   d. To increase crystallinity

8. Why must the monomers of a degradable polymer be biocompatible for medical applications?
   a. The biocompatibility of all polymers is determined by the biocompatibility of its monomers.
   b. Biodegradable polymers will break down to monomers in vivo.
   c. Biocompatible monomers are safe for the workers who handle them during synthesis.
   d. Biocompatible monomers are environmentally friendly.

9. Which of following schematic polymers could be a thermoplastic elastomer?

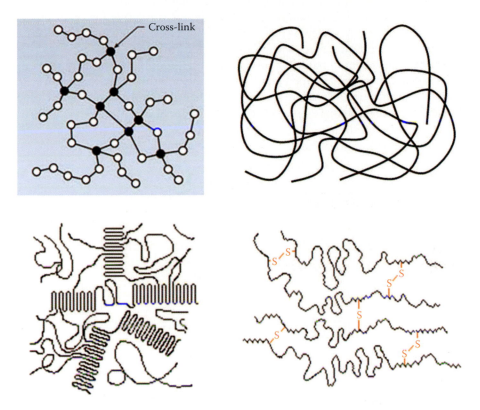

10. Which of the aforementioned schematic polymers is a thermoset elastomer?
11. Which of the aforementioned schematic polymers is a thermoplastic?

PROBLEMS AND EXERCISES

1. Describe the common feature and differences between polymers and the other two types of materials (metal and ceramic) in terms of building blocks and networks.
2. What is a functional group? List five functional groups.
3. The chemical bonding between C—C on polymer chains is covalent. Covalent bonds are typically rigid and lack tolerance to any deformation that attempts to change their bonding direction. Discuss how the rigid covalent C—C bonds in the backbone allow for the flexibility of polymer chains?
4. Discuss why polymers can never be fully crystallized, while all metals can.
5. At small strains, Equation 8.3 can be linearized to give Equation 8.4. Compute the errors caused by the approximation, when $\varepsilon = 5\%$, 10%, and 15%.
6. A composite is made of poly(glycerol sebacate) (PGS) and 10 vol.% of Bioglass® particles. The Young's modulus of the highly cross-linked PGS is 1.5 MPa at small strain (up to 10%). Calculate the Young's modulus of the aforementioned composite.

7. List polymer strengthening methods. Address the following questions:
   a. What is the common mechanism of polymer deformation?
   b. What is the common nature of all polymer strengthening and hardening methods?
   c. What is the common mechanism of metal deformation?
   d. What is the common nature of all metal strengthening and hardening methods?
8. Discuss the difference between step- and chain-growth polymerization.
9. What is esterification? What are polyesters? What is hydrolysis?
10. Describe the selection principles of implant polymers.
11. Describe steric hindrance.
12. Rank the following bonding according to their chemical stabilities:

$$C-C, C-F, C-Si, Si-O, C-O, C-N$$

13. Describe the strategies of tuning degradation of polymers.

ADVANCED TOPIC: POLYMERS AND POLYMER SCAFFOLDS FOR SOFT TISSUE ENGINEERING

Polymers

Polymers are the major type of materials used in soft tissue engineering. Selected biopolymers are listed in Table 8.6. They can be naturally occurring or synthetic. Detailed reviews are available in the literature [1–5].

Naturally Occurring Polymers   Natural extracellular matrices of soft tissues are composed of various collagens. Hence much research effort has been focused on naturally occurring polymers such as collagen [6,7] and chitosan [8] for many tissue engineering applications. Theoretically, naturally occurring polymers should not cause foreign body/material responses when implanted in human tissue, depending on how they are processed. In their native state, they provide a substrate for cellular attachment, proliferation, and differentiation in living tissue. So these polymers are a favorite substrate for tissue engineering [1,9]. Table 8.7 presents major naturally occurring polymers, their sources, and applications. Among them, collagen, fibrin, gelatin, and alginate have been extensively investigated for myocardial tissue engineering [10,11].

Synthetic Polymers   Although naturally occurring polymers possess advantages in terms of tissue compatibility, their poor mechanical properties and variable physical properties with different sources of the protein matrices have hampered their progress with the approaches listed earlier. Concerns have also arisen regarding immunogenic problems associated with the introduction of foreign collagen [12].

Following on from efforts to develop naturally occurring polymers as scaffold materials, attention has shifted more toward synthetic polymers, which have now become essential materials for tissue engineering. This is not only due to their excellent processing characteristics, which can ensure their off-the-shelf availability, but because of their excellent biocompatibility and biodegradability [12,13]. Synthetic polymers have predictable and reproducible mechanical and physical properties (e.g., tensile strength, elastic modulus, and degradation rate), and can be manufactured with great precision. Although they are unfamiliar to cells, causing problems such as persistent inflammatory

Table 8.6
Selected Polymeric Biomaterials for Tissue Engineering

Biomaterial	Abbreviation
1. *Synthetic Polymers*	
Bulk biodegradable polymers	
Aliphatic polyesters	
Poly(lactic acid)	PLA
Poly(D-lactic acid)	PDLA
Poly(L-lactic acid)	PLLA
Poly(D,L-lactic acid)	PDLLA
Poly(glycolic acid)	PGA
Poly(lactic-*co*-glycolic acid)	PLGA
Poly(ε-caprolactone)	PCL
Poly(hydroxyalkanoate)	PHA
Poly(3- or 4-hydroxybutyrate)	PHB
Poly(3-hydroxyoctanoate)	PHO
Poly(3-hydroxyvalerate)	PHV
Poly (*p*-dioxanone)	PPD or PDS
Poly(propylene fumarate)	PPF
Poly(1,3-trimethylene carbonate)	PTMC
Poly(glycerol-sebacate)	PGS
Poly(ester urethane)	PEU
Surface bioerodible polymers	
Poly(ortho ester)	POE
Poly(anhydride)	PA
Poly(phosphazene)	PPHOS
Polyurethane	PU
Nondegradable polymers	
Poly(tetrafluoroethylene)	PTFE
Poly(ethylene terephthalate)	PET
Poly(propylene)	PP
Poly(methyl methacrylate)	PMMA
Poly(*N*-isopropylacrylamide)	PNIPAAm
2. *Natural Degradable Polymers*	
Polysaccharides	
Hyaluronan	HyA
Alginate	
Chitosan	
Starch	
Proteins	
Collagen	
Gelatin	
Fibrin	

Sources: Seal, B.L. et al., Mater. Sci. Eng. R Rep., 34(4–5), 147, 2001; Atala, A. and Lanza, R.P., Methods of Tissue Engineering, Academic Press, San Diego, CA, 2002; Gunatillak, P.A. and Adhikari, R., Eur. Cell Mater., 5, 1, 2003; Garlotta, D., J. Polym. Environ., 9, 63, 2001; Nugent, H.M. and Edelman, E.R., Circ. Res., 92(10), 1068, 2003.

Table 8.7

List of Naturally Occurring Polymers, Their Sources, and Main Application Fields

Polymer	Source	Main Application Fields
Collagen	Tendons and ligament	Multiple applications, including cardiac and bone tissue engineering
Collagen-GAG (Alginate) Copolymers		Artificial skin grafts for skin replacement
Albumin	In blood	Transporting protein, used as coating to form a thromboresistant surface
Hyaluronic acid	In the ECM of all higher animals	An important starting material for preparation of new biocompatible and biodegradable polymers that have applications in drug delivery and tissue engineering, including cardiac tissue engineering
Fibrinogen-fibrin	Purified from plasma in blood	Multiple applications, including cardiac tissue engineering
Gelatin	Extracted from the collagen of animal connective tissue	Multiple applications, including cardiac tissue engineering
Chitosan	Shells of shrimp and crabs	Multiple applications, including cardiac tissue engineering
Matrigel™ (gelatinous protein mixture)	Mouse tumor cells	Myocardial tissue regeneration
Alginate	Abundant in the cell walls of brown algae	Multiple applications, including cardiac tissue engineering
Polyhydroxyalkanoates	By fermentation	Cardiovascular and bone tissue engineering

Source: Atala, A. and Lanza, R.P., Methods of Tissue Engineering, Academic Press, San Diego, CA, 2002.

reactions, erosion, or mismatched compliance, they may be replaced in vivo in a timely fashion by native extracellular matrices, formed by cells which integrate with them, or cells seeded within the implanted material. It has been proposed that an ideal tissue engineered substitute should be made from a synthetic polymer scaffold.

Table 8.6 has listed most synthetic polymers used in tissue engineering. Table 8.8 provides selected properties of synthetic, biocompatible, and biodegradable polymers that have been intensively investigated as substrate materials, with type I collagen fibers being included for comparison. Among them, aliphatic polyesters (PLA, PGA, and PCL) have widely been applied to 3D tissue constructs.

Degradability is generally a desired characteristic in tissue engineering substrates because the second surgery to remove them (such as a heart patch) would be averted. Gradually, a substrate could be removed by the physiological systems of the host body, as exemplified by widely used biodegradable sutures. Furthermore, in many applications, 3D tissue engineering constructs cannot be removed, and the nondegradable biomaterials would act as barriers to new tissue ingrowth and blood flow. Nonetheless, a few nondegradable polymers, including PTFE and PET, have

Table 8.8

Selected Properties of Synthetic, Biodegradable Polymers Investigated as Scaffold Materials

Polymers	Melting Point, T_m (°C)	Glass Transition Point, T_g (°C)	Degradation Kinetics	Refs.
1. Bulk degradable polymers				
PDLLA	Amorphous	55–60	Sutures are absorbed completely in vivo in 12–16 months	[13,17,18]
PLLA	173–178	60–65	Sutures can be absorbed completely in vivo after 24 months	[13,17]
PGA	225–230	35–40	Sutures are absorbed completely in vivo in 6–12 months	[13,19,20]
PLGA	Amorphous	45–55	Sutures are absorbed completely in vivo in 2–12 months	[1]
PPF	<140	−20	Not available	[1,21]
PCL	58	70–72	Not available	[22–24]
PHB	177	4	Much slower than PLA, PGA, and PLGA	[26,27]
2. Surface erodible polymers				
Poly(anhydrides)	150–200		Surface erosion	[1,21,27]
Poly(ortho-esters)	30–100		Surface erosion	[1,28]
Polyphosphazene	−66–50	242	Surface erosion	[29,30]

been investigated for certain tissue engineering approaches, such as passive diastolic restraints [10] to treat congenital heart disease [14], and especially vascular tissue engineering [5,10,15].

To design a tissue engineering substrate, it is necessary to weigh up the *pros and cons* of the potential precursor materials, which are summarized in Table 8.9. None of polymers is universally suitable for all tissues. Actually no single material can provide all necessary properties required by a particular application. In these instances, a hybrid of natural and synthetic polymers designed to combine the advantages of both, such as a porous synthetic polymeric scaffold filled with naturally occurring biomolecules [16], is likely to be the most appropriate.

Fabrication of Polymer Scaffolds

Chemical Reactant Gas Foaming   Table 8.10 lists currently applied 3D polymer scaffold fabrication technologies. Polymer foaming technology has existed since the 1940s. The first polyurethane (PU) foam was invented by Zaunbrecher and Barth in 1942 [31]. The one-step process is composed of simultaneous reactions of polyurethane formation and gas generation by admixing an organic toluene diisocyanate (TDI), a hydroxyl-terminated aliphatic polyester, and water in the presence of a catalyst. Polyurethane chains were formed by the reaction of isocyanate groups with hydroxyl groups [32].

Table 8.9

Advantages and Disadvantages of Polymeric Biomaterials for Tissue Engineering

Biomaterial	Positive	Negative
Naturally occurring polymers	1. Excellent biocompatibility (no foreign body reactions) 2. Biodegradable (with a wide range of degradation rates) 3. Bioresorbable	1. Poor processability 2. Poor mechanical properties 3. Immunogenic problems (e.g., inflammatory responses) 4. Disease transfection
Bulk biodegradable synthetic polymers PLA PGA PLGA Poly(propylene fumarate)	1. Good biocompatibility 2. Biodegradable (with a wide range of degradation rates). 3. Bioresorbable 4. Off-the-shelf availability 5. Good processability 6. Good ductility	1. Inflammatory caused by acid degradation products 2. Accelerated degradation rates causing collapse of scaffolds
Surface bioerodible synthetic polymers Poly(ortho esters) Poly(anhydrides) Poly(phosphazene)	1. Good biocompatibility 2. Retention of mechanical integrity over the degradative lifetime of the device 3. Significantly enhanced tissue ingrowth into the porous scaffolds, owing to the increment in pore size 4. Good processability 5. Off-the-shelf availability	1. They cannot be completely replaced by new tissue 2. Concern associated with the long-term effects
Nondegradable synthetic polymers	1. No foreign body reactions 2. Tailorable mechanical properties 3. Good processability 4. Off-the-shelf availability	1. Second surgery is required, or 2. Concern associated with the long-term effect if they have to stay in the host organ for a lifetime

Carbon dioxide gas bubbles were formed by the reaction of diisocyanate groups with water. The reactions of this process are given in Equation 8.7 [32]:

$$n\text{HO} - \text{R} - \text{OH} \ + \ n\text{OCN} - \text{R}' - \text{NCO} \ \rightarrow \ (-\text{polyurethane} -)_n$$

$$n\text{OCN} - \text{R}' - \text{NCO} \ + \ n\text{H}_2\text{O} \ \rightarrow \ n\text{CO}_2 + (-\text{R}' - \text{NH} - \text{CO} - \text{NH}-)_n$$

(8.7)

where
  R is a polyester chain
  R' is an isocyanate residue

PU foams are highly porous and fully interconnected. A typical porous structure is shown in Figure 8.22. Although the virtually nondegradable PU foams have little direct applications as tissue scaffolds in tissue engineering, they have successfully been used as

Table 8.10

3D Fabrication Technologies of Polymer Scaffolds

Fabrication Technology	Required Properties of Materials	Available Pore Size (µm)	Porosity (%)	Architecture
Chemical reactant gas foaming	Polymerization produces gas	Large range 30–700	Large range >85%	100% interconnected macropores
Physically pressed gas foaming	Amorphous	<100	10–30	High volume of noninterconnected micropores
Gas foaming/ particle leaching	Amorphous	Micropores <50 Macropores <400	<97	Low volume of noninterconnected micropores combined with high volume of interconnected macropores
Polymer solution casting/particle leaching or melt polymer casting/ particle leaching	Soluble or melted	30–300	20–50	Spherical pores
Textile technology	Fibers	20–100	<95	
Emulsion freeze-drying	Soluble	<200	<97	High volume of interconnected micropores
Thermally induced phase separation/ freeze-drying	Soluble	<200	<97	High volume of interconnected micropores
SFF (3D printing)	Soluble	45–500	<60	100% interconnected macrospores

Sources: Hutmacher, D.W., Biomaterials, 21(24), 2529, 2000; Karageorgiou, V. and Kaplan, D., Biomaterials, 26(27), 5474, 2005.

a template in the fabrication of highly porous bioceramic scaffolds [35,36]. Biodegradable PU materials, which achieve degradability through incorporating degradable aliphatic polyesters as soft segments, have been foamed by other techniques listed in Table 8.10, such as particle leaching and textile techniques [37,38], which will be discussed in the following sections.

Physically Pressed Gas Foaming and Its Combination with Particulate Leaching This method produces highly porous matrices from thermoplastics, such as PLA, PGA, and their copolymer PLGA, using a high pressure gas (typically CO_2) technique. The advantage of gas foaming is that it avoids the use of organic solvents and high temperatures [39,40]. However, the gas foaming method typically yields a closed pore structure, which is disadvantageous in applications of cell transplantation (Figure 8.23a). Coalescence of bubbles, which is a very complex process [41,42], is generally needed in the production of scaffolds. To enable the fabrication of highly interconnective porous network, the gas forming method has been modified by combining it with particulate leaching

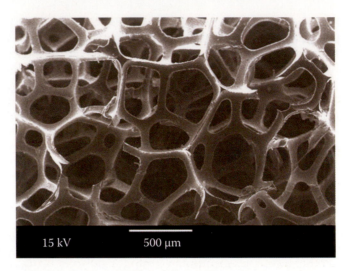

15 kV   500 μm

Figure 8.22
Macroporous structure of 60 ppi polyurethane sponge (Recticel UK, Corby).

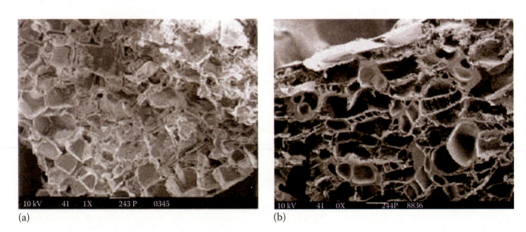

10 kV   41   1X   243 P   0345   10 kV   41   0X   244P   8836
(a)   (b)

Figure 8.23
PLGA scaffolds fabricated by the (a) gas foaming and (b) gas foaming/particulate leaching method [40,41].

(such as NaCl) [40]. The combination of high pressure gas foaming and particulate leaching techniques has significantly improved the interconnectivity of PLGA scaffolds, with porosity being 85%–97% and pore size being 250 μm (Figure 8.23b) [40].

Polymer Solution or Melt Casting/Particulate Leaching Polymer scaffolds can be constructed by mixing the polymer solution with salt or sugar particles [43,44]. A three-dimensional structure of controlled porosity is formed when salt or sugar particles are leached out into water. In the melt molding method, a fine PLGA powder is mixed with previously sieved gelatin microspheres and cast into a mold, which is heated above the melting temperature of the polymer. The PLGA/gelatin microsphere composite is subsequently removed from the mold and placed in distilled-deionized water. The gelatin, which is soluble in water, is leached out, leaving a porous PLGA scaffold with geometry identical to the shape of the mold. Using this method, it is possible to construct.

An essential requirement of this method for a scaffolding material is that the polymer must be soluble or can be melted. Hence, in principle, this technique can be applied to all thermoplastics. PU is a family of thermoplastic elastomers, which have a good processability. They can be fabricated into highly porous scaffolds by a number of foaming techniques, including salt leaching/freeze-drying [45–48]. By applying this fabrication technique, different porosities, surface-to-volume ratios, and three dimensional structures, with concomitant changes in mechanical properties can be achieved to suit a wide range of biomedical applications, including cardiovascular, musculoskeletal, and neurological tissue [49].

The main advantage of this processing technique is the ease of fabrication without the need of specialized equipment. The primary disadvantages of solution casting are (1) the limitation in the shapes (typically flat sheets and tubes are the only shapes that can formed); (2) the solubility requirements of the polymers, the challenge of producing porous elastomers, such as poly(glycerol sebacate) [50–53], remains; (3) the possible retention of toxic solvent within the polymer; and (4) the denaturation of the proteins and other molecules incorporated into the polymer by the use of solvents. The use of organic solvents to cast the polymer may decrease the activity of biomolecules (e.g., protein) [54]. The detailed processing steps can be found in protocol A of Ref. [54].

Textile Technology (Electrospinning) Electrospinning, which uses an electrical charge to draw very fine (typically on the micro- or nanoscale) fibers from a polymer solution (Figure 8.24a), has been developed to fabricate fibrous polymer scaffolds (Figure 8.24b). The fiber diameter, structure and physical properties of the nanofiber matrices can be effectively tuned by controlling various parameters that affect the electrospinning process. The nonlinear elastic deformation behavior of electrospun polymeric nanofiber mesh resembles mostly the collagen phase of a natural extracellular matrix. This, combined with excellent physical properties such as high surface area, high porosity, interconnective pores of the nanofiber matrices, well-controlled degradation rates, and biocompatibility of the base polymer, make biodegradable polymeric nanofiber matrices promising candidates for developing scaffolds for tissue engineering [55].

The electrospinning processing of chemically cross-linked elastomers is challenging. A major technical hurdle is that these polymers cannot dissolve into any solvents for

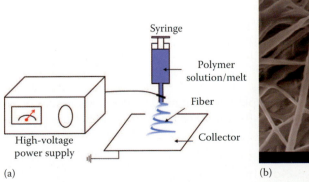
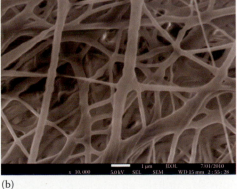

(a)

(b)

Figure 8.24
(a) Schematic illustration of electrospinning process; (b) an electrospun fibrous PLLA scaffold.

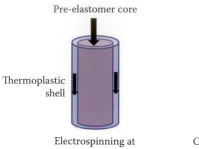

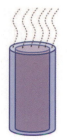

Pre-elastomer core

Thermoplastic shell

Electrospinning at room temperature

Cross-linking treatment at ~150°C

Figure 8.25
Core/shell spinning.

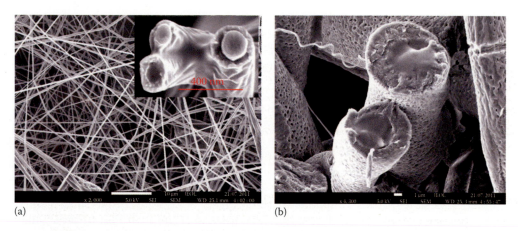

(a)   (b)

Figure 8.26
(a) Core/shell electrospun PGS/PLLA fibrous mesh and (b) the core/shell structure of the fibers. (From Xu, B. et al., Biomaterials, 34, 6306, 2013.)

electrospinning, for example, once cross-linked, and any fibers spun from uncross-linked prepolymers would be melted in subsequent cross-link treatment. Chen and coworkers have addressed this issue using a novel nanofiber fabrication technique: core/shell electrospinning (Figure 8.25). In this technique, the core is fed with a PGS non-cross-linked prepolymer, and the shell is fed with a thermoplastic. During the cross-linking process, the solid thermoplastic shell maintains the tubular shape, while the melted PPS prepolymer inside the tubes undergoes a cross-link reaction. So far, PGS has been synthesized into sheets with a printed microstructure (by lithography) [56], formed into 3D porous scaffolds (by a salt leaching technique) [57,58] and spun into fibers [59]. Most recently, researchers successfully created a muscle-like fibrous sheet with PGS using a core/shell electrospinning (Figure 8.26) [59]. This new process has produced a porous, elastomeric 3D scaffold that mechanically matches the stiffness of heart tissue [60].

Emulsion Freeze-Drying   Another method to foam polymers with variable porosity and pore size utilizes an emulsion/freeze-drying process [61]. Water is added to a solution of PLGA in methylene chloride to create an emulsion. The mixture is then homogenized, poured into a copper mold, and quenched in liquid nitrogen. After quenching,

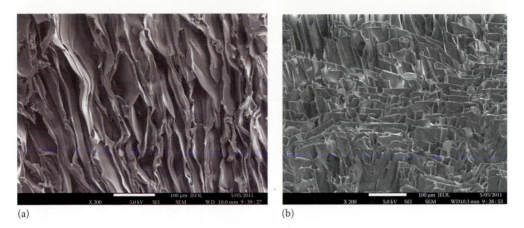

(a)   (b)

Figure 8.27
(a) Porous structure of scaffolds produced by thermally induced phase separation (TIPS)/freeze-drying. (b) Morphology on the cross section of the specimen.

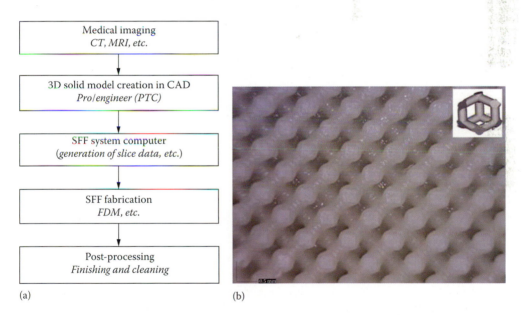

(a)   (b)

Figure 8.28
(a) Flowchart of the typical rapid prototyping (RP) process. (From Leong, K.F. et al., Biomaterials, 24(13), 2363, 2003). (b) A scaffold fabricated by the 3D printing technique. (From Chen, Q.Z., Development of bioglass(R)-ceramic scaffolds for bone tissue engineering, in Materials Department, Imperial College London, London, U.K., 2006.)

the polymer scaffold is freeze dried to remove the water and solvent. Scaffolds with porosity of up to 90% and median pore sizes in the range of 15–35 μm can be fabricated with an interconnected pore structure. In comparison to solvent casting/particulate leaching, the scaffolds produced with this method offer much higher specific pore surface area as well as the ability to make thick (>1 cm) polymer scaffolds, but the overall size of the pores is smaller [62].

Thermally Induced Phase Separation/Freeze-Drying Porous structure can also be achieved through phase-separation and evaporation. One approach to induce phase separation is to lower the temperature of the suspension of polymeric materials. The solvent is solidified first, forcing the polymer into the interstitial spaces. The frozen mixture is then lyophilized using a freeze-dryer, in which the ice solvent evaporates [63–66]. The typical porous structure of scaffolds produced by TIPS is shown in Figure 8.27. The alignment character in this porous structure is considered desirable, as it may provide a geometric cue for the regeneration of aligned muscular tissue [67].

Solid Free-Form (3D Printing) Solid free-form (SFF) techniques, also known as rapid prototyping (RP), are computer-controlled fabrication processes. They can rapidly produce highly complex 3D objects using data generated by computer aided design (CAD) systems. An image of a defect in a patient can be taken, which is used to develop a 3D CAD computer model. The computer can then reduce the model to slices or layers (Figure 8.28a). The 3D objects are constructed layer by layer using rapid prototyping techniques (Figure 8.28b) of fused deposition modeling (FDM), 3D printing (3D-P), stereo lithography, or extrusion free-forming [68].

BIBLIOGRAPHY

References for Text

1. Painter, P.C. and M.M. Coleman, *Fundamentals of Polymer Science: An Introductory Text*. Lancaster, PA: Technomic Pub. Co, 1997.
2. McCrum, N.G., C.P. Buckley, and C.B. Bucknall, *Principles of Polymer Engineering*. Oxford, U.K.: Oxford University Press, 1997, p. 1.
3. Odian, G. *Principles of Polymerization*. Hoboken, NJ: Wiley-Interscience, 2004.

Websites

http://www.chem.qmul.ac.uk/iupac/.
The International Union of Pure and Applied Chemistry: http://www.iupac.org/.

References for Advanced Topics

1. Seal, B.L., T.C. Otero, and A. Panitch, Polymeric biomaterials for tissue and organ regeneration. *Materials Science & Engineering R-Reports*, 2001;**34**(4–5):147–230.
2. Atala, A. and R.P. Lanza, *Methods of Tissue Engineering*. San Diego, CA: Academic Press, 2002.
3. Gunatillak, P.A. and R. Adhikari, Biodegradable synthetic polymers for tissue engineering. *European Cells & Materials*, 2003;**5**:1–16.
4. Garlotta, D., A literature review of poly(lactic acid). *Journal of Polymers and the Environment*, 2001;**9**:63–84.
5. Nugent, H.M. and E.R. Edelman, Tissue engineering therapy for cardiovascular disease. *Circulation Research*, 2003;**92**(10):1068–1078.
6. Yaylaoglu, M.B. et al., A novel osteochondral implant. *Biomaterials*, 1999;**20**(16):1513–1520.
7. Du, C. et al., Three-dimensional nano-HAp/collagen matrix loading with osteogenic cells in organ culture. *Journal of Biomedical Materials Research*, 1999;**44**(4):407–415.
8. Brown, C.D. and A.S. Hoffman, Modification of natural polymer: Chitosan. In *Methods of Tissue Engineering*, A. Atala and R.P. Lanza, eds. San Diego, CA: Academic Press, 2002, pp. 565–574.

9. Badylak, S.F., The extracellular matrix as a biologic scaffold material. *Biomaterials*, 2007;**28**(25):3587–3593.

10. Christman, K.L. and R.J. Lee, Biomaterials for the treatment of myocardial infarction. *Journal of the American College of Cardiology*, 2006;**48**(5):907–913.

11. Zimmermann, W.H., I. Melnychenko, and T. Eschenhagen, Engineered heart tissue for regeneration of diseased hearts. *Biomaterials*, 2004;**25**(9):1639–1647.

12. Vacanti, C.A., L.J. Bonassar, and J.P. Vacanti, Structure tissue engineering. In *Principles of Tissue Engineering*, R.P. Lanza, R. Langer, and J.P. Vacanti, eds. San Diego, CA: Academic Press, 2000, pp. 671–682.

13. Middleton, J.C. and A.J. Tipton, Synthetic biodegradable polymers as orthopedic devices. *Biomaterials*, 2000;**21**(23):2335–2346.

14. Krupnick, A.S. et al., A novel small animal model of left ventricular tissue engineering. *Journal of Heart and Lung Transplantation*, 2002;**21**(2):233–243.

15. Giraud, M.N. et al., Current state-of-the-art in myocardial tissue engineering. *Tissue Engineering*, 2007;**13**(8):1825–1836.

16. Taira, M., Y. Araki, and J. Takahashi, Scaffold consisting of poly (lactide-caprolactone) sponge, collagen gel and bone marrow stromal cells for tissue engineering. *Journal of Materials Science Letters*, 2004;**20**:1773–1774.

17. Lu, L.C. and A.G. Mikos, Poly(lactic acid). In *Polymer Data Handbook*, J.E. Mark, ed. Oxford, U.K.: Oxford Press, 1999, pp. 527–533.

18. Yang, S.F. et al., The design of scaffolds for use in tissue engineering. Part 1. Traditional factors. *Tissue Engineering*, 2001;**7**(6):679–689.

19. Lu, L.C. and A.G. Mikos, Poly(glycolic acid). In *Polymer Data Handbook*, J.E. Mark, ed. Oxford, U.K.: Oxford Press, 1999, pp. 566–569.

20. Ramakrishna, S. et al., *An Introduction to Biocomposites*. London, U.K.: Imperial College Press, 2004, p. 36.

21. Gunatillake, P.A. and R. Adhikari, Biodegradable synthetic polymers for tissue engineering. *European Cells & Materials*, 2003;**5**:1–16.

22. Iroh, J.O., Poly(epsilon-caprolactone). In *Polymer Data Handbook*, J.E. Mark, ed. Oxford, U.K.: Oxford Press, 1999, pp. 361–362.

23. Baji, A. et al., Processing methodologies for polycaprolactone-hydroxyapatite composites: A review. *Materials and Manufacturing Processes*, 2006;**21**(2):211–218.

24. Calandrelli, L. et al., Natural and synthetic hydroxyapatite filled PCL: Mechanical properties and biocompatibility analysis. *Journal of Bioactive and Compatible Polymers*, 2004;**19**(4):301–313.

25. Ramsay, B.A. et al., Biodegradability and mechanical-properties of poly-(beta-hydroxybutyrate-*co*-beta-hydroxyvalerate) starch blends. *Applied and Environmental Microbiology*, 1993;**59**(4):1242–1246.

26. Chen, G.Q. and Q. Wu, The application of polyhydroxyalkanoates as tissue engineering materials. *Biomaterials*, 2005;**26**(33):6565–6578.

27. Yoda, N., Synthesis of polyanhydrides II: New aromatic polyanhydrides with high melting points and fibre-forming properties. *Die Makromolekulare Chemie*, 2003;**32**:1–12.

28. Kellomaki, M., J. Heller, and P. Tormala, Processing and properties of two different poly (ortho esters). *Journal of Materials Science-Materials in Medicine*, 2000;**11**(6):345–355.

29. Magill, J.H., Poly(phosphazenes), bioerodible, In *Polymer Data Handbook*, J.E. Mark, ed. Oxford, U.K.: Oxford Press, 1999, pp. 746–749.

30. Laurencin, C.T. and S. Lakshmi. Polyphosphazene nanofibers for biomedical applications: Preliminary studies. In *Proceedings of NATO ASI Conference*, Antalya, Turkey, 2003.

31. Zaunbrecher, K. and H. Barth, A process for the preparation of solid or resilient nature light materials. German Patent DE936113C, filed December 15, 1942.

32. Ashida, K., *Polyurethane and Related Foams: Chemistry and Technology*. Boca Raton, FL: CRC Press/Taylor & Francis Group, 2007.

33. Hutmacher, D.W., Scaffolds in tissue engineering bone and cartilage. *Biomaterials*, 2000;**21**(24):2529–2543.

34. Karageorgiou, V. and D. Kaplan, Porosity of 3D biomaterial scaffolds and osteogenesis. *Biomaterials*, 2005;**26**(27):5474–5491.
35. Chen, Q.Z., I.D. Thompson, and A.R. Boccaccini, 45S5 Bioglass (R)-derived glass-ceramic scaffolds for bone tissue engineering. *Biomaterials*, 2006;**27**(11):2414–2425.
36. Chen, Q.Z. et al., Improved mechanical reliability of bone tissue engineering (Zirconia) scaffolds by electrospraying. *Journal of the American Ceramic Society*, 2006;**89**(5):1534–1539.
37. Hafeman, A.E. et al., Characterization of the degradation mechanisms of lysine-derived aliphatic poly(ester urethane) scaffolds. *Biomaterials*, 2011;**32**(2);419–429.
38. Guelcher, S.A. et al., Synthesis, mechanical properties, biocompatibility, and biodegradation of polyurethane networks from lysine polyisocyanates. *Biomaterials*, 2008;**29**(12):1762–1775.
39. Mooney, D.J. et al., Novel approach to fabricate porous sponges of poly(D,L-lactic-co-glycolic acid) without the use of organic solvents. *Biomaterials*, 1996;**17**(14):1417–1422.
40. Harris, L.D., B.S. Kim, and D.J. Mooney, Open pore biodegradable matrices formed with gas foaming. *Journal of Biomedical Materials Research*, 1998;**42**(3):396–402.
41. Ghosh, G., Coalescence of bubbles in liquid. *Bubble Science, Engineering and Technology*, 2009;**1**(1–2):75–87.
42. Krasovitski, B. et al., Growth and collapse of vapour bubble and shockwave emission around holmium laser beam: Theory and experiments. *Bubble Science, Engineering and Technology*, 2010;**2**(1):17–24.
43. Ma, P.X. and J.W. Choi, Biodegradable polymer scaffolds with well-defined interconnected spherical pore network. *Tissue Engineering*, 2001;**7**(1):23–33.
44. Mikos, A.G. et al., Preparation and characterization of poly(l-lactic acid) foams. *Polymer*, 1994;**35**(5):1068–1077.
45. Spaans, C.J. et al., High molecular weight polyurethanes and a polyurethane urea based on 1,4-butanediisocyanate. *Polymer Bulletin*, 1998;**41**(2):131–138.
46. Gogolewski, S. and K. Gorna, Biodegradable polyurethane cancellous bone graft substitutes in the treatment of iliac crest defects. *Journal of Biomedical Materials Research. Part A*, 2007;**80**(1):94–101.
47. Spaans, C.J. et al., A new biomedical polyurethane with a high modulus based on 1,4-butanediisocyanate and ε-caprolactone. *Journal of Materials Science. Materials in Medicine*, 1998;**9**(12):675–678.
48. Gogolewski, S., K. Gorna, and A.S. Turner, Regeneration of bicortical defects in the iliac crest of estrogen-deficient sheep, using new biodegradable polyurethane bone graft substitutes. *Journal of Biomedical Materials Research. Part A*, 2006;**77**(4):802–810.
49. Guelcher, S.A., Biodegradable polyurethanes: Synthesis and applications in regenerative medicine. *Tissue Engineering Part B: Reviews*, 2008;**14**(1):3–17.
50. Stuckey, D.J. et al., Magnetic resonance imaging evaluation of remodeling by cardiac elastomeric tissue scaffold biomaterials in a rat model of myocardial infarction. *Tissue Engineering Part A*, 2010;**16**(11):3395–3402.
51. Liang, S.L. et al., The mechanical characteristics and in vitro biocompatibility of poly(glycerol sebacate)-bioglass (R) elastomeric composites. *Biomaterials*, 2010;**31**(33):8516–8529.
52. Chen, Q.Z. et al., Elastomeric nanocomposites as cell delivery vehicles and cardiac support devices. *Soft Matter*, 2010;**6**(19):4715–4726.
53. Chen, Q.Z. et al., An elastomeric patch derived from poly(glycerol sebacate) for delivery of embryonic stem cells to the heart. *Biomaterials*, 2010;**31**(14):3885–3893.
54. Laurencin, C.T., H.H. Lu, and Y. Khan, Processing of polymer scaffolds: Polymer-ceramic composite foams. In *Methods of Tissue Engineering*, A. Atala and R.P. Lanza, eds. San Diego, CA: Academic Press, 2002, pp. 705–714.
55. Nair, L.S., S. Bhattacharyya, and C.T. Laurencin, Development of novel tissue engineering scaffolds via electrospinning. *Expert Opinion on Biological Therapy*, 2004;**4**(5):659–668.
56. Bettinger, C.J. et al., Three-dimensional microfluidic tissue-engineering scaffolds using a flexible biodegradable polymer. *Advanced Materials*, 2005;**18**(2):165–169.
57. Gao, J., P.M. Crapo, and Y.D. Wang, Macroporous elastomeric scaffolds with extensive micropores for soft tissue engineering. *Tissue Engineering*, 2006;**12**(4):917–925.

58. Sales, V.L. et al., Protein precoating of elastomeric tissue-engineering scaffolds increased cellularity, enhanced extracellular matrix protein production, and differentially regulated the phenotypes of circulating endothelial progenitor cells. *Circulation*, 2007;**116**(11):I55–I63.

59. Yi, F. and D.A. Lavan, Poly(glycerol sebacate) nanofiber scaffolds by core/shell electrospinning. *Macromolecular Bioscience*, 2008;**8**(9):803–806.

60. Xu, B. et al., Non-linear elasticity of core/shell spun PGS/PLLA fibres and their effect on cell proliferation. *Biomaterials*, 2013;**34**:6306–6317.

61. Whang, K. et al., A novel method to fabricate bioabsorbable scaffolds. *Polymer*, 1995;**36**(4):837–842.

62. Thomson, R. et al., Polymer scaffold processing. In *Principles of Tissue Engineering*, A.P. Lanza, R. Langer, and J. Vacanty, eds. Elsevier Academic Press, Burlington, MA, 2002, pp. 251–262.

63. Boccaccini, A.R. et al., Bioresorbable and bioactive composite materials based on polylactide foams filled with and coated by Bioglass (R) particles for tissue engineering applications. *Journal of Materials Science. Materials in Medicine*, 2003;**14**(5):443–450.

64. Verrier, S. et al., PDLLA/Bioglass (R) composites for soft-tissue and hard-tissue engineering: An in vitro cell biology assessment. *Biomaterials*, 2004;**25**(15):3013–3021.

65. Yin, Y.J. et al., Preparation and characterization of macroporous chitosan-gelatin beta-tricalcium phosphate composite scaffolds for bone tissue engineering. *Journal of Biomedical Materials Research. Part A*, 2003;**67A**(3):844–855.

66. Zhang, R.Y. and P.X. Ma, Poly(alpha-hydroxyl acids) hydroxyapatite porous composites for bone-tissue engineering. I. Preparation and morphology. *Journal of Biomedical Materials Research*, 1999;**44**(4):446–455.

67. Guan, J.J. et al., Preparation and characterization of highly porous, biodegradable polyurethane scaffolds for soft tissue applications. *Biomaterials*, 2005;**26**(18):3961–3971.

68. Leong, K.F., C.M. Cheah, and C.K. Chua, Solid freeform fabrication of three-dimensional scaffolds for engineering replacement tissues and organs. *Biomaterials*, 2003;**24**(13):2363–2378.

69. Chen, Q.Z., Development of bioglass(R)-ceramic scaffolds for bone tissue engineering. In *Materials Department*. London, U.K.: Imperial College London, 2006.

Further Readings

Chapter 7: Polymeric implant materials. In *Biomaterials: An Introduction*, Park, J. and R.S. Lakes, eds., 3rd edn. New York: Springer. 2007.

McCrum, N.G., C.P. Buckley, and C.B. Bucknall, *Principles of Polymer Engineering*. Oxford, U.K.: Oxford University Press, 1997, p. 1., Chapter 1.

Odian, G., *Principles of Polymerization*, Hoboken, NJ: Wiley-Interscience, 2004. pp. 1–38, Chapter 1.

Painter, P.C. and M.M. Coleman, *Fundamentals of Polymer Science: An Introductory Text*, Lancaster, PA: Technomic Pub. Co, 1997, Chapter 1.

CHAPTER 9

BIOINERT POLYMERS

LEARNING OBJECTIVES

After a careful study of this chapter, you should be able to do the following:

1. Describe strengthening/hardening mechanisms of UHMWPE
2. Describe the reason for the flexibility of polypropylene and PET
3. Describe the properties of PTFE, essential requirements of artificial blood vessels, and related challenges.
4. Describe the reason for the usage of silicone in contact lenses.
5. Describe the reason for elastomeric properties of PU
6. Describe the application of PMMA cements
7. Describe strategies to alleviate shrinkage of bone cement (and tooth fillings as well).

9.1 POLYOLEFIN

Polyolefin is a group of polymers produced from chemically unsaturated C_nH_{2n} as a monomer. Two of the simplest members are polyethylene (PE) and polypropylene (PP).

9.1.1 Polyethylene

PE is a readily crystallized thermoplastic. It is available commercially in three major grades: low, high, and ultrahigh (*ultrahigh-molecular-weight polyethylene—UHMWPE*). UHMWPE is also known as high-modulus polyethylene (HMPE) or high-performance polyethylene (HPPE). UHMWPE has extremely long chains, with a molecular mass usually between 2 and 6×10^6 g/mol. The longer chain serves to transfer load more efficiently across the polymer backbones by strengthening intermolecular interactions, resulting in a very tough material, with the highest impact strength of any thermoplastic presently made. Table 9.1 lists the properties of UHMWPE [1].

UHMWPE has over 40 years of clinical history as a successful biomaterial for use in various joint implants, including hip (Figure 6.5), knee (Figure 4.14), ankle (Figure 4.15), and shoulder (Figure 6.16) replacements [2]. It was first used clinically in 1962 by Charnley and emerged as the dominant bearing material for total hip replacements in

Table 9.1

Properties of UHMWPE

Molecular mass (10^6 g/mol)	2–6
Melting temperature (°C)	125–138
Glass transition temperature (°C)	−125
Poisson's ratio	0.46
Specific gravity	0.932–0.945
Tensile elastic modulus (GPa)	0.8–1.6
Tensile yield strength (MPa)	20–30
Tensile ultimate strength (MPa)	40–50
Tensile ultimate elongation (%)	350–525
Fracture toughness (kJ/m^2)	90
Impact strength (J/m)	>1070 (No break)
Degree of crystallinity (%)	40–75

the 1970s. After around 10 years' implantation, however, problems associated with friction and wearing of thermoplastic UHMWPE emerged in the 1980s (Figure 6.6). This is mainly due to continual reorientation of the polymer chains; hence, any hardening mechanism that can limit their movement will strengthen them and improve the wearing resistance.

In the history of UHMWPE synthesis and engineering, there have been several attempts to modify its structure to improve its clinical performance [2]. One unsuccessful attempt was to composite UHMWPE with carbon fibers. This carbon-fiber-reinforced UHMWPE was released as *Poly Two* by Zimmer in the 1970s. However, the carbon fibers had poor adhesion with the UHMWPE matrix, and its clinical performance was inferior compared to virgin UHMWPE. A second modification made by high-pressure recrystallization was released clinically as *Hylamer*™ by DePuy in the late 1980s. When gamma-irradiated in air, this material exhibited susceptibility to oxidation, also resulting in inferior clinical performance compared with virgin UHMWPE.

A major breakthrough came with the development of highly cross-linked UHMWPE in the late 1990s. The new generation of UHMWPE materials are cross-linked with gamma or electron beam radiation (50–105 kGy) and then thermally processed to improve their oxidation resistance. In 1998, highly cross-linked UHMWPE materials were introduced to orthopedics, and have rapidly become the standard of care for total hip replacements. Over the following few years, data from several centers demonstrated that highly cross-linked UHMWPE is superior to conventional thermoplastic UHMWPE for total hip replacements. Since then, highly cross-linked UHMWPE has been successfully used in all load-bearing joints. The application is currently so wide that an online repository of information and review articles related to medical grade UHMWPE, known as the UHMWPE Lexicon, was started in 2000.

To reiterate, the hardening of modern UHMWPE involves the first three mechanisms discussed in Section 8.1.9 (i.e., ultrahigh molecular weight, high crystallinity, and high cross-link density), but not by the inclusion of solid particles.

9.1.2 Polypropylene

PP belongs to a subgroup of polyolefins, *poly-alpha-olefin* (or poly-α-olefin), which are polymerized from alpha-olefins. An alpha-olefin (α-olefin) is an alkene where the

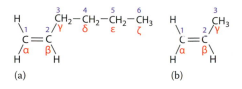

(a)   (b)

Figure 9.1
Two examples of an alpha-olefin. (From WikimediaCommons.) (a) 1-Hexene and (b) propylene.

carbon–carbon double bond starts at the α-carbon atom, that is, the double bond is between carbons 1 and 2 in the molecule (Figure 9.1a) [3]. As depicted in Section 8.1.10, one of the double carbon–carbon bonds in the unsaturated monomers is able to break and link up with other monomers to form a repeating chain. Hence, alpha-olefins can be used as comonomers to give an alkyl branched polymer, and the resultant poly-alpha-olefins have flexible alkyl branching groups on every other carbon of their polymer backbone chain [3].

Also known as polypropene, PP is the simplest poly-α-olefin (a vinyl polymer), with a methyl group –CH₃ as the branch (Figure 9.1b). It is an addition polymer and can be made from the monomer propylene (Figure 9.2). Structurally, it is similar to PE, except that every other carbon atom in the backbone chain has a methyl group attached to it (Figure 9.3). It can be atactic, isotactic, or syndiotactic. PP is unusually resistant to many chemical solvents, bases, and acids [3].

PP is a thermoplastic polymer, with most commercial forms being isotactic, with an intermediate level of crystallinity between 30% and 50%. The presence of the side methyl groups limits the crystallization, which rarely exceeds 50%–70% in isotactic materials. This is because the side alkyl groups make it very difficult for the polymer

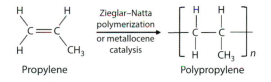

Propylene   Polypropylene

Figure 9.2
Synthesis of polypropylene.

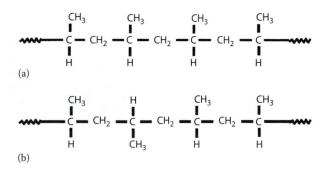

Figure 9.3
Molecular structures of (a) isotactic and (b) atactic polypropylene.

Table 9.2

Properties of Polypropylene

Melting temperature (°C)	160–170
Glass transition temperature (°C)	−20
Poisson's ratio	0.45
Density (g/cm³)	0.898–0.920
Tensile elastic modulus (GPa)	1.0–1.5
Tensile ultimate strength (MPa)	30–35
Tensile ultimate elongation (%)	400–900
Flexural elastic modulus (GPa)	1.2–1.7
Flexural strength (MPa)	37
Impact strength (J/m)	27–117
Degree of crystallinity (%)	30–60

molecules to align themselves side by side in an orderly way. This results in lower contacts between the molecules and decreases the intermolecular interactions between them. In fact, many poly-alpha-olefins do not crystallize or solidify easily and are able to remain oily, viscous liquids even at lower temperatures [4].

Table 9.2 provides some physical and mechanical properties of PP. Mechanically, PP has good flexibility due to the methyl side groups that prevent chain interactions. As a result, the chains of PP have more room to move around, such that it is more flexible than PE. PP materials typically have an exceptionally high flexural fatigue life and excellent environmental stress-cracking resistance. These properties have allowed bulk PP materials to find medical applications in finger joint prostheses (Figure 9.4). PP is also used in a wide variety of applications including packaging, labeling, textiles, stationery, containers, laboratory equipment and polymer banknotes. The textile form of PP has also been used in cardiac support device (Figure 9.5).

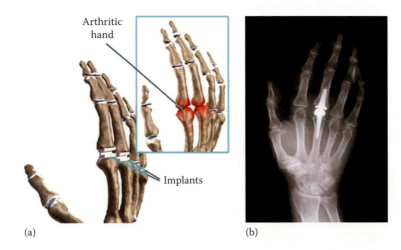

(a) (b)

Figure 9.4

Application of polypropylene in finger joint replacement. (a) Schematic illustration. (Courtesy of Randale Sechrest, Medical Multimedia Group LLC (MMG), Missoula, MT, Copyright 2002. Reproduced with permission.) (b) X-ray image of a finger joint implant.

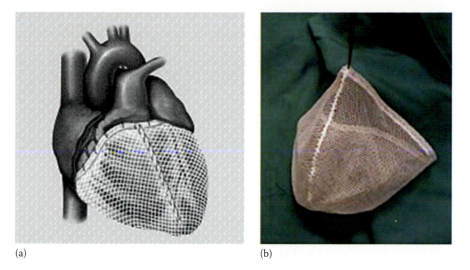

(a)   (b)

Figure 9.5
Cardiac support device (CSD). (a) Implanted in position and (b) appearance prior to surgery. The high flexibility of polypropylene and poly(ethylene terephthalate), as well as textile structure, ensures the comfort of the CSD. (Reprinted by permission from Macmillan Publishers Ltd. on behalf of Cancer Research U.K., Nat. Clin. Pract. Cardiovasc. Med., 3, 507, Copyright 2006.)

9.2 POLY(ETHYLENE TEREPHTHALATE)

Poly(ethylene terephthalate), commonly abbreviated PET, PETE, or the obsolete PETP or PET-P, is a thermoplastic polymer of the polyester family. Its monomer is bis-β hydroxyterephthalate, $C_{10}H_8O_4$ (Figure 9.6), which has nothing to do with ethylene. Polymerization is through a polycondensation reaction of the monomers, with water as the by-product. This polymer can be completely amorphous (transparent) or semicrystalline. The semicrystalline material might appear transparent (particle size <500 nm) or opaque and white (particle size up to a few microns) depending on its crystal structure [5].

Table 9.3 provides some physical and mechanical properties of PET. Similar to the role of the methyl side group in PP, the large benzyl group in the main chain lowers contacts between the molecules and decreases their intermolecular interactions. As a result, PET also shows a good flexibility, compared with PE.

PET makes up about 18% of the world polymer production and is the third-most-produced polymer; PE and PP are first and second, respectively [5]. PET has also been used widely to produce food-grade containers, as well as fibers, with the majority of the world's PET production being for the latter (in excess of 60%). In the textile industry, PET is referred to by its common name, *polyester*, whereas *PET* is generally used in the packaging industry. Textile PET has found application in cardiac support device (Figure 9.5).

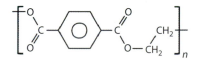

Figure 9.6
Molecular structure of poly(ethylene terephthalate) (PET).

Table 9.3

Properties of Poly(Ethylene Terephthalate)

Melting temperature (°C)	250
Glass transition temperature (°C)	70
Poisson's ratio	0.44
Density (g/cm³)	1.4–1.6
Tensile elastic modulus (GPa)	3.5–11
Tensile ultimate strength (MPa)	60–150
Tensile ultimate elongation (%)	5–70
Flexural elastic modulus (GPa)	3.5
Flexural strength (MPa)	100
Impact strength (J/m)	38

9.3   ACRYLATE POLYMER

Acrylic acid is the simplest *unsaturated carboxylic acid*, with the formula $CH_2=CHCOOH$ (Figure 9.7a). *Acrylates* are the salts and esters of acrylic acid with the formula $CH_2=CHCOOR$ (Figure 9.7b). Acrylate polymers, also referred to as *acrylics*, are a family of thermoset polymers made by the polymerization of an acrylic monomer, either acrylic acid or acrylate [6]. Two of the most common methacrylate polymers are poly(methyl acrylate) (PMA) and poly(methyl methacrylate) (PMMA) (Figure 9.8). Figure 9.9a shows the synthesis formula of thermoplastic polyacrylate. In Figure 9.9b, the synthesis formula of PMMA is illustrated.

Table 9.4 provides some physical and mechanical properties of PMMA. PMMA is a transparent, strong, and lightweight material. Its density is less than half that of silicate glasses. It also has good impact strength, higher than both silicate glasses. It has an excellent chemical resistivity (inertness) and thus is regarded as highly biocompatible in pure form [6].

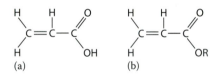

Figure 9.7
(a) Acrylic acid and (b) acrylate.

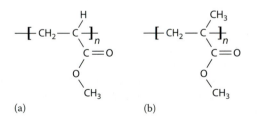

Figure 9.8
(a) Poly(methyl acrylate) is a white rubber at room temperature. (b) Poly (methyl methacrylate) (PMMA) is a strong, hard, and clear plastic.

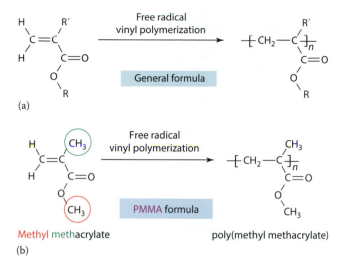

(a)

(b)

Methyl methacrylate   poly(methyl methacrylate)

Figure 9.9
Polyacrylate. (a) General reaction and (b) poly(methyl methacrylate) (PMMA).

Table 9.4

Properties of Poly(Methyl Methacrylate)

Melting temperature (°C)	160–230
Glass transition temperature (°C)	85–165
Poisson's ratio	0.35–40
Density (g/cm³)	1.17–1.20
Tensile elastic modulus (GPa)	3.0–3.5
Tensile ultimate strength (MPa)	35–80
Tensile ultimate elongation (%)	2.5–55
Flexural elastic modulus (GPa)	1.5–3.5
Flexural strength (MPa)	35–140
Impact strength (J/m)	27–65

PMMA has been used as a bone cement for hip prosthesis fixation (Figure 9.10). Bone cements are applied to anchor artificial implants (hip, knee, shoulder, and elbow joints). In addition to fixation, a special role of bone cement is to provide an elastic zone, by absorbing the locally high forces to ensure that the artificial implant remains in place over the long term. Bone cement has to be fluid before implantation and be able to *solidify* (polymerize) in situ once implanted in the body. Shrinkage during polymerization is an issue, as it causes loosening of implants, which can be alleviated by using already polymerized (i.e., solid) PMMA powder (Figure 9.11). The same strategy is also used for tooth fillings [6].

Assume the volume of a liquid of monomer is V_L (Figure 9.11a), and the volume of the material after polymerization is V_S (Figure 9.11b). Shrinkage percentage of PMMA polymer S_0 is defined as

$$S_0 = \frac{\Delta V}{V_0} = \frac{V_L - V_S}{V_L} \tag{9.1}$$

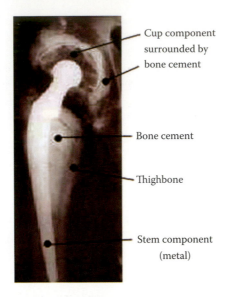

Figure 9.10
Application of PMMA bone cement in total hip replacement.

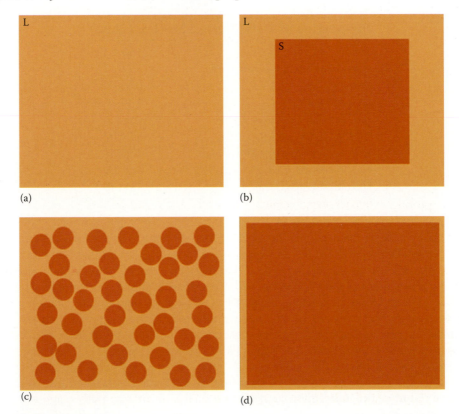

Figure 9.11
Shrinkage and its minimization of PMMA bone cement. (a) liquid monomer, (b) PMMA after polymerization, (c) PMMA powder added to monomer, and (d) level of shrinkage after polymerization. L stands for liquid and S for solid.

Table 9.5
Drawbacks of PMMA Cements

Mechanically
- It is *brittle*; it has low endurance limit and is prone to fatigue failure.
- It can be mechanically unreliable because it has entrapped *impurities* such as air and blood.
- It spawns small particles from its surface containing hard crystals of Barium sulfate which *scratch and damage the fine joint surfaces* of the artificial joint.

Biologically
- *S*mall cement particles may cause *osteolysis—bone dissolving disease*.
- It has very large surface, which may support colonization of bacteria and the development of postoperative *infections*.
- It may cause *allergy* and *anaphylactic reaction* during the operation.

and we have

$$\Delta V = S_0 V_L \tag{9.2}$$

Now, we add solid PMMA powder into the liquid monomers to a percentage P_S (Figure 9.11c). That is, in the beginning volume V_0, the volumes of solid and liquid materials are $V_0 P_S$ and $V_0(1 - P_S)$, respectively. After polymerization (Figure 9.11d), the liquid part will reduce its volume by $\Delta V = V_0(1 - P_S)S_0$, so the shrinkage percentage of the cement S_C is

$$S_C = \frac{\Delta V}{V_0} = \frac{V_0\left(1 - P_S\right)S_0}{V_0} = \left(1 - P_S\right)S_0 \tag{9.3}$$

According to Equation 9.3, the shrinkage of cement can be reduced to 40%, if we add 60% solid PMMA powder into the liquid monomer.

The product of PMMA bone cement is typically made of solid PMMA powder (mixed with catalysts, called activators) and monomer methyl methacrylate liquid. When the powder and liquid (which are separately packed as purchased) are mixed together, the monomer liquid is polymerized, which is initiated by the activator (hydrogen peroxide). The monomer liquid will wet the polymer powder particle surfaces and link them together after polymerization. The bone cement viscosity changes over time from a runny liquid into a dough-like state that can be safely applied and then finally hardens into a solid material. The set time can be tailored to help the surgeons safely apply the bone cement. PMMA cements have a number of drawbacks (Table 9.5), and its application has been reduced [6].

9.4 FLUOROCARBON POLYMERS

Polytetrafluoroethylene (PTFE) has a similar repeating unit to that of PE, except that the hydrogen atoms are replaced by fluorine atoms (Figure 9.12). PTFE is well known by the brand name Teflon®. Unlike PE, PTFE cannot be cross-linked and

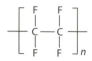

Figure 9.12
Molecular structure of polytetrafluoroethylene (PTFE).

Table 9.6
Properties of Polytetrafluoroethylene

Molecular weight of repeat unit (g/mol)	62
Melting temperature (°C)	335
Glass transition temperature (°C)	115
Poisson's ratio	0.46
Density (g/cm^3)	2.1–2.2
Tensile elastic modulus (GPa)	0.55
Tensile ultimate strength (MPa)	27
Tensile ultimate elongation (%)	300
Flexural elastic modulus (GPa)	0.50
Flexural strength (MPa)	No break
Impact strength (J/m)	190

become an elastomer because C−F bonds are very stable. Hence, PTFE is always a thermoplastic [7].

Table 9.6 provides some physical and mechanical properties of PTFE. PTFE is featured as highly chemically inert (and thus highly corrosion resistant), highly biocompatible, neither water nor oil wettable, and very flexible. It has been documented that PTFE persists at the site of reconstruction for the life of the repair. These properties make PTFE the material of choice for artificial blood vessels (Figure 9.13a), as it meets all essential requirements for this purpose, which include the following [7]:

- Biocompatibility
- Long-term durability
- Flexibility (blood vessels constantly creep and twist in the body)
- Resistance to thrombosis (blood clotting)

However, no materials are absolutely nonwettable, and thrombosis has been the biggest challenge in developing artificial blood vessels. PTFE vessels work reasonably well when their diameters are larger than 6 mm, which is the case of the application of aortic replacement (Figure 9.13b). However, most blood vessels are smaller than 6 mm in diameter, and severe thrombosis always occurs with PTFE vessels of this smaller size range. Currently, developing small-diameter blood vessels is one of the most active research areas in the field of biomaterials.

Another potential application of PTFE is as a heart patch in the surgical treatment of congenital heart disease (Figure 9.14). In certain congenital heart diseases, the heart of a newborn baby can be formed with an excessively small left ventricle. The small size may cause little problem when the baby is young, but as the baby grows, the need for oxygen increases, and the small ventricle may no longer maintain sufficient blood circulation. A potential surgical treatment is to enlarge the heart ventricle (Figure 9.14).

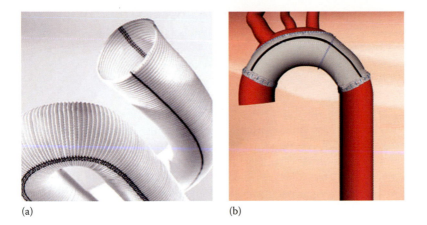

(a)   (b)

Figure 9.13
(a) Artificial vessel made of PTFE and (b) application as aorta prostheses.

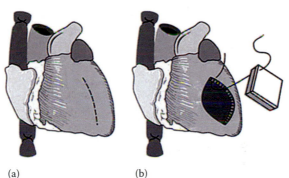

(a)   (b)

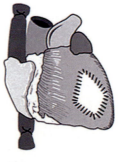

(c)

Figure 9.14
Schematic illustration of heart showing surgical procedure of PTFE heart patch implantation in rats. (a) A 6 mm midline ventriculotomy was created laterally to the left of the anterior descending artery. (b) A 4 × 4 × 2 mm³ patch was then implanted and sutured to the myocardium. (c) The restructured myocardium allows for partial enlargement of the ventricular cavity. (From Krupnick, A.S. et al., J. Heart Lung Transplant., 21, 233, 2002. Reproduced with permission of De Gruyter GmBH, J. Heart Lung Transplant., Copyright 2002.)

In brief, a long ventriculotomy is created in lateral position to the left anterior descending artery, and a properly sized artificial patch is sutured into the left ventricle to enlarge the ventricular cavity [8].

9.5   SILICONE

Silicones, more precisely called polymerized siloxanes or polysiloxanes, are mixed inorganic–organic polymers with the chemical formula $[R_2SiO]_n$, where R is an organic group such as methyl, ethyl, or phenyl [9]. A siloxane is a functional group in organo-silicon chemistry with the Si–O–Si linkage (Figure 9.15a). These polymers consist of an inorganic silicon–oxygen backbone (···–Si–O–Si–O–Si–O–···) with organic side groups attached to the silicon atoms, which are four-coordinate (Figure 9.15b). When both R groups are $-CH_3$, the polymer is called poly(dimethyl siloxane) (PDMS).

Silicones can be cross-linked via condensation curing using an acid cross-linker (Figure 9.16) or addition curing via oligomers containing vinyl groups (Figure 9.17) [9].

Table 9.7 provides some basic properties of silicone rubber. In addition, silicone rubber has the following features:

1. Si–O bonds have far lower energy than C–C bonds and so are much more stable and inert. Because of its inertness, silicone finds many applications in medical implants.
2. Generally, polysiloxane is very flexible due to large bond angles and bond lengths, when compared to those found in PE. The two side methyl groups lower contacts between the molecules, decreasing their intermolecular interactions.

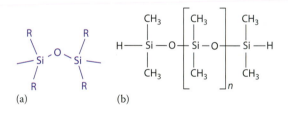
(a)   (b)

Figure 9.15
General molecular structure of (a) siloxanes and (b) polysiloxanes.

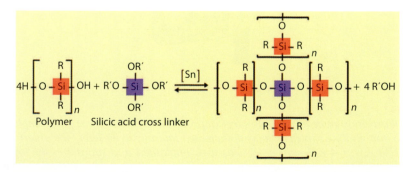

Figure 9.16
Condensation curing of silicone via an acid cross-linker.

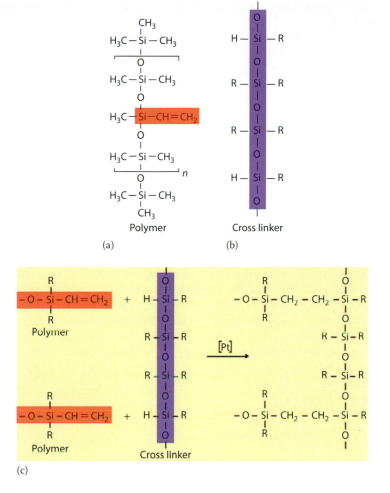

Figure 9.17
Addition curing of (a) silicone polymer using (b) oligomers containing vinyl groups, which reacts by condensation to form (c) a cross linked silicone polymer.

Table 9.7
Properties of Silicone Rubbers

Working temperature (°C)	−55 to 300
Glass transition temperature (°C)	150–200
Poisson's ratio	4.7–4.9
Density (g/cm³)	1.1–1.6
Tensile elastic modulus (GPa)	0.001–0.5
Tensile ultimate strength (MPa)	3–11
Tensile ultimate elongation (%)	100–1100
Flexural elastic modulus (GPa)	0.3–1.8
Flexural strength (MPa)	No break
Impact strength (J/m)	No break

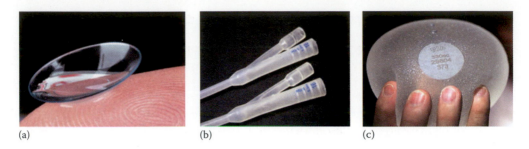

(a) (b) (c)

Figure 9.18
Applications of silicone elastomer: (a) contact lens; (b) catheters; (c) breast implant.

3. The loosely packed polymer chain network, due to the two side alkyl groups, also gives these polymers good oxygen permeability.
4. Silicon is nonwettable, a property which is desired when used in vascular grafts, but undesirable when used in contact lenses.

The high oxygen permeability of silicone is a desired property in materials used in contact lenses (Figure 9.18a). The highly hydrophobic (not wettable) nature of it also makes silicone useful for catheters (Figure 9.18b) and vascular grafts. Although silicones are typically rubber-like materials, they can also be produced in the form of a gel, for use in sealants, adhesives, and lubricants. Nowadays, breast implants (Figure 9.18c) are perhaps the most widely known surgical application of silicone.

9.6 POLYURETHANE

9.6.1 Polymer Chemistry of Polyurethanes

Polyurethane (IUPAC abbreviation PUR, but commonly abbreviated PU) is a family of copolymers in which the principal chain structure is composed of aliphatic (i.e., linear) or aromatic (cyclic/hexagonal) units R_1 and R_2, respectively, linked with polar *urethane groups* ($-NHCOO-$) (Figure 9.19):

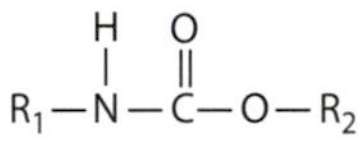

$$R_1-\overset{\overset{\displaystyle H}{|}}{N}-\overset{\overset{\displaystyle O}{\|}}{C}-O-R_2$$

Figure 9.19
Schematic diagram of a urethane monomer.

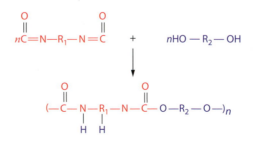

Figure 9.20
The polyaddition process in polyurethane synthesis.

R_1 is an aliphatic, aromatic, or alicyclic moiety in the isocyanate monomer (R_1–N=C=O) and R_2 is a more complex group derived from the polyol component, either *polyether* (−R−O−R′−) or *polyester* (−R−COO−R′−). Hence, the synthesis of PUs requires two essential components: *isocyanate* (typically diisocyanate O=C=N−R_1−N=C=O) and a bi- or multifunctional *polyol* with two hydroxyl (−OH) terminal groups. The principal chemical reaction involved in the synthesis of PUs is the urethane-forming reaction between isocyanate and the hydroxyl group −OH in the step growth copolymerization of diisocyanates and polyols (Figure 9.20).

PUs can be either thermoplastic or irreversibly thermoset. The use of diisocyanate and a bifunctional polyol results in thermoplastics without cross-linking, whereas the use of components with more than two functional groups (e.g., triisocyanate or a multihydroxyl polyol) will yield PUs with three-dimensional cross-linking.

9.6.2 Third Component in PU Synthesis: The Chain Extender

The direct reaction of diisocyanate with a single long-chain diol group usually produces a soft polymer with low mechanical strength. This property can be drastically changed by the addition of a so-called chain extender, which is usually a *diol* (HO−R−OH) or a *diamine* (H_2N−R−NH_2) (Figure 9.21). The chain extender is typically a shorter chain with lower molecular weight in comparison to long chain diols. A polyurethane-urea is obtained when a diamine is used (Figure 9.22a), while a polyurethane results when the diol is used (Figure 9.22b).

The chain extender is literally used to produce an *extended* sequence in the copolymer chain (Figure 9.23). These extended sequences are rigid segments that

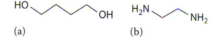

(a) (b)

Figure 9.21
Chain extenders commonly used for the synthesis of biomedical-grade polyurethanes, such as butane-diol (a) and ethane-diamine (b), characterized by having relatively shorter chains.

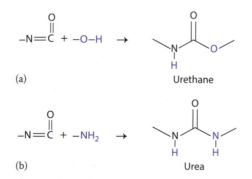

(a) Urethane

(b) Urea

Figure 9.22
Chain extension reaction occurs between isocyanate and a diol in the case of polyurethane (a) or a diamine in the case of polyurethane-urea (b).

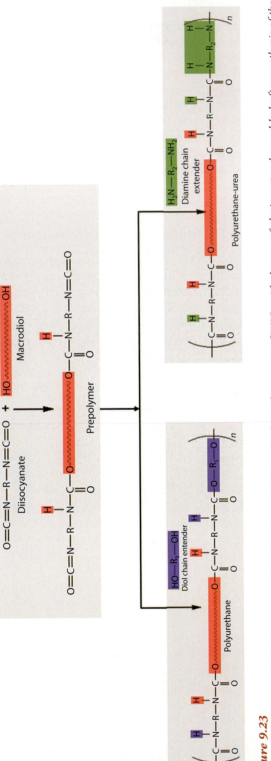

Figure 9.23

Schematic of the synthesis of a segmented polyurethane (PU) and polyurethane-urea (PUU), with the use of chain extenders added after synthesis of the prepolymer. Segmented PUs typically undergo microphase separation to form hard, crystalline domains and soft amorphous domains. The resultant polyurethanes are thus phase-segregated polymers composed of alternating dispersed soft (amorphous) segments of long-chain polyols, and hard (glassy or crystalline) segments of diisocyanate and chain extender sections (Figure 9.24).

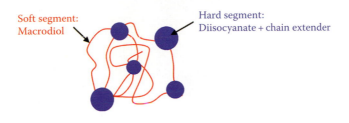

Soft segment: Macrodiol

Hard segment: Diisocyanate + chain extender

Figure 9.24
The hard segments serve as physical links between the soft segments, which results in elasticity. Other names: block copolymer, segmented copolymer.

associate with one another into three-dimensional nanophases, which act both as filler particles and physical cross-link sites to increase mechanical strength. Hence, PUs are typically synthesized from three reactant precursors: long-chain polyols (usually diols or triols), di- or triisocyanates, and chain extenders. The properties of the final polyurethane produced are primarily dependent on the chemical nature (types of diol, diamine, or isocyanine) of these three building blocks, and the relative proportions used during synthesis.

Segmented PUs typically undergo microphase separation to form hard, crystalline domains and soft amorphous domains. The resultant polyurethanes are thus phase-segregated polymers composed of alternating dispersed soft (amorphous) segments of long-chain polyols, and *hard* (glassy or crystalline) segments of diisocyanate and chain extender sections (Figure 9.24).

Under standard conditions, the amorphous domains of PU are elastomeric because the lower glass transition is lower than room temperature. The hard domains function as physical cross-links that fix each soft segment at its two ends and thus prevent the chains from flowing apart when they are stretched under applied stress. Without flow, the stretched polymer segments can then reshape elastically when stress is released. Hence, segmented PUs can exhibit rubber-like behaviors. Unlike chemical cross-links, however, these physical cross-links are not thermally stable. Subject to sufficient heat treatment, the semicrystalline hard phase can be melted as with any other thermoplastic polymer.

In short, segmented PUs are typical thermoplastic elastomers, exhibiting rubber-like mechanical properties and thermoplastic characteristics, being soluble in polar solvents and able to melt at elevated temperatures.

9.6.3 Properties and Medical Applications of PUs

PUs represent a large family of polymeric materials with an enormous diversity of chemical compositions and mechanical properties, with flexibility and moderate blood compatibility being their most prominent features. Because of this diversity, PUs are among the most extensively used synthetic polymers in biomedical applications, and remain one of the most popular groups of biomaterials applied to medical devices after half a century of use in the healthcare system [10]. Materials based on PU have played a major role in the development of durable cardiovascular devices since the 1980s, such as blood bags, vascular catheters, bladders of the left ventricle

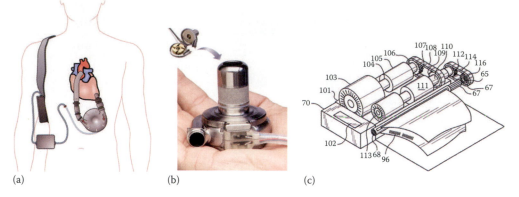

(a)   (b)   (c)

Figure 9.25

Medical applications of polyurethane in left ventricle assistant devices (LVADs). A portable LVAD worn (a), containing an implanted stator/rotor LVAD pump (b). Blood passes through this pump from the left ventricle to the aorta, while controlled by a percutaneous cable from the controller around the waist, also housed in polyurethane. An older, non-portable LVAD (c) with a continuous pump and polyurethane bladder.

assist device (LVAD) (Figure 9.25), heart valves (however not in use anymore), insulators in heart pacemakers, the total artificial heart (TAH) and small caliber grafts for vascular access and bypass surgery. Advanced topics on polyurethane as biomaterials are provided at the end of this chapter.

9.7 CHAPTER HIGHLIGHTS

1. The hardening of modern UHMWPE involves ultrahigh molecular weight, high crystallinity, and high cross-link density.
2. The side alkyl or large benzyl groups of PP or PET make it very difficult for the polymer molecules to align themselves up side by side in an orderly way. This results in lower contacts between the molecules and therefore decreased intermolecular interactions, which makes the polymer highly flexible.
3. PTFE, which is highly inert, flexible, and nonwettable by either oil or water, meets the four essential requirements on artificial blood vessels:
   Biocompatible
   • Long-term durable
   • Flexible (blood vessels constantly creep and twist in the body)
   • Resistant to thrombosis (blood clotting)
4. PTFE artificial blood vessels work reasonably well when their diameters are larger than 6 mm. However, severe thrombosis always occurs with PTFE artificial blood vessel when its diameter is 6 mm or less, which forms the biggest challenge in this field.
5. PMMA can thermoset at body temperature, and thus is applied as a bone cement. Shrinkage of bone cement and tooth fillings can be alleviated by the addition of a solid particle powder to the liquid polymer precursor.
6. The loosely packed polymer chain network of silicone due to the alkyl side chains gives these polymers good oxygen permeability, which is a necessary property of materials used in contact lens.

Table 9.8

Major Features of Bioinert Polymers and Their Applications

Polymer	Featured Properties	Major Applications
UHMWPE	Hard	Joint prosthesis
PP/PET	Flexible	Finger joint, cardiac support device
PMMA	Strong, in situ cross-linkable	Bone cement
PTFE	Flexible, nonsticky	Artificial blood vessel
Silicone	Elastic, good oxygen permeability, hydrophobic	Contact lens, blood vessel, catheter
PU	Elastic, diverse properties	Blood bag, catheter, bladder, or insulator in cardiac devices

7. PU rubber is a family of thermoplastic elastomers, in which the amorphous polymer chains are physically cross-linked to crystalline domains (precipitates).

8. Summary of bioinert polymers (Table 9.8)

ACTIVITIES

Register with UHMWPE Lexicon. Download
  Chapter 4 The origins of UHMWPE in joint replacements
  Chapter 5 Alternatives to conventional UHMWPE for hip arthroplasty

SIMPLE QUESTIONS IN CLASS

1. The superior wear-resistance of UHMWPE is NOT achieved via
   a. Cross-linking
   b. Carbon fiber reinforcement
   c. Ultrahigh molecular weight
   d. High crystallinity
2. Acrylic acid is
   a. Saturated carboxylic acid
   b. Acrylate
   c. Unsaturated carboxylic acid
   d. Alcohol
3. How can you minimize the shrinkage of PMMA bone cement?
   a. Include prepolymerized PMMA powder in liquid monomers.
   b. Reduce cross-link density.
   c. Slow down polymerization kinetics.
   d. Add an activator.
4. Currently, polytetrafluoroethylene (PTFE) is the best biomaterial for vascular applications because of (choose the best answer):
   a. Resistance to wetting
   b. Flexibility
   c. Inertness
   d. A combination of the aforementioned three properties

5. What unique property of silicone makes it the choice of material among many durable elastomers for contact lens?
   a. Chemically stabile
   b. Elastic
   c. Hydrophilic
   d. Oxygen permeable
6. Which of the following descriptions is incorrect for silicone?
   a. Chemically stabile
   b. Elastic
   c. Hydrophilic
   d. Oxygen permeable
7. Polyurethane could be
   a. Thermoset rubber
   b. Thermoplastic
   c. Chemically cross-linked elastomer
   d. Thermoplastic rubber
8. Which of the following bonding is the most stable one?
   a. C−C
   b. C−F
   c. C−O
   d. Si−O
9. Which of the following bonding is the most unstable one?
   a. C−C
   b. C−F
   c. C−O
   d. Si−O

PROBLEMS AND EXERCISES

1. Schematically demonstrate the structural difference between polyethylene (PE) and polypropylene (PP). PP has been used in the finger joint (Figure 9.4b). What mechanical property of PP makes it the biomaterial of choice for this application? Explain why PP has a better flexural fatigue resistance than PE.
2. Explain why poly(ethylene terephthalate) (PET) has a good flexibility.
3. The polymerization shrinkage of PMMA is ~1.0%. To achieve PMMA bone cement of 0.4% shrinkage, calculate the percent of PMMA powder that should be present in the bone cement mixture.
4. The polymerization shrinkage of PMMA is ~1.0%. A bone cement made of PMMA liquid and powder has a shrinkage of 0.8%. Calculate the percent of liquid and solid power components present in the bone cement.
5. The monomer of PMA shown in Figure 9.8 is not cross-linkable. Discuss what the monomer structure should be to produce cross-linkable PMA. Show your explanation with molecular structure graphs.
6. Which polymers have been used to engineer artificial blood vessels? List the essential requirements of biomaterials used as artificial blood vessels.
7. Schematically demonstrate the molecular structure of silicone. Explain why silicone has a good oxygen permeability.

8. Silicone is hydrophobic, and must be surface-modified to be hydrophilic for contact lens application. Search on Web of Science, and based on your reading, discuss how the surface of silicone has been modified to be hydrophilic.
9. Polyurethane (PU) could be either thermoplastic or rubber-like. Explain the mechanism behind the rubber behavior of PU.
10. Schematically demonstrate, based on Figures 9.16 and 9.17, the network of Silicone rubber cross-linked via condensation or addition curing.

ADVANCED TOPIC: PROPERTIES AND APPLICATIONS OF POLYURETHANE AS BIOMATERIALS

PUs remain one of the most popular groups of biomaterials applied to medical devices after half a century of use in the healthcare system [1]. These materials have played a major role in the development of durable cardiovascular devices since the 1980s, such as blood bags, vascular catheters, bladders of the left ventricle assist device (LVAD), the total artificial heart (TAH), and small caliber grafts for vascular access and bypass surgery [2]. However, they are also problematic in regard to long-term stability, manifested in failed applications as pacemaker leads and breast implant coatings [3]. During the next decade, PUs became extensively researched for their susceptibility to biodegradation. Research efforts toward understanding their biodegradation has yielded novel PUs with improved stability for long-term implantation applications, as well as an entirely new class of bioresorbable PUs. To this end, more recent attention has been paid to balancing biodegradability with the durability of PUs to achieve more tunable biomaterials.

Biocompatibility of PUs

The biocompatibility of various PUs has been intensively investigated both in vitro and in vivo for a wide range of applications, from durable medical devices (such as vascular catheters, the total artificial heart, and small-diameter vascular grafts for artificial reconstruction or bypass surgery) [3,4,8] to biodegradable implants used in tissue engineering [6]. Excellent reviews on biocompatibility of PUs can be found in three representative books: (1) *Polyurethanes in Medicine* (Lelah and Cooper, CRC Press 1986), (2) *Polyurethanes in Biomedical Applications* (Lamba et al., CRC Press, 1998), and (3) *Biomedical Applications of Polyurethanes* (Vermette et al., Eurekah.Com, 2001), as well as several specific reviews [1–3,6,9–11]. This appendix provides a summary of PU biocompatibility.

In Vitro Evaluation (Cell Culture Studies) of PUs

The cell types used to assess the biocompatibility of PUs are frequently fibroblasts and endothelial cells, which are amongst the most commonly used for cytotoxicity tests of biomaterials. Other types of cells used include specific types of leukocytes, as well as specific epithelial cells representative of those that interface with the PU materials at sites of implantation in different tissues (e.g., skin, blood vessel, tympanum, and cornea [12]). In general, PUs are recognized to have good biocompatibility, maintaining sufficient cell adhesion and proliferation rates in vitro [2,13]; however, this short-term cytocompatibility (several days) is not completely representative of the longer-term efficacy and safety of PU required in vivo (weeks to months), as discussed in the following.

In Vivo Assessment of PUs

While PUs were recognized in the 1970s and 1980s as stable materials for blood contact, and had been applied in a wide range of cardiovascular devices [3,14,15], their application in long-term implants fell under scrutiny since the failure of pacemaker leads and breast implant coatings containing PUs in the late 1980s [1]. During the next decade, the susceptibility of PUs to biodegradation was extensively researched both in vitro and in vivo, with the latter conducted by routine subcutaneous, intramuscular, and intraperitoneal implantation. Evaluations in other more specialized implantation sites, forming more complex implants, included the cardiovascular system (artificial heart [16], vascular grafts [17–22] and stents [23]), the middle ear (artificial tympanic membrane [24]), the eye (artificial intraocular lenses [25]), the digestive tract (stent-like extensions for the esophagus [26]) and digestive tract (engineered replacements for the ureter [27] and biliary ducts [28]).

In addition to mechanical failures caused by the limited biostability of PUs, the biological toxicity of degradation products of PUs was also found to be a serious problem. Aromatic diisocyanates (e.g., 4,4′-methylenediphenyl diisocyanate (MDI) and toluene diisocyanate (TDI)) have been recognized as potentially carcinogenic byproducts of PUs [29,30]. Although PUs do not degrade to isocyanates, it is likely that trace amounts of isocyanate remain unreacted within the polymer. Thus, a greater concern would be the toxicity of these and other leachates. To address this problem, aliphatic diisocyanate such as lysine diisocyanate (LDI) and 1,4-diisocyanatobutane (butyl diisocyanate, BDI), have superceded the use of aromatic diisocyanates [31–33] for the synthesis of biodegradable PUs. These polymers exhibit better blood and tissue compatibility, showing no adverse tissue reactions both in vitro and in vivo compared to those made using aromatic reactants [2,13]. PUs synthesized using LDI as the diisocyanate demonstrate no overtly harmful effects in vivo [13]. Their subcutaneous implantation in female Sprague-Dawley rats revealed that LDI-based PUs did not aggravate capsule formation, accumulation of macrophages (foreign body giant cells), or tissue necrosis [34].

Degradability of PUs

As mentioned, PUs were traditionally developed as long-term implant materials [3,35], and many attempts were made to create versions that resisted biodegradation processes [3]. Converse to this, more recent attempts have been made to enhance the biodegradability of PUs. Since the late 1990s, scientists have been utilizing the flexible chemistry and diverse mechanical properties of PU materials [5] to design degradable polymers for applications as varied as neural conduits [36], cardiac muscle engineering [37–39], and bone replacements [40]. These materials have taken advantage of processes such as hydrolytic mechanisms, and have been made with varied molecular structure to allow controlled hydrolysis rates.

DEGRADATION MECHANISMS OF POLYURETHANES

The susceptibility of PUs to biodegradation lies in soft segment components of the polymer. These segments generally dominate the degradation characteristics of PUs, with higher proportions of soft segments tending to correlate with increased degradation rate [31]. Along with the hydrolysis of ester bonds, several decomposition mechanisms have been identified in PUs used as long-term implants, including oxidation, environmental stress cracking (ESC), and enzymatic degradation [31,41], further described as follows:

1. Hydrolysis: The aliphatic ester bonds in polyester–urethanes are well known to be susceptible to hydrolysis [42].
2. Environmental stress cracking: Polyether–urethane materials are susceptible to a degradation phenomenon involving crack formation and propagation [43]. This microcracking phenomenon, known as environmental stress cracking (ESC), is believed to be due to residual polymer surface stress, which may have been introduced during the fabrication process. This could be caused by surface flaws or sensitization by reactive agents, and may not be sufficiently eliminated by annealing the materials.
3. Oxidation: In some biomedical devices, oxidative degradation can be a contributing mechanism. Implanted polyether–urethane devices that contain metallic components have been subject to bulk oxidation, initiated by corrosion products catalyzed by the aqueous ionic environment of the implant site [44,45].
4. Enzymatic degradation: PU degradation can also occur by the action of water-soluble enzymes in the physiological environment of the implant site. While enzymes have evolved biologically with highly specific affinities for particular biological substrates, some appear capable of recognizing and acting nonspecifically upon synthetic substrates in the PU polymer. Smith and colleagues found that enzymes are capable of altering the chemical structure of PU polymers [46], and although the mechanism is not certain, a mechanistic model of hydrolytic enzyme action on hydrogen-bonded sites in PUs has been proposed by Santerre and colleagues [47].
5. Mineralization/calcification: Calcification (deposition of calcium-containing apatite minerals) has also been reported to occur in cardiovascular [48] and noncardiovascular medical devices [49]. In fact, calcification is the leading macroscopic cause of failure for most prosthetic heart valves and blood pumps, limiting the functional lifetime of the device by loss of elasticity in the PU parts [50].

Among these mechanisms, ESC, oxidation, and calcification only became evident after several years of long-term implantation. For biodegradable PUs, which are designed to degrade in a relatively shorter period (several months), the effective degradation mechanism is hydrolysis with or without the assistance of enzymatic catalysis [6]. The degradation mechanisms suggested in the literature are summarized in Figure 9.26. Ester linkages are thought to hydrolyze both in vitro and in vivo, thereby yielding α-hydroxy-acid degradation products, as well as urethane and urea fragments with terminal acid groups [6].

As regards the degradation of urethane and urea fragments to free polyamines, there is currently a lack of consensus in the literature on the specific mechanism

317

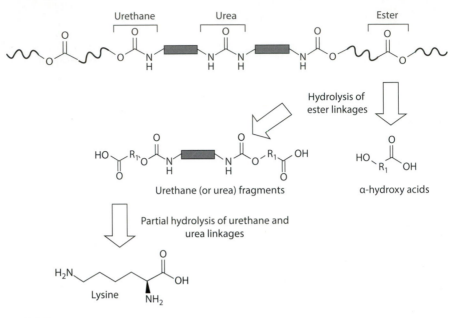

Figure 9.26
Schematic showing the sites of attack and possible by-products following breakdown of L-lysine-based poly(ester-urethane) by hydrolysis. (From Guelcher, S.A., Tissue Eng. Part B: Rev., 14, 3, 2008.)

for this. For lysine-derived polyisocyanates, hydrolysis of urethane linkages to lysine has been reported [51,52]. Hydrolysis of the ester group in lysine poly-isocyanates yields a carboxylic acid group in the polymer, which may catalyze further degradation [53]. Others have reported that urethane and urea linkages are enzymatically degradable [54]. Despite the lack of consensus regarding a specific degradation mechanism, these researchers have consistently reported that PU biomaterials prepared from lysine-derived (or other amine-derived) polyiso-cyanates are biodegradable both in vitro and in vivo to noncytotoxic products [36,40,51,52,54–56].

Biodegradable Polyurethanes Designed for Tissue Engineering and Drug Delivery

In contrast to traditional biomedical PU implants that are designed to have a long-term in vivo biostability, PUs used as tissue engineering scaffolds and drug delivery systems are designed to undergo faster hydrolytic degradation to noncytotoxic decomposition products in vivo. An immediate and frequently utilized strategy for achieving biodeg-radation of PU elastomers is to incorporate a polyester macrodiol soft segment that hydrolyzes in vitro and in vivo, such as poly(lactic acid) (PLA) or poly(glycolic acid) (PGA) [53], and polycaprolactone (PCL). Porous polyester urethane ureas (PEUUs) syn-thesized from 1,4-Diisocyanatohexane (BDI) and Poly(ε-caprolactone) PCL have been reported to be completely resorbed in rats after only 12 weeks [57]. The structures of other isocyanates and polyols used to synthesize biodegradable PU biomaterials are listed in Table 9.9.

Table 9.9

Summary of Isocyanates and Polyols Used to Synthesize Biodegradable Polyurethane Biomaterials

Isocyanates	Polyols

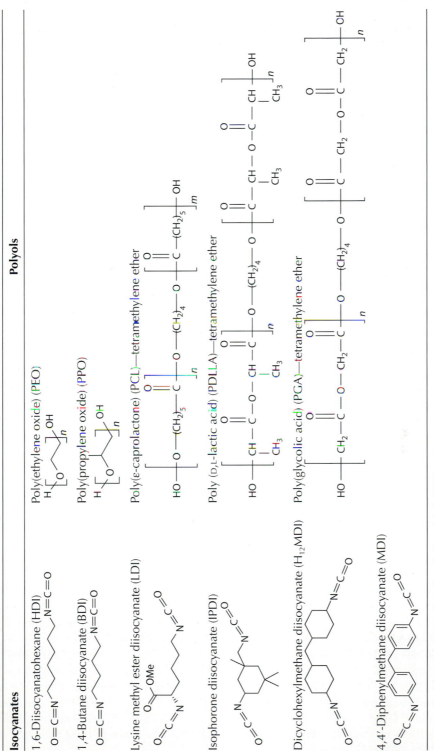

1,6-Diisocyanatohexane (HDI)

1,4-Butane diisocyanate (BDI)

Lysine methyl ester diisocyanate (LDI)

Isophorone diisocyanate (IPDI)

Dicyclohexylmethane diisocyanate (H$_{12}$MDI)

4,4'-Diphenylmethane diisocyanate (MDI)

Poly(ethylene oxide) (PEO)

Poly(propylene oxide) (PPO)

Poly(ε-caprolactone) (PCL)—tetramethylene ether

Poly (D,L-lactic acid) (PDLLA)—tetramethylene ether

Poly(glycolic acid) (PGA)—tetramethylene ether

Source: Guelcher, S.A., Tissue Eng. Part B: Rev., 14, 3, 2008.

Biodegradation of PUs can be further achieved by enhancing degradation of hard segments with the incorporation of a chain extender that is recognizable by enzymes [54,58]. PU elastomers have been synthesized from BDI, polyethylene glycol (PEG), in the form of PCL–PEG–PCL macrodiol triblock copolymers, and the synthetic peptide alanine-alanine-lysine (AAK) as a chain extender. The linkage between alanine units can be cleaved by a specific elastase. Polymers synthesized from the AAK chain extender have been observed to degrade significantly faster than those synthesized from a putrescine chain extender, and the degradation products were noncytotoxic [58].

Degradation Rates of Biodegradable PUs (Nontraditional Medical Devices)

The in vitro degradation rates of biodegradable PUs, typically in physiological solutions such as phosphate buffered saline (PBS), can be controlled by altering the composition of the polyester polyol component of these polymers [55,59–62]. PU elastomers with amorphous soft segments have been observed to degrade more rapidly than those with semicrystalline soft segments [63]. PUs with hydrophilic soft segments have been reported to exhibit increased water uptake, further enhancing the hydrolytic degradation rate [63].

In vivo evaluations have consistently demonstrated that aliphatic BDI-based PEUU elastomers degrade much faster than aromatic MDI-based PEUUs (Table 9.10). Porous PEUU synthesized from BDI and a long PCL diol (PCL2000) were almost completely absorbed at 12 weeks after implantation [57], whereas PEUU synthesized from MDI and the short-chain PCL diol (PCL350) degraded significantly more slowly, requiring longer than 24 months to be completely resorbed [64–66]. This is not surprising, as aromatic diisocyanate was historically employed for applications where degradation was not desirable, such as for pacemaker lead coverings, catheters, and wound dressings [1,35]. In contrast to the inflammation caused by biodegradable poly-L-lactic acid (PLA), poly-glycolic acid (PGA), and poly-L-lactate glycolic acid (PLGA) due to their acidic degradation products, PUs do not introduce significant pH changes in the microenvironment of their degradation and exhibit steady degradation kinetics with no significant signs of an autocatalytic effect [67].

Mechanical Properties of PUs

Besides satisfactory biocompatibility, PUs can be tailored to have a broad range of mechanical properties (Table 9.11) [42,75]. As with tuning the degradation rate, the mechanical properties can also be tuned by modifying the structure of the hard and soft segments and/or changing the relative fractions of each. Even the choice of using diamines or diols [7] as the chain extenders can alter the properties of the PUs [76]. For example, PUs prepared from 4,4′-diphenylmethane diisocyanate (MDI) and 1,4-butanediol (BDO) as hard segments, with oxypropylene-oxyethylene diol (OPOE) as soft segments, demonstrate a wide range of Young's modulus (11–1690 MPa), ultimate tensile strength (UTS) (2–60 MPa), and elongation at break (50%–570%). For this material system, these mechanical ranges are achieved by the alteration of the molar ratio of MDI/BDO to OPOE [77] (Table 9.11).

Table 9.10

Summary of the Degradation Rates of Polyurethanes

Polyurethanes	In Vivo or In Vitro	Degradation Kinetics	Refs.
Porous PEUU (~80%) synthesized from BDI and PCL (BDI/PCL2000)	In vivo: right ventricular outflow tract of rats	At 12 weeks the PEUU scaffolds were almost completely absorbed.	[57]
	In vivo: infarcted left ventricle wall surface of rats	The PEUU was largely resorbed 8 weeks after implantation.	[37]
	In vitro: release of basic fibroblast growth factor (bFGF)	Scaffolds loaded with bFGF showed slightly higher degradation rates than unloaded control scaffolds.	[68]
Porous scaffolds synthesized from BDI, PHC and PCL: 1. Polyester carbonate urethane urea (PECUU) 2. Poly(ester urethane)urea (PEUU) 3. Poly(carbonate urethane)urea (PCUU)	In vitro: PBS. In vivo: subcutaneous implants in rats	The majority of the PEUU porous scaffolds degraded over an 8-week period. Degradation rates: PCUU < PECUU < PEUU	[69]
LTI or HDI with polyester copolymer (60%–70% PCL-co-20%–30% PGA-co-10% PDLLA) and PEG (the molar ratio of polyester: PEG is 50:50)	In vitro: in enzymatic, oxidative and PBS medium	After 8 weeks of incubation, mass loss ranged from 10% to 100%, depending on both the medium and chemistry of the polymer. Generally, LTI-based polymers degrade faster than HDI-based PEUU. PEG accelerates degradation. Replacement of PGA with more PCL decreases degradation.	[70]
TMDI, with PHB and PGA-co-CL	In vivo: sciatic nerve of rats.	The molar weight decrease shows the same behavior in vivo as in vitro. A weight loss of 33%, 74%, and 88% for polymers containing 41, 17, and 8 wt.% PHB, respectively, was observed after 24 weeks by nuclear magnetic resonance (NMR) analysis. In all cases, the polymer fragments had a porous appearance with multiple surface cracks as evidenced by scanning electron microscope analysis. Guidance channels made of 8 wt.% PHB containing polymer displayed the highest degree of degradation at 24 weeks with only small polymer fragments remaining.	[36]

(Continued)

Table 9.10 (Continued)
Summary of the Degradation Rates of Polyurethanes

Polyurethanes	In Vivo or In Vitro	Degradation Kinetics	Refs.
LDI/TMDI, with PHB/HV and PCL	In vivo: subcutaneous implants in rats	After 1 year of subcutaneous implantation in rats, the molecular weight of the test polymers was reduced to about 50%, depending on the composition.	[40]
Fibrous PEUU synthesized from MDI and PCL MDI/PCL530	In vivo: infarcted left ventricle wall surface of rats.	PEUU scaffolds showed no histological signs of the degradation. Lack of cellular penetration.	[64–66]
	In vivo: rabbit and mini-pig anterior cruciate ligament (ACL) reconstruction.	MDI/PCL530 elastomers degrade very slowly. The first clear histological signs of degradation of the polymer were detected after 24 months.	[71]
Porous scaffolds synthesized from HMDI, PEO-PPO-PEO, and PCL at various ratios	In vivo: iliac crest of sheep	Degradation was observed at 24 months after implantation.	[72,73]
HDI-doped poly(1,8-octanediol citrate (POC) PEUU	In vitro: 0.05M NaCl solution	Mass loss was nearly 100% after 12–48 h incubation, depending on the synthesis conditions.	[74]

Table 9.11

Summary of the Mechanical Properties of Polyurethane Biomaterials

Polyurethanes	(Initial) Young's Modulus (MPa)	UTS (MPa)	Breaking Strain (%)	Resilience at 10% Strain (%)	Permanent Deformation (%)	Refs.
PEUU: BDI/BDA/PCL	14–78	9.2–29	660–895			[78]
PEEUU: BDI/PCL-PEG-PCL	4.6–75	8–20	325–560			[60]
PEUU: BDI/PCL	*24*	*34*	*660*	*99*		[58,69]
PECUU:BDI/PCL-polycarbonate	*9–14*	*16–21*	*667–827*	*99–100*		
PCUU: BDI/Polycarbonate	*8*	*14*	*875*	*100*		
PEUU: LDI/PCL	40	17	800		15.5	[79]
BDI/PCL	52	29	1042		12.0	
HDI/PCL	38	38	1168		18.5	
BDI·BDO·BDI·BDO·BDI/PCL	70–105	35–44	560–650			[80]
BDA/PCL	145	46.0	850		10.8	[81]
BDO/PCL	23.2	23.1	835		15.0	
BDO·BDI·BDO/PCL	70.0	45.0	560		8.9	
BDO/PCL:PLLA(50:50)	12	12	750		13.5	[82]
BDI·BDO·BDI/PCL:PLLA	60	23	640		13.5	
BDO·BDI·BDO/PCL:PLLA	62	44	560		10.0	
PEUU: MDI/PCL	6–70		16–130			[64]
LDI/PCL	*6.6–82*	*12.5–30.8*	*580–682*			[62]
LDI/PEO-PCL	*49–105*	*6–26*	*510–726*			[15]
LDI/PCL-PEO-PCL	30–300	1.3–13.5	13.8–1142			[83]
LDI/PCL	1203–1427	82–110	11			[84]
LTI/PCL						
HDI-doped POC PEUU	2.53–29.82	15.6–33.4	252–291			[74]
MDI/BDO/OPOE	11–1690	2–60	50–570			[77]

Table 9.12
Mechanical Properties of Some Human Soft Tissues

Tissue	Young's Modulus (MPa)	Strain at Break (%)	Refs.
Relaxed smooth muscle	0.006	300	[85]
Contracted smooth muscle	0.01	300	[85]
Aortic valve leaflet	15 ± 6	21 ± 12	[86]
Pericardium	20.4 ± 1.9	34.9 ± 1.1	[87]
Cerebral vein	6.85	83	[88]
Myocardium	0.2–0.5 (at the end of diastole)	>20	[89,90]

Most aliphatic diisocynate (BDI, LDI, and HDI)-based PEUUs have a Young's modulus (at small strains) and ultimate tensile strength (UTS) of several tens of MPa, and an impressively large breaking strain in the range of 100%–1000% (Table 9.11). The Young's moduli of PUs are close to the stiffness range of some soft tissues, but still significantly higher than many soft tissues (Table 9.12). Nonetheless, PUs can be processed into very thin films (10–15 μm in thickness) [38,39] and highly porous networks [37] which further enhances compliance of PUs. A major limitation of these biodegradable PEUUs is that they do not fare well in dynamic environments (such as cardiac muscle) due to the onset of permanent deformation (column 6 of Table 9.11). As such, the design and development of a soft and completely elastic material (with 100% recovery from deformation) for tissue engineering still remains a challenge.

Thermal Properties and Processability of PUs

Unlike chemical cross-linking, which renders materials insoluble and incapable of being further shaped by heat and pressure, physically cross-linked PU elastomers have a good processability [91], such that they can be easily melted around 50°C. Hence, they can be fabricated into various complicated shapes, such as fibers, sheets, and highly porous scaffolds by a number of techniques, such as extrusion [92], wet spinning [71,120], electrospinning [93–96], thermally induced phase separation (TIPS) [67], and salt leaching/freeze-drying [72,73,80,81] (Table 9.13). By applying such fabrication techniques, different porosities, surface-to-volume ratios, and three-dimensional structures can be achieved. PUs with concomitant changes in mechanical properties can in this way be designed and produced to suit a wide range of soft tissue engineering applications, including for the repair of cardiovascular, muscular, and neuronal tissues [6].

Applications of PUs in Tissue Engineering

Since the early 1990s, polyurethane elastomers have been studied for soft tissue engineering, in particular cardiovascular tissue [3,14,15]. The superelasticity of certain polyurethane elastomers has made them ideal for cardiac muscle repair [37–39]. As discussed, the Young's modulus of most PU is in the range of 2–100 MPa (Table 9.11), which is much higher than that of the heart muscle at the end of diastole; however, fabrication of PU thin films [38,39] or highly porous networks [37] allows finer tuning of compliance for specific mechanical ranges. Researchers from the University of Toronto [38,39] carried out a series of in vitro studies on the integrity of the cardiomyocytes

Table 9.13

Summary of the Thermal Properties of Polyurethane Biomaterials

Polyurethanes	M_w (kDa)	Viscosity (dL/g)	T_g (Soft Domain) (°C)	T_m (Hard Domain) (°C)	Water Contact Angle (°)	Refs.
PEUU: BDI/BDA/PCL	74.7–352.1		−54.3 to −36.5	40.2–44.7		[78]
PEUU: BDI/PCL-PEG-PCL	78.0 112.4		−53.4 to −46.6	40.5–52.8	32–68	[60]
PEUU: BDI/PCL		1.38	−54	40	80	[58,69]
PECUU: BDI/ PCL-polycarbonate		0.8–1.32	−54 to −51	16–24	76–81	
PCUU: BDI/polycarbonate		0.8	−46		73	[79]
PEUU: LDI/PCL		2.18	−52.1			
BDI/PCL		1.05	−56.7			
HDI/PCL		1.72	−51.0			
BDI·BDO·BDI·BDO·BDI/PCL		1.02–2.00	−60.4 to −54.0			[80]
BDA/PCL		3.55	−57			
BDO/PCL		3.04		19.7		[81]
BDO·BDI·BDO/PCL		2.94				
BDO/PCL-PLLA(50:50)		1.8	−9	53		[82]
BDI·BDO·BDI/PCL-PLLA		1.0	−21	51		
BDO·BDI·BDO/PCL-PLLA		2.0	−5	49		
PEUU: MDI/PCL			−48.2 to −5.5			[64]
BDI/PCL	36.1–64.4		−55 to −52	21–61	74–83	[97]
LDI/PCL	46.1–185.6		−52 to −6	43–45		[62]
LDI/PEO-PCL	120–234		−38 to −16	47–48		[15]
HDI/PEO-PCL	24.0–139.0		−51.9 to −25.5	42–45		[63]
BDI/PEG	23.4–42.8		−43 to −40	18–20		[98]
LDI·BDI/PEG			−39			

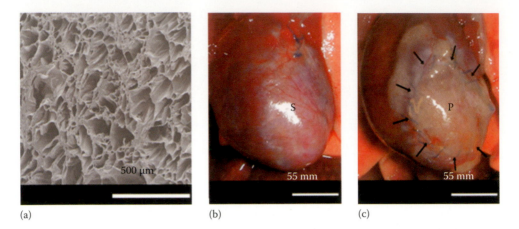

(a) (b) (c)

Figure 9.27
Images of polyester urethane urea (PEUU) and representative images of implants on cardiac tissue. SEM micrograph of PEUU material, showing porous thin-walled features. (a). Representative images of implants after 8 weeks, at the anterior view of an infarction control heart (b) and PEUU-patched infracted heart (c). Black arrows point to the implanted PEUU patch. S, the infracted scar; P, patch implanted area. (Reprinted from J. Amer. Coll. Cardiol., 49(23), Fujimoto, K.L. et al., An elastic, biodegradable cardiac patch induces contractile smooth muscle and improves cardiac remodeling and function in subacute myocardial infarction, 2292–2300, 2007, Copyright 2007, with permission from Elsevier.)

grown on thin patterned polyurethane films. Adult or embryonic stem-cell-derived cardiomyocytes were seeded onto the films and cultured for up to 4 weeks. At the end of culture, multilayered cell populations (~2–3 cell layers thick) had formed, with cardiomyocyte patterning aligning with that of the films. The cardiomyocytes were not only dense and linearly aligned, but were able to physically contract the underlying polyurethane films, as a kind of integrated and functional PU/muscle unit [38]. These results are intriguing, and indicate that PU and PEU films could be promising heart patch biomaterials, although this was not explicitly pointed out by the researchers at the time [38,39].

Another research team based at the University of Pittsburgh [37,69,99,100] report an exciting animal trial using a porous, biodegradable PU (BDI/PCL2000) heart patch (Figure 9.27). The patch was sutured to an infarcted region of rat cardiac muscle, and was later found to promote contractile smooth muscle tissue formation, improved tissue remodeling, and contractile function at the chronic stage. Similar research from Swiss and German groups [65,66,101–103] has applied a more slowly degrading PU (MDI/PCL530) as a heart patch (Table 9.14). These studies suggest that the PU heart patch approach could be a new therapeutic option against postinfarct cardiac failure.

From the point of view of degradation, PUs could be useful in tissue engineering for implants that require a longer retention time or a higher stability in the surrounding tissue environment, but eventually absorbed. This might be useful for tissues with slower healing and remodeling times, or with an inability to maintain innate structural integrity (e.g., large wounds). In addition to cardiovascular tissue engineering, PUs have proven highly versatile for the repair of other tissue types including nerves [36,104–107], blood vessels [99], and load-bearing tissue including bone [72,73,108,109], cartilage [110], fibrocartilage [111–116], and ligament [64,71], as summarized in Table 9.14.

Table 9.14

Summary of Tissue Engineering Applications of Polyurethanes

Applications/Animal Models	Polyurethane Scaffolds	Major Conclusions	Refs.
Cardiovascular TE/right ventricular outflow tract in rats	Porous (porosity ~80%) PEUU: (BDI/PCL2000)	The PEUU patch demonstrated suitable mechanical properties and biocompatible characteristics in this model, permitting cellular integration and endocardial endothelialization with minimal inflammation	[57]
Cardiovascular TE/infarcted left ventricle wall surface of rats	Porous (porosity ~80%) PEUU: (BDI/PCL2000)	Implantation of a PEUU patch onto a subacute myocardial infarction promoted contractile phenotype smooth muscle tissue formation and improved cardiac remodeling and contractile function at the chronic stage	[37]
	Fibrous PEUU: (MDI/PCL530)	Myoblasts were found throughout the seeded patches, but no sign of differentiation could be observed at 4 weeks after implantation in rats	[65]
		Myoblast-seeded polyurethane scaffolds prevent post-myocardial infarction progression toward heart failure as efficiently as direct intramyocardial injection	[66]
		Progression toward heart failure was significantly prevented for up to 6 months after injection of myoblasts and for up to 9 months following biograft implantation.	[64]
		Nevertheless, this effect vanished after 12 months, with immunohistological examinations revealing an absence of the transplanted myoblasts within the scaffold. Hence, beneficial effects of tissue engineering therapy over cell therapy for stabilization of heart function were transient	

(Continued)

Table 9.14 (*Continued*)
Summary of Tissue Engineering Applications of Polyurethanes

Applications/Animal Models	Polyurethane Scaffolds	Major Conclusions	Refs.
		Scaffolds with untransfected myoblasts also yielded smaller infarctions than injections of untransfected myoblasts	[101]
		Akt1-overexpressing skeletal myoblasts can maintain myocardial function after infarction, reduce infarction size, and induce neovascularization. Scaffold-based cell transfer does not augment this reverse remodeling capacity	
Vascular TE/small-diameter vessels—abdominal aortic interposition graft placement in rats	Fibrous PEUU: (BDI/PCL2000)	Surface treatment: Luminally modified with a nonthrombogenic, 2-methacryloyloxyethyl phosphorylcholine (MPC), a phospholipid mimicking copolymer	[99]
		The surface modified vascular graft exhibited good nonthrombogenic properties in vitro and in vivo, with patency at 8 weeks being 92% for the coated grafts compared to 40% for the noncoated grafts Mechanical properties compatible with native arterial conduits. The grafts were less compliant than rat aortas prior to implantation, then after 4 weeks in vivo they approximated native values, but subsequently became stiffer again at later time points	
Musculoskeletal TE/rabbits and mini-pigs' anterior cruciate ligament (ACL) reconstruction.	Fibrous PEUU: MDI/PCL530	Following in vivo remodeling, the grafts showed a neo-intimal tissue formation that exhibited both smooth muscle and endothelial markers as well as oriented collagen and elastin deposition Overall, a mild foreign body reaction and a mild inflammatory response were observed	[64,71]

Application	Scaffold/material	Remarks	References
Knee-joint meniscus	Porous scaffolds: MDI/PLLA or MDI/PLLA-co-PCL	Ingrowth of connective tissue in close contact with the PUUR fibers was detected in both rabbits and mini-pigs	[113–116]
		Normal fibrocartilage tissue developed inside the implants, whereas control defects only showed repair with fibrous tissue	
		After fibrocartilage had formed, vascularity decreased and was completely absent in mature fibrocartilage	
		Implantation of the porous polymer enhanced vascularity, resulting in healing of meniscal lesions extending into the avascular part. Healing by repair tissue resembling normal meniscal fibrocartilage	
	Porous scaffolds: BDI/50:50 PCL-co-PLLA	To mitigate the potential risk of releasing toxic aromatic diamines, BDI was used to replace MDI	[79,80,111,117–119]
Bone TE/iliac crest of sheep	Porous scaffolds synthesized from HMDI, PEO-PPO-PEO, and PCL at various ratios. Pore size: 300–2000 μm; porosity: 85%	At 18 and 25 months, all the defects in the ilium implanted with polyurethane bone substitutes had healed with new bone.	[72,73]
		The extent of bone healing depended on the chemical composition of the polymer from which the implant was made	
		The implants from polymers with the incorporated calcium-complexing additive were the most effective promoters of bone healing, followed by those with vitamin D, and polysaccharide-containing polymer	
		There was no bone healing in the control defects.	
Bone TE/in vitro	BDI with PCL films	Bone marrow stromal cells were cultured on rigid polymer films under osteogenic conditions for up to 21 days. This study demonstrated the suitability of this family of PEUUs for bone tissue engineering applications	[97]

(Continued)

Table 9.14 (Continued)

Summary of Tissue Engineering Applications of Polyurethanes

Applications/Animal Models	Polyurethane Scaffolds	Major Conclusions	Refs.
Bone TE/femoral condyle of rabbit	LTI with PCL-co-PGA-co-PDLLA	Extensive cellular infiltration deep to the implant, and new bone formation at 6 weeks	[120]
Cartilage/in vitro	Porous scaffolds synthesized from HMDI with PCL and ISO	Although the covalent incorporation of the isoprenoid molecule into the polyurethane chain modified the surface chemistry of the polymer, it did not affect the viability of attached chondrocytes. The change of surface characteristics and the more open pore structure of the scaffolds produced from the isoprenoid-modified polyurethane are beneficial for the seeding efficiency and the homogeneity of the tissue engineered constructs	[110]
Nerve TE/sciatic nerve of rat	Tubular polymer synthesized from TMDI with PGA-co-PCL as soft segments and PHB as hard segments	Out of 26 implanted NGCs, 23 contained regenerated tissue cables centrally located within the channel lumen and composed of numerous myelinated axons and Schwann cells The inflammatory reaction associated with the polymer degradation had not interfered with the nerve regeneration process. Macrophages and giant cells surrounded polymer material remnants, respectively	[36]

Application	Polymer/Material	Findings	References
Nerve TE/subcutaneous implants in rats	LDI/HMDI/TMDI, PHB and PGA-co-PCL	All test polymers exhibit favorable tissue compatibility. The formed capsule was 60–250 μm thick	[36,40]
Drug (vancomycin) delivery/femur and plug defects in rat	LTI	PU/drug scaffolds were biocompatible. Active drug release was maintained for up to 8 weeks at concentrations well above both the minimum inhibitory concentration (MIC) and the minimum bactericidal concentration (MBC). Locally delivered drug enhanced new bone formation in the PU scaffolds at week 4. The performance of PU (LTI) was comparable to PMMA beads in vivo. However, compared with PMMA, PUR is a biodegradable system which does not require the extra surgical removal step in clinical use	[121–126]
Drug delivery/basic fibroblast growth factor (bFGF)	Porous (porosity ~80%) PEUU synthesized from BDI and PCL (BDI/PCL2000)	The released bFGF remained bioactive over 21 days as assessed by smooth muscle mitogenicity	[68]
A potential for wide applications in soft TE/subcutaneous implants in rats	Porous scaffolds synthesized from BDI, PHC, and PCL	Noncytotoxic and to support smooth muscle cell adhesion and proliferation in vitro. In vivo toxicity assessment has not been pursued	[69]

BIBLIOGRAPHY

References for Text

1. Stein, H.L., Ultrahigh molecular weight polyethylenes (UHMWPE). *Engineered Materials Handbook*, 1998;**2**:167–171.
2. Kurtz, S.M., *The UHMWPE Biomaterials Handbook: Ultra-High Molecular Weight Polyethylene in Total Joint Replacement*, 2nd edn. Amsterdam, the Netherlands: Elsevier Academic Press, Burlington, MA, 2009.
3. Maier, C. and T. Calafut, *Polypropylene: The Definitive User's Guide and Databook*. William Andrew Inc., Norwich, New York, 1998, p. 14.
4. Moore, E.P., *Polypropylene Handbook: Polymerization, Characterization, Properties, Processing, Applications*. New York: Hanser Publishers, 1996.
5. Gupta, V.B. and Z. Bashir, Chapter 7: PET Fibers, films, and bottles. In *Handbook of Thermoplastic Polyesters*, S. Fakirov, ed. Weinheim, Germany: Wiley-VCH.
6. Jaeblon, T., Polymethylmethacrylate: Properties and contemporary uses in orthopaedics. *Journal of the American Academy of Orthopaedic Surgeons*, 2010;**18**(5):297–305.
7. Black, J. ed., Chapter 19: Thermoplatic polymer in biomedical applications: Structures, properties and processing. In *Handbook of Biomaterials Properties*. Chapman & Hall, London, UK.
8. Krupnick, A.S. et al., A novel small animal model of left ventricular tissue engineering. *Journal of Heart and Lung Transplantation*, 2002;**21**(2):233–243.
9. Lynch, D.S. and W. Lynch, *Handbook of Silicone Rubber Fabrication*. New York: Van Nostrand Reinhold Company, 1997.
10. Lelah, M.D. and S.L. Cooper, *Polyurethanes in Medicine*. Boca Raton, FL: CRC Press, 1986.

Websites

http://www.britannica.com/EBchecked/topic/468698/major-industrial-polymers.
http://www.heart.org/HEARTORG/.
http://www.nhlbi.nih.gov/health/health-topics/topics/vad/.
http://www.uhmwpe.org/.

References for Advanced Topic

1. Santerre, J.P. et al., Understanding the biodegradation of polyurethanes: From classical implants to tissue engineering materials. *Biomaterials*, 2005;**26**(35):7457–7470.
2. Zdrahala, R.J. and I.J. Zdrahala, Biomedical applications of polyurethanes: A review of past promises, present realities, and a vibrant future. *Journal of Biomaterials Applications*, 1999;**14**(1):67–90.
3. Zdrahala, R.J., Small caliber vascular grafts. 2. Polyurethanes revisited. *Journal of Biomaterials Applications*, 1996;**11**(1):37–61.
4. Aldenhoff, Y.B.J. et al., Performance of a polyurethane vascular prosthesis carrying a dipyridamole (Persantin (R)) coating on its lumenal surface. *Journal of Biomedical Materials Research*, 2001;**54**(2):224–233.
5. Tawa, T. and S. Ito, The role of hard segments of aqueous polyurethane-urea dispersion in determining the colloidal characteristics and physical properties. *Polymer Journal*, 2006;**38**(7):686–693.
6. Guelcher, S.A., Biodegradable polyurethanes: Synthesis and applications in regenerative medicine. *Tissue Engineering Part B: Reviews*, 2008;**14**(1):3–17.
7. Ilavsky, M. et al., Network formation in polyurethanes based on triisocyanate and diethanolamine derivatives. *European Polymer Journal*, 2001;**37**(5):887–896.

8. Behrend, D. and K.P. Schmitz, Polyurethane or silicone as a material for long-term implants—A critical-review. *Biomedizinische Technik*, 1993;**38**(7–8):172–178.

9. Christenson, E.M., J.M. Anderson, and A. Hittner, Biodegradation mechanisms of polyurethane elastomers. *Corrosion Engineering Science and Technology*, 2007;**42**(4):312–323.

10. Griesser, H.J., Degradation of polyurethanes in biomedical applications—A review. *Polymer Degradation and Stability*, 1991;**33**(3):329–354.

11. Szycher, M., A.M. Reed, and I.N.C. Soc Plast Engineers, Medical-grade polyurethanes: A critical review. In *ANTEC '96: Plastics—Racing into the Future*, Vols. I–III—Vol. I: Processing; Vol. II: Materials; Vol. III: Spacial Areas. Society of Petroleum Engineers, Brookfield, CT. 1996, pp. 2758–2766.

12. Marois, Y. and R. Guidoin, Biocompatibility of polyurethanes. In *Biomedical Applications of Polyurethanes*, P. Vermette et al., eds. Georgetown, TX: Landies Bioscience, 2001, pp. 77–96.

13. Fromstein, J.D. and K.A. Woodhouse, *Polyurethane Biomaterials*. London, U.K.: Informa Healthcare, 2006, pp.1–10.

14. Hinrichs, W.L.J. et al., In vivo fragmentation of microporous polyurethane-based and copolyesterether elastomer-based vascular prostheses. *Biomaterials*, 1992;**13**(9):585–593.

15. Fromstein, J.D. and K.A. Woodhouse, Elastomeric biodegradable polyurethane blends for soft tissue applications. *Journal of Biomaterials Science. Polymer Edition*, 2002;**13**(4):391–406.

16. Dostal, M. et al., Mineralization of polyurethane membranes in the total artificial-heart (tah)—A retrospective study from long-term animal-experiments. *International Journal of Artificial Organs*, 1990;**13**(8):498–502.

17. Marois, Y. et al., An albumin-coated polyester arterial graft: In vivo assessment of biocompatibility and healing characteristics. *Biomaterials*, 1996;**17**(1):3–14.

18. Marois, Y. et al., In vivo evaluation of 4 chemically processed biological grafts implanted as infrarenal arterial substitutes in dogs. *Biomaterials*, 1989;**10**(6):369–379.

19. Marois, Y. et al., In vivo evaluation of hydrophobic and fibrillar microporous polyetherurethane urea graft. *Biomaterials*, 1989;**10**(8):521–531.

20. Marois, Y. et al., Vascugraft(R) microporous polyesterurethane arterial prosthesis as a thoraco-abdominal bypass in dogs. *Biomaterials*, 1996;**17**(13):1289–1300.

21. Okoshi, T. et al., Penetrating micropores increase patency and achieve extensive endothelialization in small diameter polymer skin coated vascular grafts. *ASAIO Journal*, 1996;**42**(5):M398–M401.

22. Akiyama, N. et al., A comparison of CORVITA and expanded polytetrafluoroethylene vascular grafts implanted in the abdominal aortas of dogs. *Surgery Today: The Japanese Journal of Surgery*, 1997;**27**(9):840–845.

23. vanderGiessen, W.J. et al., Marked inflammatory sequelae to implantation of biodegradable and nonbiodegradable polymers in porcine coronary arteries. *Circulation*, 1996;**94**(7):1690–1697.

24. Bakker, D. et al., Biocompatibility of a polyether urethane, polypropylene oxide, and a polyether polyester copolymer—A qualitative and quantitative study of 3 alloplastic tympanic membrane materials in the rat middle-ear. *Journal of Biomedical Materials Research*, 1990;**24**(4):489–515.

25. Bruin, P. et al., Autoclavable highly cross-linked polyurethane networks in ophthalmology. *Biomaterials*, 1993;**14**(14):1089–1097.

26. Watkinson, A.F. et al., Esophageal-carcinoma—Initial results of palliative treatment with covered self-expanding endoprostheses. *Radiology*, 1995;**195**(3):821–827.

27. Lennon, G.M. et al., Firm versus soft double pigtail ureteral stents—A randomized blind comparative trial. *European Urology*, 1995;**28**(1):1–5.

28. Rossi, P. et al., Clinical experience with covered wallstents for biliary malignancies: 23-month follow-up. *Cardiovascular and Interventional Radiology*, 1997;**20**(6):441–447.

29. Cardy, R.H., Carcinogenicity and chronic toxicity of 2,4-toluenediamine in f344 rats. *Journal of the National Cancer Institute*, 1979;**62**(4):1107–1116.

30. Schoenta, R., Carcinogenic and chronic effects of 4,4′-diaminodiphenylmethane an epoxy-resin hardener. *Nature*, 1968;**219**(5159):1162–1163.

31. Pinchuk, L., A review of the biostability and carcinogenicity of polyurethanes in medicine and the new generation of 'biostable' polyurethanes. *Journal of Biomaterial Science. Polymer Edition*, 1994;**6**(3):225–267.

32. Gunatillake, P.A. et al., Designing biostable polyurethane elastomers for biomedical implants. *ChemInform*, 2003;**34**(41). doi:10.1002/chin.200341282.

33. Lamba, N. et al., *Polyurethanes in Biomedical Applications*. Boca Raton, FL: CRC Press, 1998, pp. 5–25.

34. Zhang, J.-Y. et al., Synthesis, biodegradability, and biocompatibility of lysine diisocyanate-glucose polymers. *Tissue Engineering*, 2002;**8**(5):771–785.

35. Lamba, N.M.K., K.A. Woodhouse, and S.L. Cooper, *Polyurethanes in Biomedcial Applications*. Boca Raton, FL: CRC Press, 1998.

36. Borkenhagen, M. et al., In vivo performance of a new biodegradable polyester urethane system used as a nerve guidance channel. *Biomaterials*, 1998;**19**(23):2155–2165.

37. Fujimoto, K.L. et al., An elastic, biodegradable cardiac patch induces contractile smooth muscle and improves cardiac remodeling and function in subacute myocardial infarction. *Journal of the American College of Cardiology*, 2007;**49**(23):2292–2300.

38. McDevitt, T.C. et al., Spatially organized layers of cardiomyocytes on biodegradable polyurethane films for myocardial repair. *Journal of Biomedical Materials Research. Part A*, 2003;**66A**(3):586–595.

39. Alperin, C., P.W. Zandstra, and K.A. Woodhouse, Polyurethane films seeded with embryonic stem cell-derived cardiomyocytes for use in cardiac tissue engineering applications. *Biomaterials*, 2005;**26**(35):7377–7386.

40. Saad, B. et al., Development of degradable polyesterurethanes for medical applications: In vitro and in vivo evaluations. *Journal of Biomedical Materials Research*, 1997;**36**(1):65–74.

41. Jayabalan, M., P.P. Lizymol, and V. Thomas, Synthesis of hydrolytically stable low elastic modulus polyurethane-urea for biomedical applications. *Polymer International*, 2000;**49**(1):88–92.

42. Stokes, K., R. McVenes, and J.M. Anderson, Polyurethane elastomer biostability. *Journal of Biomaterials Applications*, 1995;**9**(4):321–354.

43. Phillips, R.E., M.C. Smith, and R.E. Thoma, Biomedical applications of polyurethanes: Implications of failure mechanisms. *Journal of Biomaterial Application*, 1988;**3**:207–227.

44. Stokes, K. and K. Cobian, Polyether polyurethanes for implantable pacemaker leads. *Biomaterials*, 1982;**3**(4):225–231.

45. Stokes, K., R. McVenes, and J.M. Anderson, Polyurethane elastomer biostability (vol 9, pg 347, 1995). *Journal of Biomaterials Applications*, 1995;**10**(2):188–188.

46. Smith, R., C. Oliver, and D.F. Williams, The enzymaticdegradation of polymers in vitro. *Journal of Biomedical Material Research*, 1987;**21**:991–1003.

47. Santerre, J.P. et al., Interactions of hydrolytic enzymes at an aqueous polyurethane interface. In *Proteins at Interfaces II: Fundamentals and Applications*, T.A. Horbett and J.L. Brash, eds. American Chemical Society. Books Department, Washington, DC, 1995, pp. 352–370.

48. Hennig, E. et al., Calcification of artificial heart-valves made out of polyurethane. *International Journal of Artificial Organs*, 1982;**5**(1):71–71.

49. Thoma, R.J., R.E. Phillips, and M.C. Smith, Calcification and invitro degradation of poly(ether) urethanes. *Abstracts of Papers of the American Chemical Society*, 1988;**196**:141-PMSE.

50. Schoen, F.J. et al., Biomaterial-associated calcification: Pathology, mechanism, and strategies for prevention. *Journal of Biomedical Material Research*, 1988;**22**(Suppl. A1):11–36.

51. Zhang, J.Y. et al., A new peptide-based urethane polymer: Synthesis, biodegradation, and potential to support cell growth in vitro. *Biomaterials*, 2000;**21**(12):1247–1258.

52. Zhang, J.Y. et al., Synthesis, biodegradability, and biocompatibility of lysine diisocyanate-glucose polymers. *Tissue Engineering*, 2002;**8**(5):771–785.

53. Bruin, P. et al., Design and synthesis of biodegradable poly(ester-urethane) elastomer networks composed of non-toxic building-blocks. *Makromolekulare Chemie-Rapid Communications*, 1988;**9**(8):589–594.

54. Elliott, S. ct al., Identification of biodegradation products formed by ʟ-phenylalanine based segmented polyurethaneureas. *Journal of Biomaterials Science. Polymer Edition*, 2002;**13**(6):691–711.

55. Guelcher, S. et al., Synthesis, in vitro degradation, and mechanical properties of two-component poly(ester urethane)urea scaffolds: Effects of water and polyol composition. *Tissue Engineering*, 2007;**13**(9):2321–2333.

56. Guelcher, S.A. et al., Synthesis and in vitro biocompatibility of injectable polyurethane foam scaffolds. *Tissue Engineering*, 2006;**12**(5):1247–1259.

57. Fujimoto, K.L. et al., In vivo evaluation of a porous, elastic, biodegradable patch for reconstructive cardiac procedures. *Annals of Thoracic Surgery*, 2007;**83**(2):648–654.

58. Guan, J.J. and W.R. Wagner, Synthesis, characterization and cytocompatibility of polyurethaneurea elastomers with designed elastase sensitivity. *Biomacromolecules*, 2005;**6**(5):2833–2842.

59. Gorna, K. and S. Gogolewski, Preparation, degradation, and calcification of biodegradable polyurethane foams for bone graft substitutes. *Journal of Biomedical Materials Research. Part A*, 2003;**67A**(3):813–827.

60. Guan, J.J. et al., Biodegradable poly(ether ester urethane)urea elastomers based on poly(ether ester) triblock copolymers and putrescine: Synthesis, characterization and cytocompatibility. *Biomaterials*, 2004;**25**(1):85–96.

61. Storey, R.F. et al., Bioabsorbable composites. 2. Nontoxic, l-lysine-based poly(ester-urethane) matrix composites. *Polymer Composites*, 1993;**14**(1):17–25.

62. Skarja, G.A. and K.A. Woodhouse, Structure-property relationships of degradable polyurethane elastomers containing an amino acid-based chain extender. *Journal of Applied Polymer Science*, 2000;**75**(12):1522–1534.

63. Skarja, G.A. and K.A. Woodhouse, Synthesis and characterization of degradable polyurethane elastomers containing an amino acid-based chain extender. *Journal of Biomaterials Science. Polymer Edition*, 1998;**9**(3):271–295.

64. Gisselfalt, K., B. Edberg, and P. Flodin, Synthesis and properties of degradable poly(urethane urea)s to be used for ligament reconstructions. *Biomacromolecules*, 2002;**3**(5):951–958.

65. Siepe, M. et al., Construction of skeletal myoblast-based polyurethane scaffolds for myocardial repair. *Artificial Organs*, 2007;**31**(6):425–433.

66. Siepe, M. et al., Myoblast-seeded biodegradable scaffolds to prevent post-myocardial infarction evolution toward heart failure. *Journal of Thoracic and Cardiovascular Surgery*, 2006;**132**(1):124–131.

67. Guan, J. et al., Preparation and characterization of highly porous, biodegradable polyurethane scaffolds for soft tissue applications. *Biomaterials*, 2005;**26**(18):3961–3971.

68. Guan, J., J.J. Stankus, and W.R. Wagner, Biodegradable elastomeric scaffolds with basic fibroblast growth factor release. *Journal of Controlled Release*, 2007;**120**(1–2):70–78.

69. Hong, Y. et al., Tailoring the degradation kinetics of poly(ester carbonate urethane)urea thermoplastic elastomers for tissue engineering scaffolds. *Biomaterials*, 2010;**31**(15):4249–4258.

70. Hafeman, A.E. et al., Characterization of the degradation mechanisms of lysine-derived aliphatic poly(ester urethane) scaffolds. *Biomaterials*, 2011;**32**(2):419–429.

71. Liljensten, E. et al., Studies of polyurethane urea bands for ACL reconstruction. *Journal of Materials Science. Materials in Medicine*, 2002;**13**(4):351–359.

72. Gogolewski, S., K. Gorna, and A.S. Turner, Regeneration of bicortical defects in the iliac crest of estrogen-deficient sheep, using new biodegradable polyurethane bone graft substitutes. *Journal of Biomedical Materials Research. Part A*, 2006;**77A**(4):802–810.

73. Gogolewski, S. and K. Gorna, Biodegradable polyurethane cancellous bone graft substitutes in the treatment of iliac crest defects. *Journal of Biomedical Materials Research. Part A*, 2007;**80A**(1):94–101.

74. Dey, J. et al., Development of biodegradable crosslinked urethane-doped polyester elastomers. *Biomaterials*, 2008;**29**(35):4637–4649.
75. Yoda, R., Elastomers for biomedical applications. *Journal of Biomaterials Science. Polymer Edition*, 1998;**9**(6):561–626.
76. Oertel, G. and L. Abele, *Polyurethane Handbook: Chemistry, Raw Materials, Processing, Application, Properties*, 2nd edn. Munich, Germany: Hanser; Hanser/Gardner [distributor], 1994, p. xxii, 688pp.
77. Zdrahala, R.J. et al., Polyether-based thermoplastic polyurethanes. I. Effect of the hard-segment content. *Journal of Applied Polymer Science*, 1979;**24**(9):2041–2050.
78. Guan, J.J. et al., Synthesis, characterization, and cytocompatibility of efastomeric, biodegradable poly(ester-urethane)ureas based on poly(caprolactone) and putrescine. *Journal of Biomedical Materials Research*, 2002;**61**(3):493–503.
79. deGroot, J.H. et al., New biomedical polyurethane ureas with high tear strengths. *Polymer Bulletin*, 1997;**38**(2):211–218.
80. Spaans, C.J. et al., A new biomedical polyurethane with a high modulus based on 1,4-butanediisocyanate and epsilon-caprolactone. *Journal of Materials Science. Materials in Medicine*, 1998;**9**(12):675–678.
81. Spaans, C.J. et al., High molecular weight polyurethanes and a polyurethane urea based on 1,4-butanediisocyanate. *Polymer Bulletin*, 1998;**41**(2):131–138.
82. de Groot, J.H. et al., On the role of aminolysis and transesterification in the synthesis of epsilon-caprolactone and L-lactide based polyurethanes. *Polymer Bulletin*, 1998;**41**(3):299–306.
83. Abraham, G.A., A. Marcos-Fernandez, and J. San Roman, Bioresorbable poly(ester-ether urethane)s from L-lysine diisocyanate and triblock copolymers with different hydrophilic character. *Journal of Biomedical Materials Research. Part A*, 2006;**76A**(4):729–736.
84. Guelcher, S.A. et al., Synthesis, mechanical properties, biocompatibility, and biodegradation of polyurethane networks from lysine polyisocyanates. *Biomaterials*, 2008;**29**(12):1762–1775.
85. Chandran, K.B., *Cardiovascular Biomechanics*. New York: New York University Press, 1992.
86. Balguid, A. et al., The role of collagen cross-links in biomechanical behavior of human aortic heart valve leaflets—Relevance for tissue engineering. *Tissue Engineering*, 2007;**13**(7):1501–1511.
87. Lee, J. and D. Boughner, Mechanical properties of human pericardium. Differences in viscoelastic response when compared with canine pericardium. *Circulation Research*, 1985;**57**(3):475–481.
88. Monson, K.L. et al., Axial mechanical properties of fresh human cerebral blood vessels. *Journal of Biomechanical Engineering*, 2003;**125**(2):288–294.
89. Nakano, K. et al., Myocardial stiffness derived from end-systolic wall stress and logarithm of reciprocal of wall thickness: Contractility index independent of ventricular size. *Circulation*, 1990;**82**(4):1352–1361.
90. Nagueh, S.F. et al., Altered titin expression, myocardial stiffness, and left ventricular function in patients with dilated cardiomyopathy. *Circulation*, 2004;**110**(2):155–162.
91. Krol, P., Synthesis methods, chemical structures and phase structures of linear polyurethanes. Properties and applications of linear polyurethanes in polyurethane elastomers, copolymers and ionomers. *Progress in Materials Science*, 2007;**52**(6):915–1015.
92. Richardson, T.B. et al., Study of nanoreinforced shape memory polymers processed by casting and extrusion. *Polymer Composites*, 2011;**32**(3):455–463.
93. Zhuo, H.T., J.L. Hu, and S.J. Chen, Coaxial electrospun polyurethane core-shell nanofibers for shape memory and antibacterial nanomaterials. *Express Polymer Letters*, 2011;**5**(2):182–187.
94. Sambaer, W., M. Zatloukal, and D. Kimmer, 3D modeling of filtration process via polyurethane nanofiber based nonwoven filters prepared by electrospinning process. *Chemical Engineering Science*, 2011;**66**(4):613–623.

95. Stankus, J.J., J. Guan, and W.R. Wagner, Fabrication of biodegradable elastomeric scaffolds with sub-micron morphologies. *Journal of Biomedical Material Research. Part A*, 2004;**70**(4):603–614.

96. Stankus, J.J. et al., Fabrication of cell microintegrated blood vessel constructs through electrohydrodynamic atomization. *Biomaterials*, 2007;**28**(17):2738–2746.

97. Kavlock, K.D. et al., Synthesis and characterization of segmented poly(esterurethane urea) elastomers for bone tissue engineering. *Acta Biomaterialia*, 2007;**3**(4):475–484.

98. Guelcher, S.A. et al., Synthesis of biocompatible segmented polyurethanes from aliphatic diisocyanates and diurea diol chain extenders. *Acta Biomaterialia*, 2005;**1**(4):471–484.

99. Soletti, L. et al., In vivo performance of a phospholipid-coated bioerodable elastomeric graft for small-diameter vascular applications. *Journal of Biomedical Materials Research. Part A*, 2011;**96A**(2):436–448.

100. Amoroso, N.J. et al., Elastomeric electrospun polyurethane scaffolds: The interrelationship between fabrication conditions, fiber topology, and mechanical properties. *Advanced Materials*, 2011;**23**(1):106–111.

101. Siepe, M. et al., Scaffold-based transplantation of akt1-overexpressing skeletal myoblasts: Functional regeneration is associated with angiogenesis and reduced infarction size. *Tissue Engineering. Part A*, 2011;**17**(1–2):205–212.

102. Giraud, M.N. et al., Long-term evaluation of myoblast seeded patches implanted on infarcted rat hearts. *Artificial Organs*, 2010;**34**(6):E184–E192.

103. Blumenthal, B. et al., Polyurethane scaffolds seeded with genetically engineered skeletal myoblasts: A promising tool to regenerate myocardial function. *Artificial Organs*, 2010;**34**(2):E46–E54.

104. Chiono, V. et al., Poly(ester urethane) guides for peripheral nerve regeneration. *Macromolecular Bioscience*, 2011;**11**(2):245–256.

105. Wang, X.H. et al., Peroneal nerve regeneration using a unique bilayer polyurethane-collagen guide conduit. *Journal of Bioactive and Compatible Polymers*, 2009;**24**(2):109–127.

106. Pfister, L.A. et al., Nerve conduits and growth factor delivery in peripheral nerve repair. *Journal of the Peripheral Nervous System*, 2007;**12**(2):65–82.

107. Soldani, G. et al., Manufacturing and microscopical characterisation of polyurethane nerve guidance channel featuring a highly smooth internal surface. *Biomaterials*, 1998;**19**(21):1919–1924.

108. Schlickewei, C. et al., Interaction of sheep bone marrow stromal cells with biodegradable polyurethane bone substitutes. *Macromolecular Symposia*, 2007;**253**:162–171.

109. Hill, C.M. et al., Osteogenesis of osteoblast seeded polyurethane-hydroxyapatite scaffolds in nude mice. *Macromolecular Symposia*, 2007;**253**:94–97.

110. Eglin, D. et al., Farsenol-modified biodegradable polyurethanes for cartilage tissue engineering. *Journal of Biomedical Materials Research. Part A*, 2010;**92A**(1):393–408.

111. deGroot, J.H. et al., Meniscal tissue regeneration in porous 50/50 copoly(L-lactide/epsilon-caprolactone) implants. *Biomaterials*, 1997;**18**(8):613–622.

112. Klompmaker, J. et al., Meniscal repair by fibrocartilage in the dog: Characterization of the repair tissue and the role of vascularity. *Biomaterials*, 1996;**17**(17):1685–1691.

113. Klompmaker, J. et al., Meniscal replacement using a porous polymer prosthesis: A preliminary study in the dog. *Biomaterials*, 1996;**17**(12):1169–1175.

114. deGroot, J.H. et al., Use of porous polyurethanes for meniscal reconstruction and meniscal prostheses. *Biomaterials*, 1996;**17**(2):163–173.

115. Klompmaker, J. et al., Meniscal repair by fibrocartilage—An experimental-study in the dog. *Journal of Orthopaedic Research*, 1992;**10**(3):359–370.

116. Klompmaker, J. et al., Porous polymer implant for repair of meniscal lesions—A preliminary-study in dogs. *Biomaterials*, 1991;**12**(9):810–816.

117. DeGroot, J.H., H.W. Kuijper, and A.J. Pennings, A novel method for fabrication of biodegradable scaffolds with high compression moduli. *Journal of Materials Science. Materials in Medicine*, 1997;**8**(11):707–712.

118. Spaans, C.J. et al., Solvent-free fabrication of micro-porous polyurethane amide and polyurethane-urea scaffolds for repair and replacement of the knee-joint meniscus. *Biomaterials*, 2000;**21**(23):2453–2460.

119. Spaans, C.J. et al., New biodegradable polyurethane ureas, polyurethanes, and polyurethane amides for in vivo tissue engineering: Structure-properties relationships. *Abstracts of Papers of the American Chemical Society*, 2001;**222**:37-PMSE.

120. Dumas, J.E. et al., Synthesis, characterization, and remodeling of weight-bearing allograft bone/polyurethane composites in the rabbit. *Acta Biomaterialia*, 2010;**6**(7):2394–2406.

121. Yoshii, T. et al., A sustained release of lovastatin from biodegradable, elastomeric polyurethane scaffolds for enhanced bone regeneration. *Tissue Engineering. Part A*, 2010;**16**(7):2369–2379.

122. Li, B. et al., Sustained release of vancomycin from polyurethane scaffolds inhibits infection of bone wounds in a rat femoral segmental defect model. *Journal of Controlled Release*, 2010;**145**(3):221–230.

123. Hafeman, A.E. et al., Local delivery of tobramycin from injectable biodegradable polyurethane scaffolds. *Journal of Biomaterials Science. Polymer Edition*, 2010;**21**(1):95–112.

124. Li, B., J.M. Davidson, and S.A. Guelcher, The effect of the local delivery of platelet-derived growth factor from reactive two-component polyurethane scaffolds on the healing in rat skin excisional wounds. *Biomaterials*, 2009;**30**(20):3486–3494.

125. Hafeman, A.E. et al., Injectable biodegradable polyurethane scaffolds with release of platelet-derived growth factor for tissue repair and regeneration. *Pharmaceutical Research*, 2008;**25**(10):2387–2399.

126. Li, B. et al., The effects of rhBMP-2 released from biodegradable polyurethane/microsphere composite scaffolds on new bone formation in rat femora. *Biomaterials*, 2009;**30**(35):6768–6779.

Further Readings

Black, J.B. and Hastings, G., Chapter 19: Thermoplatic polymer in biomedical applications: Structures, properties and processing, Chapter 20: Biomedical elastomers. In *Handbook of Biomaterials Properties*. Chapman and Hall, London, UK, 1998.

Kurtz, S.M., Chapter 4: The origins of UHMWPE in joint replacements, Chapter 5: The Clinical performance of UHMWPE in hip replacements, Chapter 6: Alternatives to conventional UHMWPE for hip arthroplasty. In *The UHMWPE Handbook*. Elsevier Academic Press, San Diego, CA, 2004.

Mark, J.E., E. Erman, and F.R. Eirich, eds., *Science and Technology of Rubber*, 3rd edn. London, U.K.: Elsevier Academic Press, 2005.

Park, J. and R.S. Lakes, Chapter 7: Polymeric implant materials. In *Biomaterials: An Introduction*, 3rd edn. New York: Springer, 2007.

CHAPTER 10

BIORESORBABLE POLYMERS

LEARNING OBJECTIVES

After a careful study of this chapter, you should be able to do the following:

1. Describe the three biodegradation steps
2. Describe the molecular structures of PGA, PLA, PCL, and PHA
3. Describe the synthesis of polyesters and polyamides
4. Describe degradation kinetics of PLA, PGA, PLGA, PCL, and PHA; and explain the structural mechanisms for the rank of their degradation rates
5. Describe the structural mechanisms for the stress–strain curves of synthetic rubber and natural soft tissues

10.1 BIODEGRADATION OF POLYMERS

10.1.1 Degradation of Polymers

Although metals and polymers are vastly different, they share certain similarities. In principle, a piece of metal can be regarded as a giant molecule, and metal atoms are the building blocks (monomers) of the lattice (network). As described in Chapter 2, most metals or metal products corrode in an oxygenated and hydrated environment, during which the giant molecule breaks down into metal ions. This is accelerated in biological environments with higher levels of aqueous salts.

Likewise, most polymers or polymer products deteriorate under the influence of one or more environmental factors such as heat, light, or chemicals. This process is commonly called degradation or *aging*, rather than corrosion. Based on the environmental factors involved, polymer degradation is classified as (1) photo-induced degradation, (2) thermal degradation, or (3) chemical degradation. During any of these processes, long polymer chains break down to shorter segments, and as a result, the polymer loses its structural and chemical properties, resulting in cracking and chemical disintegration of products. While not desirable in terms of loss of structural integrity, they are useful in biodegradable implants. Temporary implants made from degradable biomaterials offer several benefits, compared with nondegradable implants. These include the following:

- No requirements of a second surgery of removing a temporary device after serving its purpose, for example, surgical sutures, cardiac stents, and orthopedic pins
- Elimination of chronic inflammation associated with foreign body reaction
- Ability to deliver drugs
- Potential to achieve radical treatment, that is, tissue engineering and regeneration

10.1.2 General Process of Polymer Biodegradation

Polymer degradation in biological environments is a form of chemical degradation, which is directly responsible for the resorbability of biomaterials. In order to be resorbed, synthetic polymer chains must be first *cleaved* by chemical reactions to low-molecular-weight by-products outside the cells, which are then stored or transported into cells, metabolized, and excreted (removed) by the physiological system (Figure 10.1). The products of polymer chain cleavage directly determine the biocompatibility of a polymer implant.

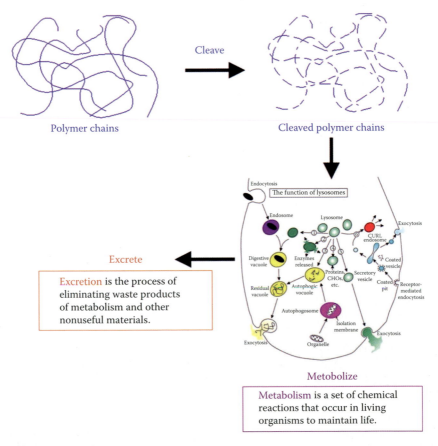

Figure 10.1
An overview of biodegradation process of a polymer in the body.

The low-molecular-weight by-products can then be processed by *metabolism*, which refers to the set of chemical reactions that occur within the cells of living organisms. These processes involve intracellular enzyme-catalyzed reactions that allow organisms to derive chemical energy from simple molecules (e.g., carbohydrates, amino acids, lipids), digested from food nutrients, enabling tissues to maintain their structures, and respond to their environments. A substance necessary for or taking part in a metabolic process is called *metabolite*.

Metabolic turnover results in the production of waste products (e.g., surplus metabolites, ammonium/urea, aqueous ions, dissolved gases), which are then discharged from the body by *excretion*. A substance produced by metabolism is also called a *metabolite*. All tissues release these metabolites, with the rate depending on the type of tissue and activity of cell division. The circulation then carries the molecules to the liver for further detoxification, followed by filtration through the kidneys to produce *urine*, which is discharged through the urethra. In short, the biodegradation of polymers proceeds in three major steps [1]:

$$\text{Cleavage} \rightarrow \text{Metabolism} \rightarrow \text{Excretion.}$$

Excess break-down products unable to be fully metabolized may be stored in tissues, causing progressive cytotoxicity and cell death. For instance, the PMMA debris released from total hip replacement due to wearing of the line component kills macrophages, resulting in aseptic loosening (Figure 3.11).

10.1.3 Cleavage of Polymer Chains

This step is typically initiated by *abiotic* mechanisms, which refers to chemical breakdown that does not involve biological attack. In an abiotic decomposition process, a polymer is converted to simpler products by either *hydrolysis* or *oxidation*, and thus, the rate of an abiotic process is determined by the physical accessibility of the polymer structure to water and oxygen molecules. Abiotic mechanisms proceed in a slow, diffusive manner. Hence, crystallinity and cross-link density of polyesters strongly influence the rate of hydrolysis, with the amorphous regions degrading prior to the degradation of the crystalline and cross-linked regions, due to their impermeability to water and oxygen.

A *biotic* degradation process refers to the metabolic breakdown of materials into simpler components by *living organisms*. Hydrolysis mediated by hydrolase enzymes following the colonization of cells on the surface of the polymer is one type of biotic mechanism. A biotic degradation process always proceeds on polymer surfaces in a layer-by-layer manner, because a polymer chain network is too dense to allow immigration of enzymes or cells [1].

It should be emphasized that being a catalyst, an enzyme accelerates the rate of a chemical reaction via reducing its energy barrier, rather than changing the reaction mechanism. Hence, both abiotic and biotic hydrolysis are the same chemical reaction, resulting in the same polymer cleavage products, except that the latter increases the reaction rate at a polymer surface, where the enzyme acts as a catalyst.

10.1.3.1 Hydrolyzable Polymers

In Chapter 8 (Section 8.2.2), we learned that the biostability of polymers is primarily determined by the chemical bonding on the backbone and steric interference. Bonds such as C−C, C−F, C−Si, and Si−O are strong

341

bonds, giving polymers long durability. Since the cleavage of polymers proceeds via hydrolysis and oxidation, hydrolyzable groups along the main chains are critical for a polymer to be biodegradable. Such functional groups include ester, amide, enamine, urea, and urethane (Figure 10.2). Representative polymers include polyesters, polyanhydrides, polycarbonates, polyamides, and poly(amino acids) (Figure 10.3). Other factors, the presence of suitable substituents, correct stereo-configuration, acidity of the environment, and conformational flexibility, also contribute to the biodegradability of polymers [1].

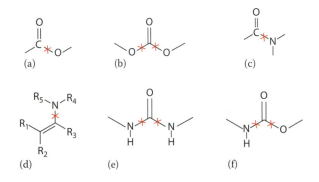

Figure 10.2
Hydrolyzable groups and bonds (X). (a) Ester group; (b) carbonate group; (c) amide; (d) enamine; (e) urea; (f) urethane.

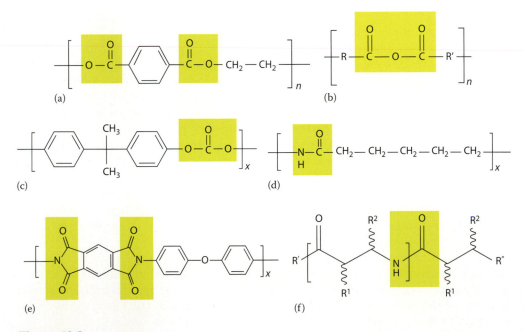

Figure 10.3
Representative hydrolysable polymers: (a) polyester; (b) polyanhydride; (c) polycarbonate; (d) polyamide; (e) polyimide (Adapted from Cowie, Blackie, J.M.G., Polymers: Chemistry & Physics of Modern Materials, 2nd edition, Chapman & Hall, London, UK, 1991, http://chem.chem. rochester.edu/~chem421/classify.htm.); (f) Poly(amino acid).

10.2   POLYESTERS: PGA, PLA, AND PCL

10.2.1   Esters

An ester is the molecule formed from the reaction of a carboxylic acid (−COOH group) and a hydroxyl (−OH) compound, alcohol (Figure 10.4). The preparation of an ester is known as an *esterification* reaction.

Carboxylic acids and their ester derivatives are abundant in foods. A fatty acid is a carboxylic acid often with a long unbranched *aliphatic* (linear, nonaromatic, no ring in the chain) tail, which is either saturated or unsaturated. An example is oleic acid, $CH_3(CH_2)_7CH=CH(CH_2)_7COOH$ (Figure 10.5a). All fats are derived from glycerol and fatty acids. The molecules are called *triglycerides*, which are triesters of glycerol (Figure 10.5b). Fats may be solid (Figure 10.6a) or liquid (Figure 10.6b) at room temperature, primarily depending on their molecular weight. Esters with low molecular weight are commonly used as fragrances and found in essential oils (Figure 10.6c). Phosphoesters form the backbone of DNA molecules.

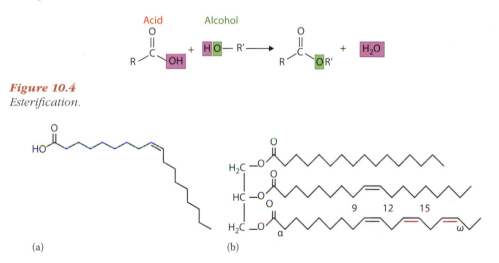

Figure 10.4
Esterification.

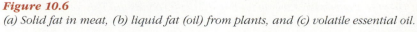

(a)   (b)

Figure 10.5
Molecular structures of (a) a fatty acid (oleic acid) (From Kaneko F et al., Phys. Chem. B 101, 1803, 1997.) and (b) a triglyceride, comprising of three long chain fatty acids liked to a glycerol molecule. (From Wolfgang, S., Seoul, Korea, 2005, public domain. http://upload.wikimedia.org/ wikipedia/commons/b/be/Fat_triglyceride_shorthand_formula.PNG).

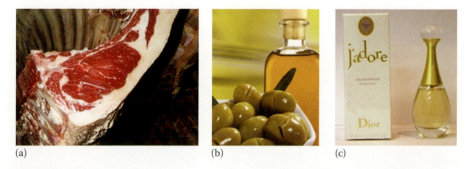

(a)   (b)   (c)

Figure 10.6
(a) Solid fat in meat, (b) liquid fat (oil) from plants, and (c) volatile essential oil.

10.2.2   Synthesis of PGA, PLA, and PCL

Polyesters represent a category of polymers which contain the ester functional group ($-$COO$-$) in their main chain. Poly(glycolic acid) (PGA) (or polyglycolide), poly(lactic acid) (PLA) (or polylactide), poly (ε-caprolactone) (PCL), and their copolymers are the most frequently utilized synthetic polymers in medical devices to date. PGA and PLA are derived from renewable resources [1].

PGA is the simplest linear, aliphatic polyester, and can be prepared from glycolic acid by means of polycondensation or from cyclic di-ester (known as *glycolide*) by means of ring-opening polymerization in the presence of a metal catalyst (Figure 10.7). Glycolic acid is found in sugar crops, and glycolide is obtained by heating and dehydrating glycolic acid.

Similar to PGA, PLA can be produced from lactic acid by means of polycondensation or cyclic di-ester (known as *lactide*) by means of ring-opening polymerization (Figure 10.8). Structurally, PLA is similar to PGA, only that each carbon atom in the backbone chain has a methyl group ($-$CH$_3$) attached to it. Lactic acid is known as milk acid. In animals, lactate (ester of lactic acid) is constantly produced during normal metabolism and exercise, similar to the fermentation reaction in yeast. This acid is also found in corn starch, tapioca roots, chips or starch, or sugarcane. Lactide is obtained by heating and dehydrating lactic acid.

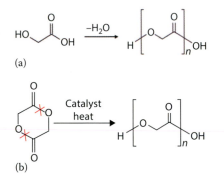

Figure 10.7
Synthesis of PGA: (a) polycondensation from glycolic acid; (b) ring-opening (either of the two crossed bonds) polymerization from glycolide.

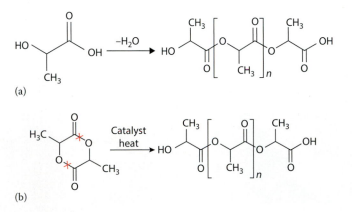

Figure 10.8
Synthesis of PLA. The ring is opened at either of the crossed CO–O bonds. (a) Polycondensation of lactic acid. (b) Ring-opening (either of the two crossed bonds) polymerization of lactide.

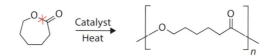

Figure 10.9
Ring-opening polymerization of PCL.

PCL is also prepared by ring-opening polymerization of ε-caprolactone using a metal catalyst (Figure 10.9). The most common industrial route to produce PGA, PLA, and their copolymers is the ring-opening polymerization of cyclic monomers, typically catalyzed by tin octoate [Sn(Oct)$_2$], and the copolymers of PLA and PGA with PCL are all produced by ring-opening polymerization of their cyclic monomers.

10.2.3 Properties of PGA, PLA, and PCL

These saturated, aliphatic polyesters are thermoplastic. PLA exists in three forms: L-PLA (PLLA), D-PLA (PDLA), and racemic mixture of D,L-PLA (PDLLA). PLLA and PGA are practically crystalline, whereas PDLLA and PLGA are intrinsically amorphous due to the chain stereo-irregularity. Selected physical and mechanical properties of these three polyesters are given in Table 10.1.

10.2.4 Degradation of Polyesters

In general, polyesters are characterized by their hydrolytic instability owing to the presence of the ester linkage in their backbone. PGA, for example, is naturally degraded in the body by hydrolysis and is absorbed as water-soluble monomers. The hydrolysis of crystallized polyesters takes place in two steps, during which the polymer is converted back to its monomer. First, water diffuses into the amorphous (noncrystalline) regions of the polymer matrix, cleaving the ester bonds. The second step starts after the amorphous regions have been eroded, exposing the crystalline portion of the polymer to hydrolytic attack. Upon collapse of the crystalline regions, the polymer chains dissolve.

When implanted into the body, polyesters are always hydrolyzed under the mediation of cellular enzymes, especially those with esterase activity. Under enzymatic mediation, polyesters always degrade faster than in an enzyme-free environment, such as in vitro.

Studies on sutures have shown that PGA is completely resorbed by the body in a time frame of 4–6 months, while PLA needs a much longer time to be completely resorbed, typically 2 years (Table 10.2). However, the copolymers and blends of PGA

Table 10.1

Selected Physical and Mechanical Properties of PLA, PGA, PLGA, and PCL (Bulk Materials)

Polymers	T_m (°C)	T_g (°C)	Crystallinity (%)	Young's Modulus (GPa)	Ultimate Tensile Strength (MPa)
PGA	220–230	35–40	45–55	7–10	70
PLLA	170–180	60–65	30–40	3–16	30–80
PDLLA	Amorphous	55–60	0	1–4	30–50
PLGA	Amorphous	45–55	0	1–4	30–50
PCL	60	−70	40–50	0.3–0.4	10–15

Table 10.2

Biodegradable Rates of PGA, PLA, PLGA, PCL, and P3HB

Polymers	Degradation Kinetics
PDLLA	Sutures are resorbed completely in vivo in 12–18 months
PLLA	Sutures can be resorbed completely in vivo after 24 months
PGA	Sutures are resorbed completely in vivo in 4–6 months
PLGA	Sutures are resorbed completely in vivo in 2–12 weeks
PCL	Time to be resorbed is typically 2–3 years
P3HB	Slower than PLA, PGA, and PLGA

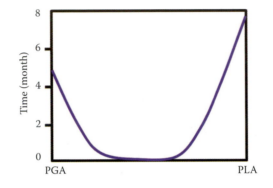

Figure 10.10
In vivo degradation rates of PGA, PLA, and their copolymers.

and PLA can be resorbed completely within several weeks, much faster than either homopolymer alone (Figure 10.10). The degradation rate of PCL is generally slower than both PGA and PLA. To summarize, these polyesters can be ranked in the following order, in terms of degradation kinetics, from faster to slower:

$$\underrightarrow{\text{PGLA} > \text{PGA} > \text{PDLLA} > \text{PLLA} > \text{PCL} > \text{P3HB}}_{\text{Degradation rate decreasing}}$$

For P3HB, readers are referred to Section 9.3.

The aforementioned rank of degradation rates can be explained by what we have learnt in Chapter 8: that the steric hindrance of side chains and crystallinity both affect the hydrolysis rate (water attack) with the former being the primary factor. First, the side chains ($-CH_3$) on PLA (Figure 10.8) shield the ester bonds from the attack of water molecules, and this steric hindrance effect is responsible for the slow degradation of PLA, compared with PGA, even though the latter is more crystalline. Second, the amorphous structure of PDLLA makes the polymer degrade faster than its partially crystalline PLLA counterpart. Third, in the copolymer of PLA and PGA, the PGA segments are in an amorphous state and thus degrade faster than its crystalline state in pure PGA, which explains why PLGA degrades faster than either PGA or PLA alone. Last, PCL polymer chains are primarily composed of chemically inert and hydrophobic $-(CH_2)_5$ segments (Figure 10.9) with only one ester bond for every five $-CH_2$ blocks. That is, PCL contains much fewer hydrolysable functional groups compared with PLA and PGA chains, and this makes the PCL polymer degrade the most slowly.

10.2.5 Biocompatibility of Polyesters

The toxicity of degradable polymers arises from their biodegradation products. The degradation products of PGA, PLA, and PCL are their monomers, that is, glycolic acid, lactic acid, or primelic acid. These chemicals are natural metabolic by-products in the body and can still reenter the tricarboxylic acid cycle (Krebs cycle)* once converted to pyruvic acid, after which they are further broken down to water and carbon dioxide (as HCO^{3-}), which is expelled as gas in the lungs, or as ions with water in the urine. However, excess acidic products are also associated with inflammation at surgical sites—an issue especially when the polymers are used to deliver cells.

10.2.6 Biomedical Applications of PGA, PLA, and PCL

The medical application of PGA began in 1962 when it was used to develop the first synthetic resorbable suture. By then it was marketed under the trade name of Dexon™. Today it is sold as Surgicryl™. The material in VICRYL™ (polyglactin 910) suture is actually a copolymer of 90% PGA and 10% PLA. The suture is coated with N-laurin and L-lysine, which render the thread extremely smooth, soft, and safe for knotting. It is also coated with magnesium stearate and finally sterilized with ethylene oxide gas. The degradation of Polyglactin 910 is completed between 60 and 90 days. It is commonly used for subcutaneous sutures, intracutaneous closures, abdominal and thoracic surgeries.

The traditional role of PGA as a biodegradable suture material has led to its evaluation in other biomedical fields. Implantable medical devices have been produced with PGA, including anastomosis rings, pins, rods, plates, and screws. It has also been explored as a controlled drug delivery system and tissue engineering scaffold (Figure 10.11). Dermagraft® is a cryopreserved human fibroblast-derived dermal substitute; it is composed of fibroblasts, extracellular matrix, and a bioabsorbable scaffold (polyglactin). This product is limited to treating full-thickness burns (Figure 10.12) and diabetic foot ulcers.

10.3 POLYESTERS: PHA

10.3.1 Synthesis of PHAs

Poly(hydroxyalkanoates) (PHAs) (Figure 10.13) are naturally occurring polyesters produced by a variety of bacteria, usually under artificial laboratory conditions of limiting nutrients (e.g., ammonium, potassium, sulfate, magnesium, and phosphate) but excess carbon source. This unbalanced nutrient supply leads to intracellular storage of excess nutrients, which accumulate as PHA granules that can account for up to 90% of the cells' dry weight. To date, over 150 hydroxyalkanoate units with different R-pendant groups have been isolated from bacterial sources [1].

10.3.2 Biocompatibility of PHAs

Like other biological polymers, PHAs intrinsically have excellent biocompatibility, and naturally occurring P3HB has been found as a ubiquitous component of the cellular membranes of animals. The presence of relatively large amounts of low-molecular-weight

---

* *A series of chemical reactions used by multicellular organisms to generate energy through the oxidation of acetate derived from carbohydrates, fats, and amino acids into carbon dioxide.*

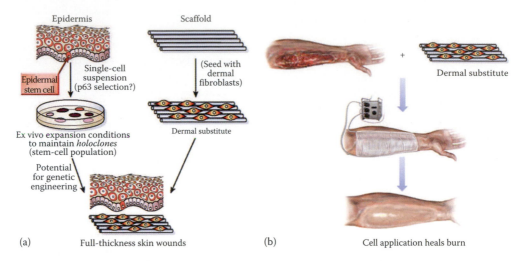

(a) Full-thickness skin wounds   **(b)** Cell application heals burn

Figure 10.11

Skin tissue engineering. (a) Step one: Patient cells are harvested, expanded, and loaded on synthetic scaffold. (b) Step two: the artificial dermal substitute is applied to skin wounds to enhance healing, prevent dehydration, and minimize infection. (http://www.ptei.org/interior.php?pageID=115.) (a) (Reprinted by permission from Macmillan Publishers Ltd., Nature, Bianco, P. and Robey, P.G., Stem cells in tissue engineering, 414(6859):118–121, copyright 2001.) (b) (Courtesy of Gerlach, J.C., McGowan Institute for Regenerative Medicine, Pittsburgh, PA, reproduced with permission.)

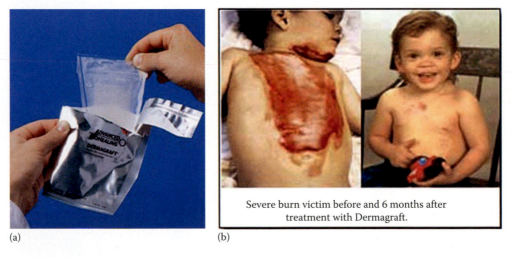

Severe burn victim before and 6 months after treatment with Dermagraft.

(a)   (b)

Figure 10.12

(a) A skin substitute product: Dermagraft and (b) case of successful restoration after its application.

P3HB in human blood and the fact that the degradation product, 3 hydroxybutyric acid (3HB), is a natural human metabolite present in the brain, heart, lung, liver, kidney, and muscle tissue as well as excreted matter serve as evidence of the potential for P3HB to integrate with and be processed by these tissues. The toxicity of a PHA product is caused by the bacterial synthesis, as well as the fabrication process, rather than the PHA material itself. Hence, PHA products have long been under intensive and rigorous evaluation both in vitro and in vivo.

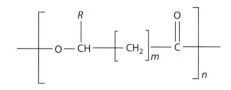

Figure 10.13
Chemical structures of polyhydroxyalkanoates (PHAs). In this single segment, m can take on a value of 1, 2, or 3, yet m = 1 is most common; n can range from 100 to several thousands, and R can represent a variable. When R = CH$_3$ and m = 1, the structure represents poly (3-hydroxybutyrate) (P3HB). When R = H and m = 2, the structure becomes poly (4-hydroxybutyrate) (P4HB). When R = H and m = 0, the structure is PGA. When R = CH$_3$ and m = 0, the structure is PLA. PHAs refer to the structures with nonzero m.

10.3.3 Biodegradation Rates

Although bacterial sources of P3HB are amorphous, up to 50% crystallization occurs upon retrieval from the bacteria. The degradation kinetics of this variety of PHAs is generally slower than that of PLA/PGA/PLGA, owing to the crystalline structure, the steric hindrance of the R side chain, and the chemically inert segments of $(CH_2)_m$.

10.3.4 Properties of PHAs

The availability of over 150 different types of PHAs offers an extraordinarily wide selection of physical and mechanical properties (Table 10.3) from crystalline (brittle) polymers to rubber-like elastomers. This variety is imparted by the ability to manipulate the length of the side chains and the distance between ester linkages in the polymer backbone. PHAs with short side chains tend to be more crystalline and hard, whereas PHAs with longer side chains are generally soft and flexible, showing typical elastomeric behavior. Since their T_g is below room temperature, PHAs can have properties resembling either thermoplastic polymers (P3HB) or thermoplastic elastomers (P4HB), depending on the level of crystallinity.

10.3.5 Medical Applications of PHAs

PHAs have also been explored as tissue engineering scaffold materials. Because of their slow degradation characteristics, these polymers could be used in tissue engineering as implants that require longer retention times and higher stability in the surrounding environment, but which eventually resorb.

Table 10.3
Thermal and Mechanical Properties of some PHAs

Polymer	T_g (°C)	T_m (°C)	Young's Modulus (GPa)	Ultimate Tensile Strength (MPa)	Elongation at Beak (%)
P3HB	4–10	175–185	2.5–4	35–60	2–60
P4HB	−47	61	0.05–0.23	35–50	>1000

10.4 ELASTOMERIC POLYESTER: POLY(POLYOL SEBACATE)

10.4.1 Synthesis of Poly(Polyol Sebacate)

Poly(polyol sebacate) (PPS) is a family of cross-linked polyester elastomers, developed for medical applications at MIT [2]. PPS is synthesized from a polyol (an alcohol containing multiple hydroxyl groups) and sebacic acid. A subclass of polyols is represented by the sugar alcohols, which are commonly used in the food industry. Glycerol, maltitol, sorbitol, and xylitol represent the most common types (Table 10.4). Sebacic acid is a dicarboxylic, a naturally occurring chemical derived from castor oil. In the industrial sector, sebacic acid derivatives have been used as plasticizers, aromatics, antiseptics, cosmetics, and drug coatings. Poly(sebacic acid), for example, is surface erodible and is used in drug delivery where a constant erosion rate is required. One such application is in intracranial devices for the treatment of cancer.

Usually, the synthesis of PPS involves polycondensation (esterification) between carboxylic acids and alcohol groups (Figure 10.14). The primary $-OH$ groups at the two ends of polyol monomers react first with the carboxylic acid groups, forming polymer chains at the early stage of polymerization (Figure 10.14a). At later stages there is a deficiency of primary alcohol groups in the reaction system so that the secondary $-OH$ groups (toward the middle of the polyol monomers) then react with the $-COOH$ groups to form ester links and eventually cross-links between the polymer chains (Figure 10.14b).

Table 10.4
Some Common Types of Sugar Alcohols and Their Structures

Sugar Alcohol	Molecular Structure	PPS Polymer
Glycol (2-carbon)		PES
Glycerol (3-carbon)		PGS
Erythritol (4-carbon)		PErS
Xylitol (5-carbon)		PXS
Mannitol (6-carbon)		PMS
Sorbitol (6-carbon)		PSS

Source: Chen, Q.Z. et al., Prog. Polym. Sci., 38, 584, 2013.

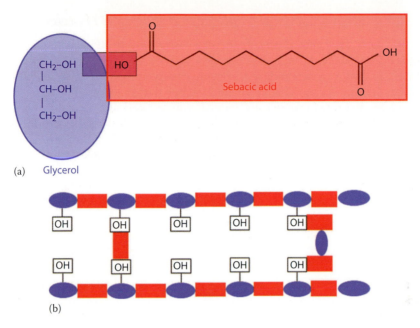

(a) Glycerol

(b)

Figure 10.14
Chemical cross-linking of PGS monomers (a) occurs at the hydroxyl groups on the sebacic acid backbones (b) to form a networked elastomer.

10.4.2   Biodegradation and Biocompatibility of PPS

PPS polymers are rapidly degraded in vivo, over several weeks, in a layer-by-layer, enzyme-mediated process. Their degradation products, polyol and sebacic acid, are both endogenous monomers found in human metabolites. As a metabolic intermediate in the mammalian carbohydrate metabolism, glycerol and xylitol enters the metabolic pathway slowly without causing rapid fluctuations of blood glucose levels. Hence, PPSs generally have little toxicity to the body tissues. In vivo applications of PGS in myocardial tissue engineering [4] consistently show little foreign body response in terms of acute or chronicle inflammation.

10.4.3   Mechanical Properties of PPS Polymers

Compared with PGA, PLA, PCL, and PHA materials, all of which have Young's modulus at the GPa level, PPS members are relatively soft, with Young's modulus in the order of MPa and UTS being only several MPa (Table 10.5).

Table 10.5
Mechanical Properties of Poly(Polyol Sebacate) (PPS) and Their Copolymers

Polymer	Young's Modulus (MPa)	UTS (MPa)	Elongation at Beak (%)	Resilience (%)
PGS	<1.5	<1.5	40–700	>98
PXS	<5.5	<2.5	30–700	>98
PSS	<3.0	<1.2	65–200	>98

10.4.4 Stress–Strain Curves of Synthetic and Biological Elastomers

Soft PPS polymers show typical elastomeric stress–strain curves (Figure 10.15a). The initial part of this curve, where the stiffness decreases with increasing load (*deformation softening*) (Figure 10.15b), can be predicted from thermodynamic theory, by considering the rubber as an entropy spring. This treatment assumes that all extension occurs via *conformational changes* (i.e., as opposed to bond stretching) and also assumes that the chain is composed of a series of joined links that are equally likely to lie in any direction. If N is the number of chain segments per unit volume and λ is the *extension ratio* (defined to be L/L_0, where L and L_0 are the initial and final length of the rubber, respectively), then the nominal stress for a rubber loaded in uniaxial tension is predicted to be as follows:

$$\sigma = kTN\left[\lambda - \frac{1}{\lambda^2}\right]. \tag{10.1}$$

where

    k is the Boltzmann constant
    T is the temperature

This gives the blue stress–strain curve of the form in Figure 10.15b.

At lower extensions (stages 1 and 2) (Figure 10.16), the theoretical stress-extension curve is fairly similar to the S-shaped curves obtained experimentally. At extensions of $\lambda = 4$ the experimental and theoretical curves diverge, with much larger stiffness seen experimentally than predicted theoretically. This occurs because at larger extensions the assumptions of the model are no longer valid: the polymer chains are mostly aligned with the applied stress and so applying higher stress stretches strong intramolecular bonds (stage 3).

If a material contains prealigned fibers, its stress–strain curve will start from stage 2. Without the initial stage 1, the shape of stress–strain curve is J-shaped. This explains why biological soft tissues (e.g., muscles), which are constructed of aligned fibers, all exhibit J-shaped stress–strain curves (Figure 10.17). Actually, many biological tissues are like prestressed rubbery materials, that is, they are already under tension in their neutral position, which also explains their J-shaped behavior. It must be emphasized that a biological mechanism also contributes to the abrupt increase in the J-shape stress–strain curve of

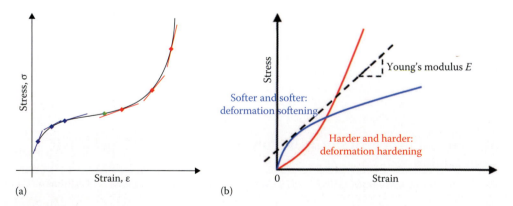

(a)   (b)

Figure 10.15
(a) A typical stress–strain curve of an elastomer; (b) deformation softening and deformation hardening curve.

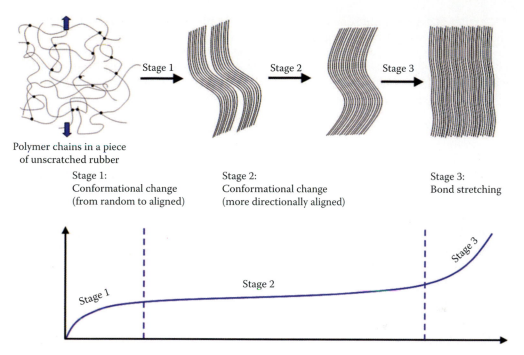

Stage 1:
Conformational change
(from random to aligned)

Stage 2:
Conformational change
(more directionally aligned)

Stage 3:
Bond stretching

Figure 10.16
Structural changes in elastomeric polymers at different stages of a stress–strain curve.

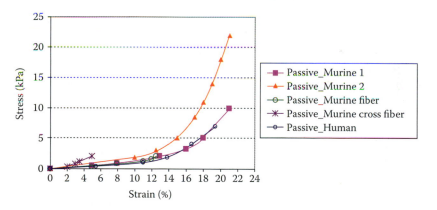

Figure 10.17
Stress–strain curves of heart muscle.

muscle in vivo, which involves calcium ions flowing in and out muscle cells during contraction, resulting in shortening and stiffening of the bulk muscle.

A similar effect occurs in materials that contain stiff fibers in a soft matrix. Initially, the stress acts only against the soft matrix, but with time the fibers align in the direction of the stress. When the further tension works against the stiffer fibers, the material become strong. This effect is observed in arterial walls, where the collagen fibers act as the stiffer fibers. The curves in Figure 10.17 represent passively stretched muscle under ex-vivo conditions, which are less resistant to strain than contracted, functional muscle in vivo. At higher stresses, stiffening is more related the aligned proteins within muscle fibres (see advanced topics).

Textile materials represent a nonbiological example of materials with J-shaped stress–strain curves. Knitted materials and woven fabrics pulled at 45° to the warp and weft have J-shaped curves. This is the mechanical reason why textile structure is used in cardiac support devices (Figure 8.5). In this case, the J-shaped stress–strain curve of textile materials is designed to be as close as possible to that of heart muscle, which is stiffer and less pliable than standard muscle fibers, owing to the more complex, cross-linked histology of cardiac muscle fibers.

10.5 POLYETHER: POLY(ETHYLENE GLYCOL)

10.5.1 Synthesis of PEG

Poly(ethylene glycol) (PEG) is the most commercially important type of polyether, with the formula being $H-(O-CH_2-CH_2)_n-OH$ (Figure 10.18). PEG is typically produced by the interaction of ethylene oxide with ethylene glycol, or ethylene glycol oligomers, catalyzed by acidic or basic catalysts:

$$HOCH_2CH_2OH + n(CH_2CH_2O) \rightarrow HO(CH_2CH_2O)_{n+1}H$$

10.5.2 Applications of PEG

PEGs are liquids or low-melting solids, depending on their molecular weights. PEG is highly water-soluble, can form hydrogels and is nontoxic, making it ideal for a wide range of pharmaceutical and food-based applications. PEG is used as an excipient in many pharmaceutical products, with lower-molecular-weight variants used as solvents in oral liquids and soft capsules, whereas solid high-molecular-weight variants are used as ointment bases, tablet binders, film coatings, and lubricants. PEG is also used in lubricating eye drops and more viscous products, including as a base in skin creams and lubricants. PEG is also used in a number of toothpastes as a dispersant and an antifoaming agent in food.

10.6 POLYAMIDE

10.6.1 Synthesis of Polyamides

A polyamide can occur naturally (such as proteins), and can be made artificially, with examples being nylons. The amide link, also known as a *peptide bond*, is produced from the condensation reaction of an amino group and a carboxylic acid group, where a small molecule, usually water, is eliminated. The amino and carboxylic acid group can be present on the same monomer (Figure 10.19a), or the polymer can be constituted of two different bifunctional monomers, one with two amino groups and the other with two carboxylic acid groups (Figure 10.19b). Amino acids are an example of single monomers (if the difference between *R* groups is ignored) reacting with identical molecules to form a poly(amino acid), known as *polypeptide*.

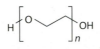

Figure 10.18
Molecular structure of PEG.

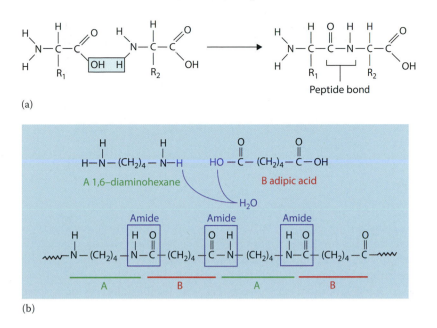

(a)

(b)

Figure 10.19
Polycondensation of polyamide: (a) polypeptide and (b) nylon.

10.6.2   Stability of Peptide Bonds in Aqueous Solution at pH 7

Similar to the ester bond, the peptide bond is thermodynamically unstable with respect to its hydrolysis products, having a tendency to be hydrolyzed. Kinetically, the rate of peptide bond hydrolysis under physiological conditions is very slow; the half-time for the reaction can be years. Thus, the peptide bond is stable in aqueous solution in a physiological timescale, and its hydrolysis is almost impossible without enzyme activity. Being thermodynamically unstable but kinetically stable is the feature of all biological polymers, that is, proteins, DNA, RNA, and polysaccharides. These two features figure prominently in the regulation of macromolecular metabolism.

10.7   SURFACE-ERODIBLE POLYMERS

There is a family of hydrophobic polymers that undergo a heterogeneous hydrolysis process that is predominantly confined to the polymer–water interface. This property is referred to as surface-eroding as opposed to bulk degrading behavior. In a surface-erodible material, the polymer chains contain hydrolysable groups and tend to break down in an aqueous environment. But the hydrophobic property of the polymer, and crystallized or cross-linked network structure make water molecules difficult to diffuse into the bulk polymer. Hence, erosion occurs on the surface, layer by layer. Examples of surface-erodible polymers are polyurethane, poly(anhydride), poly(ortho ester), and poly(phosphazene).

Whether a degradation process is surface erosion (layer by layer) or bulk degradation depends on the competition between diffusion kinetics in the network and the cleavage rate of polymer chains. If the rate of diffusion is much slower than the rate of cleavage of polymer chains, then surface erosion dominates the degradation process. If the rate of diffusion is much greater than the rate of cleavage of polymer chains, then bulk degradation dominates.

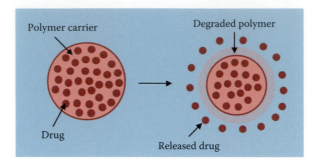

Figure 10.20
Controlled drug release.

These surface-eroding polymers have been used as drug delivery vehicles (Figure 10.20) and artificial scaffolds for tissue engineering. Their surface-eroding characteristics offer three key advantages over bulk degradation when used as biomaterials, especially in bone tissue engineering scaffolds: (1) retention of mechanical integrity over the degradation lifetime of the device; (2) minimal toxic effects (e.g., low local acidity) owing to lower solubility and concentration of degradation products; and (3) enhanced tissue ingrowth into the porous scaffolds over time, owing to the increase in pore size as the erosion proceeds.

10.8 BIOLOGICAL POLYMERS

As introduced in Chapter 1, biomaterials encompass biological materials. Biomacromolecules can be classified into four groups:

1. Polysaccharides (polymers with carbohydrate monomers)
2. Proteins (polymers with amino acid monomers)
3. Lipids (i.e., fatty acids = short chain hydrocarbons, with mixed saturated and unsaturated C−C bonds, sometimes with trimester cross-links)
4. Polynucleic acids (i.e., DNA, RNA—purine and pyrimdine polymers)

More discussions on these biomacromolecules will be provided in the Advanced Topic section of this chapter and in Chapter 16.

10.9 CHAPTER HIGHLIGHTS

1. The biodegradation of polymers proceeds in three major steps:

$$\text{Cleavage} \rightarrow \text{Metabolism} \rightarrow \text{Excretion.}$$

2. Cleavage is initiated by abiotic mechanisms, which include hydrolysis and/or oxidation. The kinetics of an abiotic process is determined by the physical accessibility of the polymer structure to water or oxygen molecules. Abiotic mechanisms proceed in a diffuse manner.
3. Biodegradation rates of chemical bonds in polymers:
   - C−C, C−H, C−F, Si−O: physiologically inert
   - HN−CO, peptide bond: hydrolyzable but very slowly, virtually impossible without enzyme activity
   - CO−O, ester bond: hydrolysis proceeds without enzyme activity, though can be accelerated by enzyme-mediation

356

4. A rank of some polyesters, in terms of degradation kinetics, from faster to slow:

$$\underrightarrow{\underline{\text{PGLA} > \text{PGA} > \text{PDLLA} > \text{PLLA} > \text{PCL} > \text{P3HB}}_{\text{Degradation rate decreasing}}}$$

which can be explained by the steric hindrance of side chains and crystallinity of these polymers.

5. The degradation product of these polyesters is their monomers, that is, glycolic acid, lactic acids, or primelic acid. These chemicals are natural metabolites in the body and can be excreted by the physiological system.

6. The stress–strain curves of elastomers show three stages:

   Stage 1: The initial convex shape of the stress–strain curves is due to the change in conformation of polymer chains, from completely random tangling toward aligning in the direction of the stress.

   Stage 2: During the plateau stage, the polymer chains are aligned more closely toward the direction of the stress, a process called progressive recruitment of strain-resistant components. This process requires little further force.

   Stage 3: Once the polymer chains are aligned well along the external stress direction, the stress stretches directly against the chemical bonds on the polymer chains, resulting in abrupt rising of stress.

7. Biological tissues are prealigned fibrous rubbery materials. So their stress–strain curves start with stage 2, showing J-shaped behavior.

SIMPLE QUESTIONS IN CLASS

1. Which of the following bonding is hydrolyzable?
   a. C−O
   b. C−C
   c. C−F
   d. C−H
2. Which of the following polymers is amorphous?
   a. PLLA
   b. PCL
   c. PGA
   d. PDLLA
3. In general, poly(lactic acids) (PLA) degrades more slowly than poly(glycolic acid) (PGA), because of the
   a. High crystallinity of PLA
   b. Steric interference in PLA chain (e.g., water access to the ester)
   c. High molecular weight of PLA
   d. Stable chemical bonds in the chain of PLA
4. The mechanism of cross-linking in poly(glycerol sebacate) (PGS) is
   a. Physical cross-linking by hard blocks
   b. Chemical cross-linking between carbon and carbon on backbone, as in PE
   c. Chemical ester bonding between glycerol and sebacic acid
   d. Hydrogen bonding

5. Which of the following polymers is partially crystalline?
   a. PDLLA
   b. PLGA
   c. PLLA
   d. Cross-linked PGS
6. Which of the following materials' degradation *must* involve enzymes?
   a. PLA
   b. PGA
   c. Polypeptides
   d. Bioglass
7. Which of the following polymers degrade most slowly?
   a. P3HB
   b. PLA
   c. PGA
   d. PCL
8. Natural elastic muscles show J-shaped curves. Why?
   a. Natural collagens are softer than synthetic rubbers.
   b. Polymer chains in muscles are well-aligned, and there is no *conformational stretching* stage that occurs in randomly structural synthetic polymers.
   c. Calcium ions transport in and out of muscle cells.
   d. Both b and c.

PROBLEMS AND EXERCISES

1. List four potential benefits of biodegradable polymers.
2. Describe the general biodegradation mechanisms of synthetic polymers.
3. Rank PGA, PLA, and PLGA in terms of their degradation kinetics, from the fastest (1) to the slowest (3). Explain the reasons for the order.
4. Among PLA, PGA, PCL, and P3HB, which one degrades most slowly? Explain your answer.
5. What are the typical shapes of the stress–strain curves of synthetic elastomers and muscles? Describe the mechanisms behind the two types of curves.
6. Briefly describe the deformation mechanisms at each of the different stages in the S-shaped stress–strain curve exhibited by some synthetic polymers.

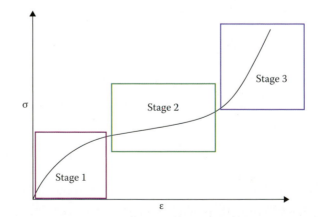

7. Briefly describe the in vitro deformation mechanisms at each of the different stages in the J-shaped stress–strain curve exhibited by some muscles.

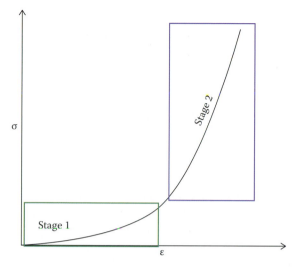

8. Briefly describe the in vivo deformation mechanisms at each of the different stages in the J-shaped stress–strain curve exhibited by some muscles.
9. Schematically show the molecular structure of xylitol and sebacic acid. To produce a very soft, fast degradable elastomer from these two monomers, what molar ratios would you use? To produce a rigid and slowly degradable elastomer from these two monomers, what molar ratios would you use? Discuss and explain your answers.
10. A cyclic stress–strain curve of an elastomeric poly(glycerol sebacate) (PGS) fibrous mash is given in the following. Compute the resilience of this material.

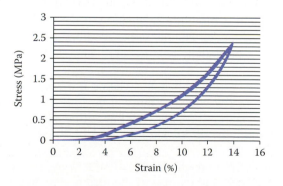

LABORATORY PRACTICE 4

Mechanical properties of synthetic polymers (PGS) and biological tissue (muscle).

ADVANCED TOPIC: NATURAL POLYMERS: RESILIN, SILK, AND GLUTEN

Molecular Structure of Proteins

Proteins are organic compounds made of amino acids linked to form a linear chain (Figure 10.18a). The 22 naturally occurring amino acids can be linked together in varying sequences to form a vast variety of protein structures, both structural (e.g., fibrous structures) and functional (e.g., enzymes, ligands and receptors, antibodies). In this section, three natural proteins, resilin, silk, and gluten, are reviewed as biomaterials, focusing on their biocompatibility, biodegradability, mechanical properties, and applications.

Resilin

Biological Function of Resilin   Resilin is an elastomeric protein found in many insects. It is the most efficient naturally occurring elastomeric protein known in terms of resilience. The contraction and efficient manipulation of resilin enables the organism to generate mechanical energy and carry out organized and sophisticated movements, such as flight and jumping [1] using a form of nearly perfect mechanical spring motion by insects [2].

Biocompatibility and Biodegradability of Resilin   Mouse fibroblast NIH 3T3 fibroblasts seeded on synthetic resilin-like elastomer (RLP12) gels spread with well-formed and organized stress fibers, indicating good cytocompatibility and cell adhesion [3]. Although resilin is insoluble in all solvents due to the chemical resistance of peptide bonds, it is readily digested by all the proteolytic enzymes tested so far [4]. The digestion of 10 mg locust resilin takes less than 1 day by 3 mg subtilisin in 3 mL of 0.2 M phosphate buffer, pH 8.0 at 30°C.

Mechanical Properties of Resilin   There are two reasons for the popularity of resilin as an alternative elastomeric material. First, the resilience of the resilin isolated from locust tendon has been reported to be 97%—only 3% of stored energy is lost as heat [5]. Second, resilin consists of a three-dimensional (3D) network with thermally agitated and randomly kinked molecular chains, stably cross-linked by dityrosine and trityrosine [6], which makes it potentially able to serve as a stable, deformable network in cells and tissue [4].

Resilin will be rubbery only when the chains are solvating or the temperature reaches a certain level, below which resilin will become glassy and solid [7]. At room temperature, hydrated resilin is a rubber with low stiffness and high extensibility, demonstrating a Young's modulus of 50–300 kPa, UTS of 60–300 kPa, and elongation at break of 250%–300% [4].

Since large amounts of pure resilin from natural sources are very difficult to obtain, Elvin and colleagues cloned and expressed the resilin gene to produce a soluble protein followed by photo cross-linking it to form an extremely resilient rubbery hydrogel, rec-1 resilin [3]. Recently, these researchers also isolated the gene from *Drosophila melanogaster* and inserted it into *Escherichia coli* bacteria to make pro-resilin, followed by cross-linking the pro-resilin into a rubbery solid. The material behaved exactly like resilin with 90%–92% resilience and could be stretched to three times its original shape. The material was concluded as having great potential in making replacements for intervertebral discs, which are highly resistant to compressive strain, but essentially fibrous in structure [8]. In addition to this, Guokui and colleagues synthesized recombinant *Drosophila melanogaster* resilin cross-linked with chitin (*N*-acetylglucosamine), a rigid sugar derived from arthropod shell, in order to generate a material with more resilient mechanical properties [9].

Applications of Resilin in Tissue Engineering   Artificial titin has been made by cross-linking the protein domains of resilin to mimic the natural protein that is made of regions with different mechanical properties. The resulting biomaterials had high resilience at low strain and shock absorbance at high strain, similar to the passive elastic properties of muscle. The application of this new muscle-mimetic biomaterial as scaffolds and the matrix for artificial muscles remains to be exploited [10].

Although resilin has shown good cytocompatibility, and is subject to proteolytic enzyme degradation, much further information is needed on its biocompatibility. Like elastin, resilin is soft and elastic. The application of this new muscle-mimetic biomaterial as scaffolds and the matrix for artificial muscles remains to be developed.

Spider and Silkworm Silk

Functions of Silk   Natural silk fibers are produced by arthropods such as silkworms, for example, *Bombyx mori* (also called silk moth), *Anthereae pernyi* (Chinese tussach moth), and spiders. Silkworms and spiders produce a variety of structural silk polymers, which have evolved to function in air rather than in aqueous media, and whose mechanical properties range from rubber-like to extremely rigid [11]. Silkworms construct cocoons from silk fibers for protection during their metamorphosis into butterflies or moths [12]. Spiders use their silk to make webs, which function as nets to suspend themselves and catch insects, or as nests or cocoons for protection for their offspring [11].

Biocompatibility of Silk: Cellular Attachment and Spreading   In general, cell attachment on natural silk is poor, as observed in cultures of dermal fibroblasts, endothelial cells, keratinocytes, Schwann cells, and mesenchymal stem cells [13–17]. This is related to the amino acid sequence of silk proteins and its influence on secondary and tertiary structure, protein origin (natural or recombinant), and also the processing conditions (the use of organic or aqueous solvents, sterilization, etc.).

Significant research efforts have been devoted to improving cell attachment to silk surfaces via both chemical and genetic approaches. These include (1) plasma treatment of surfaces [17]; (2) synthesis of hybrid matrices composed of silk proteins and ECM proteins such as collagen, laminin, and fibronectin [18–22]; (3) coating silk fibers with collagen I, fibronectin III, laminin, or elastin [23]; and (4) the decoration of silk proteins with RGD motifs (tri-peptide arginine-glycine-aspartic acid; the adhesion motif for integrins present in fibronectin III), either by chemical cross-linking or by genetic engineering [24–27]. Covalent decoration of fibroin proteins (*B. mori*) has been achieved by coupling the synthetic peptide GRGDS with carboxyl groups from aspartic and glutamic acid residues of the protein [24,27–29]. One of the advantages of a protein-based material is the possibility to genetically engineer the primary sequence of the proteins, which allows the generation of structurally defined proteins. Genetic engineering allows the incorporation of the RGD sequence in recombinant silk proteins, which has been demonstrated for a spider silk-like protein [30] and fibroin synthesized by transgenic *B. mori* silkworms [22,31,32].

The attachment and spreading of various cells (e.g., human buccal keratinocytes, epidermal keratinocytes, human mesenchymal stem cells, and gingival fibroblasts) have been improved on hybrid and coated silk-based scaffolds compared with those cells cultured on unmodified silk nanofibers [33–37]. Cultivation of fibroblasts on films made of genetically engineered silk proteins has also revealed improved cell adherence [22].

Biocompatibility of Silk—In Vitro Evaluation There is a long-standing concern regarding the biocompatibility of natural silk, primarily due to the heterologous nature of these peptides (fibroin and seracin), a similar issue to fibrin and fibrillin. Silk-based materials have been analyzed in vitro using different cell types [13,15,31,38] (Table 10.6). The reason for the controversial results on biocompatibility is that silk can be extracted by various methods that result in silk exhibiting different physical and biological properties. Also, there may be several sources of toxicity of silk-based materials (e.g., degummed silk [16]), which are unclear as yet, including the presence of residual organic solvents used during silk protein processing. HFIP (1,1,1,3,3,3-hexafluoro-2-propanol) used in silk processing [39], for example, may cause cell death. Another reason for an increase in cell mortality could be related to the lack of attachment and cell–cell adhesion, which could induce cellular apoptosis as mentioned previously [40]. Hence, there is a need for improving the techniques of silk processing. Owing to the presence of β-sheets within silk-based materials, there is the potential for cross-linking of amyloidogenic peptides, which might be toxic and could induce neurodegenerative diseases such as Alzheimer's disease or Parkinson's disease [41,42].

Biocompatibility of Silk: In Vivo Assessment Although toxicity of sericin has not been reported, evidence exists in humans that sericin can induce a strong allergic response [50–53] (Table 10.7). Consequently, sericin is removed (and replaced by gelatin) in silkworm silk products intended to be used in medicine [65]. The immune response induced by fibroin has been extensively studied, revealing that the presence of fibroin leads to an extremely low (or complete absence of) immune response [57–61]. Long-term in vivo experiments (carried out with *B. mori* 3D fibroin scaffolds over the duration of 1 year in Lewis rats) concerning the expression of some modulators of acute inflammation demonstrated that the induction of cytokines was, in general, low (i.e., without chronic inflammation) [62]. Interestingly, the silk-material processing conditions were shown to be important for inducing cytokine production, further suggesting that residual solvent molecules within the scaffolds may be partly responsible for the immune response [62].

There are few in vivo studies on the efficacy of implanted spider silk scaffolds. In one study, spider-silk scaffolds were found to be well tolerated over a 2-month implantation [63]. In another study, however, spider-silk proteins were reported to induce severe inflammation and massive infiltration of leukocytes in the case of a subcutaneous implantation of sterilized spider egg-sac silk in rats [64]. Furthermore, there is also concern over amyloid formation [41,42].

Biodegradability of Silk Silks degrade via both enzymatic and nonenzymatic hydrolysis processes, as summarized in Table 10.8 [12]. Silkworm silk generally degrades faster in the presence of an enzyme than in an enzyme-free environment. However, the few available in vivo degradation studies [62] indicate that fibroin does not seem to degrade faster in vivo than in vitro via enzyme-free degradation (2 months) [66]. It has been pointed out by Leal-Egana and Scheibel [12] that in vitro biodegradation of silk matrices

Table 10.6

Biocompatibility of Silk-Based Biomaterials In Vitro

Material	Cell Type	Major Results	Refs.
Silkworm silk/ sericin	Mouse MC3T3 osteoblasts	Sericin coating improved cell adhesion, proliferation, calcium deposition, and specific alkaline phosphatase activity, compared with noncoated Ti alloy implants	[43]
Silkworm silk/ natural sericin	Human endothelial cells (HMEC-1 line)	Sericin and silk-conditioned medium had no negative effect on cell proliferation	[16]
Silkworm silk/ fibroin	L929 murine fibroblasts	After 24 h of incubation, cells showed an improved spreading on fibroin films in comparison with films made of collagen. After 7 days of cell culture, the viability and proliferation of cells on fibroin films was much higher than on either uncoated or collagen-coated plates.	[15]
Degummed silkworm or spider silks	Human endothelial cells (HMEC-1 line)	Endothelial cells exposed to the silks showed lower rates of proliferation and metabolism than nonexposed cells. The toxicity of the silk was negligible after thorough enzymatic treatment of the fibers with trypsin. It is proposed that the silk contained one or more cytotoxic components, which needed to be removed prior to medical use.	[16,44]
Silkworm silk/ fibroin scaffolds	Human outgrowth endothelial cells Primary human osteoblasts	Evaluated at 1 and 4 weeks of culture, progressing maturation of the tissue construct with culture time under culture conditions designed for outgrowth endothelial cells.	[38]
Sericin silk (SS)	Mouse fibroblasts	SS from all extraction methods had no toxicity to cells at concentrations up to 40 μg/mL after 24 h incubation. At higher concentrations, heat-degraded SS was the least toxic to cells and activated the highest collagen production, while urea-extracted SS showed the lowest cell viability and collagen production. SS from urea extraction was severely harmful to cells at concentrations higher than 100 μg/mL.	[45–47]

(Continued)

363

Table 10.6 (Continued)

Biocompatibility of Silk-Based Biomaterials In Vitro

Material	Cell Type	Major Results	Refs.
Sericin and fibroin	RAW 264.7 Murine macrophage	Silk fibers were largely immunologically inert in short- and long-term culture with macrophages while insoluble fibroin particles induced significant TNF release. Soluble sericin proteins extracted from native silk fibers did not induce significant macrophage activation. The low level of inflammatory potential of silk fibers makes them promising candidates in future biomedical applications.	[48]

may not be directly correlated with in vivo conditions where the microenvironment of the tissue presents factors that could substantially modify the silk surfaces and their physicochemical properties and/or biological reactivity. Proteases used in vitro, such as mycolysin, protease XIV, trypsin, and α- chymotrypsin, clearly do not represent the complex arrays of proteases in the environment of an implant, such as metalloproteases [113].

The biodegradation rates of silk are greatly influenced by their processing procedures. For example, fibroin scaffolds prepared from the all-aqueous process degrade to completion between 2 and 6 months in vivo in a rat model, while those prepared from organic solvent (hexafluoroisopropanol (HFIP) degrade relatively slowly, with remnants of fibroin from *B. mori* scaffolds observable for more than 1 year after implantation [62]. In addition, blending other materials (such as chitosan) with silk proteins has been shown to facilitate matrix degradation and improve cell infiltration [111]. Despite the very few studies of spider silk biodegradation, it is apparent that spider silk degrades much more slowly than silkworm silk [63].

Mechanical Properties of Silkworm Silk   Silkworm silk is not stretchy at all, having a modulus of 6–9 GPa, ultimate tensile strength of ~1 GPa, and rupture elongation of ~10%. The pure silk should not be labeled as elastic protein. Soft tissues and organs of the human body present values of Young's moduli between 1 and 200 kPa. Although it is possible to prepare scaffolds of silk with elastic moduli higher than 400 kPa (Table 10.9), silkworm silk-based materials are more suitable for the generation of stiff and/or moderately stiff implants (e.g., bone or ligament), rather than for regeneration of soft organs, such as muscle [12].

Efforts have been invested to develop recombinant fibroin–elastin copolymers [76,77]. Non-cross-linked recombinant silk–elastin-like protein copolymer films exceed the properties of native aortic elastin, attaining an ultimate tensile strength of 2.5 MPa, Young's modulus of 1.3 MPa, extensibility of 190%, and resilience of 86% after 10 cycles of mechanical preconditioning. These mechanical properties of methanol treated non-cross-linked films are very comparable to those of native elastin from bovine ligament, which is reported to display a Young's modulus of 1.1 MPa, ultimate tensile strength of 2 MPa, and deformability of 150% [77]. After glutaraldehyde cross-linking, the deformability increases to 245%, and ultimate tensile strength to 5.4 MPa [77].

Table 10.7

Biocompatibility of Silk-Based Biomaterials In Vivo

Material	Animal Model	Major Comments	Refs.
Sericin	Rat/excised wound	Wound-healing tests with creams containing sericin (8% w/v) did not induce hypersensitivity or other systemic responses in tests with rats.	[49]
Sericin	Human	A mild reaction to surgical sutures after thyroid surgery is common and is characterized by local edema and inflammation around the surgical scar.	[50–54]
Sericin (*B. mori*)	Human	Allergenic in humans at very low concentrations (0.003 units/mg), inducing type I allergic responses, upregulating levels of IgE, and producing asthma or rhinitis.	[12,53,55]
Fibroin	Mice/subcutaneous tissue/15 days	The silk showed long-lasting biocompatibility, inducing a mild foreign body response with no fibrosis, and efficiently guiding reticular connective tissue engineering.	[56]
	Rabbit/distal femurs/12 weeks	Silk fibroin hydrogel or scaffold accelerated bone remodeling processes, compared with control groups.	[57,58]
	Rabbit/calvaria/ 12 weeks	The silk fibroin nanofiber membrane was shown to possess good biocompatibility with enhanced bone regeneration and no evidence of any inflammatory reaction.	[59]
	Mice/cranial defects	No inflammation was observed.	[60]
	Mice/bladder/70 days	Silk scaffolds supported significant increases in bladder capacity and voided volume while maintaining similar degrees of compliance relative to the control group.	[61]
	Nude and Lewis rat/ short-term (2 months) long-term (1 year)	Throughout the period of implantation, all scaffolds were well tolerated by the host animals and immune responses to the implants were mild.	[62]
Spider-silk	Mice/subcutaneous/ 2 months	The rS1/9 scaffolds implanted were well tolerated. Over a 2-month period, the scaffolds promoted an ingrowth of de novo formed vascularized connective tissue elements and nerve fibers.	[63]
Spider egg-sac silk	Rats/subcutaneously/ 7 weeks	The silk induced severe inflammation and massive infiltration of leukocytes when subcutaneously implanted in rats.	[64]

Table 10.8
Degradation of Silk-Based Biomaterials In Vitro or In Vivo

Silk-Based Material	In Vitro: Enzyme/ Concentration; or In Vivo: Animal Model	Incubation Time	Degradation Rate	Refs.
Silk fibroin coating	0.05 M sodium phosphate buffer/0	15 days	60%–70%	[34,65]
Silk fibroin yarns	0.05 M sodium phosphate buffer/0	77 days	~100%	[66]
Silk fibroin/ carboxymethyl chitin films	Protease mycolysin– pronase (EC 3.4.24.31)/ 4 U mg^{-1}	2 days	20%–90%	[67]
Silk/keratin gelified in water or formic acid	Trypsin/5 U/mL	22 days	20%–95%	[68]
Silk fibroin sheets	Protease XIV/ 1 U/mL	15 days	30%	[65]
Silk fibroin fibers	Protease XIV/ 1 U/mL	42 days	30%	[66]
Silk scaffolds 4% (dried/ methanol treated)	Protease XIV/ 0.2 U/mL	10 days	0%	[69]
Silk scaffolds 6%–8% (dried/methanol treated)	Protease XIV/ 0.2 U/mL	22 days	20%–30%	[69]
Silk fibroin (coating polyester prosthesis)	Protease XIV/ 1 U/mL	15 days	30%	[34]
Silk fibroin (coating polyester prosthesis)	Collagenase IA/ 1 U/mL	15 days	70%	[34]
Silk fibroin sheets	Collagenase IA/ 1 U/mL	15 days	50%	[65]
Silk fibroin (coating polyester prosthesis)	α-Chymotrypsin/ 1 U/mL	15 days	55%	[34]
Silk fibroin sheets	α-Chymotrypsin/ 1 U/mL	15 days	70%	[70]
Silk fibroin scaffold prepared in aqueous process	Nude and Lewis rat/short-term (2 months) long-term (1 year)	2–6 months	100%	[62]
Silk fibroin scaffold prepared from organic solvent (hexafluoroisopropanol (HFIP)		1 year	Remnants of fibroin are observable.	[62]

(Continued)

Table 10.8 (Continued)
Degradation of Silk-Based Biomaterials In Vitro or In Vivo

Silk-Based Material	In Vitro: Enzyme/ Concentration; or In Vivo: Animal Model	Incubation Time	Degradation Rate	Refs.
SeriFascia™ surgical mesh (silk fibroin) Mersilene mesh (made of nonabsorbable polyester, poly (ethylene terephthalate)	1 cm diameter abdominal wall defect was made in 36 Sprague–Dawley rats/up to 94 days	30 and 94 days	A significant 33% and 57% reduction of SeriFascia suture mass was observed at 30 and 94 days, respectively. SeriFascia surgical mesh initially absorbed at an ideal rate that supported recovery of load-bearing by the host repair tissue.	[71,72]
Spider silk: Spidroin 1 (rS1/9)	Phosphate buffer Oxidizing environment	11 weeks 11 weeks	Stable. Starting to degrade.	[63]

Source: Leal-Egana, A. and Scheibel, T., Biotechnol. Appl. Biochem., 55, 155, 2010.

Mechanical Properties of Spider Silk   Viscid and dragline silks are two types of silks that are the best studied. For spiders that use an orb-type web, viscid silk forms the glue-covered catching spiral, while dragline silk is used as safety line to anchor the frame of the web. Typical stress–strain curves of these two silks are shown in Figure 10.21.

Viscid Silk   Like elastin and resilin, viscid silk has a low initial stiffness, E_{init} = 3 MPa, and a high elongation at break, ε_{max} = 2.5. However, it is much stronger than elastin or resilin, having tensile strength of 450 MPa, which makes it the strongest elastomeric material yet known. The superelastic behavior of viscid silk is unexpected for an elastic protein because viscid silk fibers function in air and other elastomeric proteins are brittle polymeric glasses in dried air [11]. The difference for spider's viscid silk is that the molecular mobility in its protein network is maintained by the presence of low-molecular-weight organic compounds in the glue [86]. These compounds can absorb water from the air, penetrate the silk network, and thus plasticize the silk proteins [87]. In addition, water absorbed into the glue layer keeps the glue sticky for its role in prey capture.

Dragline Silk   In contrast to the viscid silk, the dragline silk is not very stretchy, having an initial modulus of 10 GPa, ultimate tensile strength of 1.1 GPa, and rupture elongation of 30%. It is not clear if the label of *elastic protein* is suitable for dragline silk, as its resilience is low, typically 30%–40% [84,88], with the mechanical properties of dragline silk strongly affected by the working environment, and the fiber thickness differences. Like most polymers, dragline silk shows dramatic increases in strength and toughness when strain rate is increased (Figure 10.22). When dragline is immersed in water, it swells and is transformed into a rubber-like elastic material (Figure 10.23). Figure 10.24 provides an overview of mechanical properties of the elastic proteins reviewed in Section 10.4.

Table 10.9

Mechanical Properties of Silk and Silk-Based Materials

Silk	Material from	Young's Modulus	UTS	Elongation at Break (%)	Resilience (%)	Refs.
Silkworm:						
Native silk (from raw *B. mori* silk)	Fiber	8.5 GPa				[73]
Sericin-free silk (from raw *B. mori* silk)	Fiber	6 GPa				[73]
Silk fibroin	Fibers	5 GPa	300 MPa	20		[74]
Silk fibroin	Fibers	2 GPa	300 MPa	40		[75]
Fibroin and recombinant human tropoelastin	Film	2–9 MPa			68–97	[76]
Recombinant silk–elastin-like protein copolymer	Film					[77]
Fibroin hydrogel (isolated from cocoons of *B. mori*)	Hydrogel (4%–16% w/v)	0.5–4.0 MPa				[78]
Fibroin hydrogel 10% blends with poly(vinyl alcohol at different ratios (isolated from cocoons of *B. mori*)	Hydrogel	57–175 MPa				[71]
Fibroin 5.8% scaffolds, freeze-drying procedure with different treatments (isolated from cocoons of *B. mori*)	Porous scaffold	0.01–0.17 MPa				[79]
Fibroin 6% scaffolds, freeze-drying/lyophilization procedure (isolated from cocoons of *B. mori*)	Porous scaffold	0.4 MPa				[80]
Spider silk:						
Viscid silk (from *Araneus diadematus*)	Fiber	Initial *E*: 3 MPa	450 MPa	250	30–40	[81]
Dragline silk (from *Araneus diadematus*)	Fiber	10 GPa	1.1 GPa	30	30–40	[82–85]

Sources: Gosline, J. et al., *Philos. Trans. R. Soc. Lond. B Biol. Sci.*, 357(1418), 121, 2002; Leal-Egaña, A. and Scheibel, T., *Biotechnol. Appl. Biochem.*, 55, 155, 2010.

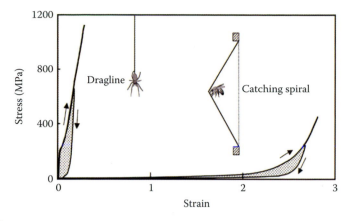

Figure 10.21
Stress–strain curves and overlaid stress–strain cycles for dragline and viscid silks from the spider Araneus diadematus. (From Gosline, J.M. et al., J. Exp. Biol., 202(23), 3295, 1999. Copyright 1999, reprinted with permission of the Company of Biologists Ltd.)

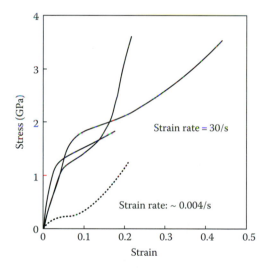

Figure 10.22
The effect of strain rate on the mechanical properties of dragline silk from Araneus diadematus. (Reprinted from Gosline, J.M. et al., Phil. Trans. Roy. Soc. Lond. B Biol. Sci., 357(1418), 121–132, 2002. Copyright 2002 by permission of the Royal Society.)

Applications of Silk in Tissue Engineering   The applications of silk fibroin as tissue engineering materials have widely been investigated with many types of tissues and organs, including bone, cartilage, ligament, vascular tissue, skin, nerve, and ocular tissues, as listed in Table 10.10. Although reversible outcomes have been reported [89], the majority of data, especially the long-term in vivo trials [72,73] and clinical follow-up reports [90], demonstrate that silk fibroin causes little or no foreign body effects and is thus a worthy candidate for tissue engineering exploration [91]. However, significant questions concerning the effects of various processing and fabrication conditions on the biomaterial fibroin, when implanted in vivo, and on the phenotype of important

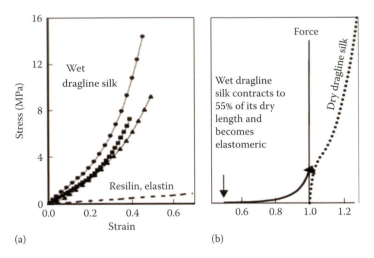

(a)   (b)

Figure 10.23

The effect of water on the mechanical properties of dragline silk. The stress–strain curves compare the material properties of wet dragline silk compared with the rubber-like proteins elastin and resilin (a). The change in the force–elongation behavior of dragline silk that occurs when it is immersed in water (b). The initial stiffness for wet dragline silk is ~10 MPa. (Reprinted from Gosline, J.M. et al., Phil. Trans. Roy. Soc. Lond. B Biol. Sci., 357(1418), 121–132, 2002. Copyright 2002 by permission of the Royal Society.)

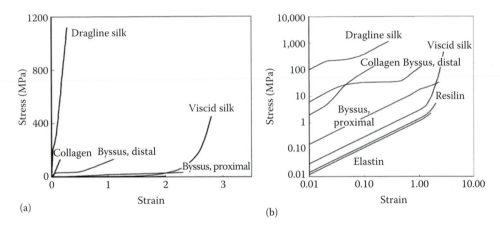

(a)   (b)

Figure 10.24

Stress–strain curves for seven elastic proteins. The plot is dominated by superstrong spider silks; as a consequence, the curves for the rubber-like proteins, elastin and resilin, are indistinguishable from the strain axis and have been left unlabeled (a). Stress–strain curves for the seven elastic proteins from (a) are plotted on logarithmic axes (b) to reveal the full diversity of their mechanical properties [11]. Byssus represents fibrous proteins that hold together mussel shells. (Reprinted from Gosline, J.M. et al., Phil. Trans. Roy. Soc. Lond. B Biol. Sci., 357(1418), 121–132, 2002. Copyright 2002 by permission of the Royal Society.)

cell types [91] remain to be determined. Since silk fibroins are essentially not elastic proteins, we will not discuss their applications in further detail. Interested readers can refer to a recent review on this topic [92].

In contrast to the extensive investigation of silk fibroin, there are very few reports on the application of spider silk in tissue engineering, as shown in Table 10.10.

Table 10.10

Applications of Silk in Tissue Engineering

Material	Type of Tissue Engineered	Animal Model/ Implantation Duration	Major Results	Refs.
Silkworm (*Bombyx marl*) fibroin sponge	Cartilage	Rabbit knee joints/12 weeks	Cartilage was regenerated in large defects on rabbit knee joints within the sponge, which resembles hyaline cartilage at 12 weeks after implantation.	[101]
Fibroin sponge/apatite composite	Bone	Rat mandibular bone/8 weeks	Silk scaffold, which was premineralized in vitro, can serve as a potential substrate for bMSCs to construct tissue-engineered bone for mandibular bony defects.	[102–104]
Fibroin scaffold	Ligament	Rat primary fascial defect/90 days	Although a higher grade of neovascularization was observed in silk scaffold, the silk explants induced a strong foreign body reaction showed a remarkable higher number of foreign body giant cells that characteristically spread from the periphery into implants. Polypropylene (PP) explants showed a more moderate foreign body reaction.	[89]
Knitted fibroin silk mesh	Ligament	Pig anterior cruciate ligament (ACL)/24 weeks	Histology observation showed that MSCs were distributed throughout the regenerated ligament and exhibited fibroblast morphology. The key ligament ECM components including collagen I, collagen III, and tenascin-C were produced prominently. The tensile strength of regenerated ligament also met the mechanical requirements.	[35,105]
Pure fibroin silk	Ligament	Dog knees, anterior cruciate ligament (ACL)/6 weeks	The onset of an inflammatory tissue reaction was seen in both the silk scaffold and the composite silk scaffold groups	[106]

(Continued)

Table 10.10

Applications of Silk in Tissue Engineering

Material	Type of Tissue Engineered	Animal Model/ Implantation Duration	Major Results	Refs.
Silk-collagen-hyaluronan hybrid material			Monocytes presented in the silk composite scaffold, and giant cells were absent in all cases. Granulation tissue consisting of fibroblasts, lymphocytes, monocytes, and collagen fibers and the formation of new blood vessels were observed in hybrid scaffolds. No reparative tissues, such as blood vessels, collagen, and cells were observed in the silk scaffold-grafted group. These results suggest that the hybrid substrate, rather than the pure silk one, is biocompatible in vitro and enhances new blood vessel and cell migration in vivo.	[73]
Silk fibroin scaffold	Ligament	Goat anterior cruciate ligament (ACL)/12 months	The initial positive clinical, gross pathologic, histologic, and mechanical results demonstrate the potential of this scaffold.	[107]
Electrospun fibroin silk using an all aqueous process	Small-diameter vessel	In vitro	Human endothelial cells and smooth muscle cells were successfully cultured on the electrospun silk.	[108, 109]
Tubular electrospun silk fibroin scaffolds	Small-diameter vessel	In vitro Human coronary artery smooth muscle cells and human aortic endothelial cells were sequentially seeded onto the luminal surface of the tubular scaffolds and cultivated under physiological pulsatile flow	The results demonstrate the successful integration of vascular cells into silk electrospun tubular scaffolds as a step toward the development of tissue-engineered vascular grafts similar to native vessels in terms of vascular cell outcomes and mechanical properties.	

Material	Tissue type	Model/duration	Findings	Reference
Silk-fibroin-based mat	Peripheral nerve	In vitro/Schwann cells	The electrospun fibroin mats supported the survival and growth of the Schwann cells.	[110]
PLGA-silk fibroin-collagen	Nerve	In vitro/Schwann cells	50% PLGA, 25% silk fibroin, and 25% collagen is more suitable for nerve tissue engineering compared to PLGA nanofibrous scaffolds.	[111, 112]
Silk fibroin conduit	Peripheral nerve	Lewis rats sciatic nerve defect/8 weeks	There were a greater number of proximal spouts and distal connections within the silk guide than in collagen guides. In addition to tailorable degradation rates, our silk conduits possess a favorable immunogenicity and remyelination capacity for nerve repair.	[113]
Spider silk: Decellularized vein grafts filled with spider silk fibers	Peripheral nerve	Used as a guiding material to bridge a 6.0 cm tibial nerve defect in adult sheep/6 and 10 months	Spider silk enhances Schwann cell migration, axonal regrowth, and remyelination including electrophysiological recovery in a long-distance peripheral nerve gap model resulting in functional recovery.	[100]
Genetically engineered *Nephila clavipes* spidroin 1 (rS1/9)	Skin	Subcutaneously into Balb/c mice/2 months	The rS1/9 scaffolds implanted were well tolerated. Over a 2-month period, the scaffolds promoted an ingrowth of de novo formed vascularized connective tissue elements and nerve fibers.	[63]
Porous silk fibroin films	Skin	Rat/14 days	Angiogenesis of the material films underwent initiation (day 5–7), followed by a rapid growth (day 7–13) and remodeling period (after the day 13).	[114]
Porous silk fibroin scaffolds	Skin	Rat/18 days	Inflammatory cells disappeared in the scaffold within 7 days.	[115]

(Continued)

Table 10.10 (Continued)

Applications of Silk in Tissue Engineering

Material	Type of Tissue Engineered	Animal Model/ Implantation Duration	Major Results	Refs.
			At day 18 after implantation new tissues formed in the scaffolds whose structure was almost equal to normal skin structure where proportional distribution of functional blood vessels could be found.	
			In summary, the silk scaffold significantly promoted the skin recovery from full thickness detect, compared with PVA.	
SeriFascia surgical mesh (silk fibroin) Mersilene mesh (made of nonabsorbable polyester, poly (ethylene terephthalate)	Skin	1 cm diameter abdominal wall defect was made in 36 Sprague–Dawley rats/94 days	Significantly greater tissue ingrowth observed in the SeriFascia surgical mesh group. SeriFascia surgical mesh initially bioresorbed at an ideal rate that supported the transfer of load-bearing responsibility to developing host repair tissue.	[72]
Silk fibroin–chitosan (SFCS)	Skin	Skin defect in male mice/4 weeks	Human adipose-derived stem cells seeded on a silk fibroin–chitosan scaffold enhance wound healing and show differentiation into fibrovascular, endothelial, and epithelial components of restored tissue.	[116]
DermaSilk® Knitted silk garments	Skin	Human/on eczema severity and pruritus in patients with atopic dermatitis/random, double blind/28 days	The decrease in pruritus values between day 0 and day 28 was greater for the DermaSilk group. This study demonstrates the importance of including the AEM 5772/5 finish to the specially knitted silk for a long-term improvement of atopic eczema symptoms.	[90]

Silk fibroin	Eye/corneal	In vitro	Human and rabbit corneal fibroblast proliferation, alignment, and corneal extracellular matrix expression on these films in both 2D and 3D cultures were demonstrated.	[117]
Silk fibroin	Eye/corneal	In vitro Culturing endothelial layer	Successful growth of primary human corneal endothelial cells on coated fibroin.	[118]
		In vitro Culturing human tympanic membrane cells (hTMC)	The silk substrate supports epithelial/keratinocyte phenotype and cell adhesion, with hTMC more proliferative than on the PET membranes.	[119–121]
Silk fibroin (SF)	Drug delivery	In vitro stage	Growth factor loaded SF scaffolds were suggested for the tissue engineering of bone and cartilage, as well as for vascular and nerve regeneration devices and wound-healing products. SF matrices were proposed for oral, transmucosal, and ocular drug delivery.	[122–125]

Source: Kon'kov, A.S. et al., Appl. Biochem. Microbiol., 46(8), 739, 2010.

The possibility of using recombinant spidroins as a base for biomedical constructs is discussed in previous reviews [93,94]. Spidroins and composite materials have been used for designing microcapsules [95,96], water-insoluble gels [97], and spongy 3D structures supporting cell adhesion and proliferation [63,64,98]. The 3D matrices fabricated from natural spidroins of the spider *Araneus diadematus* have also been used for obtaining artificial cartilage tissue, which supports the growth and adhesion of chondrocytes as effectively as the matrices from fibroin [99].

Elastic spider silk from genus *Nephila* spiders was reported to be successfully applied as a guiding material to bridge a 6.0 cm tibial nerve defect in adult sheep for 6–10 months [100], showing enhanced Schwann cell migration, axonal regrowth, and remyelination, as well as electrophysiological recovery in a long-distance peripheral nerve gap model. In another study, the recombinant analogue of natural spidroin produced by *Nephila clavipes* was fabricated into 3D porous constructs using the salt-leaching technique [63]. The scaffolds implanted subcutaneously into mice over a 2-month period were well tolerated, with the promotion of ingrowth and newly formed vascularized connective tissue and nerve fibers [63]. Further studies are needed to explore the possibility of applying genetic engineering approaches to obtain recombinant spider silk protein analogues, which in the future will widen the choice of biopolymers of this kind.

Gluten

Gluten in Food and Biocompatibility   Driven by the huge concern over the environment, renewable agriculture-derived materials have gained increasing attention over the past several years, as sustainable alternatives to replace the use of petroleum and natural gas products in biomaterial processing. Among various plant polymers, wheat proteins (starch and gluten) have been explored as biomaterials [126,127], due to their excellent biocompatibility [128]. Gluten (from Latin gluten *glue*) is a protein composite of a gliadin and glutelin, which co-exist with starch in the endosperm of wheat and related plant species. In contrast to the active research on starch-based biomaterials [129], there are few research reports on the use of gluten for biomedical applications [126,127], though gluten has been actively investigated as food packing materials [130]. Major limitations of gluten materials (fibers or films) include their high cost, poor mechanical properties, and hydrolytic stability [127,131,132], compared to the synthetic polymer-based materials.

The cytotoxicity of gliadin is another reason that wheat proteins have not been used in tissue engineering. Gliadins are some of the best examples of food-derived pathogens. People with gluten-sensitive enteropathy (celiac disease) are sensitive to α, β, and γ gliadins [133]. Those with wheat-dependent (WD) exercise-induced anaphylaxis, WD uticaria and Baker's asthma are sensitive to ω-gliadins [133]. Hence, gluten-free foods are developed for patients with celiac disease [134].

Biodegradability of Gluten   The biodegradation of gluten has mostly been studied in farmland soils. Although these data are not entirely indicative of the degradation kinetics of these materials under physiological conditions within tissues, they could be used as qualitative indicator of an aqueous environment. In general, wheat proteins degrade much more rapidly than synthetic polymers, being completely absorbed in about 1 month. Soy protein–gluten films, for example, degrade with 50% weight loss in about 10 days, and 95% weight loss in 30 days in simulated farmland soil conditions [135]. Wheat-gluten-based materials plasticized with glycerol were reported to be fully degraded after 36 days in aerobic fermentation (catalyzed by bacteria) and within 50 days in farmland soil [136]. A series of chemically cross-linked wheat-gluten-based natural polymers were shown to reach 93%–100% biodegradation within 22 days [137], a slower rate compared with uncross-linked equivalents. In another study where gluten films were developed as biomaterials for tissue engineering, gliadin and glutenin films experienced about 50% and 90% weight loss, respectively, under aqueous conditions (pH 7.2) for 15 days at 37°C [127].

Mechanical Properties of Gluten   A major limitation of the wheat gluten materials is their relatively poor mechanical properties. Wheat gluten is brittle in dry conditions (Figure 10.25) [127] and difficult to process without adding plasticizers [138,139]. In Figure 10.25, the 100% gluten fibers attain a Young's modulus of 5 GPa, UTS of 125 MPa, and elongation at break of 24%. The maximal elastic strain is about 1% or below.

Plasticized gluten can be elastic, evidenced by the fact that gluten gives elasticity to bread dough and helps it keep in shape. Glycerol and water are two most frequently used plasticizers. Plasticized gluten shows a typical rubber deformation behavior (Figure 10.26) [140], with a maximal elongation being about 200%. It is because of this property that gluten is labeled as an elastic protein [141].

Applications of Gluten in Tissue Engineering   Gluten has also been investigated as a drug delivery vehicle [132]. In another study, wheat gluten films were developed for application in tissue engineering [127]. To the best knowledge of the authors, there are no formal reports on the in vitro and in vivo evaluation of gluten as yet.

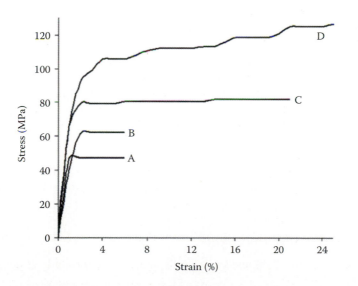

Figure 10.25

Effect of drawing and dry heating of the solid fibers (annealing) on the stress–strain behavior of 100% wheat gluten fibers: undrawn and unheated fibers (A); undrawn heated fibers (125°C for 90 min) (B); drawn and unheated fibers (about 250% of the initial length) (C); and drawn and annealed fibers (about 250%, 125°C for 90 min) (D). (From Reddy, N. and Yang, Y.Q., Biomacromolecules, 8(2), 638, 2007.)

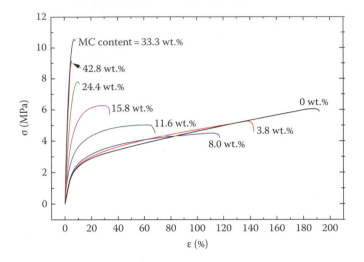

Figure 10.26
Stress–strain relationship of wheat gluten/methylcellulose/glycerol composites with various meth-ylcellulose contents as indicated. Note: the 0 wt.% samples are made of plasticized gluten with no addition of methylcellulose. (From Song, Y.H. and Zheng, Q., Ind. Crop Prod., 29(2–3), 446, 2009.)

BIBLIOGRAPHY

References for Text

1. Scott, G., *Degradable Polymers: Principles and Applications,* Kluwer Academic Publishers, Dordrecht, the Netherlands, 2002.
2. Wang, Y.D., G.A. Ameer, B.J. Sheppard, and R. Langer, A tough biodegradable elastomer. *Nature Biotechnology*, 2002;**20**:602–606.
3. Chen, Q.Z., S.L. Liang, and G.A. Thouas. Elastomeric biomaterials for tissue engineering. *Progress in Polymer Science*, 2013;**38**:584–671.
4. Stuckey, D.J. et al., Magnetic resonance imaging evaluation of remodeling by cardiac elastomeric tissue scaffold biomaterials in a rat model of myocardial infarction. *Tissue Engineering Part A*, 2010;**16**:3395–3402.

Websites

http://ceramics.org/about-us/international-ceramic-societies.
http://virtuallaboratory.colorado.edu/Biofundamentals/lectureNotes/Topic3–4_Peptide%20 bonds.htm.

References for the Advanced Topics

1. Nairn, K.M. et al., A synthetic resilin is largely unstructured. *Biophysical Journal*, 2008;**95**(7):3358–3365.
2. Weis-Fogh, T., Elasticity in arthropod locomotion: A neglected subject, illustrated by the wing system of insects. *Proceedings XVth International Congress of Zoology*, 1959;**4**:393–395.
3. Charati, M.B. et al., Hydrophilic elastomeric biomaterials based on resilin-like polypeptides. *Soft Matter*, 2009;**5**(18):3412–3416.
4. Weis-Fogh, T., A rubber-like protein in insect cuticle. *The Journal of Experimental Biology*, 1960;**37**(4):889–907.

5. Weis-Fogh, T., Thermodynamic properties of resilin, a rubber-like protein. *Journal of Molecular Biology*, 1961;**3**(5):520–531.
6. Andersen, S.O., The cross-links in resilin identified as dityrosine and trityrosine. *Biochimica et Biophysica Acta*, 1964;**93**:213–215.
7. McCartney, J.E., Heat contraction of elastic tissue. *Experimental Physiology*, 1913;**7**(2):103–114.
8. Elvin, C.M. et al., Synthesis and properties of crosslinked recombinant pro-resilin. *Nature*, 2005;**437**(7061):999–1002.
9. Qin, G. et al., Expression, cross-linking, and characterization of recombinant chitin binding resilin. *Biomacromolecules*, 2009;**10**(12):3227–3234.
10. Lv, S. et al., Designed biomaterials to mimic the mechanical properties of muscles. *Nature*, 2010;**465**(7294):69–73.
11. Gosline, J. et al., Elastic proteins: biological roles and mechanical properties. *Philosophical Transactions of the Royal Society of London. Series B, Biological Sciences*, 2002;**357**(1418):121–132.
12. Leal-Egana, A. and T. Scheibel, Silk-based materials for biomedical applications. *Biotechnology and Applied Biochemistry*, 2010;**55**:155–167.
13. Seo, Y.K. et al., Correlation between scaffold in vivo biocompatibility and in vitro cell compatibility using mesenchymal and mononuclear cell cultures. *Cell Biology and Toxicology*, 2009;**25**(5):513–522.
14. Mandal, B.B. and S.C. Kundu, Cell proliferation and migration in silk fibroin 3D scaffolds. *Biomaterials*, 2009;**30**(15):2956–2965.
15. Acharya, C., S.K. Ghosh, and S.C. Kundu, Silk fibroin protein from mulberry and non-mulberry silkworms: Cytotoxicity, biocompatibility and kinetics of L929 murine fibroblast adhesion. *Journal of Materials Science. Materials in Medicine*, 2008;**19**(8):2827–2836.
16. Hakımi, O. et al., Modulation of cell growth on exposure to silkworm and spider silk fibers. *Journal of Biomedical Materials Research. Part A*, 2010;**92A**(4):1366–1372.
17. Jeong, L. et al., Plasma-treated silk fibroin nanofibers for skin regeneration. *International Journal of Biological Macromolecules*, 2009;**44**(3):222–228.
18. Lu, Q. et al., Cytocompatibility and blood compatibility of multifunctional fibroin/collagen/heparin scaffolds. *Biomaterials*, 2007;**28**(14):2306–2313.
19. Asakura, T. et al., Production and characterization of a silk-like hybrid protein, based on the polyalanine region of *Samia cynthia* ricini silk fibroin and a cell adhesive region derived from fibronectin. *Biomaterials*, 2004;**25**(4):617–624.
20. Cirillo, B., M. Morra, and G. Catapano, Adhesion and function of rat liver cells adherent to silk fibroin/collagen blend films. *International Journal of Artificial Organs*, 2004;**27**(1):60–68.
21. Adachi, T. et al., Generation of hybrid transgenic silkworms that express *Bombyx mori* prolyl-hydroxylase alpha-subunits and human collagens in posterior silk glands: Production of cocoons that contained collagens with hydroxylated proline residues. *Journal of Biotechnology*, 2006;**126**(2):205–219.
22. Yanagisawa, S. et al., Improving cell-adhesive properties of recombinant *Bombyx mori* silk by incorporation of collagen or fibronectin derived peptides produced by transgenic silkworms. *Biomacromolecules*, 2007;**8**(11):3487–3492.
23. Tamatani, S. et al., Histological interaction of cultured endothelial cells and endovascular embolic materials coated with extracellular matrix. *Journal of Neurosurgery*, 1997;**86**(1):109–112.
24. Sofia, S. et al., Functionalized silk-based biomaterials for bone formation. *Journal of Biomedical Materials Research*, 2001;**54**(1):139–148.
25. Chen, J.S. et al., Human bone marrow stromal cell and ligament fibroblast responses on RGD-modified silk fibers. *Journal of Biomedical Materials Research. Part A*, 2003;**67A**(2):559–570.
26. Altman, G.H. et al., Silk-based biomaterials. *Biomaterials*, 2003;**24**(3):401–416.
27. Kambe, Y. et al., Effects of RGDS sequence genetically interfused in the silk fibroin light chain protein on chondrocyte adhesion and cartilage synthesis. *Biomaterials*, 2010;**31**(29):7503–7511.

28. Kim, J.W. et al., Effect of RGDS and KRSR peptides immobilized on silk fibroin nanofibrous mats for cell adhesion and proliferation. *Macromolecular Research*, 2010;**18**(5):442–448.

29. Kambe, Y. et al., Effect of RGDS-expressing fibroin dose on initial adhesive force of a single chondrocyte. *Bio-medical Materials and Engineering*, 2010;**20**(6):309–316.

30. Bini, E. et al., RGD-functionalized bioengineered spider dragline silk biomaterial. *Biomacromolecules*, 2006;**7**(11):3139–3145.

31. Morgan, A.W. et al., Characterization and optimization of RGD-containing silk blends to support osteoblastic differentiation. *Biomaterials*, 2008;**29**(16):2556–2563.

32. Yang, M. et al., Silklike materials constructed from sequences of *Bombyx mori* silk fibroin, fibronectin, and elastin. *Journal of Biomedical Materials Research. Part A*, 2008;**84A**(2):353–363.

33. Min, B.M. et al., Formation of silk fibroin matrices with different texture and its cellular response to normal human keratinocytes. *International Journal of Biological Macromolecules*, 2004;**34**(5):281–288.

34. Huang, F.H., L.Z. Sun, and J. Zheng, In vitro and in vivo characterization of a silk fibroin-coated polyester vascular prosthesis. *Artificial Organs*, 2008;**32**(12):932–941.

35. Fan, H.B. et al., In vivo study of anterior cruciate ligament regeneration using mesenchymal stem cells and silk scaffold. *Biomaterials*, 2008;**29**(23):3324–3337.

36. Meinel, L. et al., Engineering cartilage-like tissue using human mesenchymal stem cells and silk protein scaffolds. *Biotechnology and Bioengineering*, 2004;**88**(3):379–391.

37. Meinel, L. et al., Engineering bone-like tissue in vitro using human bone marrow stem cells and silk scaffolds. *Journal of Biomedical Materials Research. Part A*, 2004;**71A**(1):25–34.

38. Fuchs, S. et al., Dynamic processes involved in the pre-vascularization of silk fibroin constructs for bone regeneration using outgrowth endothelial cells. *Biomaterials*, 2009;**30**(7):1329–1338.

39. Teule, F. et al., A protocol for the production of recombinant spider silk-like proteins for artificial fiber spinning. *Nature Protocols*, 2009;**4**(3):341–355.

40. Reddig, P.J. and R.L. Juliano, Clinging to life: Cell to matrix adhesion and cell survival. *Cancer and Metastasis Reviews*, 2005;**24**(3):425–439.

41. Westermark, P., K. Lundmark, and G.T. Westermark, Fibrils from designed non-amyloid-related synthetic peptides induce AA-amyloidosis during inflammation in an animal model. *PLoS One*, 2009;**4**(6):e6041.

42. Lundmark, K. et al., Protein fibrils in nature can enhance amyloid protein A amyloidosis in mice: Cross-seeding as a disease mechanism. *Proceedings of the National Academy of Sciences of the United States of America*, 2005;**102**(17):6098–6102.

43. Meinel, L. et al., The inflammatory responses to silk films in vitro and in vivo. *Biomaterials*, 2005;**26**(2):147–155.

44. Hakimi, O. et al., Spider and mulberry silkworm silks as compatible biomaterials. *Composites Part B-Engineering*, 2007;**38**(3):324–337.

45. Thitiwuthikiat, P., P. Aramwit, and S. Kanokpanont, Effect of Thai silk sericin and its extraction methods on L929 mouse fibroblast cell viability. In *Functionalized and Sensing Materials*, S. Suttiruengwong and W. Sricharussin, eds., Trans Tech Publications Limited, Dümpten, Switzerland, 2010, pp. 385–388.

46. Aramwit, P. et al., The effect of sericin from various extraction methods on cell viability and collagen production. *International Journal of Molecular Sciences*, 2010;**11**(5):2200–2211.

47. Aramwit, P. et al., The effect of sericin with variable amino-acid content from different silk strains on the production of collagen and nitric oxide. *Journal of Biomaterials Science. Polymer Edition*, 2009;**20**(9):1295–1306.

48. Panilaitis, B. et al., Macrophage responses to silk. *Biomaterials*, 2003;**24**(18):3079–3085.

49. Aramwit, P. and A. Sangcakul, The effects of sericin cream on wound healing in rats. *Bioscience Biotechnology and Biochemistry*, 2007;**71**(10):2473–2477.

50. Brown, S.F. and M. Coleman, Severe immediate reactions to biologicals caused by silk allergy. *Journal of the American Medical Association*, 1957;**165**(17):2178–2180.

51. Wuthrich, B. et al., Wild silk asthma—Still a current inhalative allergy. *Schweizerische Medizinische Wochenschrift*, 1985;**115**(40):1387–1393.
52. Hollander, D.H., Interstitial cystitis and silk allergy. *Medical Hypotheses*, 1994;**43**(3):155–156.
53. Wen, Z.M. et al., Partial characterization of the silk allergens in mulberry silk extract. *Journal of Investigational Allergology & Clinical Immunology*, 1996;**6**(4):237–241.
54. Hocwald, E. et al., Adverse reaction to surgical sutures in thyroid surgery. *Head and Neck*, 2003;**25**(1):77–81.
55. Singh, K.P. and R.S. Jayasomu, *Bombyx mori*—A review of its potential as a medicinal insect. *Pharmaceutical Biology*, 2002;**40**(1):28–32.
56. Dal Pra, I. et al., De novo engineering of reticular connective tissue in vivo by silk fibroin nonwoven materials. *Biomaterials*, 2005;**26**(14):1987–1999.
57. Fini, M. et al., The healing of confined critical size cancellous defects in the presence of silk fibroin hydrogel. *Biomaterials*, 2005;**26**(17):3527–3536.
58. Meinel, L. et al., Silk based biomaterials to heal critical sized femur defects. *Bone*, 2006;**39**(4):922–931.
59. Kim, K.H. et al., Biological efficacy of silk fibroin nanofiber membranes for guided bone regeneration. *Journal of Biotechnology*, 2005;**120**(3):327–339.
60. Karageorgiou, V. et al., Porous silk fibroin 3-D scaffolds for delivery of bone morpho-genetic protein-2 in vitro and in vivo. *Journal of Biomedical Materials Research. Part A*, 2006;**78A**(2):324–334.
61. Mauney, J.R. et al., Evaluation of gel spun silk-based biomaterials in a murine model of bladder augmentation. *Biomaterials*, 2011;**32**(3):808–818.
62. Wang, Y. et al., In vivo degradation of three-dimensional silk fibroin scaffolds. *Biomaterials*, 2008;**29**(24–25):3415–3428.
63. Moisenovich, M.M. et al., In vitro and in vivo biocompatibility studies of a recombi-nant analogue of spidroin 1 scaffolds. *Journal of Biomedical Materials Research. Part A*, 2011;**96A**(1):125–131.
64. Gellynck, K. et al., Biocompatibility and biodegradability of spider egg sac silk. *Journal of Materials Science. Materials in Medicine*, 2008;**19**(8):2963–2970.
65. Li, M.Z., M. Ogiso, and N. Minoura, Enzymatic degradation behavior of porous silk fibroin sheets. *Biomaterials*, 2003;**24**(2):357–365.
66. Horan, R.L. et al., In vitro degradation of silk fibroin. *Biomaterials*, 2005;**26**(17):3385–3393.
67. Wongpanit, P., Y. Tabata, and R. Rujiravanit, Miscibility and biodegradability of silk fibroin/carboxymethyl chitin blend films. *Macromolecular Bioscience*, 2007;7(12):1258–1271.
68. Vasconcelos, A., G. Freddi, and A. Cavaco-Paulo, Biodegradable materials based on silk fibroin and keratin. *Biomacromolecules*, 2008;**9**(4):1299–1305.
69. Kim, U.J. et al., Three-dimensional aqueous-derived biomaterial scaffolds from silk fibroin. *Biomaterials*, 2005;**26**(15):2775–2785.
70. Li, M.Z. et al., Structure and properties of silk fibroin-poly(vinyl alcohol) gel. *International Journal of Biological Macromolecules*, 2002;**30**(2):89–94.
71. Horan, R.L. et al., Biological and biomechanical assessment of a long-term bioresorbable silk-derived surgical mesh in an abdominal body wall defect model. *Hernia*, 2009;**3**(2):189–199.
72. Altman, G.H. et al., The use of long-term bioresorbable scaffolds for anterior cruciate ligament repair. *Journal of the American Academy of Orthopaedic Surgeons*, 2008;**16**(4):177–187.
73. Liu, H.F. et al., Modification of sericin-free silk fibers for ligament tissue engineering application. *Journal of Biomedical Materials Research. Part B, Applied Biomaterials*, 2007;**82B**(1):129–138.
74. Tsukada, M. et al., Physical-properties of silk fibers treated with ethylene-glycol diglycidyl ether by the pad batch method. *Journal of Applied Polymer Science*, 1993;**50**(10):1841–1849.
75. Freddi, G. et al., Chemical-structure and physical-properties of *Antheraea-assama* silk. *Journal of Applied Polymer Science*, 1994;**52**(6):775–781.
76. Hu, X.A. et al., Biomaterials derived from silk-tropoelastin protein systems. *Biomaterials*, 2010;**31**(32):8121–8131.

77. Teng, W.B., J. Cappello, and X.Y. Wu, Recombinant silk-elastinlike protein polymer displays elasticity comparable to elastin. *Biomacromolecules*, 2009;**10**(11):3028–3036.

78. Kim, U.J. et al., Structure and properties of silk hydrogels. *Biomacromolecules*, 2004;**5**(3):786–792.

79. Nazarov, R., H.J. Jin, and D.L. Kaplan, Porous 3-D scaffolds from regenerated silk fibroin. *Biomacromolecules*, 2004;**5**(3):718–726.

80. Hu, K. et al., Preparation of fibroin/recombinant human-like collagen scaffold to promote fibroblasts compatibility. *Journal of Biomedical Materials Research. Part A*, 2008;**84A**(2):483–490.

81. Gosline, J.M. et al., Elastomeric network models for the frame and viscid silks from the orb web of the spider *Araneus-diadematus*. In *Silk Polymers: Materials Science and Biotechnology*, D. Kaplan et al., eds., American Chemical Society, New York, 1994, pp. 328–341.

82. Gosline, J.M., M.W. Denny, and M.E. Demont, Spider silk as rubber. *Nature*, 1984;**309**(5968):551–552.

83. Gosline, J.M., M.E. Demont, and M.W. Denny, The structure and properties of spider silk. *Endeavour*, 1986;**10**(1):37–43.

84. Gosline, J.M. et al., The mechanical design of spider silks: From fibroin sequence to mechanical function. *Journal of Experimental Biology*, 1999;**202**(23):3295–3303.

85. Guerette, P.A. et al., Silk properties determined by gland-specific expression of a spider fibroin gene family. *Science*, 1996;**272**(5258):112–115.

86. Vollrath, F. et al., Compounds in the droplets of the orb spiders viscid spiral. *Nature*, 1990;**345**(6275):526–528.

87. Townley, M.A. et al., Comparative-study of orb web hygroscopicity and adhesive spiral composition in 3 araneid spiders. *Journal of Experimental Zoology*, 1991;**259**(2):154–165.

88. Shao, Z.Z. and F. Vollrath, The effect of solvents on the contraction and mechanical properties of spider silk. *Polymer*, 1999;**40**(7):1799–1806.

89. Spelzini, F. et al., Tensile strength and host response towards silk and type I polypropylene implants used for augmentation of fascial repair in a rat model. *Gynecologic and Obstetric Investigation*, 2007;**63**(3):155–162.

90. Stinco, G., F. Piccirillo, and F. Valent, A randomized double-blind study to investigate the clinical efficacy of adding a non-migrating antimicrobial to a special silk fabric in the treatment of atopic dermatitis. *Dermatology*, 2008;**217**(3):191–195.

91. Harkin, D.G. et al., Silk fibroin in ocular tissue reconstruction. *Biomaterials*, 2011;**32**(10):2445–2458.

92. Kon'kov, A.S., O.L. Pustovalova, and I.I. Agapov, Biocompatible materials from regenerated silk for tissue engineering and medicinal therapy. *Applied Biochemistry and Microbiology*, 2010;**46**(8):739–744.

93. Rabotyagova, O.S., P. Cebe, and D.L. Kaplan, Self-assembly of genetically engineered spider silk block copolymers. *Biomacromolecules*, 2009;**10**(2):229–236.

94. Kluge, J.A. et al., Spider silks and their applications. *Trends in Biotechnology*, 2008;**26**(5):244–251.

95. Hermanson, K.D. et al., Permeability of silk microcapsules made by the interfacial adsorption of protein. *Physical Chemistry Chemical Physics*, 2007;**9**(48):6442–6446.

96. Hermanson, K.D. et al., Engineered microcapsules fabricated from reconstituted spider silk. *Advanced Materials*, 2007;**19**(14):1810–1815.

97. Rammensee, S. et al., Rheological characterization of hydrogels formed by recombinantly produced spider silk. *Applied Physics A: Materials Science & Processing*, 2006;**82**(2):261–264.

98. Chen, X., Z.Z. Shao, and F. Vollrath, The spinning processes for spider silk. *Soft Matter*, 2006;**2**(6):448–451.

99. Gellynck, K. et al., Silkworm and spider silk scaffolds for chondrocyte support. *Journal of Materials Science. Materials in Medicine*, 2008;**19**(11):3399–3409.

100. Radtke, C. et al., Spider silk constructs enhance axonal regeneration and remyelination in long nerve defects in sheep. *PLoS One*, 2011;**6**(2):e16990.

101. Shangkai, C. et al., Transplantation of allogeneic chondrocytes cultured in fibroin sponge and stirring chamber to promote cartilage regeneration. *Tissue Engineering*, 2007;**13**(3):483–492.
102. Kim, H.J. et al., Bone tissue engineering with premineralized silk scaffolds. *Bone*, 2008;**42**(6):1226–1234.
103. Zhao, J. et al., Apatite-coated silk fibroin scaffolds to healing mandibular border defects in canines. *Bone*, 2009;**45**(3):517–527.
104. Jiang, X.Q. et al., Mandibular repair in rats with premineralized silk scaffolds and BMP-2-modified bMSCs. *Biomaterials*, 2009;**30**(27):4522–4532.
105. Liu, H.F. et al., In vivo study of ACL regeneration using silk scaffolds in a pig model. In *13th International Conference on Biomedical Engineering*, Vols. 1–3, C.T. Lim and J.C.H. Goh, eds., Springer, Switzerland, 2009, pp. 1512–1514.
106. Seo, Y.K. et al., Increase in cell migration and angiogenesis in a composite silk scaffold for tissue-engineered ligaments. *Journal of Orthopaedic Research*, 2009;**27**(4):495–503.
107. Soffer, L. et al., Silk-based electrospun tubular scaffolds for tissue-engineered vascular grafts. *Journal of Biomaterials Science. Polymer Edition*, 2008;**19**(5):653–664.
108. Zhang, X.H. et al., Dynamic culture conditions to generate silk-based tissue-engineered vascular grafts. *Biomaterials*, 2009;**30**(19):3213–3223.
109. Zhang, X.H., C.B. Baughman, and D.L. Kaplan, In vitro evaluation of electrospun silk fibroin scaffolds for vascular cell growth. *Biomaterials*, 2008;**29**(14):2217–2227.
110. Xu, S.Q. et al., In vitro biocompatibility of electrospun silk fibroin mats with Schwann cells. *Journal of Applied Polymer Science*, 2011;**119**(6):3490–3494.
111. Wang, G.L. et al., Electrospun PLGA-silk fibroin-collagen nanofibrous scaffolds for nerve tissue engineering. *In Vitro Cellular & Developmental Biology. Animal*, 2011;**47**(3):234–240.
112. Wei, Y. et al., Schwann-like cell differentiation of rat adipose-derived stem cells by indirect co-culture with Schwann cells in vitro. *Cell Proliferation*, 2010;**43**(6):606–616.
113. Ghaznavi, A.M. et al., Silk fibroin conduits: A cellular and functional assessment of peripheral nerve repair. *Annals of Plastic Surgery*, 2011;**66**(3):273–279.
114. Zhan, K.H. et al., Characterization of angiogenesis during skin wound repair by porous silk fibroin film. In *Silk: Inheritance and Innovation—Modern Silk Road*, L. Bai and G.Q. Chen, eds., Trans Tech Publications Limited, Dümpten, Switzerland, 2011, pp. 181–185.
115. Guan, G.P. et al., Promoted dermis healing from full-thickness skin defect by porous silk fibroin scaffolds (PSFSs). *Bio-medical Materials and Engineering*, 2010;**20**(5):295–308.
116. Altman, A.M. et al., IFATS collection: Human adipose-derived stem cells seeded on a silk fibroin-chitosan scaffold enhance wound repair in a murine soft tissue injury model. *Stem Cells*, 2009;**27**(1):250–258.
117. Lawrence, B.D. et al., Silk film biomaterials for cornea tissue engineering. *Biomaterials*, 2009;**30**(7):1299–1308.
118. Madden, P.W. et al., Human corneal endothelial cell growth on a silk fibroin membrane. *Biomaterials*, 2011;**32**(17):4076–4084.
119. Ghassemifar, R. et al., Advancing towards a tissue-engineered tympanic membrane: Silk fibroin as a substratum for growing human eardrum keratinocytes. *Journal of Biomaterials Applications*, 2010;**24**(7):591–606.
120. Chirila, T.V. et al., *Bombyx mori* silk fibroin membranes as potential substrata for epithelial constructs used in the management of ocular surface disorders. *Tissue Engineering Part A*, 2008;**14**(7):1203–1211.
121. Chirila, T. et al., Silk as substratum for cell attachment and proliferation, In *Pricm 6: Sixth Pacific Rim International Conference on Advanced Materials and Processing*, Pts. 1–3, Y.W. Chang, N.J. Kim, and C.S. Lee, eds., Trans Tech Publications Limited, Dümpten, Switzerland, 2007, pp. 1549–1552.
122. Wenk, E., H.P. Merkle, and L. Meinel, Silk fibroin as a vehicle for drug delivery applications. *Journal of Controlled Release*, 2011;**150**(2):128–141.
123. Wenk, E. et al., Microporous silk fibroin scaffolds embedding PLGA microparticles for controlled growth factor delivery in tissue engineering. *Biomaterials*, 2009;**30**(13):2571–2581.

124. Wenk, E. et al., Silk fibroin spheres as a platform for controlled drug delivery. *Journal of Controlled Release*, 2008;**132**(1):26–34.
125. Wang, X.Q. et al., Silk microspheres for encapsulation and controlled release. *Journal of Controlled Release*, 2007;**117**(3):360–370.
126. Venkatraman, S., F. Boey, and L.L. Lao, Implanted cardiovascular polymers: Natural, synthetic and bio-inspired. *Progress in Polymer Science*, 2008;**33**(9):853–874.
127. Reddy, N. and Y.Q. Yang, Novel protein fibers from wheat gluten. *Biomacromolecules*, 2007;**8**(2):638–643.
128. Reddy, N. and Y.Q. Yang, Potential and properties of plant proteins for tissue engineering applications. In *13th International Conference on Biomedical Engineering*, Vols. 1–3, C.T. Lim and J.C.H. Goh, eds., Springer, Switzerland, 2009, pp. 1282–1284.
129. Rodrigues, M.T. et al., Tissue-engineered constructs based on SPCL scaffolds cultured with goat marrow cells: Functionality in femoral defects. *Journal of Tissue Engineering and Regenerative Medicine*, 2011;**5**(1):41–49.
130. Domenek, S., M.H. Morel, and S. Guilbert, Wheat gluten based biomaterials: Environmental performance, degradability and physical modifications. In *Gluten Proteins*, D. Lafiandra, S. Masci, and R. Dovidio, eds., The Royal Society of Chemistry, Cambridge, UK, 2004, pp. 443–446.
131. Vaz, C.M. et al., Casein and soybean protein-based thermoplastics and composites as alternative biodegradable polymers for biomedical applications. *Journal of Biomedical Materials Research. Part A*, 2003;**65A**(1):60–70.
132. Liu, X.M. et al., Microspheres of corn protein, zein, for an ivermectin drug delivery system. *Biomaterials*, 2005;**26**(1):109–115.
133. Stenman, S.M. et al., Enzymatic detoxification of gluten by germinating wheat proteases: Implications for new treatment of celiac disease. *Annals of Medicine*, 2009;**41**(5):390–400.
134. Di Cagno, R. et al., Gluten-free sourdough wheat baked goods appear safe for young celiac patients: A pilot study. *Journal of Pediatric Gastroenterology and Nutrition*, 2010;**51**(6):777–783.
135. Park, S.K., N.S. Hettiarachchy, and L. Were, Degradation behavior of soy protein-wheat gluten films in simulated soil conditions. *Journal of Agricultural and Food Chemistry*, 2000;**48**(7):3027–3031.
136. Domenek, S. et al., Biodegradability of wheat gluten based bioplastics. *Chemosphere*, 2004;**54**(4):551–559.
137. Zhang, X.Q. et al., Biodegradation of chemically modified wheat gluten-based natural polymer materials. *Polymer Degradation and Stability*, 2010;**95**(12):2309–2317.
138. Gomez-Martinez, D. et al., Modelling of pyrolysis and combustion of gluten-glycerol-based bioplastics. *Bioresource Technology*, 2011;**102**(10):6246–6253.
139. Kurniawan, L., G.G. Qiao, and X.Q. Zhang, Chemical modification of wheat protein-based natural polymers: Grafting and cross-linking reactions with poly(ethylene oxide) diglycidyl ether and ethyl diamine. *Biomacromolecules*, 2007;**8**(9):2909–2915.
140. Song, Y.H. and Q. Zheng, Structure and properties of methylcellulose microfiber reinforced wheat gluten based green composites. *Industrial Crops and Products*, 2009;**29**(2–3):446–454.
141. Shewry, P.R. et al., *Elastomeric Proteins Structures, Biomechanical Properties, and Biological Roles*. Cambridge University Press: Cambridge, U.K., 2003.
142. Bianco, P. and Robey, P.G., Stem cells in tissue engineering, *Nature*, 2001;**414**(6859):118–121.

Further Readings

Park, J. and R.S. Lakes, *Biomaterials: An Introduction*, 3rd edn. New York: Springer, 2007.
Scott, G. *Degradable Polymers: Principles and Applications,* Kluwer Academic Publishers, Dordrecht, the Netherlands, 2002.

CHAPTER 11

COMPOSITE BIOMATERIALS

LEARNING OBJECTIVES

After a careful study of this chapter, you should be able to do the following:

1. Describe the rationale behind the development of composites, using specific samples
2. Convert wt.% and vol.% of fibers in composites
3. Predict Young's modulus of fiber composites, using the Voigt model or Shear-Lag model
4. Describe the constituents of bone, dentin, and enamel and their hierarchical structures
5. Be familiar with two dental composites: resin-based composite and glass–ionomer composite

11.1   OVERVIEW OF COMPOSITES

Composite materials have been known in various forms throughout the history of mankind. Clay–straw composites have been known for more than 5000 years, whereby natural fibers produced from various plants were mixed with clay in water and used as a composite to make bricks for walls and shelters (Figure 11.1). In this application, the polymer constituent (natural fibers) toughens the ceramic matrix (clay), improving the mechanical integrity of the clay, which would otherwise develop many cracks during the mud-drying process (slurry of the composite).

The history of modern composites probably began in the 1930s when a strong plastic mold was successfully made using fiberglass materials, produced by Owens Corning Fiberglass Company, and phenolic resin. These reinforced plastic dies soon became the standard for prototype parts.

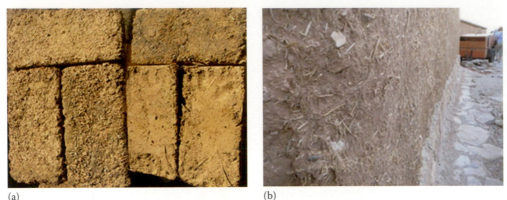

(a)   (b)

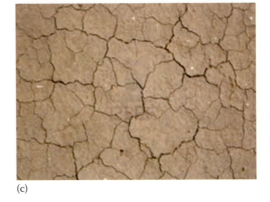

(c)

Figure 11.1
Composite of natural fibers (straw) and clay used in walls: (a) Bricks of clay–straw; (b) a wall coated with composite made of clay and dried straw; (c) without the toughening effect of fibrous fillers, cracks develop in clay during the drying process.

The use of composite materials is motivated by the idea that by combining two or more distinct materials, a new material can be engineered with the desired combination of properties (e.g., lightness, strength), with the desirable material properties that either material alone cannot offer. The advantage of composite materials is the large scope for tailoring their structure to suit the service conditions.

11.1.1   Definition of Composites

In most textbooks of materials science and engineering and topic books on composites, composite materials are defined as physical combinations of two or more of the three basic materials classes: metals, ceramics, and polymers. However, the boundary of composite materials has been expanded to cover any material made from two or more constituent materials with vastly different physical or chemical properties, where the individual components remain separate and distinct within the finished structure. According to this expanded definition, a polymer blend made of a soft amorphous matrix embedded with hard resin particles is called a composite.

Glass–ceramic, which is made of an amorphous glass strengthened with a hard crystalline phase (such as $CaSiO_3$), is thus called a composite. Perlitic steel, which combines hard brittle cementite (FeC_3) with soft ductile ferrite (α-Fe), can also be appropriately regarded as a composite, as done by many researchers to this day.

11.1.2 Classification of Composites

Composite materials can be classified in a number of ways. The following two ways are most frequently used in industry [1]:

1. Grouping according to the fiber shape
   a. *Particulate-reinforced*: The composites are strengthened by dispersed particles (Figure 11.2a).
   b. *Monofilament/fiber-reinforced*: The composites contain continuous (aligned) or short (aligned or random) fibers (Figure 11.2b,c).
   c. *Multifilament/structural-reinforced*: The composites are laminates, sandwiched panels (Figure 11.2d), or a woven porous network (Figure 11.2e through f). Cellular solids (foams, such as wood) are those in which the *inclusions* are voids, filled with air or liquid.

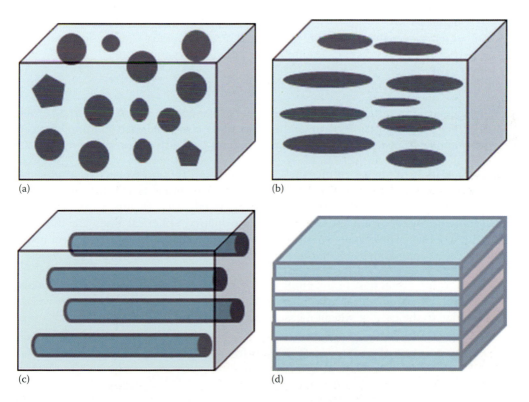

(a)   (b)

(c)   (d)

Figure 11.2
Fiber architectures (the arrangement and distribution of fibers): (a) particles; (b) short fibers; (c) ply: a unidirectional lamina; (d) laminate: a stack of laminae;   *(Continued)*

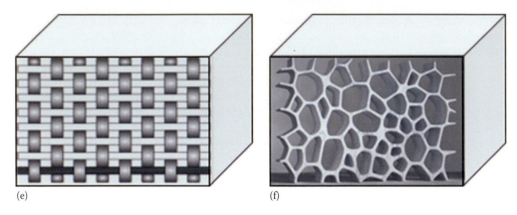

(e)   (f)

Figure 11.2 (Continued)
Fiber architectures (the arrangement and distribution of fibers): (e) woven: braided and knitted fiber arrangements; (f) porous.

  2. Grouping according to the nature of the matrix
    a. *Polymer–matrix composite (PMC)*: They are mostly widely used in industrial applications. They are usually reinforced with aligned ceramic fibers, such as glass or carbon.
    b. *Metal–matrix composite (MMC)*: Commercial usage of MMC is still rather limited.
    c. *Ceramic–matrix composite (CMC)*: The development of CMC is slow, partly because these composites are rather difficult to manufacture.

11.1.3 General Structure–Property Relationship

The mechanical properties of a composite material depend on the *shape* of the second particles, the *volume fraction* occupied by them, and on the *interface bonding* between the constituents [1]. Anisotropy is often an important property of composite materials.

11.1.3.1 Effects of Shape Stiff platelet inclusions are the most effective in creating a stiff composite, followed by fibers. The least effective geometry for stiff inclusions is the spherical particle, even if the particles are perfectly rigid (Figure 11.3). When the inclusions are more compliant (softer) than the matrix, spherical ones are the least harmful, whereas platelet ones are the most harmful mechanically. Soft spherical inclusions are used intentionally as crack stoppers to enhance the toughness of polymers.

11.1.3.2 Volume Fraction of a Composite The preparation of composite materials, especially those particle-reinforced ones, is frequently conducted based on the weight fraction, due to the ease of weight measurement of a powder. However, the mechanical

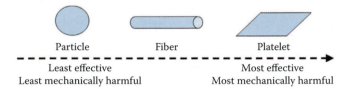

Figure 11.3
Effects of fibers on mechanical properties of composites.

properties of composites are directly linked with the volume fraction of composite materials. Hence, it is necessary to convert weight fraction to volume fraction, and vice versa. The conversion equations between volume and weight fractions are given as follows:

$$
\begin{cases}
v_f = \dfrac{w_f/\rho_f}{w_f/\rho_f + w_m/\rho_m} \\[3mm]
w_f = \dfrac{v_f\rho_f}{v_f\rho_f + v_m\rho_m}
\end{cases}, \tag{11.1}
$$

where

w_f and w_m are the weight fractions of fiber and matrix
v_f and v_m are the volume fractions of fiber and matrix
ρ_f and ρ_m are the density of fiber and matrix

The volume fraction of a composite is often measurable from their geometric arrangement. In a long-fiber (ply) arrangement (Figure 11.4), the volume fraction of fibers, f, is given:

$$
\begin{cases}
f = \dfrac{\pi}{2\sqrt{3}}\left(\dfrac{r}{R}\right)^2 & \text{(hexagonal)} \\[3mm]
f = \dfrac{\pi}{4}\left(\dfrac{r}{R}\right)^2 & \text{(square)}
\end{cases} \tag{11.2}
$$

The maximum value of f is

$$
\begin{cases}
f_{max} = 0.907 & \text{(hexagonal)} \\[2mm]
f_{max} = 0.785 & \text{(square)}
\end{cases} \tag{11.3}
$$

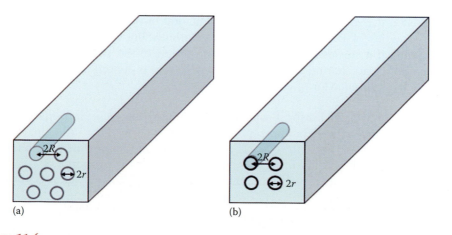

(a) (b)

Figure 11.4
Two fiber arrangements in composites: (a) hexagonal; (b) cubic.

However, *the practical limit for a commercial composite is 0.7*, beyond which composites are technically impossible.

For short fibers, the characterization is more complicated, involving fiber orientation and length distribution [1]. The fiber orientation distributions in three dimensions can be presented with (1) (α, β) method, (2) Fourier transform, or (3) pole figure (texture). The fiber length distributions can be measured using (1) an indirect method involving physical property measurement, (2) direct methods by dissolving the matrix, or (3) microscopy. Two average lengths of fibers are as follows:

3. Number average fiber length: $L_N = \dfrac{\sum N_i L_i}{\sum N_i}$

4. Weight (or volume) average fiber length: $L_W = \dfrac{\sum W_i L_i}{\sum W_i} = \dfrac{\sum V_i L_i}{\sum V_i}$

The length distribution based on weight (or volume) is more meaningful in practice.

11.1.3.3 Effect of Volume Fraction: The Concept of Load Transfer

The stress in a composite may vary sharply from point to point, but the proportion of the external load borne by each of the individual constituents can be gauged by volume-averaging the load within them:

$$f_{matrix}\overline{\sigma}_{matrix} + f_{fiber}\overline{\sigma}_{fiber} = \sigma_A \tag{11.4}$$

where

f_{matrix} and f_{fiber} are the volume fractions of fiber and matrix

$\overline{\sigma}_{matrix}$ and $\overline{\sigma}_{fiber}$ are the volume-averaged matrix and fiber stresses in a composite under an external applied stress σ_A, containing reinforcement at a volume fraction of f_{fiber}

The proportion of the load carried by the fiber and reminder by the matrix is independent of the applied load and is an important characteristic of the composite materials. It depends on the volume fraction, shape, orientation of the reinforcement and on the elastic properties of both constituents. The reinforcement may be regarded as acting efficiently if it carries a relatively high proportion of the externally applied load. Analysis of the load sharing that occurs in a composite is central to an understanding of the mechanical behavior of composite materials.

11.1.3.4 Prediction of Elastic Properties of Composites

It is important in practice to predict mechanical parameters of composites from their individual components. In this section, we only discuss axial Young's modulus E in fiber-reinforced composites. First, the axial stiffness is the most important property. Second, fiber composites often appear in natural composites. The coordinate system is chosen as follows (Figure 11.5):

- *Axial* Young's modulus of long-fiber composites

    Voigt model (equal strain): $E_{axial} = f_{matrix}E_{matrix} + f_{fiber}E_{fiber}$ (11.5)

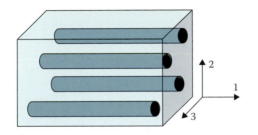

Figure 11.5
Coordinate system of fiber composites.

This equation is valid to a high degree of precision, providing the fibers are long enough for the *equal strain assumption* to apply. This model assumes that the matrix and fibers are strained equally.

- The axial Young's modulus of short-fiber composites is well predicted by the Shear-Lag model:

$$E_{axial} = f_{fiber} E_{fiber} \left(1 - \frac{\tan b(ns)}{ns} \right) + f_{matrix} E_{matrix} \qquad (11.6)$$

where
$s = L/r$
L is the fiber half-length
r is the fiber radius
n is typically about 0.1 for polymer–matrix composites

11.1.3.5 Interface Bonding Interfacial bonding between fibers and matrix is established via the following mechanisms:

- Interdiffusion and chemical reaction
- Electrostatic attraction
- Mechanical keying: caused by the roughness of the two surfaces
- Residual stresses

The first mechanism is used in the dental composite, glass–ionomer composite (GIC) (Section 11.3).

11.2 NATURAL COMPOSITES: BONE

Natural composites include bone, tooth (dentin and enamel), and cartilage. Natural foams include lung, cancellous bone, and wood, which can also be treated as composites. Overall, natural composites exhibit complex, hierarchical structures in which particulate, porous, and fibrous structural features are seen on different microscales, and in different locations, depending on the function (Figure 11.6). As shown, a typical long bone, for example, comprises of compact bone (dense, aligned matrix, mostly inorganic) and spongy bone (also called trabecular or cancellous bone, a porous matrix created by struts called trabelculae, with pores occupied by marrow and blood vessels) (Figure 11.6a). A tooth comprises of enamel (the strongest hard tissue of the body), dentin (similar to compact bone), and pulp (soft tissue) (Figure 11.6b).

Mechanically, most of the stresses are carried by the outer compact bone and the spongy bone at the two epiphysis ends. The inorganic fibers (i.e., bone minerals)

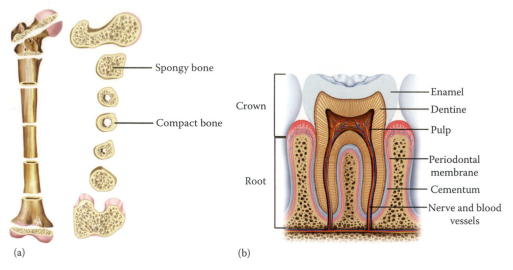

(a)   (b)

Figure 11.6
Anatomic structure of (a) long bone and (b) tooth.

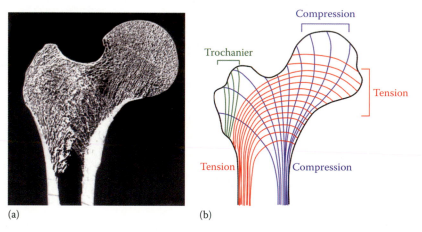

(a)   (b)

Figure 11.7
(a) Microstructure of cancellous bone showing alignment of trabeculae. (From Glimcher, M.J., Rev. Mineral. Geochem., 64, 223, 2006. Copyright 2006, reprinted with permission from the Mineralogy Society of America, Chantilly, VA.) (b) Diagram of stress field inside cancellous bone of the femoral head.

within the compact bone and the spongy bone at high-stress areas (e.g., femoral head) form directionally along stress–strain conduction regions, distributing the forces evenly within the bone (Figure 11.7). A similar structural principle is used in aeroplane fuselage composites, where different layers of fiberglass or carbon-fiber are aligned in different directions, depending on the local stresses and function of the panel.

11.2.1 Constituents of Bone, Dentin, and Enamel (Human)

11.2.1.1 Inorganic Constituents of Bone
Approximately, 70 wt.% of bone is composed of inorganic substances. Almost all of this inorganic substance is hydroxyapatite, which is essentially composed of calcium, phosphorus, oxygen, and hydrogen.

Hydroxyapatite contains no vitamins, fatty acids, enzymes, proteins, or carbohydrates but is a major source of calcium and phosphorus.

11.2.1.2 Organic Constituents of Bone Approximately, 30 wt.% of bone is composed of organic materials (on a dry weight basis). Of this amount nearly 95 wt.% is collagen, a mostly fibrous protein. In other words, up to one-third of bone is collagen with a tiny fraction of other compounds.

11.2.1.3 Constituents of Dentine and Enamel The composition of dentin is similar to bone, comprising ~70 wt.% apatite and ~30 wt.% collagen. Enamel contains a significantly high level of apatite, the weight percentage of apatite in dried enamel being ~97 wt.%.

11.2.2 Volume Fraction of Apatite in Bone, Dentin, and Enamel

The density of hydroxyapatite is 2.8–3.16 g/cm³, and that of dried collagen varies from 1.3 to 1.4 g/cm³. According to the calculation using Equation 11.1, the volumetric contents of apatite and proteins in dry bone (i.e., bone + collagen) are nearly equal, that is, ~50 vol.%. Considering that there is ~10 vol.% of water and pores in bone, the volumetric contents of apatite and organics in fresh bone are both ~45 vol.%.

The same can be said for enamel, where the volume percentage of apatite in dried enamel is 93 vol.%, according to the calculation using Equation 11.1. Considering that there is ~3 vol.% water in enamel, the content of apatite in living enamel is ~90 vol.%. Table 11.1 summarizes the weight and volume fractions of apatite and proteins in these three hard tissues.

11.2.3 Prediction of Stiffness of Bone, Dentin, and Enamel

Bone can be more or less considered a short-fiber-reinforced composite. The bone apatite crystals are very small and platelet-shaped (length ≈ 200–600 Å, width ≈ 100–200 Å, thickness ≈ 20–50 Å) [2], as illustrated in Figure 11.8.

The aspect ratio of the apatite platelets, $s = L/r$, is typically taken to be 25 in bone [2]. Hence, $\tanh(ns)/ns \approx 0.40$, and Equation 10.6 would become

$$E_1 = 0.60 f_{\text{fiber}} E_{\text{fiber}} + f_{\text{matrix}} E_{\text{matrix}}. \tag{11.7}$$

Table 11.1
Constituents of Cortical Bone, Dentin, and Enamel (Human)

	Water or Pores	Collagen	Apatite
Dried cortical and dentin		33 wt.%	67 wt.%
		50 vol.%	50 vol.%
Fresh cortical and dentin	10 vol.%	45 vol.%	45 vol.%
Dried enamel		3 wt.%	97 wt.%
		7 vol.%	93 vol.%
Fresh enamel	3 vol.%	7 vol.%	90 vol.%

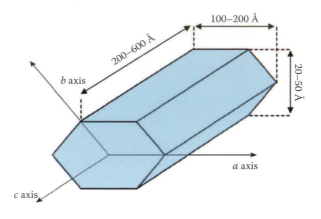

Figure 11.8
Apatite crystal of bone. (From Kothawz, S.P. and Guzelsun, N., J. Theory Biol., 219, 269, 2002.)

To include the effect of water and pores in fresh bone, this equation needs to be further modified. Based on the rule of mixture, we have the following:

$$E_1 = 0.60 f_{\text{apatite}} E_{\text{apatite}} + f_{\text{collagen}} E_{\text{collagen}} + f_{\text{water-pore}} E_{\text{water-pore}}. \qquad (11.8)$$

The Young's modulus of collagen, noncarbonated apatite, and carbonated apatite are given in Table 11.2. Using Equation 11.8 of the Shear-Lag model, the Young's modulus of bone, dentin, and enamel can be calculated. Note that $E_{\text{water-pore}} \approx 0$.

The theoretical Young's modulus of bone and dentin predicted from carbonated hydroxyapatite (Table 11.3) fall within the range of experimental values, but the Young's modulus of bone or dentin predicted based on nonsubstituted apatite are outside the range of experimental values. This indicates that the apatite in bone and dentin are always carbonated.

The theoretical values of Young's modulus of enamel fall in the lower range of the experimental data when the prediction is made based on the carbonated apatite, and

Table 11.2
Young's Modulus of Apatite and Collagen

	Young's Modulus (GPa)
Collagens (wet)	0.1–1.0
Carbonated apatite	55–80
Nonsubstituted hydroxyapatite	110–130

Table 11.3
Young's Modulus of Bone, Dentine, and Enamels

Fresh Tissues	Young's Modulus (GPa)	
	Experimental Data	Theoretical Prediction Using Shear-Lag Model
Bone/dentine	10–30	15–22 (if apatite is carbonated)
		30–35 (if apatite is not carbonated)
Enamel	35–80	30–45 (if apatite is carbonated)
		60–70 (if apatite is not carbonated)

fall in the upper range when based on nonsubstituted apatite. This indicates that the improved strength of enamel, compared with those of cortical bone and dentin, is the result of both an increased content of apatite in this tissue and a reduced degree of carbonation in apatite.

11.3   DENTAL COMPOSITES

A dental filling composite (white fillings) is typically composed of an acrylate–resin matrix, such as bisphenol A-glycidyl methacrylate (Bis-GMA) and urethane dimethacrylate (UDMA), as well as an inorganic filler, typically SiO_2-based glass ceramics. The filler gives the composite wear resistance and translucency, while alleviating shrinkage. The development of white fillings has primarily been driven by their improved aesthetics (Figure 5.3). Unlike black-colored amalgam which fills a hole with poor aesthetic qualities, composite cavity restorations restore the tooth close to its original physical state and appearance. However, time to failure is still longer for amalgam, and it remains to be superior over resin-based composites in terms of long-term success rates.

11.3.1   Management of Shrinkage

In general, a successful result cannot be guaranteed when using resin-based composites for posterior restorations. This is due to polymerization shrinkage, which is still regarded as the primary negative characteristic of composite resins. Polymerization of dimethacrylate-based composites is always accompanied by substantial volumetric shrinkage in the range of 2%–6%, with the stress associated with the shrinkage resulting in cracks (Figure 11.9).

Shrinkage stress is proportional to Young's modulus E of a material. Hence, soft materials (smaller E) show reduced shrinkage stress. A softer liner which has a relatively low elastic modulus can absorb shrinkage energy at interfaces. Therefore, glass–ionomer composite, *sandwich technique*, provides significant clinical advantages. The glass–ionomer is used as a liner and base (Figure 11.10).

Polyacrylate (resin) composite filling

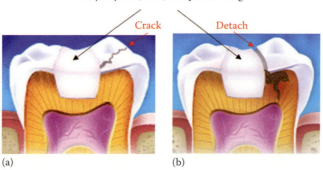

(a)   (b)

Figure 11.9
Schematic illustrations of (a) a crack in the host tooth and (b) detachment between tooth filling and the host tooth caused by polymerization shrinkage.

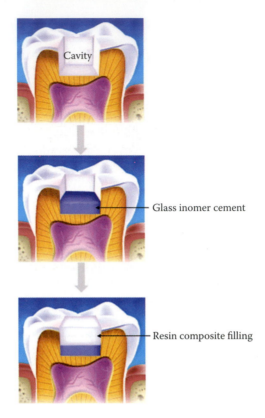

Figure 11.10
Schematic illustration of sandwich technique of using glass–ionomer composite (GIC).

11.3.2 Glass–Ionomer Cement

These materials are based on the acid–base reaction of silicate glass powder and poly-acrylic acid liquid. The liquid is an aqueous solution of polyacrylic acid at a concentration of 40%–50%. Typical percentages of the glass powder are as follows:

- Silica 42%
- Alumina 28%
- Aluminum fluoride 2%
- Calcium fluoride 16%
- Sodium fluoride 9%
- Aluminum phosphate 3%

When the powder and liquid are mixed together, an acid–base reaction occurs on the surface of the glass particles, causing them to partially dissolve (Figure 11.11). The chemical adhesion between poly(acrylic acid) and glass particles makes GIC much less brittle than either the resin–matrix or glass-filler material alone. GIC also has a bone-bonding ability, with bonding between the cement and hard dental tissues achieved through an ionic exchange at the interface.

The function of GIC is similar to that of bone cement. GIC and PMMA act together to serve as a cement to assist the adhesion of implants and host tissues. While PMMA alone cannot replace metal implants that are strong and tough, GIC alone also cannot replace the resin-based composite fillings that have good wear resistance.

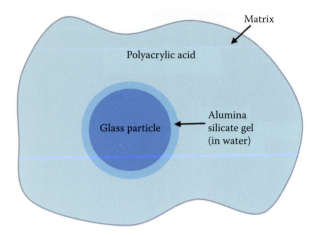

Figure 11.11
Chemical adhesion of glass particles with the resin–matrix in glass–ionomer cement.

11.4 ARTIFICIAL BONE

Since natural bone is basically a polymer–ceramic composite, it is logical to develop ceramic-reinforced polymer–matrix composites as artificial bone. Almost all possible combinations of previously described polymeric biomaterials (PLA, PGA, PCL, PMMA, etc.) and bioceramics (hydroxyapatite, calcium phosphates, bioactive glasses, etc.) have been explored. No matter which materials or processing techniques have been used, none of the currently developed artificial bone has been shown to be comparable with natural bone, which is light, strong, and tough.

Bone is neither as strong as many metals and ceramics, nor as tough as many elastomers and thermoplastics. But it simply has a superb combination of strength and toughness, which has not been fully replicated in any synthetic polymer–matrix composites. The challenges are twofold. First, with the traditional fabrication techniques, strengthening of almost all synthetic materials can only be achieved by sacrificing toughness (Figure 11.12). Second, the structure of natural bone is highly hierarchical micro- (Figures 11.6 and 11.7) and nanostructure (Figure 11.13). If the simple structures illustrated in Figure 11.2 could provide the body with appropriate properties

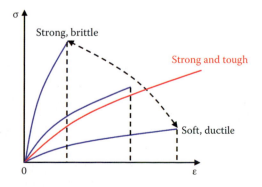

Figure 11.12
Antagonistic mechanical properties (strength–toughness).

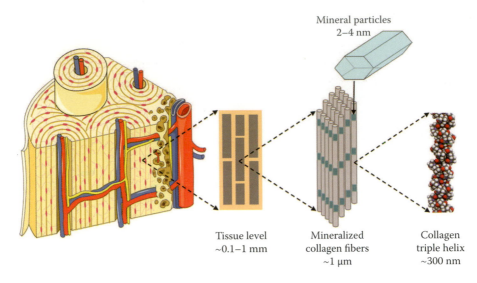

Figure 11.13
Highly hierarchical composite structure of natural bone.

and functions, nature would unlikely have to evolve such complicated bone structure. Hence, to develop biomimetic techniques that are able to fabricate the nanostructure in natural bone tissue perhaps is the best way to address the challenge.

11.5 CHAPTER HIGHLIGHTS

1. Conservation between wt.% and vol.% of fibers in a composite:

$$\begin{cases} v_f = \dfrac{w_f/\rho_f}{w_f/\rho_f + w_m/\rho_m} \\[2ex] w_f = \dfrac{v_f\rho_f}{v_f\rho_f + v_m\rho_m} \end{cases}.$$

2. To predict mechanical properties of long-fiber composites using Voigt model (equal strain):

$$E_{axial} = v_{matrix}E_{matrix} + v_{fiber}E_{fiber}.$$

3. To predict mechanical properties of short-fiber composites using the Shear-Lag model (equal strain):

$$E_{axial} = f_{fiber}E_{fiber}\left(1 - \frac{\tan h(ns)}{ns}\right) + f_{matrix}E_{matrix}.$$

4. Dental composites include resin-based composite fillings and GIC.
5. Natural bone has a highly hierarchical micro- and nanostructure, which renders bone a unique combination of properties: that of being light, strong, and tough. An artificial composite has yet to be developed that can compare with natural bone.

LABORATORY PRACTICE 5

1. Mechanical testing of pork femoral bone OR
2. Scanning electron microscope characterization of apatite crystals in a pork bone (collagen is burnt off at 200°C)

SIMPLE QUESTIONS IN CLASS

1. Which of the following is most effective in strengthening the matrix of a composite?
   a. Particles
   b. Platelets
   c. Fibers
   d. A mixture of all three
2. Cortical and cancellous bones are, respectively,
   a. Porous and dense
   b. Compact and spongy
   c. Spongy and compact
   d. Dense and porous
3. Which of the following hard tissues is strongest?
   a. Cortical
   b. Spongy
   c. Dentin
   d. Enamel
4. Enamel is stronger than dentin and compact bone, primarily because
   a. The hydroxyapatite in enamel is less carbonated and thus more crystallized.
   b. Enamel contains a higher percentage of minerals.
   c. Enamel contains less water.
   d. The hydroxylapatite in dentin and enamel is less crystallized.
5. Glass–ionomer composite (GIC) is much less brittle than resin-based composite tooth fillings, but has a similar strength to the latter. The reason for this is
   a. Flexibility of the matrix in GIC
   b. Small shrinkage of GIC
   c. Small volume fraction of glass filler in GIC
   d. Chemical bonding between the filler and polymer–matrix of GIC
6. Glass–ionomer composite (GIC) provides significant clinical advantages in addressing the detachment problem caused by the shrinkage of resin-based composite tooth fillings. This improvement is achieved primarily by
   a. Softness (i.e., low stiffness) of GIC
   b. Small shrinkage of GIC
   c. Bone-bonding ability of GIC
   d. Chemical bonding between the filler and polymer–matrix of GIC
7. In which of the following scenarios could high strength and toughness be achieved concurrently?
   a. Add hard filler into thermoplastics
   b. Add ceramic fillers into metals
   c. Add ceramic fillers into elastomers
   d. Alloy metals with strong metal elements

8. No matter what materials are used, artificial bone is rather disappointing, with no successful development of man-made bone that can compete with natural bone. The major challenge is
   a. How to achieve both strength and toughness
   b. How to achieve excellent biocompatibility
   c. How to synthesize the highly hierarchical structure of bone
   d. How to achieve good bonding to natural bone

PROBLEMS AND EXERCISES

1. Prove with your calculation that the maximal volume fraction of a hexagonal- or square-distributed fiber-reinforced composite is

$$\begin{cases} f_{max} = 0.907 \quad \text{(hexagonal)} \\ f_{max} = 0.785 \quad \text{(square)} \end{cases}$$

2. Describe the compositional, structural, and mechanical difference between dentin, enamel, and cortical bone?
3. Freshly dissected cortical bone contains ~10 vol.% water. Dried cortical bone contains ~70 wt.% minerals and ~30 wt.% collagen proteins. The density of carbonated hydroxyapatite is ~2.8 g/cm³, and the density of dried collagen is ~1.3 g/cm³.
   a. Calculate the volume percentage of minerals and proteins (each) in dehydrated bone.
   b. Calculate the volume percentage of minerals and proteins (each) in hydrated bone.
4. Wet bone contains HA (41.6 vol.%), protein (38.4 vol.%), and water (20 vol.%). The Young's modulus of carbonated apatite is 54 GPa. The Young's modulus of collagen proteins is 1.25 GPa. Calculate the axial Young's modulus of cortical bone.
5. Water corresponds to ~20 vol.% of the some bone in mammals. On a dry weight basis, approximately 70 wt.% of the bone is composed of carbonated apatite. The density of apatite is ~3.0 g/cm³. The density of dry collagens is ~1.2 g/cm³.
   a. Calculate the volume percentages of hydroxylapatite and collagen in dry bone.
   b. Calculate the volume percentages of water, HA, and collagen in bone in vivo.
6. Water corresponds to ~3 vol.% of enamel. On a dry weight basis, ~97 wt.% of the enamel is composed of hydroxylapatite. The density of hydroxyapatite is ~3.0 g/cm³. The density of proteins in vitro (i.e., dried) is ~1.0 g/cm³. Calculate the volume percentages of apatite and collagen in enamel in vivo.
7. The Young's modules of carbonated apatite and collagens are given in the following:

Components	Young's Modulus (GPa)
Collagen	1.25
Carbonated apatite	55–80
Noncarbonated apatite	110–130

a. Calculate the axial Young's modulus of cortical bone (in vivo), using the Shear-Lag model and the volume percentages from Exercise 3.
b. Discuss whether the apatite in cortical bone and dentin is carbonated or not.
c. Calculate the axial Young's modulus of enamel (in vivo), using the Shear-Lag model and the volume percentages from Exercise 6.
d. Briefly discuss whether the apatite in enamel is carbonated or not.
8. Three elastomer composites are made of elastomer (as matrix) filled with bioceramic powder. The density of the elastomer and bioceramic is 1.1 and 2.8 g/cm^3, respectively. The Young's modulus of the elastomer and bioceramic is 0.2 and 35 GPa, respectively. The weight percentage of the bioceramic powder in the three materials is, respectively, 1%, 5%, and 10%. Calculate
a. the volume percentage of each composite;
b. The Young's modulus of each composite.
Table and graphically demonstrate your data.
9. If the aforementioned composite is reinforced by long fibers of the same bioceramics, calculate the axial Young's modulus of the three composites. Table and graphically demonstrate your data.
10. If the aforementioned composite is reinforced by short fibers of the same bioceramics, with an aspect ratio being 10, 25, 50, or 100, calculate the axial Young's modulus of the 12 composites. Table and graphically demonstrate your data.
11. Compare the results of Exercise 8–10, and discuss how the shape of bioceramic filler influences the reinforcement efficiency.

ADVANCED TOPIC: DEVELOPMENT OF ARTIFICIAL BONE: COMPOSITES AND SCAFFOLDS

Polymer–Matrix Bioceramic-Filled Composites and Scaffolds

As mentioned previously, from a biological perspective it is a natural strategy to combine polymers and ceramics to fabricate biomaterials for bone repair and substitution, because native bone is the combination of a naturally occurring polymer and biological apatite. From the materials science point of view, composite materials can capitalize on their advantages and minimize their shortcomings. For instance, since the release of acidic degradation from polymers is involved in inflammatory reactions [1–3], the basic degradation of calcium phosphate or bioactive glasses would buffer the acidic by-products of polymers and may thereby help to avoid the formation of an unfavorable environment for cells due to a decreased pH. Mechanically, bioceramics are much stronger than polymers and play a critical role in providing mechanical stability to constructs prior to synthesis of new bone matrix by cells. However, ceramics and glasses are very brittle and sensitive to flaws. Ceramic and glass materials have been combined with various polymers to form composite biomaterials for the treatment of bone defects. Table 11.4 lists the different types and mechanical properties of polymer–matrix ceramic/glass composites designed as biomedical devices or scaffold materials for bone repair.

In general, all these synthetic composites have good biocompatibility. For instance, the combination of TCP and PLA in a composite possesses the osteoconductivity of β-TCP and the degradability of PLA [4]. PLGA and HA were reported to combine the

Table 11.4
Biocomposites Designed for Bone Repair

Ceramic/Polymer		Percentage of Ceramic (%)	Strength (MPa)	Modulus (GPa)	Maximal Strain (%)	Toughness (kJ/m²)	Refs.
HA fiber	PDLLA	2–10.5 (vol.)	45	2			[21]
HA	PLLA	10–70 (wt.)	50–60	6–13	0.7–2.3		[20]
	PLGA	40–85 (vol.)	22	1		5.29	[22–24]
	Chitosan	40–85 (vol.)	12	2		0.092	[23]
	Chitosan+PLGA	40–85 (vol.)	43	2.5		9.77	[23]
	PPhos	85–95 (wt.)					[25]
	Collagen	50–72 (wt.)					[26]
β-TCP	PLLA-co-PEH	75 (wt.)	51	5			[4,27]
AW	PE	10–50 (vol.)	18–28	1–6			[28–30]
Ca$_3$(CO$_3$)$_2$	PLLA	30 (wt.)	50	3–6			[31]
Human cortical bone		70 (wt.)	50–150 (tensile) 130–180 (compressive)	10–30		2	[32–35]

degradability of PLGA with the bioactivity of HA, fostering cell proliferation and differentiation as well as mineral formation [5–7]. Furthermore, the composites of bioactive glass-PLA were observed to form calcium phosphate layers on their surfaces and support rapid and abundant growth of human osteoblasts and osteoblast-like cells when cultured in vitro [8–19].

A comparison between dense composites and cortical bone indicates that the most promising synthetic composite seems to be HA fiber-reinforced PLA composite [20], which can exhibit mechanical properties close to the lower ranges of cortical bone.

Fabrication of Composite Scaffolds

Polymer–matrix bioceramic-reinforced composites are an important group of biomaterials for tissue-engineering applications [36,37]. Among the technologies in Table 11.5, solution casting with/without particle leaching [15,18,19,38] and thermally induced phase separation (TIPS) combined with freeze-drying [9–12,39,40] have been applied to the fabrication of polymer–ceramic composite scaffolds. In addition there are two other methods: microsphere-sintering and foam-coating, which are developed for the combination of ceramic and polymeric materials, as listed in Table 11.5. This section briefly introduces the processing techniques of polymer–ceramic composite scaffolds.

Solution Casting/Particle Leaching and Microsphere Packing   Polymer–ceramic constructs can be fabricated by the solution-casting method. The polymer microspheres are at first formed from traditional water oil/water emulsions. Polymer–ceramic scaffolds can then be constructed by mixing solvent, salt or sugar particles, ceramic granules, and prehardened microspheres [15,18,19,38,41]. A three-dimensional (3D) structure of controlled porosity is formed based on this method combined with particle leaching and microsphere packing.

Thermally Induced Phase Separation/Freeze-Drying   Porous structure can also be achieved through phase separation and evaporation. One approach to induce phase separation is to lower the temperature of the suspension of polymer and ceramic materials. The solvent is solidified first, forcing the polymer and ceramic mixture into the interstitial spaces. The frozen mixture is then lyophilized using a freeze-dryer, in which the ice solvent evaporates [8,12,39,40].

Microsphere-Sintering   In this process, microspheres of a ceramic and polymer composite are synthesized first, using the emulsion/solvent evaporation technique. Sintering the composite microspheres together yields a 3D, porous scaffold [42,43].

Foam-Coating   An alternative approach to address the combination of polymeric and ceramic materials is to coat bioactive ceramics onto polymeric foams [44,45]. The inverse method, namely, polymer-coated ceramic scaffolds, has also been investigated [46–48]. A tough scaffold has been achieved through bioglass-based scaffolds coated with poly(glycrol sebacate) [46].

Biomaterials: A Basic Introduction

Table 11.5
Fabrication Methods of Three-Dimensional Porous Composite Scaffolds

Fabrication Technique	Biocomposite Ceramic	Polymer	Percentage of Ceramic (%)	Porosity (%)	Pore Size (µm)	Refs.
Solvent casting/particle leaching	HA	PLGA	60–75 (wt.)	81–91	800–1800	[38]
	Bioglass®	PLLA	20–50 (wt.)	77–80	~100 (macro) ~10 (micro)	[15]
	Phosphate glass	PLA-PDLLA	40 (wt.)	93–97		[18]
	A/W	PDLLA	20–40 (wt.)	85.5–95.2	98–154	[19]
Thermally induce phase separation/freeze-drying	β-TCP	Chitosan-Gelatin	10–70 (wt.)		322–355	[39]
	HA	PLLA	50 (wt.)	85–95	100 × 300	[40]
	Bioglass	PDLLA	5–29 (wt.)	94	~100 (macro) 10–50 (micro)	[9–12,17,50]
Microsphere/sintering	Amorphous CaP	PLGA	28–75 (wt.)	75	>100	[42,43]
	Bioglass	PLGA	75 (wt.)	43	89	[14]
Polymer foam/ceramic coating	HA	PLGA	40–85 (vol.)			[23,24]
	Bioglass	PDLLA				[44,45,51]
Ceramic foam/polymer coating	HA foam	PDLLA				[47,48]
	Bioglass	PGS				[46]

Source: Chen, Q.Z., Development of Bioglass(R)-Ceramic Scaffolds for Bone Tissue Engineering, Imperial College London, London, U.K., 2006.

BIBLIOGRAPHY

References for Text

1. Hull, D. and T.W. Clyne, *An Introduction to Composite Materials*, Cambridge University Press, 1996.
2. Kothawz, S.P. and N. Guzelsun, Modeling the tensile mechanical behavior of bone along the longitudinal direction. *Journal of Theoretical Biology*, 2002;**219**:269–279.

Websites

http://www.asc-composites.org/.
http://www.escm.eu.org/.
http://www.iom3.org/content/british-composites-society.

References for the Advanced Topic

1. Bergsma, E.J., F.R. Rozema, R.R.M. Bos, and W.C. Debruijn, Foreign-body reactions to resorbable poly(L-lactide) bone plates and screws used for the fixation of unstable zygomatic fractures. *Journal of Oral and Maxillofacial Surgery*, 1993;**51**:666–670.
2. Bergsma, J.E., W.C. Debruijn, F.R. Rozema, R.R.M. Bos, and G. Boering, Late degradation tissue-response to poly(L-lactide) bone plates and screws. *Biomaterials*, 1995;**16**:25–31.
3. Temenoff, J.S., L. Lu, and A.G. Mikos, Bone tissue engineering using synthetic biodegradable polymer scaffolds. In *Bone Engineering*, J.E. Davies, ed. Toronto, Ontario, Canada: EM Squared, 2000, pp. 455–462.
4. Kikuchi, M., J. Tanaka, Y. Koyama, and K. Takakuda, Cell culture test of TCP/CPLA composite. *Journal of Biomedical Materials Research*, 1999;**48**:108–110.
5. Attawia, M.A., K.M. Herbert, and C.T. Laurencin, Osteoblast-like cell adherence and migration through 3-dimensional porous polymer matrices. *Biochemical and Biophysical Research Communications*, 1995;**213**:639–644.
6. Laurencin, C.T., M.A. Attawia, H.E. Elgendy, and K.M. Herbert, Tissue engineered bone-regeneration using degradable polymers: The formation of mineralized matrices. *Bone*, 1996;**19**:S93–S99.
7. Devin, J.E., M.A. Attawia, and C.T. Laurencin, Three-dimensional degradable porous polymer-ceramic matrices for use in bone repair. *Journal of Biomaterials Science. Polymer Edition*, 1996;**7**:661–669.
8. Boccaccini, A.R., I. Notingher, V. Maquet, and R. Jerome, Bioresorbable and bioactive composite materials based on polylactide foams filled with and coated by Bioglass (R) particles for tissue engineering applications. *Journal of Materials Science. Materials in Medicine*, 2003;**14**:443–450.
9. Maquet, V., A.R. Boccaccini, L. Pravata, I. Notingher, and R. Jerome, Preparation, characterization, and in vitro degradation of bioresorbable and bioactive composites based on Bioglass (R)-filled polylactide foams. *Journal of Biomedical Materials Research. Part A*, 2003;**66A**:335–346.
10. Maquet, V., A.R. Boccaccini, L. Pravata, I. Notingher, and R. Jerome, Porous poly(alpha-hydroxyacid)/Bioglass (R) composite scaffolds for bone tissue engineering. I: Preparation and in vitro characterisation. *Biomaterials*, 2004;**25**:4185–4194.
11. Blaker, J.J., J.E. Gough, V. Maquet, I. Notingher, and A.R. Boccaccini, In vitro evaluation of novel bioactive composites based on Bioglass (R)-filled polylactide foams for bone tissue engineering scaffolds. *Journal of Biomedical Materials Research. Part A*, 2003;**67A**:1401–1411.
12. Verrier, S., J.J. Blaker, V. Maquet, L.L. Hench, and A.R. Boccaccini, PDLLA/Bioglass (R) composites for soft-tissue and hard-tissue engineering: An in vitro cell biology assessment. *Biomaterials*, 2004;**25**:3013–3021.

13. Stamboulis, A.G., A.R. Boccaccini, and L.L. Hench, Novel biodegradable polymer/bioactive glass composites for tissue engineering applications. *Advanced Engineering Materials*, 2002;**4**:105–109.

14. Lu, H.H., S.F. El-Amin, K.D. Scott, and C.T. Laurencin, Three-dimensional, bioactive, biodegradable, polymer-bioactive glass composite scaffolds with improved mechanical properties support collagen synthesis and mineralization of human osteoblast-like cells in vitro. *Journal of Biomedical Materials Research. Part A*, 2003;**64A**:465–474.

15. Zhang, K., Y.B. Wang, M.A. Hillmyer, and L.F. Francis, Processing and properties of porous poly(L-lactide)/bioactive glass composites. *Biomaterials*, 2004;**25**:2489–2500.

16. Blaker, J.J., R.M. Day, V. Maquet, and A.R. Boccaccini, Novel bioresorbable poly(lactide-co-glycolide) (PLGA) and PLGA/Bioglass((R)) composite tubular foam scaffolds for tissue engineering applications. In *Advanced Materials Forum II*, R. Martins, E. Fortunato, I. Ferreira, and C. Dias, eds., Trans Tech Publications, Uetikon, Zurich, Switzerland, 2004, pp. 415–419.

17. Blaker, J.J., V. Maquet, R. Jerome, A.R. Boccaccini, and S.N. Nazhat, Mechanical properties of highly porous PDLLA/Bioglass (R) composite foams as scaffolds for bone tissue engineering. *Acta Biomaterialia*, 2005;**1**:643–652.

18. Navarro, M., M.P. Ginebra, J.A. Planell, S. Zeppetelli, and L. Ambrosio, Development and cell response of a new biodegradable composite scaffold for guided bone regeneration. *Journal of Materials Science. Materials in Medicine*, 2004;**15**:419–422.

19. Li, H.Y. and J. Chang, Preparation and characterization of bioactive and biodegradable Wollastonite/poly(D,L-lactic acid) composite scaffolds. *Journal of Materials Science. Materials in Medicine*, 2004;**15**:1089–1095.

20. Kasuga, T., Y. Ota, M. Nogami, and Y. Abe, Preparation and mechanical properties of poly-lactic acid composites containing hydroxyapatite fibers. *Biomaterials*, 2001;**22**:19–23.

21. Deng, X.M., J.Y. Hao, and C.S. Wang, Preparation and mechanical properties of nanocomposites of poly(D,L-lactide) with Ca-deficient hydroxyapatite nanocrystals. *Biomaterials*, 2001;**22**:2867–2873.

22. Xu, H.H.K. and C.G. Simon, Self-hardening calcium phosphate cement-mesh composite: Reinforcement, macropores, and cell response. *Journal of Biomedical Materials Research. Part A*, 2004;**69A**:267–278.

23. Xu, H.H.K., J.B. Quinn, S. Takagi, and L.C. Chow, Synergistic reinforcement of in situ hardening calcium phosphate composite scaffold for bone tissue engineering. *Biomaterials*, 2004;**25**:1029–1037.

24. Xu, H.H.K. and C.G. Jr. Simon, Self-hardening calcium phosphate composite scaffold for bone tissue engineering. *Journal of Orthopaedic Research*, 2004;**22**:535–543.

25. Greish, Y.E., J.D. Bender, S. Lakshmi, P.W. Brown, H.R. Allcock, and C.T. Laurencin, Low temperature formation of hydroxyapatite-poly(alkyl oxybenzoate)phosphazene composites for biomedical applications. *Biomaterials*, 2005;**26**:1–9.

26. Rodrigues, C.V.M. et al., Characterization of a bovine collagen-hydroxyapatite composite scaffold for bone tissue engineering. *Biomaterials*, 2003;**24**:4987–4997.

27. Peter, S.J., S.T. Miller, G.M. Zhu, A.W. Yasko, and A.G. Mikos, In vivo degradation of a poly(propylene fumarate) beta-tricalcium phosphate injectable composite scaffold. *Journal of Biomedical Materials Research*, 1998;**41**:1–7.

28. Juhasz, J.A. et al., Mechanical properties of glass-ceramic A-W—Polyethylene composites: Effect of filler content. *Bioceramics*, 2003;**15**:947–950. Uetikon, Zurich, Switzerland: Trans Tech Publications Ltd.

29. Juhasz, J.A. et al., Apatite-forming ability of glass-ceramic apatite-wollastonite—Polyethylene composites: Effect of filler content. *Journal of Materials Science. Materials in Medicine*, 2003;**14**:489–495.

30. Juhasz, J.A. et al., Mechanical properties of glass-ceramic A-W-polyethylene composites: Effect of filler content and particle size. *Biomaterials*, 2004;**25**:949–955.

31. Kasuga, T., H. Maeda, K. Kato, M. Nogami, K. Hata, and M. Ueda, Preparation of poly(lactic acid) composites containing calcium carbonate (vaterite). *Biomaterials*, 2003;**24**:3247–3253.

32. Nalla, R.K., J.H. Kinney, and R.O. Ritchie, Mechanistic fracture criteria for the failure of human cortical bone. *Nature Materials*, 2003;**2**:164–168.

33. Zioupos, P. and J.D. Currey, Changes in the stiffness, strength, and toughness of human cortical bone with age. *Bone*, 1998;**22**:57–66.

34. Keaveny, T.M. and W.C. Hayes. Mechanical properties of cortical and trabecular bone. In *Bone: A Treatise*, Vol. 7: Bone Growth, B.K. Hall, ed. Boca Raton, FL: CRC Press, 1993, pp. 285–344.

35. Moore, W.R., S.E. Graves, and G.I. Bain, Synthetic bone graft substitutes. *Australian and New Zealand Journal of Surgery*, 2001;**71**:354–361.

36. Liang, S.L., W.D. Cook, G.A. Thouas, and Q.Z. Chen, The mechanical characteristics and in vitro biocompatibility of poly(glycerol sebacate)-Bioglass (R) elastomeric composites. *Biomaterials*, 2010;**31**:8516–8529.

37. Chen, Q.Z. et al., Elastomeric nanocomposites as cell delivery vehicles and cardiac support devices. *Soft Matter*, 2010;**6**:4715–4726.

38. Guan, L.M. and J.E. Davies, Preparation and characterization of a highly macroporous biodegradable composite tissue engineering scaffold. *Journal of Biomedical Materials Research. Part A*, 2004;**71A**:480–487.

39. Yin, Y.J., F. Ye, J.F. Cui, F.J. Zhang, X.L. Li, and K.D. Yao, Preparation and characterization of macroporous chitosan-gelatin beta-tricalcium phosphate composite scaffolds for bone tissue engineering. *Journal of Biomedical Materials Research. Part A*, 2003;**67A**:844–855.

40. Zhang, R.Y. and P.X. Ma, Poly(alpha-hydroxyl acids) hydroxyapatite porous composites for bone-tissue engineering. I. Preparation and morphology. *Journal of Biomedical Materials Research*, 1999;**44**:446–455.

41. Ma, P.X. and J.W. Choi, Biodegradable polymer scaffolds with well-defined interconnected spherical pore network. *Tissue Engineering*, 2001;**7**:23–33.

42. Khan, Y.M., D.S. Katti, and C.T. Laurencin, Novel polymer-synthesized ceramic composite-based system for bone repair: An in vitro evaluation. *Journal of Biomedical Materials Research. Part A*, 2004;**69A**:728–737.

43. Ambrosio, A.M.A., J.S. Sahota, Y. Khan, and C.T. Laurencin, A novel amorphous calcium phosphate polymer ceramic for bone repair: 1. Synthesis and characterization. *Journal of Biomedical Materials Research*, 2001;**58**:295–301.

44. Roether, J.A., A.R. Boccaccini, L.L. Hench, V. Maquet, S. Gautier, and R. Jerome, Development and in vitro characterisation of novel bioresorbable and bioactive composite materials based on polylactide foams and Bioglass (R) for tissue engineering applications. *Biomaterials*, 2002;**23**:3871–3878.

45. Gough, J.E., M. Arumugam, J. Blaker, and A.R. Boccaccini, Bioglass (R) coated poly(DL-lactide) foams for tissue engineering scaffolds. *Materialwissenschaft und Werkstofftechnik*, 2003;**34**:654–661.

46. Chen, Q.Z., J.M.W. Quinn, G.A. Thouas, X.A. Zhou, and P.A. Komesaroff, Bone-like elastomer-toughened scaffolds with degradability kinetics matching healing rates of injured bone. *Advanced Engineering Materials*, 2010;**12**:B642–B648.

47. Miao, X., G. Lim, K.H. Loh, and A.R. Boccaccini, Preparation and characterisation of calcium phosphate bone cement. *Materials Processing Properties Performance (MP3)*, 2004;**3**:319–324.

48. Kim, H.W., J.C. Knowles, and H.E. Kim, Hydroxyapatite porous scaffold engineered with biological polymer hybrid coating for antibiotic Vancomycin release. *Journal of Materials Science. Materials in Medicine*, 2005;**16**:189–195.

49. Chen, Q.Z., *Development of Bioglass(R)-Ceramic Scaffolds for Bone Tissue Engineering*. London, U.K.: Imperial College London, 2006.

50. Boccaccini, A.R. and J.J. Blaker, Bioactive composite materials for tissue engineering scaffolds. *Expert Review of Medical Devices*, 2005;**2**:303–317.

51. Tamai, N. et al., Novel hydroxyapatite ceramics with an interconnective porous structure exhibit superior osteoconduction in vivo. *Journal of Biomedical Materials Research*, 2002;**59**:110–117.

52. Glimcher, M.J., *Reviews in Mineralogy and Geochemistry*, 2006;**64**:223–282.

Further Readings

Chapter 8: Composite as biomaterials. In *Biomaterials: An Introduction*, Park, J. and R.S. Lakes, eds., 3rd edn. New York: Springer, 2007.

Chapter 10: Biomaterials for dental applications. In *Handbook of Materials for Medical Devices*, Davies, J.R. ed. Americal Society for Metals (ASM) International, Materials Park, OH, 2003.

Craig, R.G. and J.M. Powers, eds., *Restorative Dental Materials*, 11th edn. St. Louis, MO: Mosby Inc (an affiliate of Elsevier Science), 2002.

Hull, D. and T.W. Clyne, *An Introduction to Composite Materials*, Chapters 1–6, Cambridge University Press, 1996.

MEDICAL SCIENCE

CHAPTER 12

MEDICINE AND MEDICAL SCIENCE

LEARNING OBJECTIVES

After a careful study of this chapter, you should be able to do the following:

1. Describe the generic relationship between medicine and medical science, and appreciate its similarity to the relation between materials science and materials engineering.
2. Appreciate the big picture of medical science, and the similar approaches to those in materials science.
3. Appreciate that structure–function relationships exist in organisms as in materials.
4. Appreciate the learning goals of Part II of this book.

12.1 MEDICINE AND MEDICAL SCIENCE

The relationship between medicine (an applied science) and medical science (basic science) is similar to that between materials engineering (an applied science) and materials science (basic science) (Chapter 1). *Medicine* is the applied science encompassing all health care practices evolved to maintain and restore health by the diagnosis, prevention, and treatment of illness in human beings. *Medical science*, as the basic science of medicine, is about the principles of how the human body works and the mechanisms of diseases, aiming to find new ways to cure or treat disease by developing advanced diagnostic tools or new therapeutic strategies. Throughout human history, many principles of medicine were established based on their direct clinical application, especially in the case of pharmacology and surgery. Empirical knowledge in medicine has led to foundations in the theoretical system, medical science. At the same time, medical sciences have evolved independently and systematically, based on laboratory experimentation and discoveries from animal and cell/tissue-based models. Contemporary medicine applies medical science and technology to diagnose and treat injury and disease. Today, it is the advances in medical science and technology that enhance medical practices in the health care system, with constant feedback to engineering to continually improve the technology.

411

12.2   MEDICAL SCIENCE VERSUS MATERIALS SCIENCE

As introduced in Chapter 1, materials science is the study of the relationship between structures and properties of materials. Likewise, medical science is essentially the study of a relationship between structures and functions of biological matter. Like materials that exhibit structure on more than one length scale (Figure 1.2), all biological systems demonstrate highly complex, self-assembled hierarchical structures (Figure 12.1). Atoms are chemically bonded to become biomolecules (e.g., lipids, peptides, nucleotides, and metabolites), which are organized to form larger structural and/or functional macromolecules. Larger functional biomolecules can have specialized signaling roles (e.g., enzymes, hormones, and binding proteins). Structural biomolecules form larger nanoscale structures (e.g., membranes, fibrous cytoskeleton, and extracellular matrix). Some of these form the components of larger microscale structures including organelles, which form compartments in cells that contain functional moieties. Cells, which are composed of various types of organelles, are the basic building blocks of living tissues of all organs. The body survives on the functions of its organs.

Anatomy is the study of the body's structure. Each part of the body performs a specific function, much like it has been *engineered* for a particular role. These roles are a complex combination of static (e.g., skeletal support, organ containment) and dynamic roles (such as digestion, respiration, circulation, reproduction). Physiology is the study of the functions of organs and how the functions of the body work toward performing a specific task. Hence, anatomy is highly integrated with physiology. While the link between structure and function is always present, it is not always well understood. This complexity is still the subject of many ongoing areas of research.

Anatomy can further be divided into macroscopic (or gross) anatomy and microscopic anatomy. Gross anatomy involves the study of relatively large structures and features visible to the unaided eye, typically organs (Figure 12.2). Gross anatomy is equivalent to macrostructure study in materials science. There are many ways to approach gross anatomy:

- Surface anatomy
- Regional anatomy
- Systemic anatomy
- Developmental anatomy
- Comparative anatomy
- Medical anatomy
- Radiographic anatomy
- Surgical anatomy

In this book, we adopt systemic anatomy as our approach. In the human body, there are 11 organ systems:

1. Integumentary (Skin)
2. Muscular
3. Skeletal
4. Nervous
5. Endocrine
6. Cardiovascular (circulatory)
7. Lymphatic
8. Respiratory

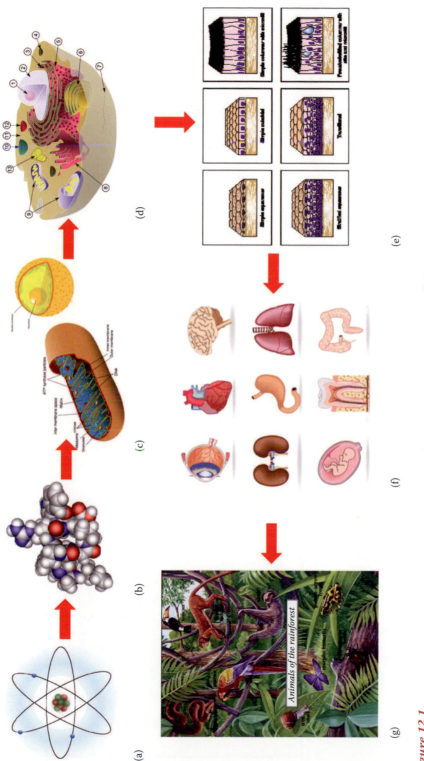

Figure 12.1

Multilevel structures in organisms: (a) atoms, (b) molecules, (c) organelles, (d) cells, (e) tissues, (f) organs, and (g) organisms. (d: From https://gcps. desire2learn.com/d2l/lor/viewer/viewFile.d2lfile/6605/4821/animal%20cell.jpg).

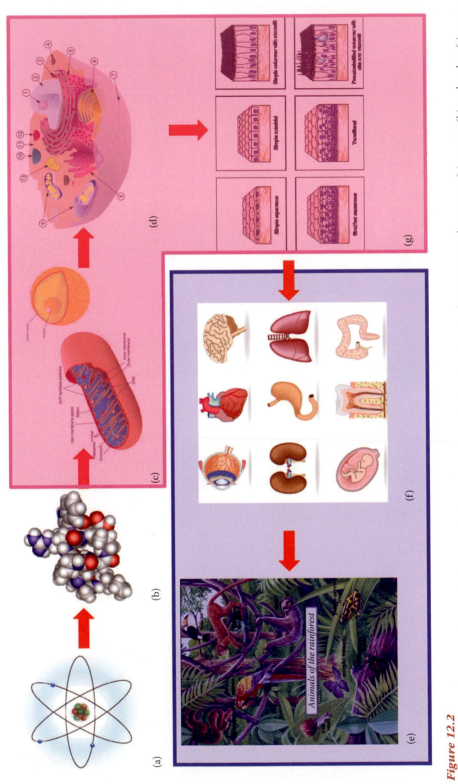

Figure 12.2
Macro– (gross) and microanatomy, which are equivalent to macro– and microstructure studies in materials science: (a) atoms, (b) molecules, (c) organelles, (d) cells, (e) organisms, (f) organs, and (g) tissues. (c and d: From the CreationWikiCommon.)

9. Digestive
10. Urinary
11. Reproductive

Microanatomy can be subdivided into two specialties, which are concerned with micro-scopic structures in cells (i.e., cytology) or organ tissues (i.e., histology), respectively. Cytology involves the analysis of the internal structure of individual cells. Histology is a study of tissues, groups of specialized cells, and cell products that work together to perform specific functions (Figure 12.2). Microanatomy is equivalent to the microstruc-ture study in materials science.

In addition to anatomy, histology, and cell biology (cytology), medical science cov-ers more than 20 subjects, as listed in Table 12.1. However, these three subjects are the most fundamental knowledge, based on which other subjects of medical science have been established. Hence, anatomy, histology, and cell biology forms the primary content of Part II of this book.

Table 12.1
Major Subjects of Medical Science

Subjects	Study Objectives
Anatomy	The structure of organisms
Biochemistry	The chemical substances and processes occurring in living organisms
Biomechanics	The structure and function of biological systems by means of the methods of mechanics
Biophysics	Biological systems by use of the methods of physics and physical chemistry
Cytology	The microscopic structure and function of individual cells
Embryology	The early development of organisms
Endocrinology	Hormones and their effect throughout the body of animals
Epidemiology	The demographics of disease processes and epidemics
Genetics	Genes, and their role in biological inheritance
Histology	The microscopic structures of biological tissues
Immunology	The immune system, which includes the innate and adaptive immune system in humans, the body's defense system
Medical physics	The applications of physics principles in medicine
Medical statistics	The application of statistics to biomedical fields
Microbiology	Microorganisms, including protozoa, bacteria, fungi, and viruses
Molecular biology	Molecular underpinnings of the process of replication, transcription, and translation of the genetic material
Neuroscience	The nervous system. A main focus of neuroscience is the biology and physiology of the human brain and spinal cord
Pathology	Diseases and disorders—the causes, progression, and resolution at all levels of structure and function, from cells to systems
Pharmacology	Drugs and their actions
Physiology	The normal functioning of the body and the underlying regulatory mechanisms
Radiobiology	The interactions between ionizing radiation and living organisms
Toxicology	Hazardous effects of drugs and poisons

12.3   LEARNING GOALS OF PART II

Part II is designed for students to achieve three goals:

Goal 1

Be familiar with basic medical terms, appreciate basic medical concepts, to be able to communicate effectively with the medical community

Learning a science, especially medical science, is also a process of learning a scientific language. Unless you know the names and their meanings, you will have trouble saying what you mean; you will have trouble understanding what others are saying; and you will not be able to communicate well. In the field of medical science, an immense range of scientific terminology has been created and routinely used. This is similar to the level of nomenclature used in chemical structures, as outlined by IUPAC (e.g., dextro- and levo-, zwitterion). Medical terms largely originate from Latin or Greek, to describe the main features of the object or process. In some cases, however, these terms can be inhibitory to understanding the meaning of the process by the lay person, patients, or even scientists from other fields. This is due to some processes having similar sounding roots, and some used as jargon among medical practitioners.

For example:

Sub = below
Cutis = skin
Subcutaneous = below the skin
Myo = muscle
Cardium = heart
Myocardium = muscle of the heart
Epi = above
Staxis = dripping
Epistaxis = commonly called blood nose
Peri = around
Stallein = to place
Peristalsis = radial muscle contractions of digestion

Note: epistaxis and peristalsis sound very similar, but mean very different processes. Furthermore, the first is a type of pathology, while the second is part of routine physiology in the body.

Goal 2

Be aware of the most threatening human diseases and potential applications of biomaterials

It is important, especially for engineering students, to clearly understand the fundamentals of health care in the practice of medicine, that is, the body heals itself. In medical treatment, practitioners support a patient's vital functions by optimizing the environment most conductive to healing. Basically, physicians attempt to neutralize hostile factors and at the same time enhance the supply of oxygen and nutrients that the body needs for the healing process. Surgeons eliminate hostile factors through excising the necrotic or malign tissue that is the source of unfavorable chemical agents, reconstruct tissue through the suture of the remaining tissue, auto-/allo-/xeno-transplantation, or implantation of prosthesis, and manipulate the local environment to help the body heal itself by, for example, medication and blood supply. Hence, *the application of biomaterial implant is an option only when the body cannot heal itself.* In many clinical scenarios, the applications of biomaterials are limited as an alternative treatment when no standard or conventional treatments can help. As such, it is important to be aware of the most threatening diseases, as these are the scenarios when artificial tissue or organs made of biomaterials could find applications.

Another limit on the application of biomaterials lies in the fact that besides physical (especially mechanical) support, biomaterials have no other biological functions, although can have biological side effects (e.g., cytotoxicity, metabolic degradation products). In some cases, biomaterials can replace biological materials, the major function of which is mechanical, and their other biological aspects can essentially be ignored. For example, in teeth or bone, the function is largely mechanical such that dentists and orthopedists can use metal implants to restore the mechanical function of the damaged tissues. In many other cases, however, the biological functionality of the tissues or organs is so dynamic that it is meaningless to replace them with biomaterials, for example, the spinal cord or brain [1].

Goal 3

Understand physical properties of biological tissues

The study of the relationships between the structure and physical properties of biological matter is as important as that of the biomaterials designed for their repair or replacement. However, traditionally this subject has been laid aside by most medical practitioners and researchers in biologically oriented disciplines. This is due to the fact that workers in those fields are concerned with the biochemical and physiological aspects of function rather than the physical properties of tissues as, in a sense, biomaterials in themselves [1]. Up to now, this research sub-discipline has remained poorly explored, although awareness will increase as improvements are progressively made in understanding how physical properties of tissues play critical roles in their biological functions.

12.4   CHAPTER HIGHLIGHTS

1. As materials science is the basic science of materials engineering (an applied science), medical science is the basic science of medicine, which is the application of science encompassing all health care practices evolved to maintain and restore health by the diagnosis, prevention, and treatment of illness in human beings.
2. The link between structure and property/function is always present, but not always understood. Materials science is the study of the relationship between structures and properties of materials. Medical science is essentially the study of a relationship between structures and functions of biological substance.
3. Macro (gross) anatomy is equivalent to the macrostructure study in materials science. Microanatomy, covering histology and cytology, is equivalent to the microstructure study in materials science.
4. Three learning goals:
   a. Ability to communicate effectively with the medical community
   b. Be aware of the most threatening human diseases and potential applications of biomaterials
   c. Understand materials properties of biological tissues, and biological effects of biomaterials

ACTIVITY

Visit: http://en.wikipedia.org/wiki/List_of_medical_roots,_suffixes_and_prefixes

Search Images on Google using the following keywords:

Gray's anatomy muscles
Gray's anatomy brain
Gray's anatomy heart
Gray's anatomy bone

BIBLIOGRAPHY

Reference

1. Park, J. and R.S. Lakes, Chapter 1: Introduction. In *Biomaterials: An Introduction*, 3rd edn. New York: Springer Science & Business Media LLC, 2007.

Websites

http://en.wikipedia.org/wiki/List_of_images_and_subjects_in_Gray's_Anatomy.
http://www.bartleby.com/107/.
This site provides excellent digitalized images of the 1918 edition of Gray's Anatomy. The Bartleby.com edition of Gray's Anatomy of the Human Body features 1,247 vibrant engravings, many in color from the classic 1918 publication, as well as a subject index with 13,000 entries ranging from the Antrum of Highmore to the Zonule of Zinn.
http://education.yahoo.com/reference/gray/.
http://en.wikipedia.org/wiki/Category:Gray%27s_Anatomy-related_lists.
http://en.wikipedia.org/wiki/List_of_human_anatomical_features.
http://en.wikipedia.org/wiki/Muscular_system.
http://www.innerbody.com/.
To see detailed human anatomy charts and gather in-depth anatomy information.
http://www.imaios.com/en/e-Anatomy.
E-anatomy is an anatomy e-learning website. More than 1,500 slices from normal CT and MR exams were selected in order to cover the entire sectional anatomy of the human body.
http://www.sciencekids.co.nz/pictures/humanbody.html.
http://msjensen.cehd.umn.edu/webanatomy/.
A collection of study aids for entry-level anatomy and physiology students.
http://www.nlm.nih.gov/research/visible/visible_human.html
Produced by the National Library of Medicine. Contains complete, anatomically detailed, 3D representations of the normal male and female human bodies. Acquisition of transverse CT, MR, and cryosection images of representative male and female cadavers has been completed. The male was sectioned at 1 mm intervals, the female at one-third of a millimeter intervals.
http://www.instantanatomy.net/about.html
InstantAnantomy offers illustrations of the human body to aid the learning of human anatomy with diagrams, podcasts, and revision questions.
http://www.nlm.nih.gov/exhibition/historicalanatomies/home.html
Histological Anatomy: Digital project designed to give Internet users access to high-quality images from important anatomical atlases in the National Library of Medicine collection. The project offers selected images from NLM's atlas collection, not the entire books, with an emphasis on images and not texts.
http://www.eskeletons.org/

From University of Texas, Austin. It offers a unique set of digitized versions of skeletons in 2D and 3D in full color, animations, and much supplemental information. The user can navigate through the various regions of the skeleton and view all orientations of each element along with muscle and joint information. *eSkeletons* enables you to view the bones of both human and nonhuman primates.

http://sig.biostr.washington.edu/projects/da/

Produced by the Structural Informatics Group at the University of Washington, Seattle. This site provides access to interactive atlases of brain neuroanatomy, thoracic viscera, and knee.

http://www.cellsalive.com/

Cells Alive!: Provides basic cell biology, microbiology, and immunology videos, micrographs, and diagrams. The images are available for use in lectures and handouts and for other nonprofit educational use.

http://lane.stanford.edu/biomed-resources/bassett/index.html

Digitized version of the Stanford School of Medicine's world-renowned Bassett collection of human dissection. The Bassett Collection contains some of the most meticulously detailed dissections ever done.

http://library.med.utah.edu/WebPath/HISTHTML/NEURANAT/NEURANCA.html

The atlases include brain and spinal cord images and MRIs of the brain. Content is freely available for nonprofit use by health science educators.

https://histo.life.illinois.edu/histo/atlas/index.php

Produced by College of Medicine, University of Illinois. Over 1,000, labeled, histological images with accompanying functional descriptions. Interactive features allow the user to change magnification and examine areas of interest in great detail. Some images have interactive identification features.

http://www.anatomyatlases.org/

Anatomy Atlases is an anatomy digital health sciences library curated by Ronald A Bergman, PhD. It is written for and intended primarily for use by Medical Students, Residents, Fellows, or Attending Physicians studying anatomy.

http://link.library.utoronto.ca/anatomia/application/index.cfm

This collection features approximately 4,500 full page plates and other significant illustrations of human anatomy selected from the Jason A. Hannah and Academy of Medicine collections in the history of medicine at the Thomas Fisher Rare Book Library, University of Toronto. Each illustration has been fully indexed using medical subject headings (MeSH), and techniques of illustration, artists, and engravers have been identified whenever possible.

Noncommercial, educational, interactive links

http://www.getbodysmart.com/

GetBodySmart provides excellent illustrations with quizzes.

http://medtropolis.com/virtual-body/

Virtual Body is an awesome site. If you are studying any of the body systems, you do not want to miss this site. So much interactivity!

Commercial websites of stock-photos

http://www.canstockphoto.com/images-photos/anatomy.html
http://www.123rf.com/stock-photo/anatomy.html
http://www.matton.com/images/single/healthcare___medicine/medical_anatomy.html
http://www.stockfreeimages.com/7020056/Anatomy.html
http://www.gettyimages.com.au/creative/anatomy-stock-photos

Some interactive links:

- 3D human anatomy from Google labs, click here
- 3D human anatomy and physiology by *GetBodySmart* subject area:

Skeletal system
Muscle tissue physiology

Muscular system
Nervous system
Circulatory (cardiovascular) system
Respiratory system
Urinary system
Histology
Anatomy and physiology quizzes

- *Virtual Body*: This is an awesome site. If you are studying any of the body systems, you do not want to miss this site. So much interactivity!!!
- *Zygote* provides 3D polygonal models for animators and illustrators to create high-quality animations and renderings. The models are detailed, and organized so that you can quickly and efficiently work with exactly what you need.
- *Online Ebooks of Anatomy*—branch of biology concerned with the study of body structure of various organisms, including humans, click here
- *Inner body*: To see detailed human anatomy charts and gather in-depth anatomy information
- *Human Anatomy* for your mobile, download here
- Atlas Anatomi grant, download here (http://gallery.mobile9.com/f/495023/)
- *Atlas of Human Anatomy* (http://www.anatomyatlases.org/atlasofanatomy/index.shtml). This atlas is translated from the original atlas entitled "Handbuch der Anatomie des Menschen," which was published in 1841 in Leipzig, Germany. The author of this atlas was Professor Dr. Carl Ernest Bock, who lived from 1809 to 1874.
- *Instant anatomy*: Website with illustrations of the human body to aid the learning of human anatomy with diagrams, podcasts, and revision questions
- *e-Anatomy*: Human anatomy, medical imaging, and illustrations
- *Anatomy ebooks*: By Jones Quain, Richard Quain, William Sharpey, and Joseph Leidy on Google Books

Read Online:

1. *Online 3D Human Anatomy Maps my maps*
2. *List Of Free Web*: About Journal of Medicine articles and ebooks online

IMAGE LINKS

http://www.neuro.utah.edu/related_links/image_links.html
Many of the images in these collections are free to use for educational purposes; however, you *must* cite the original author. For citing and copyright information, please click on the "FairUseinfo" link.

General Health Sciences Images | *Anatomy* | *Embryology* | *Histology* | *Neuroanatomy* | *General Images* | *Animations*

General Health Sciences Images:

- *Bristol BioMed Image Archive—external link*, a collection of medical, dental, and veterinary images for use in teaching (FairUseinfo—*external link*)
- *CDC's Public Health Image Library—external link*, contains illustrations, photographs, and audiovisuals (FairUseinfo)

- *Eccles Multimedia Catalog—external link*, contains images, illustrations, animations, videos, and sounds related to the health sciences. (FairUseinfo—*external link*)
- *HEAL, Health Education Assets Library—external link* provides educators with high-quality and free multimedia materials (such as images and videos) to augment health sciences education. (FairUseinfo—*external link*)
- *Medical Graphics, Photography, University of Utah Health Sciences Logos—external link* (FairUseinfo—*external link*)
- National Library of Medicine—History of Medicine Division—*external link,* This system provides access to the nearly 60,000 images in the prints and photographs collection of the History of Medicine Division (HMD) of the US National Library of Medicine (NLM). The collection includes portraits, pictures of institutions, caricatures, genre scenes, and graphic art in a variety of media, illustrating the social and historical aspects of medicine. (FairUseinfo—*external link*)
- *National Science Foundation Image Library—external link* (FairUseinfo—*external link*)

Anatomy

- *Gray's Anatomy—external link*, illustrations (FairUseinfo—*external link*)
- *Slice of Life—external link*—By Suzanne Stensaas and O.E. Millhouse, The Digital Slice of Life is a cooperative project with the *Slice of Life* office—*external link*, KUED Media Solutions—*external link*, and the *Knowledge Weavers Project—external link.*

Embryology

- *Alpha Scientists in Reproductive Medicine—external link*, an IHR infertility website that has *given permission for us to use their embryology images for education.* Alpha Scientists is a nonprofit organization which provides an international forum for scientists in reproductive medicine.
- *Embryo Images—Normal & Abnormal Mammalian Development—external link*— This site is an online tutorial developed by Drs Kathleen K Sulik and Peter R Bream Jr with the assistance of Mr Tim Poe and Ms Kiran Bindra. This tutorial uses scanning electron micrographs (SEMs) to teach mammalian embryology. *There are also line drawings that require specific permission for use. We are allowed to use Dr. Sulik's images for educational purposes.*
- *The Multidimensional Human Embryo—external link* is a collaboration funded by the National Institute of Child Health and Human Development (NICHD) to produce and make available over the Internet a three-dimensional image reference of the human embryo based on magnetic resonance imaging. *The collection of images is intended to serve students, researchers, clinicians, and the general public interested in studying and teaching human development. Our "faculty can use this material without any licensing fees if they link directly to the Web site."*—We thank Dr. Bradley R. Smith for permission.

Histology

- *Blue Histology—external link*—school of anatomy and human biology, The University of Western Australia (FairUseinfo—*external link*)
- *Blood Line—external link*—the online resource for hematology education and news (FairUseinfo—*external link*)
- The Jay Doc Histo Web—*external link*—designed for University of Kansas medical students. Includes tissue slides of cell structure, epithelia, glands, nervous system, muscles, connective tissue, cartilage, bone, vascular system, blood, lymphoid system, skin, respiratory system, gastrointestinal system, eye and ear, endocrine system, urinary system, male and female reproductive system, and histopathology. (FairUseinfo—*external link*)
- *Patho Pic Pathology Image Database—external link*—Beautiful pathology images (FairUseInfo—*external link*)
- *University of Delaware's Histology Images—external link*—This website contains color histology images, compressed histology images, cell and tissue ultrastructure images, labeled illustrations, and three-dimensional models. *Dr. Roger C. Wagner has given us permission to use these images for education.*
- *USC's General Histology Images—external link*—There are 836 photomicrographs of histologic sections in this site. (FairUseinfo—*external link*)
- USC's Oral Histology Images—There are 429 photomicrographs of histologic sections in this site. (FairUseinfo—*external link*)

Neuroanatomy

- *Atlases of the Brain—external link*, contains images of the coronal brain, brain stem, spinal cord, MRI axial, MRI coronal, and MRI sagittal (FairUseinfo—*external link*)
- *The Neuro-Ophthalmology Virtual Education Library (NOVEL)—external link*—This project aims to create a model for the development of digital collections through academic library and professional society partnerships using electronic publishing technologies and a collaboration between the Spencer S. Eccles Health Sciences Library and the North American Neuro-Ophthalology Society (NANOS). (FairUseinfo—*external link*)
- *Synapse Web—external link*, images and tools (Fair Use info—*external link*)
- *Brain Maps—external link*—BrainMaps.org is a digital brain atlas based on high-resolution images of serial sections of monkey brains that is fully integrated with a high-speed database server for querying and retrieving data about primate brain structure and function over the Internet. (FairUseinfo—*external link*)

General Images and Media:

- *FreePhoto.com—external link* (FairUseinfo—*external link*)
- *Internet Archive—external link*, a website containing multiple media types for academic and research use. (FairUseinfo—*external link*)
- *New York Public Library Picture Collection—external link, The Picture Collection Online* is an image resource site for those who seek knowledge and inspiration from visual materials. It is a collection of 30,000 digitized images

from books, magazines, and newspapers, as well as original photographs, prints, and postcards, mostly created before 1923. (FairUseinfo—*external link*)

- *NOAA Photo Library—external link* (FairUseinfo—*external link*)
- *Open Photo—external link*, a public domain general photo library (FairUseinfo—*external link*)
- *University of Utah Photo Bank—external link* (FairUseinfo—*external link*)
- *U.S. Fish & Wildlife Service National Image Library—external link* (FairUseinfo—*external link*)
- The Whole Brain Atlas—*external link* includes still pictures and movies (*.html and *.mpg files) of the brain. The website has received favorable reviews from MedWorld Bestsites, Neurosciences on the Internet, and Medical Matrix. The creators allow use and distribution of these materials for educational purposes as long as proper credit is provided. (FairUseinfo—*external link*)

Animations

- *Brain Atlas: Striatal System—external link*
- *Embryological Modeling Research Group—external link*
- *Hyper Heart—external link*: An interactive animation/movie developed for Dr. Blumenthal's pharmacology course detailing bloodflow, aortic/ventricular volumes, and pressures present in a normal cardiac cycle.
- *Oculucephalic Reflex—external link*
- *Pathway Quizzes in Neuroanatomy—external link*
- *Voluntary Control of Facial Muscles*

SIMPLE QUESTIONS IN CLASS

1. *Cardiomyocyte* means
   a. Calcium in muscle
   b. Heart muscle cycling
   c. Heart muscle cell
   d. Heart beating
2. The relation between gross anatomy and histology is similar to that between
   a. Atomic physics and molecular physics
   b. Macrostructure and microstructure studies in materials science
   c. Microstructure and properties of materials
   d. Structure and function of functional materials

PROBLEMS AND EXERCISES

1. Find out about and compare what each of the following roots means:
   a. Arthro-, athero-, and arterio-
   b. Meso-, meta-, and mero-
   c. Narco-, naso-, necro, and neo-
   d. -osis, osseo-, and ossi-
   e. -plasia, -plasty, and -plegia
   f. -stalsis, -stasis, and staxis

2. Explain what each of the following medical branches is about:
   a. Biochemistry
   b. Anatomy
   c. Histology
   d. Physiology
   e. Pathology
   f. Cytology
   g. Immunology
   h. Epidemiology

CHAPTER 13

HUMAN ANATOMY AND DISEASES I

Integumentary, Skeletal, Muscular, Nervous, and Endocrine Systems

LEARNING OBJECTIVES

After a careful study of this chapter, you should be able to do the following:

1. Be familiar with gross structures of skin, bone, muscle, nerve, and endocrine systems
2. Describe the regenerative ability of each organ or tissue
3. Describe the characteristics of stem cells
4. Describe the major clinic issues of each system, and current or potential applications of biomaterials

13.1 INTEGUMENTARY SYSTEM [1,2]

13.1.1 Gross Anatomy of Skin

The integumentary system refers to skin, which consists of the integument proper (cutaneous membrane) and its derivatives (accessory structures). The integument proper is the outermost covering of the whole body, a continuous structure covering the bone, muscles, and internal organs. The cutaneous membrane includes the outer cellular epidermis layer and deeper dermis, as listed in Table 13.1. The epidermis consists of a layer of cells joined at their edges to form a continuous sheet (epithelium) (Figure 13.1). The dermis layer consists of connective tissue (readers are referred to Chapter 18 for

Table 13.1

Gross Anatomy of Skin

- The cutaneous membrane, including
  - Superficial epidermis ⎫
  - Dermis ⎬ skin
  - Hypodermis (subcutaneous layer)
- Accessory structures, including
  - Hair follicles with smooth muscle
  - Exocrine glands
  - Nerves
  - Nails

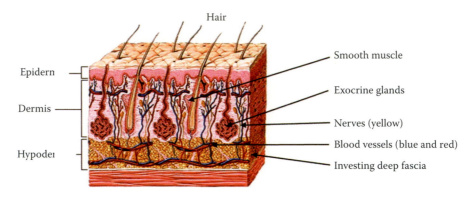

Figure 13.1
The integument and related structures.

more details), and it cushions the body from stress and strain. Beneath the dermis is the subcutaneous layer, which is known as the investing deep fascia, a type of fibrous ligament-like tissue involved in anchoring the skin to the body (connective tissue). The integumentary accessories include structural elements: hairs, nails, and various glands of the skin (Figure 13.1). The structure of the skin is also maintained by collagen and elastin networks that reside within the epidermis.

Functional elements of the skin include smooth muscle connected to the hairs, nerve endings which give the sense of touch, and a blood supply. Importantly, epithelium and connective tissue are two of the *four basic tissue types*, along with muscle and nervous tissue. You will find in Chapter 18 that all tissues fall into these four basic categories, and most organs and organ systems have more than one type. The integumentary system, as well as muscle and nerve, contains all four tissue types.

13.1.2 Functions of Skin

The skin has several functions:

- The skin covers and protects the body from abrasion, bacterial attack, ultraviolet radiation, water, and dehydration.
- It helps maintain temperature (heat loss via sweat production and evaporation).
- Its vessels serve as a blood reservoir for the body, and provide nutrients to the epithelial cell layers.

- The skin produces vitamin D required for calcium metabolism.
- Its nerve endings are essential in detecting environmental stimuli (e.g., heat, pressure, pain).

13.1.3 Regenerative Ability of the Skin and Stem Cells

The skin is one of the most regenerative organs in the body. It can self-repair effectively even after considerable damage has occurred, unless damage is so severe that only partial restoration can occur. Small populations of progenitor cells residing in the epidermis are able to regenerate the damaged cell layers and connective matrix. These include fibroblasts (cells that maintain the collagen and elastin networks), keratinocytes (cells that maintain the waterproof keratin layer on the outer epidermis), and epidermal stem cells. Other progenitor cells come from *adipose (fat) tissue* (Figure 13.2) and bone marrow.

So, all cells have a specific role in a particular organ system. This is called *cell specialization*, and specialized cells are assigned to a specific anatomical location, playing their required roles, undergoing regeneration from within the tissue itself. These subpopulations were established during early organ formation, and typically cannot move to another location to perform another role.

Progenitor cells are types of *stem cells*, cells characterized by the ability to reproduce themselves and to differentiate into a diverse range of specialized cell types. Stem cells are broadly categorized into two classes:

1. *Embryonic stem cells (ESC)* exist in a developing embryo, not yet specialized, but gradually becoming adult tissues as the organism forms. They can differentiate into all of the specialized embryonic tissues that form all of the major tissue types.
2. *Somatic (adult) stem cells* present in adult organs. Like in the skin, these stem cells act as a repair system for the body, replenishing specialized cells, but also maintaining the normal turnover of cell populations in blood, skin, bone, or intestinal tissues. Bone marrow and adipose tissue are the best known sources of adult stem cells; the latter are restricted to blood cell lineages (e.g., leukocytes, erythrocytes).

Readers are referred to Chapter 16, where stem cells are discussed in greater detail.

13.1.4 Threatening Skin Injury: Burns

Although there are a number of diseases associated with the skin, this organ normally does not develop as threatening diseases as many other internal organs, such as heart

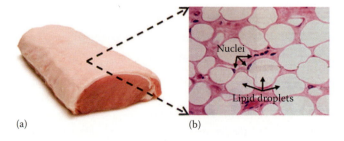

(a)   (b)

Figure 13.2
(a) Fat as we see with naked eyes and (b) the microstructure of adipose tissue.

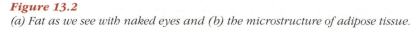

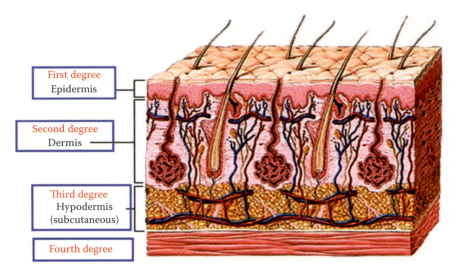

First degree
Epidermis

Second degree
Dermis

Third degree
Hypodermis
(subcutaneous)

Fourth degree

Figure 13.3
Traditional classification system of burns: first-, second-, third-, or fourth-degree.

and lung, due to its excellent regenerative ability, as well as the ease of visual diagnosis. Severe burns are common injuries that threaten this system, caused by a range of external stimuli such as heat, electricity, chemicals, friction, or radiation.

Burns can be classified by depth, mechanism of injury, extent, and associated injuries. The most commonly used classification is based on the depth of injury. The traditional system of classifying burns categorizes them as first-, second-, third-, or fourth-degree (Figure 13.3). This system is now being replaced by one reflecting the need for surgical intervention (Table 13.2). Today, the burn depths are described either

- Superficial
- Superficial partial-thickness
- Deep partial-thickness
- Full-thickness

Compared with the tradition classification of 1–4 grades, the modern nomenclatures listed earlier serve the purpose to guide treatment and predict outcome. Full-thickness, or third-degree, burn injuries usually require hospitalization and surgical treatment, including skin grafting, which is only required if the burn does not prove fatal. Autografting (transplanting from one area of the patient's body to another) is the

Table 13.2
Traditional and Current Classifications of Burns

Traditional	Current	Injury Depth
First-degree	Superficial thickness	Epidermis involvement
Second-degree	Partial thickness—superficial	Superficial (papillary) dermis
Second-degree	Partial thickness—deep	Deep (reticular) dermis
Third- or Fourth-degree	*Full thickness*[a]	*Dermis and underlying tissue and possibly muscle or bone*

[a] *Skin grafting is needed.*

standard procedure in this case. Due to the limited availability of sufficient skin from burned patients, artificial skin is desired.

13.1.5 Applications of Biomaterials in Full-Thickness Burns

As described in Chapter 10, a PGLA-based polymer has been used to fabricate Dermagraft®, which is a cryopreserved human fibroblast-derived dermal substitute composed of fibroblasts, extracellular matrix from skin tissue, and a bioresorbable scaffold (polyglactin) (Figure 10.11). This product has been reported to have successfully been applied in the treatment of full-thickness burns (Figure 10.12).

However, the major drawback of Dermagraft is that time-consuming and complex cultivation procedures are needed to produce sufficient amounts of autologous keratinocyte epithelial sheets. The time is such that it is possible to miss the critical period for treatment, and the complex cultivation procedures could cause complications or introduce infections. An off-the-shelf product that can be applied topically in a more practical time frame is yet to be developed. This may be remedied by the use of decellularized biomaterials, which can be stored for long periods.

13.2 SKELETAL SYSTEM [1,2]

13.2.1 Gross Anatomy of Skeleton

13.2.1.1 Two Subskeletons   The skeleton provides a rigid support or framework for the human body, protecting the vital organs (heart, lung, brain, liver) and enabling body movement. It is basically a combination of bones joined together by ligaments and other connective tissue. Bone is also called *osseous tissue*, by definition a type of connective tissue. The skeletal system consists of two major subdivisions (Figure 13.4):

- The *axial skeleton*, including
  - The skull
  - The vertebral column
  - The thoracic cage

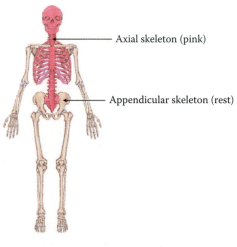

Figure 13.4
The axial and appendicular skeleton.

- The appendicular skeleton, composed of
  - Upper limbs
  - Lower limbs
  - The pectoral girdles
  - The pelvic girdle

13.2.1.2 Types of Bones The adult human body has 206 bones in total. There are five types of bones in the human body according to the shape of the bone. These are long bones, short bones, flat bones, irregular bones, and sesamoid bones (embedded within a tendon, not joined by ligaments to another bone) (Figure 13.5).

13.2.1.3 Gross Structure of an Individual Long Bone The two ends and the middle part of a long bone are defined as (Figure 13.6):

1. *Diaphysis (shaft)*: The shaft is the central portion of a long bone.
2. *Epiphysis (end)*: The ends of long bones are made up mainly of *cancellous (spongy) bone* tissue, although in growing immature bones a thin plate of cartilage exists between the epiphysis and diaphysis.

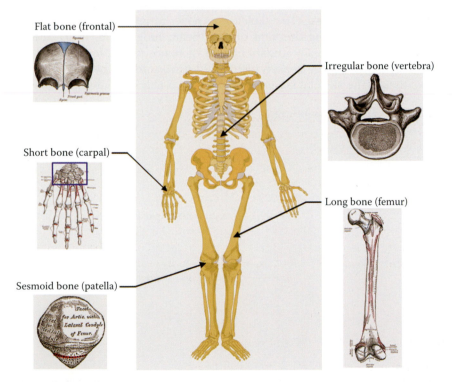

Figure 13.5
Five types of bones in the human body. (The skeleton is from the WikimediaCommons, http://commons.wikimedia.org/ and the examples of five types of bones are Gray's Anatomy on http://www.bartleby.com.)

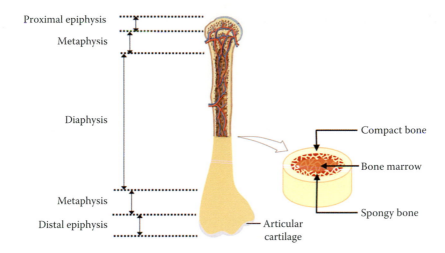

Proximal epiphysis
Metaphysis
Diaphysis
Metaphysis
Distal epiphysis
Articular cartilage
Compact bone
Bone marrow
Spongy bone

Figure 13.6
Parts of a long bone.

If we view the cross section of an individual bone, we see the following (Figure 13.6):

1. *Cortex* is the outer layer of the individual bone. It is made up of *compact (dense) bone* tissue. The cortex of the shaft region is thickened as required by applied physical stresses.
2. *Medulla* is the central portion of the individual bone. It consists of *cancellous (spongy) bone* tissue. In long bones, the medulla includes a space without intervening bony tissue, called the *medullary* or *marrow cavity*.

13.2.1.4 Articulations and Articular Cartilage Joints are also called *articulations*, enabling movement between adjacent bones, where two or more bones meet. They may be in direct contact or separated by cartilage or fluid. An *articular cartilage* covers each area where a bone contacts another bone. This articular cartilage is made up of fibrous tissue and provides a smooth surface for motions (Figure 13.7).

Other nonarticular (static) joints are made from long and short ligaments, which form rigid connections between bones. These joints are static, with some flexibility, and generally restricted to the axial skeleton. Examples include joints between skull bones (sutures), between teeth and jaw bones (periodontal ligaments), and between vertebrae of the spinal column. Hand (carpal) and foot (tarsal) bones near the wrist and ankle joints are also rigid, with many bones fitting together like pieces of a jigsaw puzzle.

13.2.2 Functions of Bone

The human skeleton serves the following functions:

- Support and protect body tissues and organs
- Provide sites for muscle attachment and work with muscles to perform movement
- Produce red blood cells (in bone marrow)
- Store mineral salts

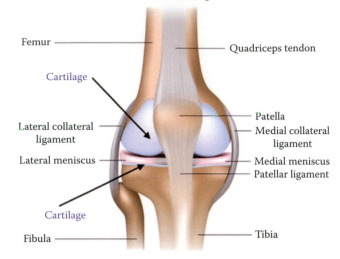

Anterior view of the right knee

Figure 13.7
Anatomy of synovial joint.

The optimal combination of strength and toughness in bone is the result of its con-stituents, as well as the hierarchy structure, which are 68 wt.% of inorganic mineral (hydroxyapatite), 30 wt.% of organic collagen, and 2 wt.% of osteocytes. Hydroxyapatite is strong, and thus tolerates compression. Collagen fibers are tough and flexible, and thus tolerate stretching, twisting, and bending. Without collagen, bone would be too brittle to maintain integrity when impacted by an external force. Without hydroxyapa-tite, the collagen simply bends out of the way when compressed.

13.2.3   Development of Bone

The formation of human skeleton starts in the early fetus, but the early form is not of bony material. Bones do however form in the location they will eventually occupy, and will have the general shape of the adult bones they will later become. There are two types of bones according to the modes of bone formation (or osteogenesis): *membranous bones* and *cartilaginous bones*, both involving the differentiation of a preexisting mesenchymal tissue (later-stage migratory types of embryonic stem cells) into bone tissue.

1. The direct conversion of mesenchymal tissue into bone is called *intramembra-nous ossification* (Figure 13.8). This process occurs primarily in the bones of the skull (Figure 13.9).
2. In other cases, such as the long bones, the mesenchymal cells differentiate into cartilage, and this cartilage is later replaced by bone, a process called *endochondral ossification*. This extremely complicated process starts from the development of cartilage tissue, which is then calcified to form spongy (cancel-lous) bone, and later increases in density to form compact bone (Figure 13.10).

13.2.4   Regenerative Capacity of Bone

Bone has an excellent ability to regenerate due to the existence of osteoprogenitor cells (osteoblasts, residual mesenchymal cells) in the *periosteum* (Figure 13.11). Stem cells are also present in the bone marrow (Figure 13.6) (hemopoietic stem cells, also called

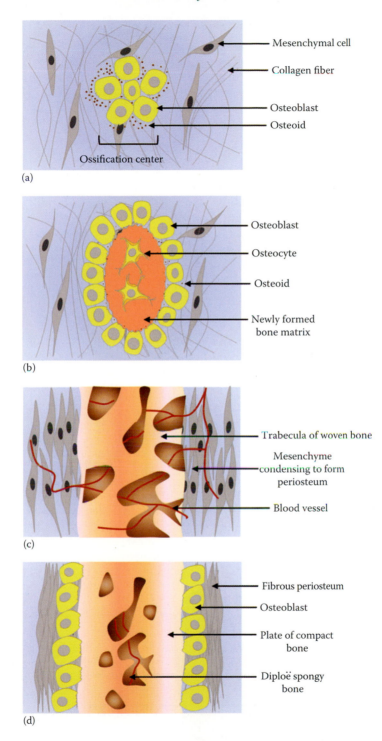

Figure 13.8
Intramembranous ossification. (a) An ossification center appears in the fibrous connective tissue membrane. (b) Bone matrix (osteoid) is secreted within the fibrous membrane. (c) Woven bone and periosteum form. (d) A bone collar of compact bone forms and red marrow appears.

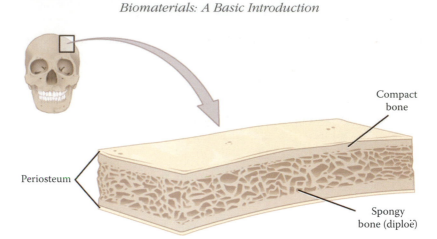

Figure 13.9
Structure of flat bone in the skull. (From the WikimediaCommons, http://commons.wikimedia.org/.)

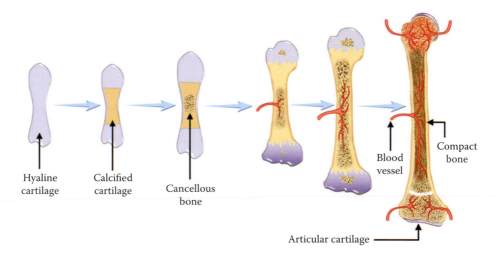
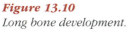

Figure 13.10
Long bone development.

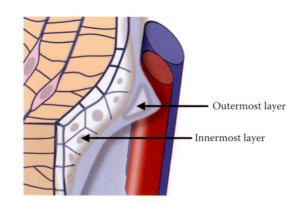

Figure 13.11
Periosteum and the innermost layer of osteoprogenior cells.

bone marrow stem cells, also originating from residual mesenchyme). The periosteum covers the bone surface not already covered by the articular cartilage, comprising of the innermost cellular layer and the outer fibrous layer.

The innermost layer is where the bone-forming (osteogenic) osteoblasts reside, remaining in a quiescent state under normal growth conditions. When an injury such as a fracture occurs to a bone, osteoblasts begin to increase their proliferation rate, differentiating into mature bone cells (osteocytes). The outermost layer is a type of fibrous connective tissue layer, containing collagen fibers, sensory nerve fibers, and blood vessels that supply the inner layer and medulla. The vessels are also involved in the clotting process during the acute phase of fracture repair, when a fibrous clot forms, gradually replaced with collagen by fibroblasts brought in by new vessels. This collagen eventually forms a random fibrous network, which eventually calcifies (~6 weeks) and remodels to form the aligned layers of compact bone (~3 months).

13.2.5 The Most Common Bone Disease: Osteoporosis

Bone disease is a condition that damages the skeleton and makes bones weak and prone to fractures. Although weak bones are not necessarily caused by aging, aging is the major reason for bone weakening. The most common bone disease is *osteoporosis*, which is characterized by low bone mass and deterioration of bone structure. This health issue continues to grow with the increase of aging populations (Figure 13.12). Worldwide, osteoporosis causes more than 8.9 million fractures annually, resulting in an osteoporotic fracture every 3 s. Worldwide, 1 in 3 women and

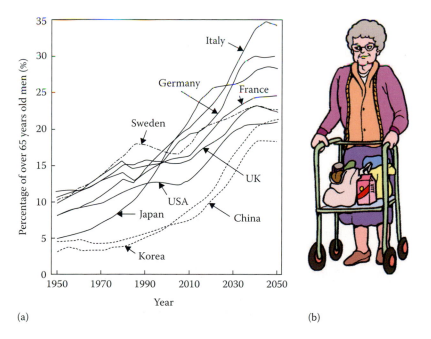

(a)   (b)

Figure 13.12
(a) Trend of aging population and (b) the associated osteoporosis issue, especially in the bones at the load-bearing sites. (With kind permission from Springer Science+Business Media: Metallurg. Mater. Trans. A, Recent metallic materials for biomedical applications, 33, 2002, 477, Niinomi, M., 2, copyright 2007.)

435

1 in 5 men aged over 50 will experience osteoporotic fractures. Osteoporosis is estimated to affect 200 million women worldwide—approximately one-tenth of women aged 60, one-fifth of women aged 70, two-fifths of women aged 80, and two-thirds of women aged 90.

Osteoporosis is mainly caused by lack of dietary minerals (e.g., calcium, fluoride), and lack of load bearing on the skeleton. Cyclic load bearing is actually transduced into micro- and nanoscale signals that stimulate osteocytes, even during low-impact movement such as walking. Thus, low-impact exercise is actually preventative against loss of bone density.

13.2.6   Applications of Biomaterials in Skeleton System

As mentioned at the beginning of Section 13.2, the primary function of the skeleton is to provide a mechanical framework to the human body. This explains why orthopedics is the largest section of medicine in terms of usage of biomaterial devices, especially metallic implants. Various applications of biomaterials in orthopedics have been described in Chapters 4 through 11. Briefly, these include short-term temporary internal fixation devices (e.g., pins, nail, screws, and plates; Figure 4.8), long-term temporary internal fixation devices (e.g., spinal cord correction devices; Figure 4.1a), permanent implants (e.g., total joint replacements; Figures 4.14 and 4.15), bone fillers (Figure 7.4a,b), tooth restorations (Figures 5.1, 5.3, and 11.9), bone cements (Figure 9.10), and innovative bone-tissue-engineering scaffolds (Figure 7.4d).

A major challenge in the application of biomaterials to treat bone diseases is associated mostly with total hip replacement (THR), resulting from erosion and fracture of the femoral head, a very common procedure in aged patients. The success rate of THR prosthesis after 20 years implantation is only around 60%–70%. The failure rate (30%–40%) is unsatisfactorily high since the life span of patients is often longer than 20 years after joint replacement implantation. Also, if prosthetic failure occurs, it is extremely difficult to remove the ruptured implants from patients, due to their permanent design. Therefore, innovative treatment strategies for bone tissue engineering are highly desirable, to enable bone regeneration in parallel with mechanical joint support.

13.3   MUSCULAR SYSTEM [1,2]

The skeletal and muscular systems are structurally and functionally interdependent. They are often considered to be a single musculoskeletal system.

13.3.1   Gross Anatomy of Muscle

When talking about muscle, most people will immediately consider skeletal muscle (Figure 13.13a). There are actually three types of muscular tissue in the body (Figure 13.13b):

1. Skeletal muscle
2. Cardiac muscle
3. Smooth muscle

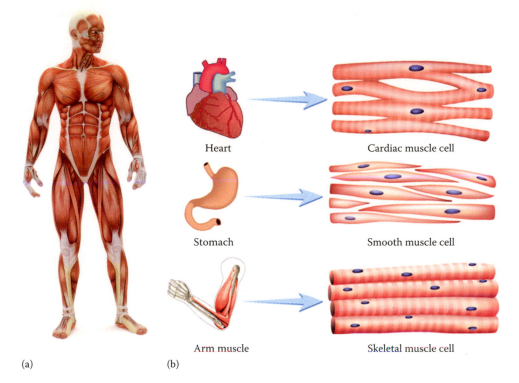

Heart   Cardiac muscle cell

Stomach   Smooth muscle cell

Arm muscle   Skeletal muscle cell

(a)   (b)

Figure 13.13
(a) Skeletal muscle and (b) three types of muscles.

These muscle tissues share four basic characters:

1. Excitability
2. Contractility
3. Extensibility
4. Elasticity

13.3.2   Skeletal Muscle

Each skeletal muscle is an individual organ of the human body. Each is attached to bones by connective tissues, having an origin and an insertion point of tendons (bundles of collagen fibers) as well as its own individual blood and nerve supply. A typical muscle, such as one which controls a joint (e.g., quadriceps over the knee joint) will contract, bringing the point of insertion toward the point of origin, using the joint as a leverage point. Their motion is voluntary, being controlled by the so-called motor nerves, which contract the muscle at the will of the individual. There are also finer sensory nerves within muscle controlling reflexes, pain, and stretch.

Structurally, skeletal muscle is characterized by striations (Figure 13.13b) referring to bands of protein that run perpendicular to the fibers that run along the muscle. The striations form anchorage points against which the contractile proteins within the muscle cells exert tension, in units called sarcomeres. Many muscle cells are joined in parallel, to form individual fibrils, which in turn are bundled together in the hundreds to form a single muscle fiber. In cross section, a muscle can be seen as having several fibers. Functionally, a single muscle contraction involves millions of sarcomere proteins under the control of calcium signaling, triggered by a nerve stimulus.

Skeletal muscle has limited regenerative ability, although there are progenitor cells (called satellite cells) in this tissue. *Muscular atrophy* is the most common muscular disease. Because muscles and nerves (neurons) supplying muscle operate as a functional unit, disease of both systems results in muscular atrophy and paralysis. Diseases and disorders that result from direct abnormalities of the muscles are called *primary muscle diseases*; those that can be traced as symptoms or manifestations of disorders of nerves or other systems are not properly classified as primary muscle diseases.

13.3.3 Cardiac Muscle

Like skeletal muscle, cardiac muscle is striated, but is characterized by extensive branching between cardiac muscle cells (cardiomyocytes), rather than independent myocytes (Figure 13.13b). Cardiac muscle operates on an involuntary basis, by cyclic firing of automatic motor nerves in the midbrain, assisted by automatic firing at specific points (nodes) around the heart. This results in cardiomyocytes contracting in a simultaneous wave to create a single heartbeat. The branching of cardiomyocytes enables a high level of connectivity between them, enabling calcium signals to fire simultaneously. This causes the muscle wall (*myocardium*) to contract at once, thereby rapidly changing the chamber volume, creating a pump that maintains constant blood circulation.

The myocardium itself is relatively thick, made up of mostly muscle fibers, but also strengthened by a network of collagen fibers. In terms of repair of the damaged heart, such as during cardiac enlargement in people with morbid obesity and/or cardiovascular disease, *the myocardium has virtually no regenerative capacity. Heart disease is the number one killer of human beings.* Readers are referred to Chapter 14 for more discussion topics on tissue-engineering approaches to repairing heart muscle.

13.3.4 Smooth (Visceral) Muscle

Smooth muscle is similar to cardiac muscle, in that it is involuntary but, as its name suggests, has no striations. Smooth muscle makes up the muscular component of various internal organs (*viscera*) of the thorax and abdomen. Organs include the gastrointestinal tract (digestive system), respiratory tract (lungs, bronchi, diaphragm, trachea), male and female reproductive tract (e.g., uterus, Fallopian tube), and the urinary system (e.g., bladder, ureters). Within these organs, smooth muscle is mainly in the form of circular bands of muscle (e.g., sphincters) that contract tubular structures (e.g., major arteries and other vessels (Figure 13.14)) and the digestive system (Figure 13.15), allowing transport of contents by cyclic waves of contractility.

Smooth muscle also forms a component of the walls of larger chambers, including the muscle wall of the uterus (*myometrium*) and the bladder. Elsewhere in the body, microscopic smooth muscle is also found adjacent to hair follicles of the skin and ciliary muscles of the eye.

Unlike the skeletal and cardiac muscle, *smooth muscle has excellent regenerative ability.* The most common disease associated with blood vessels is *thrombosis*, which

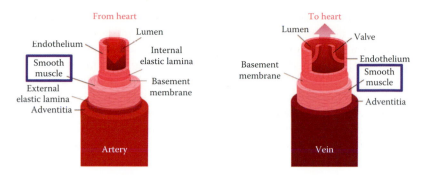

Figure 13.14
Three major layers of a blood vessel, the smooth muscle forms the middle layer.

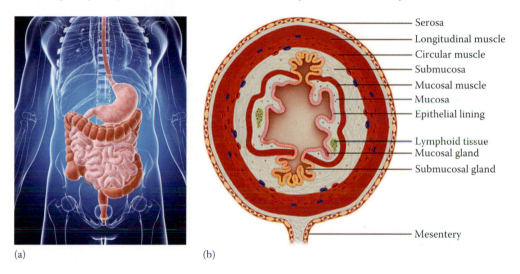

(a)   (b)

Figure 13.15
(a) Various gastrointestinal tracts in the body and (b) their cross-sectional structure. (From Virtualmedicalcentre.com, http://www.myvmc.com/anatomy/gastrointestinal-system/.)

however is not a problem of the muscular layer. The muscle in blood vessel renders the vessel with the elastic and flexible mechanical properties. Since the major function of blood vessels is to provide a physical tube for blood circulation, biomaterials find several applications here. Artificial blood vessels made of PTFE have successfully been used to repair/replace the aorta (Figure 9.13), which has a relatively large diameter compared with other blood vessels, although thrombosis remains a critical challenge in this area.

The most threatening disease of other viscera (such as gastrointestinal tract and respiratory tract) is *cancer*, a condition of uncontrolled cell division of normal tissues. The function of gastrointestinal tracts is to digest food we eat, a complex biochemical process. As such, these organs cannot be entirely replaced by any biomaterials, except for some structural elements, such as the connective tissue. The standard surgical treatment for cancer in these organs is to remove the tumor and adjacent tissues, and reconnect the rest of tracts or ducts by suturing. Fortunately, the excellent regenerative ability these organs increases the chances of recovery of the remaining parts. This is another example demonstrating the limit of biomaterials application, as discussed in Chapter 12. The application of biomaterials is limited to the replacement of a biological tissue or organ, with primarily mechanical roles (e.g., bladder).

13.3.5   Regenerative Ability and Cancer Susceptibility

Among the three types of muscles, skeletal and heart muscles have little regenerative capacity, while the smooth muscle is characterized as regenerative. It is common knowledge that the former two muscles have little cancer susceptibility, while the latter does. In general, however, muscle is less likely to form cancers than epithelial or glandular tissues, because of the higher rates of cell division in the latter. In the digestive tract, for example, a tumor may form in either of these tissues, due to abnormally high proliferation of intestinal epithelium, which is normally replaced on a daily basis, whereas the smooth muscle stays intact over a lifetime. However, a localized tumor can affect the function of the muscle by compression or displacement, thereby affecting organ function.

As a general rule, good regeneration ability is always coupled with increased cancer susceptibility. This is because the regeneration process of a tissue involves more active tissue maintenance, resulting from high levels of cell division. Dividing cells are more likely to respond to chemical or radiation carcinogens than nondividing cells. As a result, cancer rates are highest in regenerative tissues where frequent stem cell division keeps pace with the regeneration of damaged or lost tissue. Less actively dividing tissues (e.g., neural and muscle tissues), where stem cell divisions do not normally occur, are therefore less likely to form cancers. This concept will be further discussed in Chapter 16.

13.4   NERVOUS SYSTEM [1,2]

13.4.1   Gross Anatomy of the Nervous System

The nervous system is perhaps the most complex cellular system in the body. It is basically a center for data processing and signaling both voluntary and automatic functions in all tissues and organs. The system is an integrated network of neural tissue (Figure 13.16a), comprising two subsystems: the central nervous system (CNS) made of the brain and the spinal cord (Figure 13.16b) and the peripheral nervous system (PNS), including all of the neural tissue outside the CNS. The PNS is the signal transduction network, made up of both sensory and motor nerve fibers, which connect directly to the brain via the spinal cord, from which specific segments branch out to specific tissues.

The *brain* is considered one of the six vital organs of the body (Table 13.3), which are essential to life and without which the body will not survive. It is made up of a solid mass of more than 15 different kinds of nerve cells (neuron), the basic functional unit of the brain, arranged in highly organized, interconnected layers called the cerebral cortex. Here, most of the data processing of thought, decision making, sensory awareness, and coordination of movement take place. Central control of the endocrine and circadian rhythms also take place here. Neurons are further organized in functional units called centers, with their cell bodies in dense regions called gray matter, which are bridged by millions of shorter fibers (axons) arranged in parallel

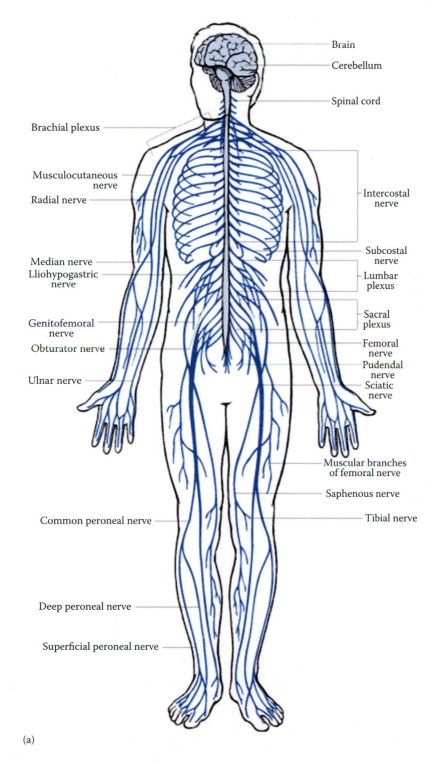

Brain

Cerebellum

Spinal cord

Brachial plexus

Musculocutaneous nerve

Radial nerve

Intercostal nerve

Subcostal nerve

Median nerve

Lliohypogastric nerve

Lumbar plexus

Sacral plexus

Genitofemoral nerve

Obturator nerve

Femoral nerve

Pudendal nerve

Ulnar nerve

Sciatic nerve

Muscular branches of femoral nerve

Saphenous nerve

Common peroneal nerve

Tibial nerve

Deep peroneal nerve

Superficial peroneal nerve

(a)

Figure 13.16

(a) The nervous system of the human body and   *(Continued)*

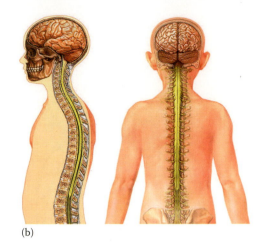

(b)

Figure 13.16 (Continued)
(b) central nervous system.

Table 13.3
Six Vital Organs and Their Major Functions

Organs	Major Functions
Brain	Control of all body systems; control of movement and integration of sensory input; feedback and data processing for thought and decision making; center for endocrine system
Heart	To pump blood, maintaining blood pressure to meet demand of tissue for vital nutrients
Lungs	Absorb oxygen from air, remove CO_2 from metabolic processes; control of humidification
Kidneys	Filter toxic elements; filter ions and maintain blood levels of aqueous species (e.g., protein, metabolites); control of water balance; control of blood pressure; control stress response via adrenalin
Liver	Removal of blood waste products; regulation of fatty acid digestion
Pancreas	Regulate blood glucose levels using insulin; other digestive roles

tracts (white matter) (Figure 13.17). Cell bodies in the gray matter produce much finer fibers called dendrites, which are interconnected at nanoscale junctions called synapses, where nerve impulses occur, and where a bulk of the signaling for data processing happens. The brain is also highly vascular, with highly dense capillary networks that provide a rich blood supply and keep the neural tissue oxygenated at all times.

Cortical neurons connect to tissues in distant parts of the body via the PNS, using much longer nerve fibers. These are organized directionally as white matter within the *spinal cord*, alongside corresponding gray matter (Figure 13.18), from which the spinal nerves emanate. Spinal nerves are involved in finer tuning of motor function by feedback loops (reflexes) and coordination with automatic functions (so-called autonomic nerves) controlling the other major organ systems, as well as muscles and skin. Amazingly, incoming sensory and outgoing motor signals are located in separate tracts, in either the front or rear of the cord. Thus, the CNS communicates with and

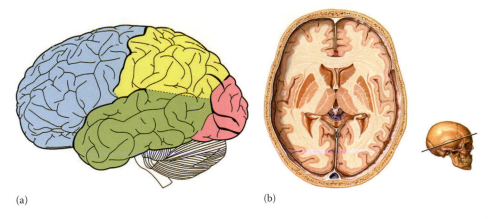

(a)   (b)

Figure 13.17
(a) Brain, a reproduction of Gray's Anatomy. (From the WikimediaCommons, http://commons. wikimedia.org/.) (b) Nerve tissues located in the cranial cavity.

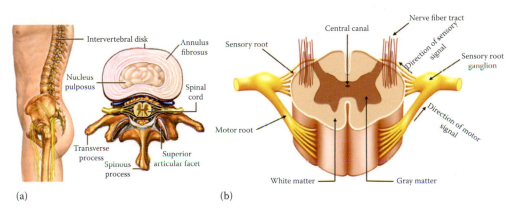

(a)   (b)

Figure 13.18
(a) The cross section of spinal cord and (b) the nerve tissue of gray matter.

coordinates responses to and from stimuli occurring in the PNS, via the spinal cord, in highly localized and discrete areas, with defined boundaries (Figure 13.19).

13.4.2   Regenerative Capacity of the PNS and CNS

Nerve cells cannot reproduce by cell division, but they do have limited ability to regenerate by axonal sprouting under certain conditions (Figure 13.20), especially in the PNS. In this process, the region around the damaged ends of the axon is first cleaned by macrophages, a specialized type of white blood cell involved in the removal of cellular debris. Then the axon reconnects with the head, rebranching and reconnecting to form new synapses. Proliferating Schwann cells, which insulate the axons, also participate in the repair of damaged peripheral nerves.

In contrast, the CNS has very limited regenerative ability, which until recently was believed to be nonexistent, due to the establishment of brain structure and maintenance of neuron populations during childhood. Regenerative failure is primarily attributable to the formation of structural barriers to axonal extension and reconnection,

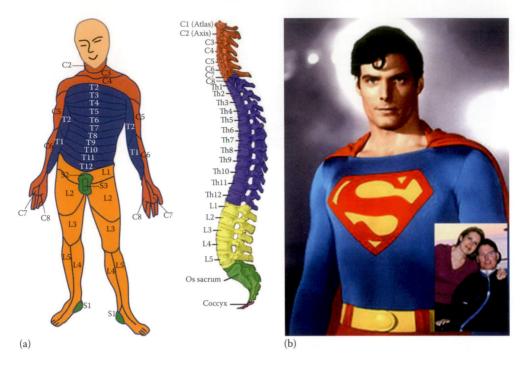

(a)   (b)

Figure 13.19
(a) A spinal nerve chart showing the connection between spinal cord nerve and muscle groups of the human body. (b) Broken spinal cord at C1 led to the tragedy of Superman actor Christopher Reeve.

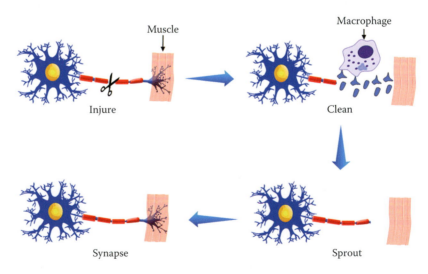

Figure 13.20
Axonal sprouting of an injured nerve cell.

in the form of *scar tissue* composed of astrocytes and connective tissue. While astrocytes undergo reactivation at these sites, and attempt to infiltrate and encourage neurons to regrow, the new branches are blocked from reaching their synaptic targets. There is currently no treatment available to restore nerve function in diseased or damaged CNS.

13.4.3 Nerve Disorders: Degeneration of Brain

Many nerve disorders result from a genetic mutation that can be inherited within families, or can occur spontaneously as a result of chemical or biological toxins (e.g., radiation). They result in damage to the neurons themselves, which leads to problems with performing routine tasks. Two of the most common diseases are Alzheimer's disease and Parkinson's disease. The former is characterized by a loss of processing ability in the brain, resulting in gradual memory loss, while the latter results in uncontrolled motor functions. Degenerative nerve diseases can be serious or life-threatening, and most of them have no cure and/or defined cause at yet, although improvements in diagnostic technology have improved the early detection of tissue damage.

13.4.4 Surgical Reconnection of PNS

For a small-gap injury, the end-to-end reconnection approach is effective if the disconnected fiber ends are directly adjacent to each other, and can be reconnected without tension. Currently, the standard method to bridge a large gap of a damaged nerve is autologous grafting (Figure 13.21). The definitions of grafting types are given in Table 13.4.

13.4.5 Application of Biomaterials and Challenges to Nerve Damage

Currently, the application of biomaterials for the treatment of nerve damage and disorders is largely in the research stage.

13.4.5.1 Nerve-Bridging Device For a large nerve defect, an autologous nerve graft that is harvested from another site in the body is commonly used to span the injury site. Disadvantages of this technique include loss of function at the donor site and the need for multiple surgeries. There are several FDA-approved nerve-bridging

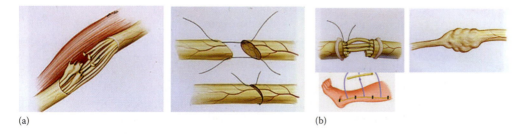

(a)   (b)

Figure 13.21
(a) End-to-end reconnection of small gap injury. (b) Autologous grafting to bridge a large gap.

Table 13.4
Definition of Autologous, Isologous, Allologous (Homologous), Xenologous

Nomenclature	Definition
Autograft	Tissue/organ transplanted from one part of the body to another of the same individual
Isograft	Transplantation of histocompatible tissue between genetically identical individuals, such as monozygotic twins
Allograft/homograft	Tissue/organ transplanted from a donor to a recipient of the same species, with the same blood type
Xenograft	Transplantation from one species to another (e.g., pigs to humans)

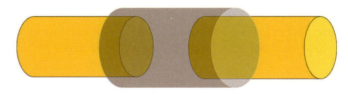

Figure 13.22
Nerve-bridging device.

devices (Figure 13.22) commercially available for relatively *short (several millimeter) nerve defects*. For example: NeuraGen™ Nerve Guide (a type I collagen tube), and SaluBridge™ Nerve Cuff.

13.4.5.2 Nonbiodegradable Artificial Nerve Grafts   Because of its inert and elastic properties, silicon tubing was one of the first and most frequently used synthetic materials for nerve grafts. In vivo intubation of regenerating nerves, however, has often led to long-term complications including fibrosis and chronic nerve compression, requiring surgical removal of the conduit.

13.4.5.3 Neural Tissue Engineering: To Address Major PN Injuries   The concept of nerve tissue engineering is illustrated in Figure 13.23. It aims to use a biomaterial tubing to create a chemically and structurally suitable environment that enhances host nerve tissue to grow. Polyglactin grafts result in poor nerve regeneration due to inflammation, and better results have been obtained with PLA-*co*-PCL, PGA, and poly(organo) phosphazine conduits. A microporous PGA mesh coated with cross-linked collagen to promote tissue proliferation has also successfully supported nerve regeneration.

13.4.5.4 Biomaterials for Drug or Cell Delivery   As depicted in Figure 10.20, another application of biomaterials in nervous system repair, especially for the treatment of CNS problems, is as a vehicle to deliver drugs or cells to the CNS. The methods of drug delivery include local administration at the damage site, or systemic administration through blood circulation, which is typical in the treatment of brain diseases. In systemic administration, drug particles have to travel a long distance before reaching the targeted tissue, and might lose their bioactivity or release kinetics.

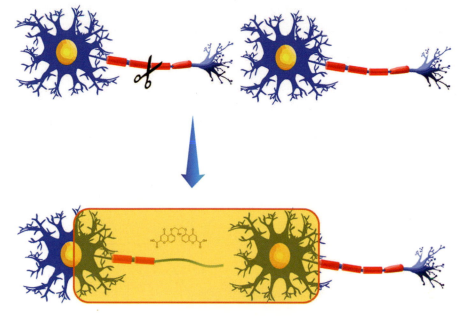

Figure 13.23
Tissue-engineering concept. (Image based on work originally published in Cukjati, D. et al., Med. Biol. Eng. Comput., 39(2), 263, 2001.)

Furthermore, they may not be able to cross the blood–brain barrier. Hence, coating of drug particles (delivery vehicles, carriers) is needed to engineer an appropriate tissue response.

13.5   ENDOCRINE SYSTEM

13.5.1   *Gross Anatomy of the Endocrine System*

The endocrine system consists of a system of several organs glands (Figure 13.24), which are involved in the production and release of hormones into interstitial fluids and the bloodstream. The primary organs of this system include the following:

- Hypothalamus
- Pituitary (gland)
- Pineal (gland)
- Thyroid (gland)
- Parathyroid (gland)
- Thymus
- Pancreas
- Adrenal (gland)
- Ovaries (female)
- Testes

Hormones are long-range signaling proteins that target other tissues, binding to receptors to stimulate a specific function. The glands listed earlier and in Figure 13.23 are the largest and most well defined, and can also signal to smaller glands such as the exocrine

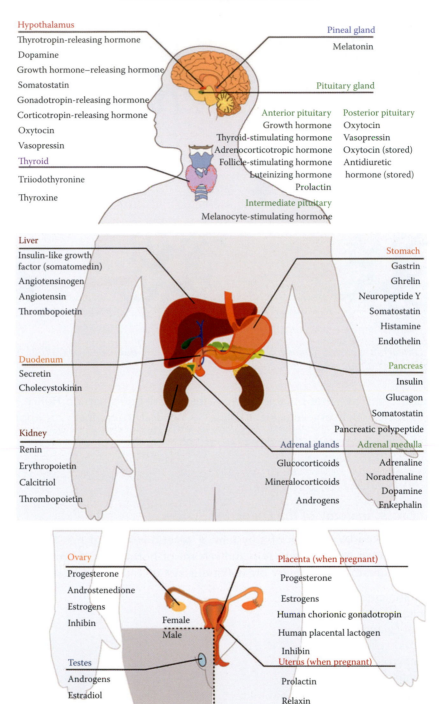

Hypothalamus
Thyrotropin-releasing hormone
Dopamine
Growth hormone–releasing hormone
Somatostatin
Gonadotropin-releasing hormone
Corticotropin-releasing hormone
Oxytocin
Vasopressin

Thyroid
Triiodothyronine
Thyroxine

Pineal gland
Melatonin

Pituitary gland

Anterior pituitary
Growth hormone
Thyroid-stimulating hormone
Adrenocorticotropic hormone
Follicle-stimulating hormone
Luteinizing hormone
Prolactin

Posterior pituitary
Oxytocin
Vasopressin
Oxytocin (stored)
Antidiuretic
hormone (stored)

Intermediate pituitary
Melanocyte-stimulating hormone

Liver
Insulin-like growth
factor (somatomedin)
Angiotensinogen
Angiotensin
Thrombopoietin

Duodenum
Secretin
Cholecystokinin

Kidney
Renin
Erythropoietin
Calcitriol
Thrombopoietin

Stomach
Gastrin
Ghrelin
Neuropeptide Y
Somatostatin
Histamine
Endothelin

Pancreas
Insulin
Glucagon
Somatostatin
Pancreatic polypeptide

Adrenal glands
Glucocorticoids
Mineralocorticoids
Androgens

Adrenal medulla
Adrenaline
Noradrenaline
Dopamine
Enkephalin

Ovary
Progesterone
Androstenedione
Estrogens
Inhibin

Female
Male

Testes
Androgens
Estradiol
Inhibin

Placenta (when pregnant)
Progesterone
Estrogens
Human chorionic gonadotropin
Human placental lactogen
Inhibin
Uterus (when pregnant)
Prolactin
Relaxin

Figure 13.24
The organs of the endocrine system and secreted hormones. Note: The stomach is not an endo-crine organ but responds closely to stimulation of apetite via the listed hormones. (From the WikimediaCommons, http://commons.wikimedia.org/.)

glands (e.g., sweat glands in skin). In addition to the aforementioned specialized endocrine organs, many others (e.g., the kidney, liver, and gonads) have secondary endocrine functions. The kidney, for example, secretes endocrine hormones such as erythropoietin and renin, which control red blood cell production and blood pressure, respectively.

13.5.2   Functions of the Endocrine System

The major functions of this system include hormone signaling for the following:

1. Regulation of routine organ homeostasis (temperature, osmotic pressure, blood pressure, fluid balance etc.)
2. Regulation and coordination of metabolism in all organs
3. Maintenance of daily and monthly cycles (e.g., menstrual cycle, cortisol cycle)
4. Acute tissue and system responses to external stresses
5. Regulation of male and female reproduction

Peripheral endocrine organs are highly specialized to manufacture local hormones in response to other central hormones produced by the hypothalamus and pituitary glands in the brain. Additional control by local nerve stimulation results in controlled secretion of hormones into the bloodstream, controlling metabolic activities of many different tissues and organs simultaneously. An excellent example is the secretion of adrenalin upon sudden sensory stimulation, such as shock. This hormone has immediate effects on blood vessels, autonomic nerves, and smooth muscle.

13.5.3   Cellular/Molecular Therapies and Application of Biomaterials

Cellular and molecular therapies are used to address pathological problems at the cellular and biochemical levels. In this regard, biomaterials can be used as drug/cell delivery vehicles. Pancreatic tissue engineering is a good example of this, with the main focus to restore the insulin-secreting ability of the pancreas in diabetics. The direct implantation of insulin-producing pancreatic islets (clusters of islet cells) into diabetics is an obvious approach. This procedure involves obtaining islets from a compatible donor pancreas, the patient's own pancreas, or those derived from stem cells. Pancreatic islet implantation is considered by many scientists to be a better alternative than pancreas organ transplant; however, successful implantation had not yet been achieved clinically, due to attack of the implanted cells by the immune system of the diabetic patient. Several groups have therefore sought to use natural polymers to encapsulate islet cells to protect them from attack. The polymer alginate is commonly used; however, collagen, chitosan, gelatin, and agarose have also been tested.

13.6   CHAPTER HIGHLIGHTS

1. Two primary layers of skin—epidermis and dermis (note: hypodermis is not included as a layer of skin):
   a. The *epidermis*, which provides waterproofing and serves as a barrier to infection;
   b. The *dermis*, which serves as a location for the appendages of skin.
2. Application of artificial skin in the treatment of full-thickness burns.
3. Two skeleton subdivisions: axial skeleton and appendicular skeleton.

4. Five types of bones according to the shape of bones: long bones, short bones, flat bones, irregular bones, and sesmoid bones.

5. Two types of bones according to the modes of bone formation (or osteogenesis): membranous bones and cartilaginous bones.

6. Parts of long bone: shafts and ends; cortical (dense) bone and cancellous (spongy) bone.

7. Osteoporosis in the aging population is one important clinical issues, and the application of biomaterials in artificial joints.

8. The skin and bone can regenerate effectively, because stem cells persist in these tissues, and replacing dead cells that have been lost during routine cell division and tissue maintenance.

9. Stem cells are those that can renew themselves and can differentiate into a diverse range of specialized cell types.

10. Three types of muscles:
    a. Skeletal muscle: voluntary movement, limited regenerative ability
    b. Cardiac muscle: automatic movement, very limited regenerative ability
    c. Smooth muscle: automatic movement, regenerative

11. Two subsystems of the nervous system:
    a. Central nervous system (CNS) has a very limited regenerative ability. Regenerative failure is attributable to a structural barrier. A potential application of biomaterials is a drug delivery vehicle and/or scaffold.
    b. Peripheral nervous system (PNS) has regenerative ability, via axonal sprouting and bridging. Biomaterials could be applied as nerve-bridging devices in these nerves.

12. Endocrine system regulates a wide range of homeostatic function, such as metabolism; hormones secreted by glands into the bloodstream; controlled by the brain.

13. Diabetes epidemic (pancreas): biomaterials could be used as drug/cell delivery vehicle to replace missing insulin or insulin-secreting cells.

14. Two major strategies to apply biomaterials:
    a. Biomaterial implants could potentially play a major role for the restoration of physical tissue injury or loss.
    b. In cellular and molecular therapies, biomaterials could be used as drug/cell delivery vehicles as well as just scaffold structures.

ACTIVITIES

Study online via the links given on the list of websites, or find more online sources for your self-studies.

SIMPLE QUESTIONS IN CLASS

1. *Integumentary system* stands for
   a. Digestive system
   b. Skin system
   c. Bone system
   d. Internal system

2. Fill the text to the boxes to identify each region:

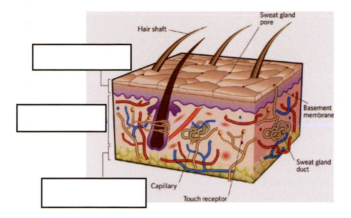

Dermis
Hypodermis
Epidermis

3. What degree of burn needs skin grafting?
   a. Superficial
   b. Superficial partial-thickness
   c. Deep partial-thickness
   d. Full-thickness

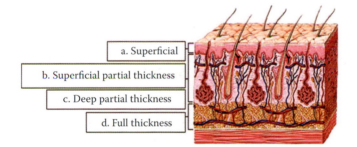

4. Which description about artificial skin, Dermagraft®, is *not* true?
   a. Dermagraft is designed to be a permanent skin graft.
   b. Dermagraft is a copolymer of PLA and PGA.
   c. Dermagraft was applied with some major problems.
   d. The application of Dermagraft is combined with cell therapy.

5. *Osseous tissue* stands for
   a. Skin
   b. Bone
   c. Skeletal muscle
   d. Nerve

6. *Osteocyte* means
   a. Bone tissue
   b. Bone collagen
   c. Bone cell
   d. Bone mineral

7. Which of the following tissues has the least regenerative ability?
   a. Bone
   b. Cartilage
   c. Skin
   d. Hair

8. Bone diseases are not as threatening as those of other vital organs, such as heart and lungs. What pathological scenario presents the number one application of biomaterials in orthopedics, and is anticipated to continue to grow?
   a. Fracture caused by traffic accidents
   b. Osteoporosis due to ageing
   c. Bone cancer
   d. Osteoarthritis

9. A muscle cell is a muscle
   a. Fibril
   b. Filament
   c. Fiber
   d. Protein

10. Among the three types of muscles, which one is voluntary?
    a. Skeletal muscle
    b. Smooth muscle
    c. Cardiac muscle

11. Among the three types of muscles, which one has an extremely limited regenerative ability?
    a. Skeletal muscle
    b. Smooth muscle
    c. Cardiac muscle

12. The central nervous system (CNS) includes
    a. All nerves in the central cavity of vertebrate
    b. Spinal cord
    c. Brain
    d. Brain and spinal cord

13. Which (between a and b) represents the direction of neuron synapses in the peripheral nerve network of the lower legs?

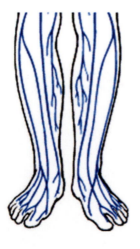 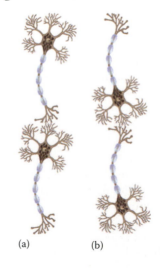

(a)　　　　　(b)

14. Which represents the correct regeneration (sprouting) scenario of the injured PNS nerve fibres shown below?

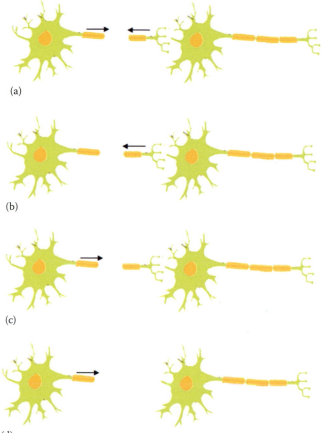

(a)

(b)

(c)

(d)

15. Currently, surgical reconstruction using biomaterial devices can be applied to which of the following tissue damage or disease conditions?
    a. Nerves in brain
    b. Nerve fibers in peripheral nerve system (PNS)
    c. Diabetes (pancreas)
    d. Nerves in the spinal cord

16. Currently, surgical reconstruction using biomaterial devices **cannot** be applied to which of the following tissue damage or disease conditions?
    a. Broken bone
    b. Nerve fibers in peripheral nerve system (PNS)
    c. Diabetes (pancreas)
    d. Blood vessels

17. Name a typical medical device, and its biomaterial, that is used to treat each of the following organ damage conditions:
    a. Bone fracture
    b. Burn
    c. Nerve damage in PNS
    d. Heart attack

PROBLEMS AND EXERCISES

1. Describe the two major characteristics of stem cells.
2. Name five regenerative organs. What is the common mechanism of regenerative ability of regenerative tissues or organs?
3. What are the major functions of somatic (adult) stem cells?
4. Discuss the current standard treatments of large bone defects.
5. List 10 orthopedic implants and the application of biomaterials in these medical devices.
6. Describe the major features of the three types of muscles.
7. Discuss the regenerative abilities of the three muscle tissues.
8. The nervous system can be subdivided into two subsystems. What are they?
9. Neurons cannot divide by mitosis. How is a neuron fiber reconstructed in the peripheral nerve system (PNS) with surgical manipulation? Why cannot neurons in the central nerve system (CNS) regenerate?
10. Discuss the current standard treatments of nerve injuries.
11. Discuss the potential strategy of treatments of nerve injuries using biomaterials.
12. Explain why biomaterials find many applications in the skeletal system, but few in the endocrine system.

ADVANCED TOPIC: BIOMATERIAL CHALLENGES IN BONE TISSUE ENGINEERING

Tissue engineering is essentially a technique for imitating nature. Natural tissues consist of three components: cells, signaling systems (e.g., growth factors) and extracellular matrix (ECM). The ECM forms a scaffold for its cells. Hence, the engineered tissue construct is an artificial scaffold populated with living cells and signaling molecules. A huge effort has been invested in bone tissue engineering, which is often thought to be the most advanced subarea in the field of tissue engineering. Nonetheless, no matter what types of biomaterials and fabrication techniques have been used, the utilization of artificial scaffolds to engineer bone tissue has been rather disappointing, with no successful and routinely used clinical examples of human applications to date [1].

An Ideal Scaffolding Material Should Be Mechanically Strong and Yet Biodegradable

To engineer bone tissue, which is hard and functions to support the body, the scaffold material must be equally strong and tough. Ideally, the scaffold needs to be degradable, as this would prevent the detrimental effects of a persisting foreign substance and allow its gradual replacement with new bone. Unfortunately, mechanical strength and biodegradability, which are two essential requirements on bone tissue scaffolds, are antagonistic toward each other. In general, mechanically strong materials (e.g., crystalline hydroxylapatites, and related calcium phosphates and crystalline polymers) are virtually bioinert, whereas biodegradable materials (e.g., amorphous calcium phosphates and amorphous polymers) tend to be brittle. Clinical investigation has shown that implanted hydroxylapatites and calcium phosphates are inert, remaining within the body for as long as 6–7 years postimplantation [2].

Ideal Degradation Kinetics of Scaffolds

The degradation kinetics of bone scaffolds must be a reasonable match to the healing rates of injured bone. Excessively rapid degradation would lead to catastrophic mechanical failure of the implant under load-bearing conditions, whereas too slow an absorption process would create a barrier to the innate remodeling and fusion processes at the wound site. The time course of healing tissue exhibits three stages: lag, log, and plateau phases [3], as illustrated in Figure 13.25 (curve C1). Accordingly, the ideal degradation kinetics of scaffolds that match the healing rate of growing bone should possess three stages as well, that is, lag (a steady state), log (rapid degradation), and plateau (end of degradation) phases (C2). Unfortunately, current biomaterials degrade immediately after implantation, showing no lag phase (C3), as seen with some degradable biomaterials that are weaker than mature (cancellous) bone [4]. Otherwise, they can be virtually inert and degrade relatively slowly (C4), which is typical of more mechanically robust biomaterials [2].

Ideal Porous Structure of Biomaterials

The development of highly porous structures to provide sufficient surfaces for cells to anchor onto, without impeding the growth of new tissue, represents another technical hurdle in tissue engineering of bone, and other implant situations. Angiogenesis (the formation of new blood vessels from existing ones) is essential for the growth of new tissue, tissue repair, and wound healing. Tissue engineering relies on angiogenesis for the vascularization of these new grafts. To achieve this, in vitro (i.e., before implantation) priming of tissue constructs for vascularization is highly desirable, and for this the tissue engineering scaffolds should have an interconnected, porous structure for cell penetration and the ability to support vascular tissue ingrowth. The ideal scaffold that promotes angiogenesis of engineered tissue sufficiently has not yet been determined. Indeed, the major disadvantage of most scaffolds reported to date is that cells tend to

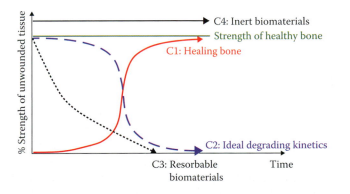

Figure 13.25
Healing rate of growing bone and degradation kinetics of biomaterials.

adhere only to the outer layer of the scaffolds [5]. This may partially explain why most scaffolds fail to vascularize, independent of their material properties [6].

Dilemmas in the Engineering of Thick Vascularized Tissue

Bone is a heavily vascularized tissue. The vascular system provides a number of critical functions, including the delivery of oxygen and nutrients, removal of waste products of metabolism, and delivery of circulating soluble factors, stem cells and progenitor cells. If the distance between the capillaries and cells exceeds 200 µm, hypoxia occurs, making local cell populations unviable. Indeed, if there is a universal message that has emerged out of past work in the tissue-engineering field, it is that angiogenesis and ingrowth of new vessels is necessary to supply the cells with oxygen, nutrients, and growth factors in engineered thick 3D tissues. This forms the greatest present challenge in the field, not just to bone, but tissue in other organs that have a 3D structure, such as CNS, skin, glands, and muscle.

The rapid growth of a new vascular system remains the major limitation in the successful introduction of tissue-engineering products to clinical practice. To achieve vascularization of tissue constructs, several approaches are currently under investigation. These include: (1) the aforementioned modification of porous structure of scaffolds; (2) the stimulation of blood vessel ingrowth from the host tissue by control over angiogenesis growth factors; and (3) the priming of tissue constructs to vascularize by loading and culturing them in vitro with vascular endothelial cells, mural cells, and/or tissue-related cells (e.g., osteoblasts). In principle, blood vessel ingrowth could form over time in implanted tissue constructs without prevascularization. However, the vascularization is in general too slow and too limited to provide sufficient vascular functions to the transplanted cells, no matter what growth factors are delivered. Research over the last several years has brought evidence that delayed vascularization is one of the major obstacles to successfully realizing the clinical use of in vitro engineered tissue and organ substitutes [6]. This explains why the successful usage of tissue-engineered constructs is currently limited to thin or avascular tissues, such as skin and cartilage.

BIBLIOGRAPHY

References for Text

1. Martini, F.H., M.J. Timmons, and R.B. Tallitsch, *Human Anatomy*, 5th edn. San Francisco, CA: Pearson/Benjamin Cummings, 2006.
2. Tate, S.S., *Anatomy and Physiology*, 8th edn. New York: McGraw Hill, 2008.
3. Gao, J., Y.M. Kim, H. Coe, B. Zern, B. Sheppard, and Y. Wang, A neuroinductive biomaterial based on dopamine. *Proc Natl Acad Sci USA*, 2006 Nov 7;**103**(45):16681–16686.

Websites

Anatomy & Physiology http://faculty.irsc.edu/FACULTY/TFischer/AP1/AP%201%20resources.htm (Fantastic website with excellent images and useful links).
Ankle (tarsal bones) http://www.prohealthsys.com/resources/grays/images/Gray576.jpg.
http://www.anatomyatlases.org/.
http://www.free-ed.net/free-ed/HealthCare/Anatomy/default.asp (Simple and concise).
http://www.innerbody.com/htm/body.html (Excellent illustrations).

Skull suture joints http://legacy.owensboro.kctcs.edu/gcaplan/anat/study%20guide/Image815.gif.
Teeth http://www.studiodentaire.com/images/en/periodontal_ligament_en.jpg.
Wrist (carpal bones) http://www.activemotionphysio.ca/media/img/1362/wrist_ganglion_anat03.jpg.

References for Advanced Topic

1. Nerem, R.M., Tissue engineering: The hope, the hype, and the future. *Tissue Engineering*, 2006;**12**(5):1143–1150.
2. Marcacci, M. et al., Stem cells associated with macroporous bioceramics for long bone repair: 6- to 7-year outcome of a pilot clinical study. *Tissue Engineering*, 2007;**13**(5):947–955.
3. Cukjati, D., S. Rebersek, and D. Miklavcic, A reliable method of determining wound healing rate. *Medical and Biological Engineering and Computing*, 2001;**39**(2):263–271.
4. Wang, Y.D., Y.M. Kim, and R. Langer, In vivo degradation characteristics of poly(glycerol sebacate). *Journal of Biomedical Materials Research. Part A*, 2003;**66A**(1):192–197.
5. Kannan, R.Y. et al., The roles of tissue engineering and vascularisation in the development of micro-vascular networks: A review. *Biomaterials*, 2005;**26**(14):1857–1875.
6. Laschke, M.W. et al., Angiogenesis in tissue engineering: Breathing life into constructed tissue substitutes. *Tissue Engineering*, 2006;**12**(8):2093–2104.
7. Niinomi, M., Recent metallic materials for biomedical applications. *Metallurg. Mater. Trans. A*, 2002;33:477.

Further Readings

Martini, F.H., M.J. Timmons, and R.B. Tallitsch, *Human Anatomy*, 5th edn. San Francisco, CA: Pearson/Benjamin Cummings, 2006. Related chapters.
Tate, S.S., *Anatomy and Physiology*, 8th edn. New York: McGraw Hill, 2008. Related chapters.

CHAPTER 14

HUMAN ANATOMY AND DISEASES II
Cardiovascular System

LEARNING OBJECTIVES

After a careful study of this chapter, you should be able to do the following:

1. Describe the three constituents: blood, heart, and vessels
2. Describe the two circuits
3. Explain why heart disease is so devastating
4. Describe key pathological mechanisms leading to heart failure after heart attack
5. Describe current treatments and their limitations
6. Appreciate potential strategies
7. Describe applications of biomaterials

14.1 ANATOMY AND FUNCTIONS OF THE CARDIOVASCULAR SYSTEM

The cardiovascular system (CVS) consists basically of three major types of organs: blood, heart, and vessels. The system provides a mechanism for the continuous and rapid transport of cells, nutrients, and waste products to and from all tissues in the body. The most important and vital of these is oxygen, supplied via lungs to all tissues and organs, and without which death can occur within minutes. Every tissue has its own blood supply and drainage, delivered from very large vessels to progressively smaller, and eventually microscopic vessels that reside deep within tissues. This forms the basis of the term *vascularized*, which describes the network of vessels throughout a living tissue that is filled with blood and under constant oxygenation, giving it its characteristic pink color as seen in surgical procedures.

Although not covered in this chapter, the CVS also includes the lymphatic system, a series of drainage vessels that removes fatty acids from the digestive system, and excess tissue fluid from outside cells. Here, we concentrate on blood transport.

14.1.1   Blood

The blood is made up of three types of cells: red blood cells, white blood cells, and platelets (Figure 14.1) suspended in a fluid called plasma, under pressure depending on which vessels they are being transported through. Plasma is composed mostly of water, with various proteins and other solutes, as listed in Table 14.1. The 1% of solutes in plasma consists of metabolites including carbohydrates (glucose, lactic acid, etc.), amino acids, and ions (e.g., Na^{2+}, K^+, Ca^{2+}, HCO^{3-}, NH^{4+}, H^+). The proteins represent a critical functional component of blood. Albumins, for example, assist in the binding and transport of growth factors and fatty acids, as well as osmotic balance. Fibrinogen on the other hand, together with a group of 12 other regulatory proteins, is involved in the clotting reaction. During this process, fibrinogen is converted to fibrin that forms a random fibrous mesh that seals the edges of ruptured vessels, trapping blood cells and thus temporarily repairing the breakage.

Red blood cells (erythrocytes) are the most common type of blood cell (99.9%) and the body's principle means of delivering oxygen to the tissues. They are smaller than most other cell types and contain very large amounts of hemoglobin. These proteins contain

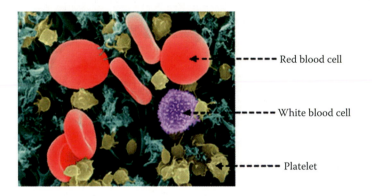

Figure 14.1
Red blood cells (red) and platelets (yellow) in the blood. The purple cell is a smaller type of white blood cell (colorized SEM image). (Courtesy of Dennis Kunkel Microscopy, Inc., Kailua, HI.)

Table 14.1
Constituents of Plasma

Components	Percentage (%)
Water	92
Plasma proteins	7
Albumin: 60%	
Globulin: 35%	
Fibrinogen: 4%	
Regulatory proteins: <1%	
Other solutes	1

porphyrin (heme) groups that bind and release oxygen in a diffusion and pH-dependent manner; the low pH outside tissues actually favors the release of oxygen. Deoxygenated porphyrins are more purple in color, whereas oxygenated porphyrins are more red, hence their red and blue depictions. Most of the lung tissue is essentially a very large surface area of vascularized membranes, which assists in oxygen diffusion into the red blood cells that have returned deoxygenated from the tissue, ready to be reoxygenated again. Owing to their small size (~6–8 μm) and discoid shape, red blood cells can access very small vessels, and pack together to flow almost in a continuous stream of cells. Their high surface-area-to-volume ratio also assists in short-range oxygen diffusion.

White blood cells (i.e., leukocytes) are cells of the immune system, defending the body against both infectious disease and foreign materials. They are of five different types, larger in size than red blood cells (up to 20 μm), and with different protective roles specific to the types. White blood cells are generally classed as either granular or agranular, depending on the density of granules (cytoplasmic particles that contain degradative enzymes). These enzymes assist in breaking down foreign particles (e.g., bacteria, viruses, particulate debris) that are consumed by the cells, such as at a wound or site of infection. The puffiness of a wound side is partly due to the increased density of white blood cells attracted to the area. On the surface of white blood cells, specific binding proteins called antibodies are able to recognize and bind to the surface of foreign objects, even foreign tissue (e.g., tissue from another species), which eventually leads to graft rejection.

Platelets (i.e., thrombocytes) (0.1%) are small, irregularly shaped 2–3 μm fragments of cells. They do not have a nucleus containing DNA like white blood cells, but still contain some cytoplasmic organelles (e.g., mitochondria). The average life span of a platelet is between 8 and 12 days. Their main role is in the formation of a blood clot (thrombus), where they strengthen the fibrin mesh, creating a layered structure that not only traps blood cells but withstands the pressure of circulating blood, especially in areas of high flow.

14.1.2 Heart

All of the tissues and fluids in the body rely on the CVS to maintain homeostasis. The proper functioning of the CVS depends on the activities of the heart, which is a hollow muscle that pumps blood throughout the blood vessels by repeated, rhythmic contractions and varies its pumping capacity depending on the needs of the peripheral tissues. The heart is one of the six vital organs (Table 13.3).

The human heart weighs 250–350 g and is about the size of a fist. It has four chambers, two superior *atria* (left and right atrium) and two inferior *ventricles* (left and right ventricle) (Figure 14.2). The atria are the receiving chambers and the ventricles are the discharging chambers. During each beating cycle, the atria contract first, forcing blood that has entered them into their respective ventricles, then the ventricles contract, pumping blood out of the heart. *Diastole* is the period of time when the heart refills with blood (Figure 14.3a). *Ventricular diastole* is the period during which the ventricles are relaxing, while *atrial diastole* is the period during which the atria are relaxing. *Systole* is the period of time when the heart contracts (Figure 14.3b). These cycles are automatic, relying on spontaneous beating of heart muscle cells, with the speed of beating controlled by the vagus nerve, a major nerve coming from brain stem (between brain and spinal cord). An important structural feature of the heart is its valves, which are actually one-way valves, allowing sequential filling of chambers, without backflow of blood.

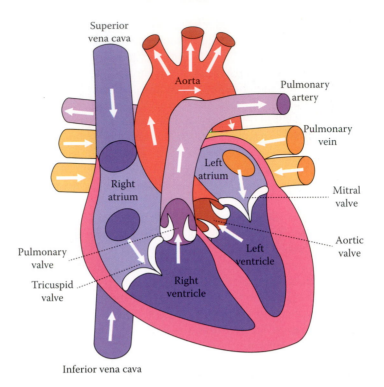

Figure 14.2
Gross structure of the heart. (Modified from the original one created by Wapcaplet and chopped by Yaddah, http://commons.wikimedia.org/.)

14.1.3 Two Circuits

The cardiovascular system consists of two closed circuits that circulate blood throughout the body in series (Figure 14.4), a pulmonary circuit and a systemic circuit. The former sends blood to the lungs; the latter supplies blood to the rest of the body.

Oxygen-depleted blood (indicated in blue) arrives into the heart from the tissues, where the *pulmonary circuit* transports it to the lungs for reoxygenation and removal of carbon dioxide. The reoxygenated blood (indicated in red) is then transported back to the heart from the lungs, where oxygen is diffused into the red blood cells. The *systemic circuit* then pumps this oxygenated blood away from the heart, out to all the tissues of the body. As the red blood cells enter these tissues, they lose oxygen and take up carbon dioxide, which is a waste gas product of metabolism in the tissue cells. The oxygen-depleted red blood cells transport the carbon dioxide back to the lungs, and we breathe it out when we exhale.

14.1.4 Blood Vessels

14.1.4.1 Arteries, Veins, and Capillaries   Blood vessels are hollow, elastic tubes that transport blood throughout the entire body. There are three major types of blood vessels: the *arteries*, which transport blood away from the heart under pressure, to supply

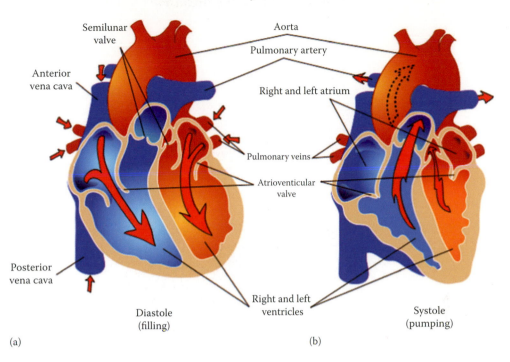

Semilunar valve

Aorta

Pulmonary artery

Anterior vena cava

Right and left atrium

Pulmonary veins

Atrioventicular valve

Posterior vena cava

Right and left ventricles

Diastole (filling)

Systole (pumping)

(a)

(b)

Figure 14.3
(a) Diastole and (b) systole. (From http://commons.wikimedia.org/produced by Mariana Ruiz Villarreal.)

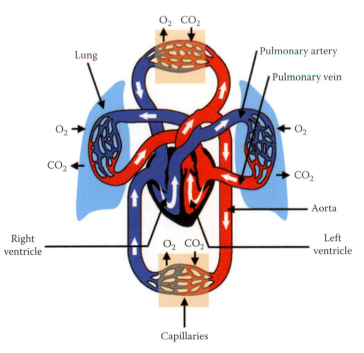

O_2 CO_2

Lung

Pulmonary artery

Pulmonary vein

O_2

O_2

CO_2

CO_2

Aorta

Right ventricle

Left ventricle

O_2 CO_2

Capillaries

Figure 14.4
The pulmonary (vertical), and systemic (horizontal) circuit. Oxygenated and oxygen-depleted blood.

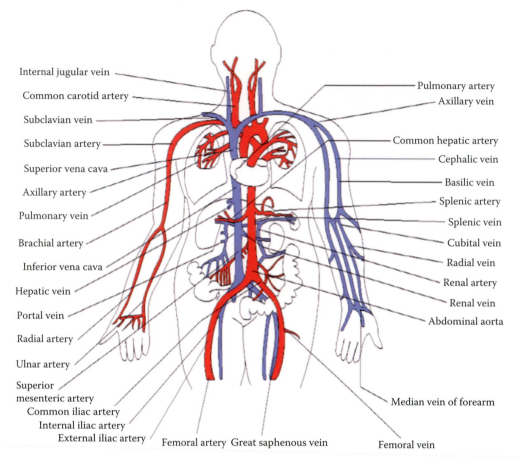

Internal jugular vein

Common carotid artery

Subclavian vein

Subclavian artery

Superior vena cava

Axillary artery

Pulmonary vein

Brachial artery

Inferior vena cava

Hepatic vein

Portal vein

Radial artery

Ulnar artery

Superior mesenteric artery

Common iliac artery

Internal iliac artery

External iliac artery

Femoral artery   Great saphenous vein

Pulmonary artery

Axillary vein

Common hepatic artery

Cephalic vein

Basilic vein

Splenic artery

Splenic vein

Cubital vein

Radial vein

Renal artery

Renal vein

Abdominal aorta

Median vein of forearm

Femoral vein

Figure 14.5
Arteries and veins in the human body.

oxygen to the tissues; the *veins*, which carry deoxygenated blood back to the heart (Figure 14.5), the *capillaries*, which are much smaller diameter, that occur in a dense 3D network within the tissues at the ends of the vascular network. These enable the exchange of water, oxygen, carbon dioxide, trace nutrients, and waste chemicals between the blood and the surrounding tissues (Figure 14.6). The capillaries also occur in lung tissue, involved mainly in oxygen diffusion, but also supplying the lung itself.

In the pulmonary circuit, oxygen-depleted blood enters the capillaries of the lungs and the oxygen-rich blood leaves these capillaries (Figure 14.6a). In the systemic circuit, the oxygen-rich blood enters the capillaries of the tissues and the oxygen-depleted blood leaves the capillaries of the same tissues (Figure 14.6b). A possible point of confusion is the red-blue indications of blood vessels (arteries and veins) and the blood itself (oxygen-rich blood and oxygen-depleted blood). The following sequential list may help:

- *Systemic veins* take deoxygenated tissue blood to the right atrium (via the vena cava)
- The right atrium drains into the right ventricle
- Right ventricle pumps the oxygen-depleted blood via the *pulmonary arteries* to the lungs

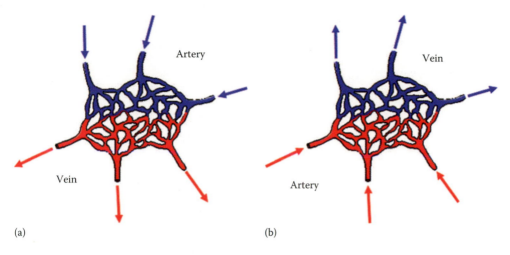

(a)   (b)

Figure 14.6
Capillaries. The red-blue color indicates oxygen-rich and oxygen-depleted blood: (a) in the pulmonary circuit (in the lungs); (b) in the systemic circuit (the rest of body).

- The *pulmonary veins* carry reoxygenated blood from the lungs back to the left atrium
- The left atrium pumps through *systemic arteries* (via the aorta) to the rest of the body

In summary, veins always enter the heart, but arteries exit the heart.

In the systemic circuit, the arteries leaving the heart are larger in diameter (e.g., aorta: ~3 cm), which gradually decrease in diameter as they branch, at particular branch points along the vascular tree. The arteries are also under active control by nerves that control smooth muscle in their walls, which can control the vessel diameter, and therefore the blood pressure in the peripheral vessels. With a single beat, the pressure of the beat itself pushes a single amount of blood down the vascular tree, further moved via a continuous wave of contraction that propagates down the vessel walls to the capillaries (hence we can feel a pulse at our wrists or major limb artery). As arteries become thinner, they gradually lose smooth muscle to form a nonelastic capillary, which might be as small as one red blood cell thick. Transport of oxygen from oxygen-rich red blood cells through these capillary *beds* (dense sponge-like networks) then becomes strictly diffusive, which is assisted by the very high surface areas of vascular walls at this scale.

Drainage of the capillary beds then empties blood from the tissues into the veins, which gradually become larger in diameter as they go back up the vascular tree, toward the heart. Veins are nonelastic and act like a blood and plasma reservoir. Because of this, gravity can have a significant effect on larger volumes of passively flowing venous blood, especially in larger veins, so veins also contain one-way valves internally, at various points along them, to prevent backflow and accumulation of deoxygenated blood near the tissues. Note that when you are dehydrated (i.e., more blood, less plasma), the veins on the outside of hands will appear more swollen.

14.1.4.2 Aorta and Coronary Arteries of the Heart

The muscular tissue of the heart is so thick that it requires its own blood supply, although around 3% can come from blood within the ventricles. The vessels that deliver oxygen-rich blood to the heart muscle are known as *coronary arteries* (Figure 14.7a), which follow the exterior surface

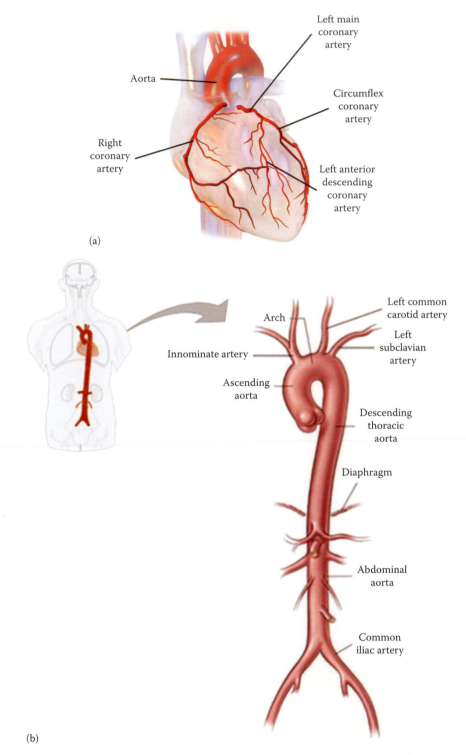

Left main
coronary
artery

Aorta

Circumflex
coronary
artery

Right
coronary
artery

Left anterior
descending
coronary
artery

(a)

Left common
carotid artery

Arch

Left
subclavian
artery

Innominate artery

Ascending
aorta

Descending
thoracic
aorta

Diaphragm

Abdominal
aorta

Common
iliac artery

(b)

Figure 14.7
(a) Aorta and coronary arteries on the heart (From the http://commons.wikimedia.org/produced by BruceBlaus) and (b) a complete aorta structure.

of the myocardium, underneath the protective pericardial membrane. These arteries are the first to branch off the aorta, the largest artery in the human body, which originates directly from the left ventricle (Figure 14.2) and extends down to the abdomen (Figure 14.7b), where it bifurcates into two smaller arteries (the common iliac arteries).

14.2   CARDIOVASCULAR DISEASE

Cardiovascular disease (CVD) describes all disorders and conditions that involve the heart and blood vessels. It is the leading cause of death and disability in both industrialized nations and the developing world, accounting for one-quarter of all deaths worldwide (Figure 14.8). Prognosis for CVD is poor, with 40% mortality within 12 months of diagnosis, and a 10% annual mortality rate thereafter. It causes significant burdens from ill health, disability, and health system costs. It is estimated that 5 million Americans, 1.8 million Britons, and 25 million people worldwide suffer from heart failure, with approximately 60,000 and 120,000 new cases diagnosed each year in the United States and the United Kingdom, respectively. The economic burden imposed by this disease has reached more than $33 billion in the United States, more than £700 million in the United Kingdom, more than $400 million in Australia annually.

There are many forms and causes of heart diseases. However, the main types of CVD in developed countries include [2] the following:

- Coronary artery disease
- Brain vessel diseases (stroke, aneurysm)
- Hypertensive heart disease (from increased blood pressure)
- Cardiomyopathy (heart muscle dysfunction)
- Rheumatic heart disease (bacterial infection)
- Peripheral vascular disease
- Congenital heart disease (inherited dysfunction)

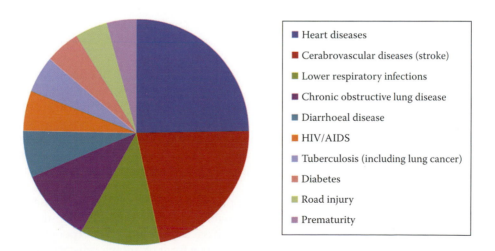

- Heart diseases
- Cerabrovascular diseases (stroke)
- Lower respiratory infections
- Chronic obstructive lung disease
- Diarrhoeal disease
- HIV/AIDS
- Tuberculosis (including lung cancer)
- Diabetes
- Road injury
- Prematurity

Figure 14.8
The 10 leading causes of death worldwide (2011). (From http://who.int/mediacentre/factsheets/fs310/en/index.html.)

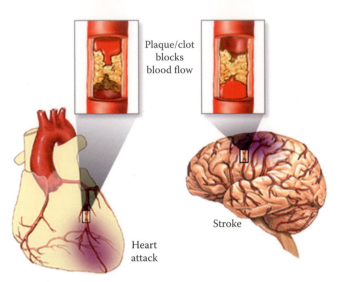

Figure 14.9
A coronary heart disease (heart attack) caused by atherosclerosis of coronary and a brain vascular disease (stroke) caused by blockage of cerebro-vessel.

A leading cause of most CVDs is atherosclerosis, which is an abnormal buildup of fats that form localized plaques inside the arteries. Atherosclerosis is most serious when it leads to reduced or blocked blood supply to the heart (causing heart attack—pain and loss of oxygenation of the muscle) (Figure 14.9) or to the brain (causing a stroke). As adults age, plaque formation can progress from simple deposit of fats within the cell that line the vessels to more complex structures made up of platelets, fibrin, and calcifications. Plaques can grow slowly and gradually restrict blood flow. If this occurs in the carotid arteries, the heart needs to work harder to keep the brain oxygenated, and if an advanced plaque (now a clot or *thrombus*) breaks apart, it can lodge in the smaller brain vessels, resulting in a stroke (Figure 14.9).

14.2.1 Coronary Artery Disease

Coronary artery disease (also known as *ischemic heart disease*) is the most common form of CVD. There are two major clinical forms, *heart attack* and *angina*. A heart attack (also known as acute *myocardial infarction*, MI) occurs when the heart blood vessel is suddenly blocked. This restricts oxygen delivery to the affected area and directly results in the local death of heart muscle cells (Figure 14.9). Heart attack is life-threatening due to the fact that the heart muscle cells (i.e., *cardiomyocytes*) virtually have no regenerative ability and that the damage of the heart muscle and its functions is permanent.

Angina is a chronic condition when a temporary loss of blood supply to the heart causes periodic, highly acute chest pain. Although angina is generally not life-threatening, people with this disease are more likely to have a heart attack or experience sudden cardiac death. Heart attacks and the most serious form of angina (unstable angina) are considered to be part of a continuum of acute coronary artery diseases, described as *acute coronary syndrome* [2].

14.2.2 Brain Vessel Diseases

Stroke occurs when an artery supplying blood to the brain either suddenly becomes blocked or begins to bleed. This may result in brain damage, leading to a sudden impairment in speaking, thinking, movement, and communication. *Stroke is often fatal.* There are two main types of stroke: a blood clot or other particles blocking a blood vessel (ischemic stroke) or the rupturing and subsequent bleeding (aneurysm) of a blood vessel (hemorrhagic stroke).

Stroke is the most common form of brain vessel (cerebrovascular) disease, which includes disorders of the blood vessels supplying the brain or its covering membranes. Transient ischemic attack is a condition related to stroke and results from a temporary blockage of the blood supply to the brain, usually lasting only a few minutes and producing stroke-like symptoms that disappear within 24 h.

14.2.3 Hypertensive Heart Disease

High blood pressure (hypertension) is a major health problem in adults, and is a major risk factor for most CVDs. Hence, it is difficult to tell apart cardiac problems associated with hypertension on its own. Nevertheless, hypertensive heart disease is a recognized condition, although it is not as likely to result in a fatality. Hypertension is more often associated with aging, Western diets leading to obesity, and chronic stressful lifestyles. The most common symptom of hypertensive heart conditions is ventricular enlargement (hypertrophy). This occurs because of increased resistance to blood flow in the peripheral circulation (see below).

14.2.4 Cardiomyopathy

Heart failure occurs when the heart is unable to maintain efficient blood flow. Typical symptoms include chronic tiredness, reduced capacity for physical activity, and shortness of breath. It is a *life-threatening condition and cannot be cured in most cases.* Heart failure can be caused by a variety of underlying conditions that impair or overload the heart, including coronary artery disease with or without an episode of acute MI (heart attack), hypertension, valvular dysfunction (damaged heart valves), general vascular dysfunction, and cardiomyopathy (primary myocardial disease). The *single most common cause of left-side cardiac failure* is ischemic heart disease with an episode of acute MI, which will eventually lead to cardiomyopathy.

Cardiomyopathy refers to a family of preexisting diseases of the heart muscle, some of which are genetic in origin, which generally result in weakening of the heart, and ultimately can lead to heart failure. This is called *intrinsic* cardiomyopathy (i.e., preexisting problems), but a majority of cardiomyopathy is *extrinsic*, caused by ischemic insult (oxygen deprivation to the heart muscle), usually after a heart attack. In this case, local muscle cell death and collagen scar formation occur at the site of ischemia.

Scar formation is a natural, protective response of the body, which occurs at sites of moderate or severe tissue damage. When tissue is under a routine mechanical stress or strain, such as constant wearing of feet or hands by shoes or tools, the affected area of tissue is thickened by stronger collagen and keratin deposition from within tissues. In more severe damage, such as a skin lesion, a fibrous clot is initially formed in the first acute phase of tissue repair, followed by a slower remodeling phase, also associated with extensive collagen formation. While the thick and stiff scar tissue serves well the purpose of mechanical protection, it is always less elastic compared to the original tissue. The compromised mechanical elasticity of scar tissue is principally of little concern in the case of passive tissue like skin, except for cosmetic reasons. However, it is a critical pathological mechanism leading to heart failure, mainly because of the dynamic nature of the heart muscle and the need for this tissue to maintain its structural integrity at all times.

Unfortunately, heart muscle damage is permanent at ischemic sites due to the very limited capacity for regeneration and replacement of dying muscle cells. Following MI, heart muscle slippage occurs (Figure 14.10), and like an overblown balloon, the weakening of the heart wall results from this slippage, leading to thinning of the wall and left-ventricular dilation (Figure 14.11). The enlargement in ventricular volume leads to

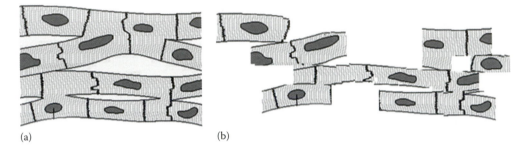

(a)   (b)

Figure 14.10
(a) Original heart muscle; (b) slippage and thinning of muscle following myocardium infarct.

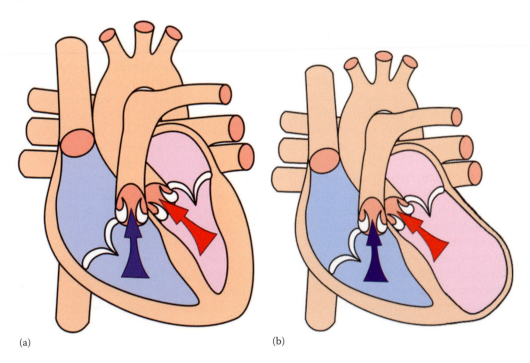

(a)   (b)

Figure 14.11
(a) Healthy heart and (b) myocardial infarct (MI) heart. (Modified from the original one created by Wapcaplet http://en.wikipedia.org/wiki/File:Heart_diastole.png.)

ventricle remodeling, during which scar formation becomes progressively worse, with increased thickening of the damaged area by recruitment of collagen. This remodeling process is initially compensatory, but the subsequent formation of a stiff but inelastic scar adds further inefficiency to the compromised mechanical pumping of the remaining ventricular muscle. The heart therefore becomes predisposed to end-stage heart failure, a condition in which the heart cannot pump sufficient amounts of blood to meet the metabolic requirements of the body.

In summary, heart failure is most frequently caused by heart attack, which starts with massive cardiomyocyte death caused by the blockage of a coronary artery. Heart muscle cells have very little ability to regenerate under such circumstances, and the permanent cell loss results in extrinsic cardiomyopathy, myocardial thinning, and ventricular dilation. Eventually, the ventricle is remodeled by the formation of inelastic collagen scar tissue. This combination of decreased contractile ability, increased stiffness, and myocardial stretching weakens the ventricle walls, resulting in increased risk of heart failure.

14.2.5 Acute Rheumatic Fever and Rheumatic Heart Disease

Acute rheumatic fever (ARF) is a condition caused by an untreated infection of group A streptococcus [3] bacteria, affecting the throat and possibly the skin. It causes inflammation throughout the body. If it recurs or is left untreated, ARF can permanently damage the heart valves, leading to rheumatic heart disease. The risk of ARF recurring is high following an initial episode. Although ARF is now a rare disease among most Australians, it still has a substantial impact on Aboriginal and Torres Strait Islander communities.

Rheumatic heart disease results in permanent damage to the heart muscle or heart valves. It often damages the heart valves by either causing them to narrow or not close properly, which causes backflow of blood and decreased cardiac output. Severe forms of the disease can result in serious incapacity or even death. Damage to the heart valve and a history of ARF are both important indicators in diagnosing rheumatic heart disease as its symptoms are common in other heart conditions.

14.2.6 Peripheral Vascular Disease

Peripheral vascular disease, also known as peripheral arterial disease, refers to the obstruction of large arteries that supply blood to the peripheral tissues, as opposed to the core circulation to the heart, abdominal organs, and brain. Two important forms of the disease are (1) atherosclerosis of the peripheral arteries and (2) abdominal aortic aneurysm. In the first case, the arteries supplying blood to the legs and feet are narrowed, potentially leading to tissue necrosis due to insufficient oxygenation, potentially leading to amputation of a limb. Abdominal aortic aneurysm is marked by abnormal widening of the descending aorta (the main artery leading from the heart) below the level of the diaphragm. This can be a life-threatening condition and surgery is necessary in some cases.

14.2.7 Congenital Heart Disease

Congenital heart disease is any disorder of the heart or central blood vessels that is present at birth. It is one of the leading causes of death in the first year of life. Symptoms may appear at birth, or sometime thereafter. They include breathlessness or a failure to attain normal growth and development. Most children with congenital heart disease are treated with surgery or catheter-based techniques, usually in infancy or early childhood.

14.3   CARDIAC PERFORMANCE: P–V LOOP

As a general practice, a diagram of a system's pressure versus volume can be used to measure the work done by the system (e.g., heat engines, various pumps, and heart) and its efficiency. Figure 14.12 represents a typical pressure–volume (P–V) loop of the beating heart, which occurs in specific stages, during successive beating and relaxing of the heart wall. When the mitral valve opens (stage 1), blood starts to fill the ventricle. When sufficient blood is filled in the heart, the ventricular wall contracts (stage 2), shrinking the ventricles and thereby ejecting blood out of the two chambers (stage 3). At the end of ejection (stage 4), the heart ventricles relax till blood fills the chamber again (stage 1).

The P–V loop has been used clinically by cardiologists to diagnose the progression of heart failure (Figure 14.13). A healthy heart beats strongly, characterized by high intraventricular pressure and large stroke volume, while a failing heart beats weakly, characterized by reduced intraventricular pressure and lower stroke volume. In the meantime, the size of the failing heart is significantly increased compared with the healthy one.

14.4   CURRENT THERAPIES FOR HEART DISEASE

Pharmacological therapies involve using drugs to target a range of different processes to prevent further heart failure, and/or minimize the damage caused by a preexisting heart failure. Some drugs target blood vessels, causing them to dilate. For example, nitrates

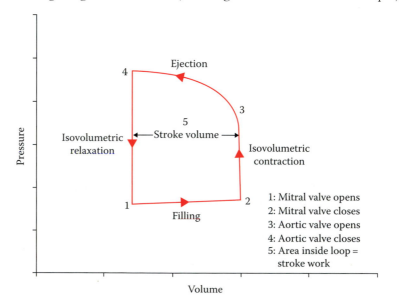

Figure 14.12
P–V loop of heart, typically stroke volume (SV) is 70 mL.

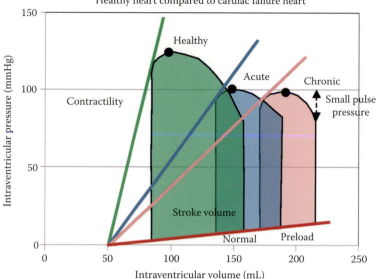

Figure 14.13
P–V loops of healthy and failing hearts. A cardiac failure heart is larger in size but has a smaller stroke volume and pulse pressure, compared to the healthy heart.

are potent dilators of the coronary arteries, which allow rapid reoxygenation of the heart muscle during angina attacks. Other drugs taken over longer periods as a chronic treatment are called β-blockers, which act to prevent heart muscle responses to adrenalin, the stress hormone that increases heart rate, thereby directly reducing cardiac workload. Angiotensin-converting enzyme (ACE) inhibitors and diuretics are perhaps the most common and effective drugs, which act to reduce systemic blood pressure, reducing the workload on the heart by giving it less pressure to pump against. Such treatments represent the current standard conservative approach in survivors of heart attacks, or those with mild symptoms of heart failure and slight limitation during ordinary activity.

Depending on the severity and urgency, interventional therapy such as bypass surgery (Figure 14.14) or implantation of pacing devices to control electrical synchrony may be required. The former is highly invasive, involving open-heart surgery, whereas the latter involves a more simple procedure of implantation of a small electrical device that generates a pulsed signal that directly controls the heart beat via small electrodes connected to the heart muscle. These approaches are now receiving widespread application, especially in patients with dramatic loss of activity.

However, both drug and interventional therapies, which do nothing about the permanent muscle cells loss, cannot adequately control disease progression to the end stage. Eventually, heart transplantation is the ultimate treatment option for end-stage heart failure. Owing to the lack of organ donors and complications associated with immune suppressive treatments, surgeons constantly look for new strategies to repair the injured heart. Table 14.2 lists currently applied or potential strategies for the treatment of heart-failure patients. Note that both bypass surgery and tissue-engineering approaches are highly invasive, involving opening of the thoracic cavity to allow access to the heart, followed by shunting of blood and temporary stoppage of the heart from pumping during the procedure.

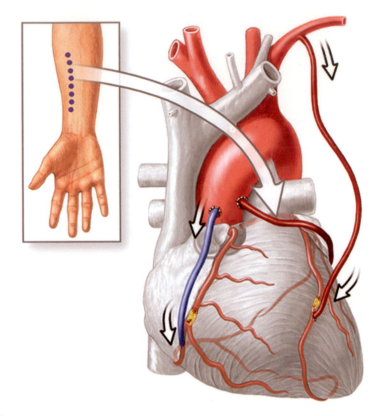

Figure 14.14
Bypass surgery involving autologous grafting of blood vessels.

Table 14.2
Strategies for the Treatment of Heart-Failure Patients

Current approaches

Pharmacological therapy

Interventional therapy

    Reduction of the heart volume

    Implantation of a pacemaker

    Bypass surgery

    Heart transplantation

Potential approaches

Tissue-engineering strategies:

    Cardiomyoplasty (active systolic assist)

    Cell-based therapy (isolated cell delivery)

    Left-ventricular restraint (passive diastolic constraint)

    Scaffold-free cell sheet implantation

    Heart patch implantation (passive diastolic constraint and cell delivery)

    3D tissue constructs (scaffold, with cells and macromolecules)

14.5 ALTERNATIVE TREATMENTS AND APPLICATION OF BIOMATERIALS

The European Commission on Health and Consumer Protection defines tissue engineering as "the persuasion of the body to heal itself through the delivery, to the appropriate site, independently or in synergy, of cells, biomolecules and supporting structures."[4] According to this definition, the surgical approaches described in the following can be all classified into the tissue-engineering category, as listed in Table 14.2.

14.5.1 Cardiomyoplasty

Cardiomyoplasty is an alternative surgical approach for treating heart failure. This procedure involves removal of sheet-like skeletal muscle from the back (Figure 14.15a) and wrapping it around the heart (Figure 14.15b), followed by pacing with electrodes and a pulse generator to induce it to contract with the heart, thereby improving cardiac pumping power. Clinical studies report that this dynamic procedure can improve left-ventricular performance, reduce cardiac dilation, and slow down disease progression [5,6]. However, quantitative hemodynamic analyses have not been consistent to determine the benefits of active systolic assist, and mortality from the operation is unacceptably high [7,8]. This has prompted the suggestion that passive* mechanical

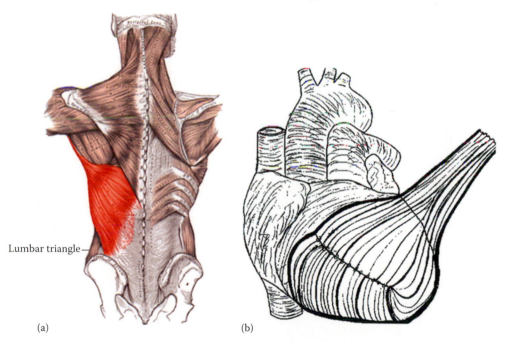

Lumbar triangle—

(a)   (b)

Figure 14.15
Cardiomyoplasty: (a) the skeletal muscle for autografting and (b) schematic image of the cardiomyoplasty wrapping technique. (a) (From http://upload.wikimedia.org/wikipedia/commons/6/6f/Latissimus_dorsi.PNG (Gray's Anatomy plates, public access).) (b) (From Bolotin, G, et al., Chest, 121(5), 1628–1633, May 2002. Reproduced with permission from the American College of Chest Physicians.)

---

* Passive mechanical properties of muscle refer to the mechanical behavior without biological stimulation. Readers are referred to Chapter 17.

constraint by the muscle wrap might halt or even reverse the negative remodeling of the dilated ailing heart. Inspired by this hypothesis, many studies have examined the use of biomaterial supports to restrain the left ventricle [9].

14.5.2 Ventricular Restraint

Marlex™ mesh (knitted polypropylene, PP) [10], Merselene™ mesh (knitted polyester) [11], Acorn CorCap™ heart mesh (knitted poly(ethylene terephthalate), PET) [12], and Myocor™ Myosplint® [12] are four representative cardiac support devices (CSD) (Figure 8.5) that have been under investigation. A typical approach of this strategy is illustrated in Figure 14.16. As shown in the diagram, the restraint provides elastic support to a compromised heart, enabling passive resistance to blood filling during diastole, while also imparting potential energy to a weaker systolic contraction. The elasticity of these devices lies in the material itself, as well as the type of knit pattern.

The mechanical working principle of the ventricle restraint is approximated by *Young–Laplace's Law*. The Young–Laplace Law relates the pressure difference across an interface between two static fluids, such as water and air, to the tension in the wall and the shape of the wall. It is a statement of normal stress balance for static fluids meeting at an interface, where the interface is treated as a surface (zero thickness), that is, assuming that the wall is very thin:

$$\Delta P = \gamma \left(\frac{1}{R_1} + \frac{1}{R_2} \right) \qquad (14.1)$$

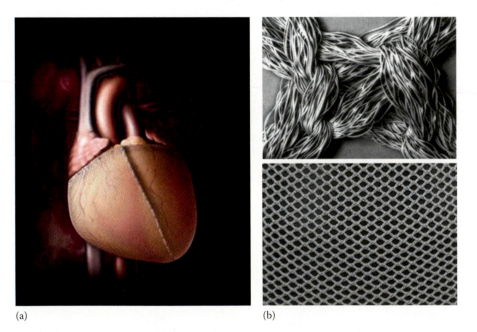

(a)   (b)

Figure 14.16
A ventricle restraint strategy offering a bridge to heart transplantation. (a) Cardiac support device by Acorn CorCap™, a typical approach of left-ventricle restraint. (b) The knitted structure of the mesh. (a) (Courtesy of Acorn Cardiovascular Inc., St. Paul, MN, 2004.) (b) (With kind permission from Springer Science+Business Media, Heart Fail. Rev., Design and features of the acorn CorCap (TM) stop cardiac support device: The concept of passive mechanical diastolic support, 10, 2005, 101, Walsh, R.G., 1, Copyright Manufactured in the Netherlands.)

where

ΔP is the pressure difference across the interface

γ is the wall tension (i.e., the force per unit length of the surface)

R_1 and R_2 are the principal radii of curvature

For a spherical container, $R_1 = R_2 = R$, which gives $\Delta P = 2\gamma/R$. For a cylindrical vessel, $R_1 = R$, $R_2 = \infty$, which gives $\Delta P = \gamma/R$. If the wall thickness is t, the stress T (i.e., the force per unit cross-sectional area) in the wall is given by $T = \gamma/t$.

The heart can be approximately treated as a cylindrical-shaped container. Hence, the Young–Laplace's Law of heart is

$$\Delta P = T \cdot t \cdot \left(\frac{1}{R} + \frac{1}{\infty} \right) = \frac{T \cdot t}{R}, \tag{14.2}$$

or

$$T = \frac{R \cdot \Delta P}{t}, \tag{14.3}$$

where the pressure difference across the wall $\Delta P = P_{\text{inside}} - P_{\text{outside}}$, as illustrated in Figure 14.17.

In the case of passive diastolic constraint (i.e., the process of blood filling into the heart, Figure 14.3), T is the stress in the heart wall, being named diastolic wall stress. Assuming that the blood pressure in the left ventricle at the end of diastole is P_{LVED}, and the supporting pressure provided by a CSD is P_{CSD}, then ΔP, which is also called *transmural pressure*, equals P_{LVED} when no CSD is applied, or $P_{\text{LVED}} - P_{\text{CSD}}$ when a CSD is implanted. Therefore, the Young–Laplace's law can be expressed by

$$\text{Maximal diastolic wall stress } T = \frac{R \cdot P_{\text{LVED}}}{t} \text{ (without a CSD)} \tag{14.4}$$

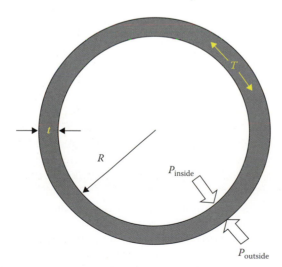

Figure 14.17
Parameters in Laplace's law. R is the radius of a cylinder-shaped ventricle, t is the thickness of the wall, T is the stress in the wall, and $\Delta P = P_{inside} - P_{outside}$.

or

$$\text{Maximal diastolic wall stress } T = \frac{R \cdot \left(P_{\text{LVED}} - P_{\text{CSD}}\right)}{t} \text{ (with a CSD)}. \qquad (14.5)$$

Myocardial infarction typically results in heart wall thinning (a reduction in t) and ventricular dilation (an increase in R and in P_{LVED} which is ΔP when no CSD is used). All these changes cause a significant increase in the heart wall stress according to Equation 14.3.

It is believed that it is the stress signal that triggers the remodeling response in the overstressed heart wall, leading to progressive structural and functional changes. Hence, in order to prevent or slow down negative ventricular remodeling, it is critical to relieve heart wall stress. This can be achieved through a heart supporting device according to Equation 14.5, as P_{CSD} provided by the CSD can effectively reduce ΔP, and thus the stress T in the heart wall.

Equation 14.15 (later in the chapter) indicates that theoretically there are no strict requirements on the mechanical properties of the biomaterials of a CSD, as long as it can provide a mechanical support at the end of diastole. Practically, however, a CSD should have optimal compliance so as to smoothly fit over the surface of heart. This compliance can be achieved, for example, through the knitting of polymer fibers (Figure 14.16b). It would also be ideal that the supporting device exhibits a nonlinear elasticity similar to that of heart muscle, such that it can reshape with the heart and thus provide mechanical support to the heart throughout the beating processes, rather than only at the end of diastole.

Although ventricular restraint has shown distinct benefits of the CSD devices in animal models over cardiomyoplasty [13], these devices have not been translated to the clinic, and there is lack of convincing evidence from Phase II trials for their clinical benefit; therefore, CSDs have not yet received the approval of the FDA [14]. It must be emphasized that a mechanical support to an injured heart is not able to compensate for any cell loss incurred, but could slow down the further progress of the disease by reducing the working load of the heart muscle. Hence, the ventricular restraint strategy is not a radical treatment. Rather, it is aimed to offer a bridge to heart transplantation. Due to lack of heart donors, many heart-failure patients might not be able to survive before a donor heart is available.

14.5.3 Stem Cell Therapy

Cell-based therapy, on the other hand, represents a radical procedure. In this approach, healthy, functional cells are injected into the infarcted region via the epicardium, coronary arteries, coronary veins, or endocardium (Figure 14.18). Studies have shown that transplantation of fetal cardiomyocytes and stem-cell-derived cardiomyocytes can result in the replacement of diseased myocardium with healthy myocardium.

Since myocardium has an extremely limited regenerative ability, the first issue in the cell therapy of its disease is the source of healthy cardiomyocytes. One concept is to draw from cells of the embryonic stage of human development, before a heart is formed. The cells at this stage have the capacity to differentiate into any tissues and organs. Embryonic stem cells will be described in detail in Chapter 16. For stem cell therapy of myocardial disease, readers are referred to the advanced topics at the end of Chapter 16.

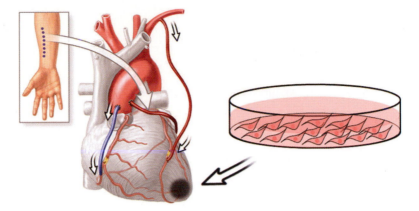

Figure 14.18
Cell therapy represents a radical treatment.

14.5.4 Combinatorial Approach: The Heart Patch

Currently, the efficiency of cell therapy is very low using current methods, due to a major loss of cells from the heart following delivery. Moreover, due to the elevated filling pressures in the beating heart, cardiac muscle slippage continues and thus negative remodeling of the infarct region occurs, unless a mechanical support is used.

The individual limitations of cell therapy and left ventricular restraint prompted the hypothesis that their combination might synergistically increase the capacity of myocardial tissue to regenerate within the body, offering a more effective clinical treatment than either strategy alone. In this approach, a *heart patch*, which is made of a polymeric material and sized to fit the infarct area, is surgically implanted. In conjunction, temporary bypass surgery is applied to transiently relieve pressure on the healing site. Furthermore, cells that are able to differentiate into cardiomyocytes, or skeletal muscle cells, are seeded directly into the patch. So this device serves the dual purpose of both a cell-delivery vehicle and a mechanical support (Figure 14.19).

Possible benefits of the proposed heart patch approach include the following:

1. The promotion of the healing of the infarcted myocardium by the implanted cells.
2. The efficiency of cell retention is improved compared to injection methods.
3. Heart wall support is increased and stress is reduced, thus preventing further left-ventricular dilation, one of the more important pathophysiological mechanisms underlying the clinical cause of progressive heart failure.
4. Heart patch biodegradability. Long-term detrimental effects associated with persisting foreign substances within the body and the need for a second operation to remove a nondegradable device are thus obviated.

To be suitable for the purposes of heart patch implementation, a biomaterial must be

- Cytocompatible, so as to be able to deliver cells
- Mechanically compatible with the heart muscle, being nonlinearly elastic, so as to not intervene the natural beating process of the host heart
- Biodegradable so as to eliminate the need of a second surgery

Up to now, heart patches made of porous polyurethane (Figure 9.27) [15], soft poly(polyol sebacte) (Figure 14.20) [16], and cell sheets (Figures 14.21 and 14.22) have been explored.

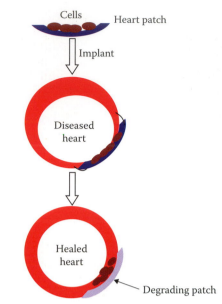

Figure 14.19

Clinical strategy of a heart patch device.

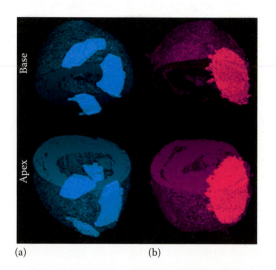

(a)   (b)

Figure 14.20

Magnetic resonance microscopy images of thermoplastic elastomer heart patches attached to the pericardium of rat hearts. Premature failure of a thermoplastic rubber: poly (ethylene terephthalate)/dimer fatty acid can be seen in green (a), while maintenance of the physical integrity of chemically cross-linked poly(glycerol sebacate) is shown in purple (b). (From Stuckey, D.J. et al., Tissue Eng. Part A, 16, 3395, 2010.)

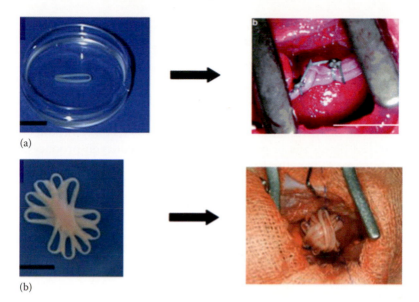

(a)

(b)

Figure 14.21
Different techniques to fix engineering heart tissue (EHT) on the recipient's heart. (a) Ring-shaped EHTs were placed around the circumference of the heart or sutured onto the heart in apical–valvular direction. (From Zimmermann, W.H. et al., Circulation, 106, 1151, 2002.) (b) Stacking EHTs were sutured on the recipient's heart. (From Zimmermann, W.H. et al., Nat. Med., 12(4), 452, 2006. Reproduced with permission from Nature Publishing Group.)

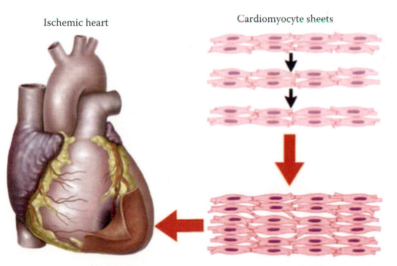

Ischemic heart

Cardiomyocyte sheets

Heart bandage

Figure 14.22
Schematic graph showing the transplantation of a myocardial cell sheet graft, also called heart bandage. (From Yang, J. et al., MRS Bull., 30, 189, 2005.)

14.6 ARTIFICIAL BLOOD VESSELS

As mentioned earlier, autologous grafting of blood vessels is the standard method of bypass surgery. The application of artificial blood vessels to small diameter (<6 mm), such as those used in bypass surgery, is hampered by the issue of thrombosis. Up to now, artificial vessels made of PTFE have only been used to substitute the aorta; however, these are also prone to thrombosis, infection, or immune rejection. One company, based at Yale University, has recently produced a bioengineered artificial blood vessel prototype made from collagen produced by endothelial cells in vitro. This natural material is able to be repopulated in vivo by the body's own cells, and is currently undergoing clinical trials (http://www.humacyte.com/products/).

14.7 CHAPTER HIGHLIGHTS

1. Three components: blood, heart, and vessels
2. Heart: two superior atria and two inferior ventricles
3. Diastole and systole
4. Two circuits: pulmonary and systemic circuits
5. Three types of blood vessels: artery, veins, and capillary
6. Aorta and coronary artery on heart
7. Why heart disease is so devastating?
   Heart is a vital organ, heart muscle cells have no regenerative ability, and heart disease is pandemic.
8. Key pathological mechanisms leading to heart failure after heart attack:
   a. Massive, permanent cell loss
   b. Ventricle dilation leading to scar formation (negative remodeling)
9. Current treatments and their limitations: Drug and surgical intervention both cannot stop the progress of the disease.
10. Alternative treatments and their limitations
    Ventricle restraint, its working principle (Young–Laplace's law)
    Cell therapy
    Combinatorial strategy
11. Applications of biomaterials:
    a. Artificial vessels: PTFE, natural polymers
    b. Cardiac supporting devices: PET, PP
    c. Pacemaker: Ti alloy, and bioinert polymers
    d. Heart patch: PU, PPS, biological tissue, collagen

ACTIVITIES

See your blood flow and heart beating at http://www.bostonscientific.com/template-data/imports/HTML/lifebeatonline/winter2007/learning.shtml.

SIMPLE QUESTIONS IN CLASS

1. Which organ does oxygen-depleted blood flows into to become oxygenated before flowing back into the left ventricle of the heart?
    a. Arm
    b. Brain
    c. Lung
    d. Vertebrate

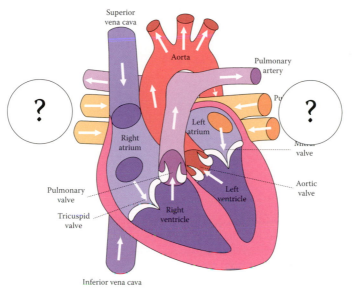

2. The pulmonary circuit (horizontal) circulates blood between
    a. Heart and arms
    b. Heart and lungs
    c. Lungs
    d. Heart and the rest of the body, except for lungs

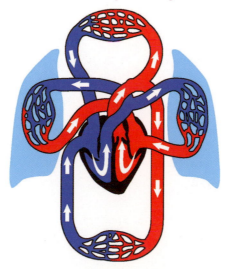

3. The systemic circuit (vertical) circulates blood between
   a. Heart and head
   b. Heart and lungs
   c. Heart and legs
   d. Heart and the rest of the body, except for lungs
4. Two key pathological mechanisms leading to heart failure after heart attack are
   a. Loss of contractility and depletion of oxygen
   b. Massive, permanent cell loss and ventricular dilation that leads to negative remodeling of heart muscle
   c. Thrombosis and high tension
   d. Loss of breathing and lack of oxygen
5. Current standard treatments of myocardial infract patients do not include
   a. Pharmaceutical therapy
   b. Surgical intervention
   c. Heart transplantation
   d. Cell therapy
6. Which disease is the number one cause of human mortality?
   a. Cancer
   b. Heart disease
   c. Osteoporosis
   d. Lung disease
7. List four current and potential medical devices, and the biomaterials used, for the treatment of cardiovascular diseases.
8. Correct the wrong labels in the following anatomical diagram of the heart:

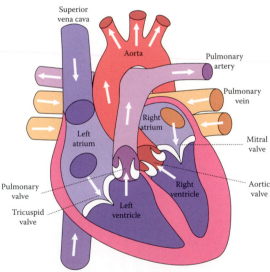

9. *Myocardial infarct* means
   a. Heart failure
   b. Heart burn
   c. Heart pain
   d. Heart attack

PROBLEMS AND EXERCISES

1. What are the three constituents of the cardiovascular system? What is the major function of the circulatory system?
2. Explain vein and artery, diastole and systole, pulmonary and systematic circuits.
3. Discuss the current standard therapies and applications of biomaterials of the following two cardiovascular diseases:
    a. Heart attack
    b. Coronary artery blockage
4. Discuss the reasons why heart disease is the most devastating disease.
5. What are the two key pathological mechanisms leading to heart failure after a heart attack?
6. Using Laplace's law, discuss why a cardiac supporting device could benefit an infarcted heart.

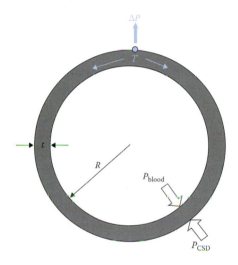

7. Discuss the advantages and disadvantages of ventral restraint and cell therapy strategies in the treatment of heart-failure patients.
8. Discuss the major issues in the cell therapy for the treatment of myocardial infarct.
9. List five applications of biomaterials in the treatment of cardiovascular diseases. Discuss the state of the art of these applications.
10. Explain active mechanical properties and passive mechanical behaviors of muscles.

BIBLIOGRAPHY

References

1. World Health Organization (WHO), http://who.int/mediacentre/factsheets/fs310/en/index.html.
2. Taylor, R.B., *Taylor's Cardiovascular Diseases: A Handbook*. New York: Springer Science + Business Media Inc., 2005.

3. Vargas, G.E. et al., Effect of nano-sized bioactive glass particles on the angiogenic properties of collagen based composites. *Journal of Materials Science. Materials in Medicine*,
   2013;**24**:1261–1269.

4. European Commission Health and Consumer Protection. Opinion on the state of
   the art concerning tissue engineering, 2001. http://ec.europa.eu/food/fs/sc/scmp/
   out37_en.pdf.

5. Chachques, J.C. et al., Study of muscular and ventricular function in dynamic cardiomyoplasty:
   A ten-year follow-up. *Journal of Heart and Lung Transplantation*, 1997;**16**(8):854–868.

6. Lorusso, R. et al., Cardiomyoplasty as an isolated procedure to treat refractory heart failure.
   European Journal of Cardio-Thoracic Surgery, 1997;**11**(2):363–371.

7. Oh, J.H., V. Badhwar, and R.C.J. Chiu, Mechanisms of dynamic cardiomyoplasty: Current
   concepts. *Journal of Cardiac Surgery*, 1996;**11**(3):194–199.

8. Eloakley, R.M. and J.C. Jarvis, Cardiomyoplasty—A critical-review of experimental and clin-
   ical-results. *Circulation*, 1994;**90**(4):2085–2090.

9. Christman, K.L. and R.J. Lee, Biomaterials for the treatment of myocardial infarction. *Journal
   of the American College of Cardiology*, 2006;**48**(5):907–913.

10. Kelley, S.T. et al., Restraining infarct expansion preserves left ventricular geometry and
    function after acute anteroapical infarction. *Circulation*, 1999;**99**(1):135–142.

11. Enomoto, Y. et al., Early ventricular restraint after myocardial infarction: Extent
    of the wrap determines the outcome of remodeling. *Annals of Thoracic Surgery*,
    2005;**79**(3):881–887.

12. Walsh, R.G., Design and features of the acorn CorCap (TM) stop cardiac support
    device: The concept of passive mechanical diastolic support. *Heart Failure Reviews*,
    2005;**10**(2):101–107.

13. Sabbah, H.N., The cardiac support device and the myosplint: Treating heart failure by tar-
    geting left ventricular size and shape. *Annals of Thoracic Surgery*, 2003;**75**(6):S13–S19.

14. www.acorncv.com/newsrelease12-08-06disputeresolutionpanelNO-FINAL.pdf.

15. Fujimoto, K.L. et al., An elastic, biodegradable cardiac patch induces contractile smooth
    muscle and improves cardiac remodeling and function in subacute myocardial infarction.
    Journal of the American College of Cardiology, 2007;**49**(23):2292–2300.

16. Stuckey, D.J. et al., Magnetic resonance imaging evaluation of remodeling by cardiac
    elastomeric tissue scaffold biomaterials in a rat model of myocardial infarction. *Tissue
    Engineering Part A*, 2010;**16**(11):3395–3402.

17. Zimmermann, W.H. et al., Cardiac grafting of engineered heart tissue in syngenic rats.
    Circulation, 2002;**106**(13):I151–I157.

18. Zimmermann, W.H. et al., Engineered heart tissue grafts improve systolic and diastolic
    function in infarcted rat hearts. *Nature Medicine*, 2006;**12**(4):452–458.

19. Yang, J., M. Yamato, and T. Okano, Cell-sheet engineering using intelligent surfaces. *MRS
    Bulletin*, 2005;**30**(3):189–193.

20. Bolotin, G. et al., *Chest*, **121**(5), 1628–1633, May 2002.

Websites

Animations of heart beating

http://www.atenmedicalart.com/anim/heart.htm.

http://www.humacyte.com/products/.

http://www.innerbody.com/anim/heart.html.

http://www.3dscience.com/Resources/3d_Heart_Model_base.php.

Heart foundations

http://www.heartfoundation.org.au/Pages/default.aspx.

http://www.heart.org/HEARTORG/.

www.bhf.org.uk/.

Human mortality
http://en.wikipedia.org/wiki/List_of_causes_of_death_by_rate.
http://www.mortality.org/.
http://www.nhlbi.nih.gov/resources/docs/2012_ChartBook_508.pdf.
http://www.who.int/en/.

Further Readings

Martini, F.H., M.J. Timmons, and R.B. Tallitsch, *Human Anatomy*, 5th edn. San Francisco, CA: Pearson/Benjamin Cummings, 2006. Related chapters.
Tate, S.S., *Anatomy and Physiology*, 8th edn. New York: McGraw Hill, 2008. Related chapters.

CHAPTER 15

HUMAN ANATOMY AND DISEASES III

Respiratory, Lymphatic, Digestive, Urinary, and Reproductive Systems

LEARNING OBJECTIVES

After a careful study of this chapter, you should be able to do the following:

1. Describe the gross anatomy of the respiratory, digestive, lymphatic, urinary, and reproductive systems
2. Describe the major health issues of these systems
3. Describe the applications of biomaterials in the treatment of problems associated with these systems

15.1   RESPIRATORY SYSTEM

15.1.1   Breathing and Respiration

Although respiration is often considered the same as breathing, the latter is actually just part of the former. Externally, *breathing* is the *mechanical process* that moves air into and out of the lungs, via either costal (thoracic) and diaphragmatic (abdominal) motion of the chest cavity, which the lungs are held into via a slight vacuum pressure. In *costal breathing*, the major structure causing the movement of the air is the rib cage, which expands and contracts the lungs within, by flexible joints at both the spinal column and the sternum (chest). In *diaphragmatic breathing*, the sheet-like muscle of the diaphragm at the bottom of the chest cavity depresses like a membrane pump, pulling the lungs down and thereby filling them with air. Both forms of breathing usually work in unison, although diaphragmatic breathing is more efficient in filling the lungs.

Oxygen from air that has been breathed into the lungs is then carried away by the blood (see last chapter), while upon breathing out, carbon dioxide is released from venous blood. *Respiration* refers to the exchange of gases between the atmosphere and the cells of the body, via the bloodstream, resulting in a complex physiological process of supply and demand. Respiration can basically be divided into two processes: (1) external respiration, the exchange of gases between the air in the lungs and blood; and (2) internal respiration, the exchange of gases between the blood and the cell populations in the body. In biochemistry and cell biology, respiration refers to the process of oxidative metabolism, where cells use oxygen to extract chemical energy from carbohydrates and amino acids. In physiology, the respiratory system refers to the major organs that supply the oxygen for respiration and systems that control this supply at times of high demand (e.g., exercise, stress responses).

15.1.2   Gross Anatomy and Functions of the Respiratory System

The respiratory system is made up of the organs involved in the breathing process, which is basically a system of transferring and conditioning the air that is taken in. This system includes the two lungs and a system of tubes (i.e., air passageways) that link the sites of gas exchange with the external environment, as illustrated in Figure 15.1 and listed in the following:

- Nose and nasal cavity
- Pharynx
- Larynx
- Trachea
- Bronchi

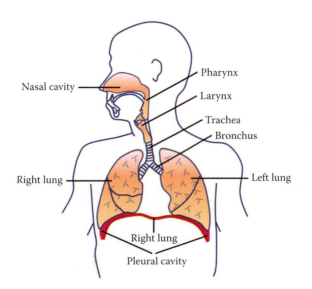

Figure 15.1
Gross anatomy of the respiratory system.

15.1.2.1 Nose, Pharynx, and Larynx (Upper Respiratory Tract) Air is able to enter either the nose or mouth; however, the nasal cavity and the pharynx in combination (the *nasopharynx*) is more specialized for conditioning the air as it is carried toward the lungs. It also has some filtering roles, via the large surface area of the membranes that produce mucus that traps and moves dust and other foreign particles before they are able to reach the lungs. The main role of these membranes is to heat and humidify the incoming air.

The *pharynx* also has other nonrespiratory roles involved in sensation of taste and smell, the latter also acting as a kind of safety barrier to prevent toxic compounds from reaching the lungs. The junction of the soft palate (roof of the mouth) and the pharynx acts as a two-way valve, allowing gas to enter the lungs, but not the digestive system, except during swallowing of food. In this case, food can enter the digestive tract via the esophagus (food tube behind the trachea) but not the lungs, because the epiglottis temporarily closes off the trachea (in front). The pharynx also contains the muscles involved in the swallowing reflex.

15.1.2.2 Trachea and Bronchi (Lower Respiratory Tract) The *trachea* is often called the windpipe in common parlance, and forms the top of the respiratory *tree*, where the vocal cords are attached, vibrating in response to exhaled air that enables speech. They also form a valve that closes off the trachea, which is activated when we hold our breath or cough, which occurs independently of swallowing (note: you can still hold your breath and swallow at the same time!). The trachea is essentially a tube, held in shape by circular rings of cartilage, which occur all the way down to the lungs. More than simply a tube, it also filters the air we breathe, via microscopic cellular finger-like projections (cilia) in the mucous membranes of it, as well as the nasopharynx above. These move in waves under autonomic nerve control away from the lungs, acting like an elevator, which helps to expel the foreign particles trapped in the mucus. Further down the lower respiratory tract, the trachea branches off into the left and right bronchus (*pl. bronchi*), two smaller air tubes that carry air directly to each lung.

Breathing starts when autonomic nerve impulses stimulate the diaphragm (Figure 15.1), causing it to contract, changing from its dome-like resting position to a flat sheet. Upon contraction, this movement enlarges the chest cavity (thorax) and pulls air like a vacuum into the lungs. When we breathe out, the diaphragm relaxes and expands once again, reducing the amount of space for the lungs and forcing air out. This forms a continuous breathing cycle, which begins before birth and continues until death. The cyclicity of breathing increases when there is extra demand on the tissues and the brain, which occurs in unison with increased heart rate as well. Hence, the respiratory system and the circulatory system work together.

15.1.3 Gross Structure and Functions of the Lungs

The rest of the lower respiratory system is made up of the lungs, the main functional organs of the respiratory system, and vital organs of the body. In the human, there are two lungs, left and right, with a cavity behind the left lung in which the heart is positioned (cardiac notch). The right lung is therefore larger in volume than the left lung, as the left lung must leave room for the heart. The left brochus also branches slightly higher because of this difference.

Structurally, both lungs are divided by large folds (fissures) into smaller compartments called pulmonary lobes (Figure 15.2). Each lobe is further partitioned into

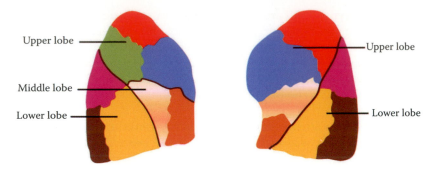

Figure 15.2
Pulmonary lobes of the lungs.

bronchopulmonary segments, like branches of a tree. The right lung is divided into three pulmonary lobes (upper (*superior*), middle (*medial*), and lower (*inferior*) and 10 bronchopulmonary segments. The left lung is divided into a superior and an inferior lobe, with a total of eight bronchopulmonary segments.

The main bronchus of each lung branches off into smaller diameter secondary (lobular) bronchi (Figure 15.3), which serve each of the pulmonary lobes. Further down the tree, the lobular bronchi branch off into yet smaller diameter tertiary (segmental) bronchi, which service the bronchopulmonary segments (Figure 15.4). Finally, at the end of each segmental tertiary bronchus branches off into smaller (1 mm diameter) bronchioles, which at this point no longer have cartilage and are thus able to remain open. Combined, it is estimated that there are around 2.4 km of airways servicing the lungs.

Air moves from the outside of the body into tiny balloon-like sacs in the lungs called alveoli (*singl. alveolus*) (Figure 15.3), which are like the leaves of the tree, serviced by the many *alveolar ducts* which terminally branch off each bronchiole. There are billions of alveoli in the adult lung, forming a three-dimensional sponge-like structure. Combined, their microscopic size produces a very large surface area equivalent to ~100 m², which is large enough to allow simple diffusion of oxygen into the pulmonary circulation. Each alveolus contains a single pulmonary arteriole and venule, which are directly apposed, so that the distance for oxygen to travel from air to a red blood cell is only a few microns.

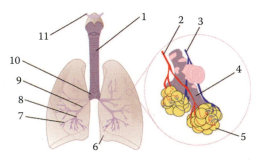

Figure 15.3
Gross structure of the lungs (blue items on the list). 1, Trachea; 2, pulmonary vein (toward the heart); 3, pulmonary artery (from the heart); 4, alveolar duct; 5, alveolus (air sac); 6, cardiac notch; 7, bronchioles; 8, tertiary bronchi; 9, secondary bronchi; 10, primary bronchi; 11, larynx. (From http://commons.wikimedia.org/ produced by Mariana Ruiz Villarreal.)

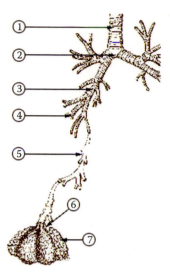

Figure 15.4
Tertiary bronchus of the lung. 1, Trachea; 2, main stem bronchus; 3, lobar bronchus; 4, segmental bronchus; 5, bronchiole; 6, alveolar duct; 7, alveolus. (From http://en.wikipedia.org/wiki/Tertiary_bronchus.)

15.1.4   Pneumocytes in Alveoli and the Regenerative Ability of Lungs

There are three major types of alveolar cells in the alveolar wall:

- Type I (*squamous alveolar*) pneumocytes are responsible for gas exchange in the alveoli and cover a majority of the alveolar surface area (more than 95%).
- Type II (*great alveolar*) pneumocytes, which secrete pulmonary surfactant to lower the surface tension of water and allow the membrane to separate, thereby increasing the capability to exchange gases.
- *Macrophages*: cells of the immune system that consume and destroy foreign materials, such as bacteria. The lungs, together with the digestive system, are the only internal organs in direct contact with the nonsterile external environment. Hence, they need a strong defense mechanism to combat foreign bodies. In the cases of the lungs, microbial particles can easily be carried passively into the alveoli in dry or wet aerosols.

The relatively good regenerative ability of lung tissue is evidenced by our capability to recover from lung infections caused by such microbial pathogens as pneumonia. Many of us have one or even more than one experience of pneumonia. Most of us survive from this disease and fully recover with the completely normal function of the lungs. Type I pneumocytes are susceptible to toxic insults and unable to replicate. In the event of damage, type II pneumocytes can proliferate and differentiate into type I cells to replace damaged type I pneumocytes. It is these stem-cell-like characteristics of type II pneumocytes that enable the lungs to regenerate to repair disease or damage.

However, if the alveolar tissue, which hosts the type II pneumocytes of the organs, is damaged, the lungs would have little ability to regenerate. Hence, the regenerative capacity of the lungs is closely dependent on the degree of damage.

15.1.5 Lung Disease: Emphysema

Lung disease is the number three cause of mortality after heart disease and cancer. Among the many types of lung diseases (also called chronic obstructive pulmonary disease (COPD)), emphysema is the most common, with a clear association with damage caused by cigarette smoking. Chronic accumulation of toxic chemicals and particles from cigarette tar causes progressive cytotoxicity, irreversibly damaging type II pneumocytes and alveolar microvessels. The main symptoms of emphysema include gradual reduction of lung capacity and inflammation, associated with chronic coughing and wheezing, and may become complicated by pulmonary hypertension and cardiac dysfunction.

Currently, the standard treatment of emphysema is aimed at relieving symptoms and preventing the disease from progressing even further. Typical management includes cessation of smoking, drug therapy (e.g., vasodilators, to improve airflow via bronchiole expansion), pulmonary rehabilitation, and oxygen therapy. These therapies afford modest rates of recovery, but do not arrest or reverse the progression of the disease.

15.1.6 New Strategy: Lung Volume Reduction Surgery

Lung volume reduction surgery (LVRS) has become an option for some emphysema patients. In this procedure, a portion of the most severely damaged lung tissue is removed (Figure 15.5), in order to ease the burden on the remaining lung tissue and chest muscles. The key rationale behind LVRS, however, is that we only use about 50% of the lungs under the normal condition, and that the unused part of lungs will be able to resume function after a resection.

Surgeons perform LVRS by removing about 20%–35% of the damaged lung. By reducing the lung size, the remaining lung and surrounding muscles (intercostal (rib) muscles and diaphragm) are able to work more efficiently. Although LVRS is a nonradical procedure, it makes breathing easier and helps patients achieve a greater quality of life.

Approximately 80% of all LVRS patients improve, with a remaining 15% showing no change. For patients with an upper lobe distribution of emphysema, bilateral staple LVRS offers a reduction in the probability of dependency on oxygen therapy (68%) or prednisone (anti-inflammatory) treatment (85%), with a 60%–70% improvement in pulmonary function. The length of time that patients benefit following LVRS is currently still being studied. For some patients the benefit lasts only 6–12 months. The typical length of benefit is 2–3 years, although some patients have experienced improvement for 5–6 years.

About 5%–10% of patients receiving bilateral staple LVRS die as a result of the surgery, with air leaks lasting at least 7 days in up to half of these cases. Other complications found in less than 5% of patients include pneumonia, arrhythmia (irregular heartbeat), heart attack, and internal bleeding.

15.1.7 Application of Biomaterials: Sealants and Bioartificial Trachea

Among a number of issues, postoperative air leakage is a major problem, mainly due to the constant positive pressure within the lung. Surgical glue is considered to be a solution. Current FDA-approved medical glues are made of either fibrin or cyanoacrylate.

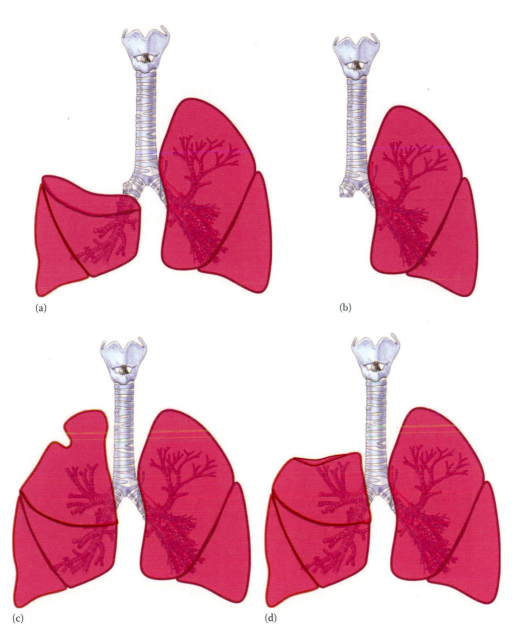

(a)

(b)

(c)

(d)

Figure 15.5

Resection in lung volume reduction surgery. (a) Lobectomy is a common surgical procedure involving removal of one lobe containing damaged cells. Removal of two lobes is called bilobectomy. (b) Pnomonectomy is most often operated for cancer or other irreversible damage of the lung that cannot be treated by removal of a smaller portion of the lung. (c) Wedge resection is often peformed to remove a small tumor, or to take a tissue sample (biopsy) for diagnostic testing. (d) Segmentectomy involves removal of a larger portion of the lung lobe than a wedge resection, but does not involve removal of the whole lobe.

Fibrin sealant, a biocompatible and biodegradable material, is a naturally occurring protein-based elastomer prepared from human blood plasma. Fibrin is involved in the clotting of blood, and is nonglobular, forming a fibrillar *mesh* that forms a hemostatic clot (in conjunction with platelets) over a wound site. Although the concerns about blood-borne virus contamination (e.g., hepatitis B, HIV-1, and parvovirus) have been eliminated by the development of complicated filtration processes, this makes the products prohibitively expensive. Synthetic sealants such as cyanoacrylates have been considered a safer, virus-free alternative. However, these sorts of sealants are relatively mechanically incompatible and nonbiodegradable, with some toxic by-products.

The regeneration of the trachea and bronchi may be a potential future application of biomaterials, since these are essentially physical tube structures. In 2008, the first clinical report of a recellularized trachea was published, which involved the removal of a trachea from a tissue donor, cellular digestion and reseeding with stem cells, then transplantation to a recipient [1]. It could also be possible to develop an artificial tracheal skeleton, similar to the cartilaginous one used here, using rapid prototyping or molding processes.

15.2   LYMPHATIC SYSTEM

15.2.1   Gross Anatomy of the Lymphatic System

As discussed in the Chapter 14, the cardiovascular system provides a constant supply of nutrients and oxygen to the tissues. Alongside the arterial and venous networks of vessels is the lymphatic system, which can also be regarded as a vascular network, although it has more protective roles in immune defense.

Between the cells of the body are spaces known as intervening (interstitial) spaces, which are filled with a clear fluid referred to as intercellular fluid or lymph. The cells continually exchange water and ions between the intercellular fluid and the plasma of the blood, with a majority of the fluid reabsorbed back into the blood vessels. The remaining fluid is drained back to the heart via the lymphatic vessels. As a drainage system, the lymphatics branch away from the tissues into progressively larger vessels, which converge at points called lymph nodes (Figure 15.6), which are small gland-like structures containing lymphocytes. There are also larger nodes, considered as lymph organs, including the spleen, thymus, and tonsils. Lymphocyte colonies play a central role in the body's defenses against viruses, bacteria, and other microorganisms; and these cells are relocated back and forth between the lymph nodes, and to the bone marrow.

Like veins, lymphatic vessels are supplied with valves to help maintain a flow of lymph in one direction only. The lymphatic vessels, to a greater or lesser extent, parallel the venous vessels along the way. The major lymph vessel in the human body is called the *thoracic duct*, which passes vertically from the abdomen up through the thorax and back into the major veins that carry blood back to the heart, in front of the neck vertebrae. The flow of lymph is also controlled in the larger vessels by smooth muscle, and the cyclic movements of breathing. Lymphatics that drain the digestive tissue of the body are also involved in removing emulsified fatty acids via the lymph.

15.2.1.1   Lymphatic Organs (the Lymphoid System)   *Tonsils* are special collections of lymphoid tissue, very similar to a cluster of lymph nodes. These are protective

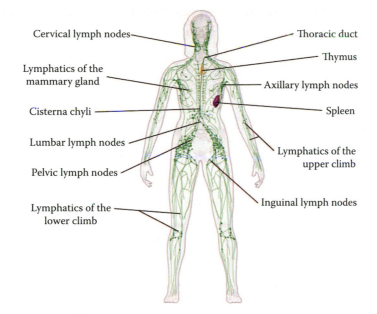

Cervical lymph nodes

Thoracic duct

Thymus

Lymphatics of the mammary gland

Axillary lymph nodes

Cisterna chyli

Spleen

Lumbar lymph nodes

Lymphatics of the upper climb

Pelvic lymph nodes

Inguinal lymph nodes

Lymphatics of the lower climb

Figure 15.6
Gross anatomy of the lymphatic system. (From http://commons.wikimedia.org/produced by Blausen.)

structures and are located primarily at the entrances of the respiratory and digestive systems. Because of this location, tonsils and other lymph nodes of the head and neck are frequently inflamed due to viral and bacterial infections, becoming swollen due to the increased proliferation of lymphocytes.

The *thymus* is another specialized type of lobular lymph node, which has a very critical role in development of the immune system in early life. The thymus is involved in a highly complex process of molecular modification of surface proteins on lymphocytes, to enable them to recognize viruses and bacteria. Once these specialized lymphocytes (also called *thymocytes*) are equipped with these proteins, they are distributed throughout the body, adapting and retaining a *memory* of the molecular composition of the infectious agent. Hence a vaccine may contain parts of bacterial proteins for the immune system to recognize, causing a temporary immune response, but thereafter returning to normal, enough to provide lymphocytes with a new molecular signal to *remember*. While removal of the thymus is not fatal, in early life it can cause severe immunodeficiency, meaning the patient is more likely to contract routine illnesses.

The *spleen* is essentially a very large lymph node, acting primarily as a blood filter and store of lymphocytes and platelets. It removes old or abnormal blood cells, and stores a range of different types of lymphocytes that participate in immune responses, and can respond to vaccines. The spleen can also store a significant population of red blood cells, which can be released in an emergency, in the case of sudden loss of blood. Processing and recycling of red blood cells is also performed by the liver and pancreas, so the spleen has a more secondary role in this process, although there have been recent reports of links between alcohol-related problems in the liver, and enlargement of the spleen.

The spleen is not a vital organ, so it is possible to remove it without jeopardizing life. Surgical removal of the spleen causes the following:

- Modest increases in circulating white blood cells and platelets
- Diminished responsiveness to some vaccines
- Increased susceptibility to infection by bacteria and protozoa

A 28-year follow-up of 740 veterans of World War II found those that had been splenectomized showed a significant excess mortality from pneumonia (6 from normally expected 1.3) and ischemic heart disease (41 from normally expected 30) but not other conditions.

15.2.2 Diseases of Lymphatic System

Lymphoma (cancer of lymphoid tissue) and *breast cancer* are two common cancers that involve the lymphatic system. Cancer cells can spread to other parts of the body through the lymphatic vessels. For example, some more invasive breast cancers that originate in the glandular tissue of the breast can spread into the lymph nodes of the chest and neck, becoming life-threatening to the heart and lungs. Another less common, but potentially life-threatening condition is a *lymphedema*, a chronic enlargement of the lymphatic vessels, caused by dysfunctional lymph nodes or blocked vessels. Very severe cases can cause massive enlargement of regions of the body (*elephantiasis*).

15.2.3 Application of Biomaterials

Except drug delivery, there are very few reports on the development of biomaterials for the treatment of disease in the lymphatic system. The following three citations provide a glimpse on the progress of biomaterials application in this system.

1. Niklason, L.E., J. Koh, and A. Solan, Tissue engineering of the lymphatic system. *Annals of the New York Academy of Sciences* 2002;**979**:27–34; discussion 35–38:

   The field of tissue engineering has seen tremendous expansion in the last decade. In the last several years, tissue-engineering strategies to treat diseases of skin, cartilage, bone, bladder, blood vessel, tendon, and other tissues have been described. However, *tissue-engineering approaches to treat diseases of the lymphatic system are currently nonexistent*. We propose that acellular tissues, either native or engineered, could be exploited as a platform for the study of lymphatic biology, and for lymphatic tissue engineering. While speculative, this type of experimental model system could prove powerful for dissecting molecular and cellular events surrounding tumor invasion of lymphatics, as well as lymphangiogenesis. Scaffolds seeded with genetically engineered lymphatic cells could also be implanted to repopulate lymphatic vasculature. In the future, the lymphatic system will surely be added to the list of tissues and organs that prove amenable to tissue-engineering therapies.

2. Hitchcock, T. and L. Niklason, Lymphatic tissue engineering: progress and prospects. *Annals of New York Academy Sciences* 2008;**1131**:44–49:

   In the last 5 years major advances have been made in the field of tissue engineering. However, while engineering of tissues from nearly every major system in the body have been studied and improved, *little has been done with the engineering of viable lymphatic tissues*. Recent advances in understanding of lymphatic biology have allowed the easy isolation of pure lymphatic cell cultures, increasing, in turn, the ability to study lymphatic biology in greater detail. This has allowed the elucidation of lymphatic properties on the structural, cellular, and molecular levels, making possible the successful development of the first lymphatic engineered tissues. Among such advances are the engineering of lymphatic capillaries, the development of a functioning bioreactor designed to culture lymph nodes *in vitro*, and in vivo growth of lymphatic organoids. However, *there has been no research on the engineering of functional lymphangions*. While the advances made in the study of lymphatic biology are encouraging, *the complexities of the system make the engineering of certain functional lymphatic tissues somewhat more difficult.*

3. Weitman, E., D. Cuzzone, and B.J. Mehrara, Tissue engineering and regeneration of lymphatic structures. *Future Oncol.* 2013;**9**(9):1365–1374. doi: 10.2217/fon.13.110:

Tissue engineering is the process by which biological structures are recreated using a combination of molecular signals, cellular components and scaffolds. Although the perceived potential of this approach to reconstruct damaged or missing tissues is seemingly limitless, application of these ideas in vivo has been more difficult than expected. However, *despite these obstacles, important advancements have been reported for a number of organ systems, including recent reports on the lymphatic system.* These advancements are important since the lymphatic system plays a central role in immune responses, regulation of inflammation, lipid absorption and interstitial fluid homeostasis. Insights obtained over the past two decades have advanced our understanding of the molecular and cellular mechanisms that govern lymphatic development and function. Utilizing this knowledge has led to important advancements in lymphatic tissue engineering....

15.3   DIGESTIVE SYSTEM

15.3.1   Gross Anatomy of the Digestive System

The human digestive system is a group of organs, functioning mostly automatically, that process solid and liquid food that we consume, to extract nutrients for tissue metabolism, growth, and normal function, and process the used and surplus materials as waste. The digestive tract itself is basically a muscular, tube-like cavity that extends from one end of the body to the other (Figure 15.7). Like the respiratory system, the digestive tract is effectively outside of the body.

The major organs involved in the human digestive system are listed as follows:

1. Mouth or oral complex
2. Pharynx
3. Esophagus
4. Stomach
5. Small intestine and associated glands (liver and pancreas)
6. Large intestine
7. Rectum
8. Anal canal and anus

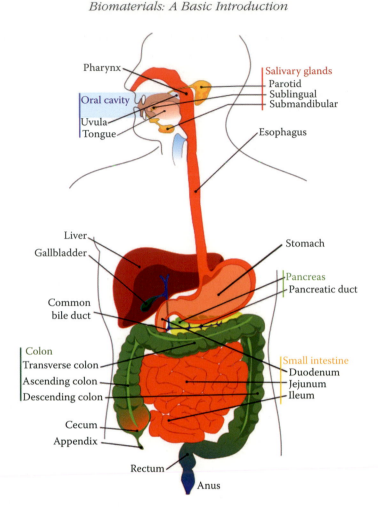

Figure 15.7
Gross anatomy of the digestive system. (From http://commons.wikimedia.org/produced by Mariana Ruiz Villarreal.)

15.3.2 Digestion: General Biochemistry of Food Breakdown

Digestion is the biochemical process by which food is converted into simpler substances that can be absorbed by the body. Each step of the digestive process occurs in a specific compartment, involved in step-by-step breakdown of food molecules (proteins, polysaccharides, fatty acids, and minerals). The first biochemical breakdown process involves the action of *digestive enzymes*, molecular catalysts that aid in the conversion of food molecules (as described for the breakdown of biomaterials in Chapter 9). Enzymes are manufactured in the salivary glands of the mouth, the lining of the stomach, the pancreas, liver, and walls of the small intestine. Digestive enzymes include some of the following enzymes:

- Amylase for starch
- Proteases for protein (e.g., trypsin, pepsin)
- Lipases for fat

In addition to the action of enzymes, hydrochloric acid secreted by the stomach plays a major role the chemical denaturation of food molecules, especially protein.

Digestion products arise from food materials as follows:

- Proteins → amino acids
- Starch (polysaccharide) → oligosaccharides (e.g., sucrose, maltose) → glucose
- Fat → Fatty acid

Digestion into these basic by-products is a bulk denaturation process. While cells in tissues are also equipped with enzymes, they require substrates in these simple forms for them to be fully metabolized, using much more complex, multistep biochemical processes.

15.3.3   Functions of Organs of the Digestive System

A common feature of the entire digestive tract is its dynamic physiology. In all compartments, food and digestive contents are in a constant state of mixing and bulk, unidirectional movement. This is mostly under muscular control, and assists the chemical and biochemical digestion processes, making them more efficient as an input–output process.

15.3.3.1   Oral Complex   The oral complex consists of the structures of the mouth, which is the first compartment of the digestive tract. Here, larger pieces of food are chewed (masticated) by physical crushing action of the teeth and jaws. Glands inside the cheeks and under the tongue secrete saliva, which moistens the food, dissolving water-soluble parts of it, while enzymes in the saliva (principally amylase) break down polysaccharides in the food. The tongue and palate (the roof of the mouth) further form a paste of the dissolved matter, which is then swallowed. The tongue is also involved in the sensation of taste, which is highly developed in humans, and is also a safety barrier against toxins, which are usually bitter or acrid, contributing to the vomiting reflex.

15.3.3.2   Pharynx and Esophagus   The pharynx is a continuation of the rear of the mouth region, immediately in front of the cervical spinal column. It is a shared passageway for both the opening to the respiratory system (trachea) and the digestive system (esophagus). The esophagus is essentially a flexible, muscular tube that passes down through the neck and chest, emptying into the stomach. During swallowing, a wave of muscular contractions begins in the rear of the pharynx, causing it to meet with the soft palate (back of the roof). Food then enters the top section of the esophagus, where the epiglottis is closed off, preventing the food from entering the respiratory tract. A more regular wave of peristaltic contraction then passes the food further down the remaining section of the esophagus to empty into the stomach.

15.3.3.3   Stomach   The stomach is a sac-like enlargement of the digestive tract specialized for the storage and bulk digestion of food that has been consumed in a large portion. The esophagus enters the stomach via a muscular opening (sphincter), which prevents the reflux of the food back upward. Since food is stored here, a person does not have to eat continuously all day. While the food is in the stomach, the digestive fluid (gastric juice) secreted from glands in the wall of the stomach (hydrochloric acid (pH ~1–3), proteases, salts) mainly digests the protein content of the food, a thick layer of mucus prevents this from happening to the stomach lining. In addition, the trilayered musculature of the walls contracts under involuntary control roughly 3 times/min,

constantly changing the volume of the compartment, to thoroughly mix the food and juices while the food is being held in the stomach. Once the food is ready, the pyloric valve of the stomach opens, and a portion of the stomach contents moves into the small intestine.

15.3.3.4 Small Intestine

The end products of digestion in the stomach enter small intestine, where most of the biochemical breakdown and nutrient absorption takes place. This compartment is perhaps the most critical, where smaller peptides, fatty acids, and some polysaccharides are further broken down into their components (e.g., polyamino acids, acylglyerols, oligosaccharides). This is also due to a combination of secretory enzymes (e.g., aminopeptidases, lipases, glycosidases, respectively), salt emulsification, and further muscular contractions (~12 cycles/min). Complete digestion results in the production of single amino acids, glucose, and colloidal fatty acids with glycerol, which are transported across the wall of the gut into the blood vessels.

Transport of these end products is performed by microscopic, brush-like structures called microvilli, produced on the surface of the cells lining the intestine. Millions of these projections enable the passive diffusion of food nutrients across an enormous surface area of cell membrane (estimated around 250 m^2, or about the size of a tennis court). These end products are then distributed to all tissues of the body, to meet the energy demands of tissue growth, repair, replacement and movement, indeed much of which occur in the small intestine itself.

15.3.3.5 Small Intestine–Associated Glands: Liver and the Pancreas

The *liver* is basically a complex biochemical factory with many functions, including detoxification, enzyme synthesis, and production of biochemicals necessary for digestion. These include aspects of carbohydrate, protein, lipid, and vitamin metabolism, as well as processes related to blood clotting and red blood cell destruction. Its digestive function is to produce a fluid called bile or gall, which is involved in salt emulsification of fats, together with lipases. The liver is a vital organ, and is crucial for survival. A large proportion of blood that carries food nutrients out of the small and large intestine passes through the liver via specialized veins (hepatic portal system). The liver processes this blood before returning it to the heart for redistribution throughout the body, detoxifying it by storing ammonium in urea, and synthesizing serum albumin. There is currently no way to compensate for the absence of liver function, although surprisingly, up to two-thirds of the liver can be removed, and still maintain satisfactory levels of vital functions.

The *pancreas* is the largest gland in the body, stretching across the posterior wall of the abdomen. When called upon, it secretes pancreatic fluid into the duodenum, at the start of the small intestine. Its duct joins the common bile duct. Pancreatic lipases are the main fatty acid processing enzymes produced by the pancreas, which function together with bile salts produced in the liver, to process fatty acids. Crucially, the pancreas is also the primary organ for producing insulin, which is the key hormone in controlling blood glucose after it has been absorbed from the small intestine, or secreted by the liver.

15.3.3.6 Large Intestine

The primary function of the large intestines is the salvaging of water, vitamins, and electrolytes. Most of the end products of digestion have already been absorbed in the small intestines. Further digestion is performed by a large population of native bacteria, which perform some fermentation roles, and produce additional vitamins. Digested food contents are first a watery fluid, which becomes

502

gradually dehydrated as it moves toward the rectum, assisted by the secretion of salt. A nearly solid mass is formed by progressive peristaltic movements, and is stored for almost a day before defecation, the evacuation of feces (waste products and indigestible matter, excess nitrogen as urea).

15.3.3.7 Rectum, Anal Canal, and Anus The rectum (Lat. *Rectum Intestinum*, meaning *straight intestine*) is an approximately 30 cm long tubular narrowing of the end of the large intestine. The structure appears wave-like from the front, and from the side, one would see that it was curved to conform the sacrum (at the lower end of the spinal column). The final storage of feces evacuation is in the rectum, which terminates in the narrow anal canal, which in the adult is about 2–4 cm in length. At the end of the anal canal is the opening called the anus. Muscles called the anal sphincters aid in the retention of feces until defecation, and open under voluntary nerve control. Venous blood draining away from lower part of the rectum does not actually enter the liver, but instead goes straight to the veins entering the heart, hence drugs supplied as suppositories are actually more quickly metabolized that injected drugs.

15.3.4 Regenerative Ability of Organs of the Digestive System

Some organs of this system have good regeneration ability, such as the stomach, small and large intestines, rectum, and liver. In fact, the liver is the most regenerative of these, capable of almost complete replacement of lost tissue. As little as a quarter to a third of residual liver can regenerate into a completely new organ in less than 8 years. This amazing ability is due to hepatocytes reentering the cell division cycle. There is also evidence of stem cells, called hepatic oval cells, which can differentiate into hepatocytes.

15.3.5 Digestive System Diseases

A prevalent disorder of the digestive system is *gastroesophageal reflux*, known as heartburn, resulting from rising up of gastric juice to the bottom end of the esophagus, which causes inflammation of the inner lining. It is caused by eating quickly, or excess fatty or acid foods, as well as problems with the esophageal sphincter. *Gastric ulcers* can occur where the mucus lining of the tract has been eroded away, causing chronic inflammation of a small area due to acid attack or bacterial infection.

Cirrhosis of the liver primarily results from excessive alcohol consumption, which results in irreversible damage to the hepatocytes, resulting in formation of scar tissue, similar to the way smoking causes lung damage and scarring in emphysema. *Gallstones* can form by crystallized deposits of bile salts produced in the liver and stored in the gall bladder, blocking the small canals that feed into the small intestine, causing intense pain and similar symptoms to heart attack. These stones are often caused by Western diets, high in fat and salt.

While some inherited disorders of the digestive system cannot be cured, many can be prevented by a diet low in fats and high in fruits and vegetables, limited alcohol consumption, and periodic medical examinations.

15.3.5.1 Cancer and Short Gut Syndrome Gastrointestinal tract cancer (also called bowel or colorectal cancer) is the most common type of cancer, mainly caused by dietary and environmental factors (e.g., alcohol, high fat diets), with some genetic component. With successful early diagnosis, the survival rate of patients with cancer of the digestive system is greater than 90%. Short bowel syndrome (SBS) is a malabsorption disorder caused by the surgical removal of more than two-thirds of the small intestine from cancer patients.

15.3.5.2 Progression of Liver Inflammation (Hepatitis) Tissue damage caused by inflammation of the liver (hepatitis) can result from alcoholism, bacterial or viral infection, fatty liver disease, or side effects of other drug treatments. Infiltration by leukocytes can sometimes result in liver enlargement, but in general there are no obvious symptoms of liver inflammation, except for failure of complete breakdown of heme proteins, which causes the characteristic yellowing of the skin and eyes (*jaundice*). Early diagnosis and treatment remains the key to successful recovery, but if left untreated, the following stages of severity can occur:

- *Fibrosis*: Depending on the degree of damage, and if left untreated, the inflamed liver begins to lay down scar tissue, which will eventually be remodeled by the regenerative hepatocytes.
- *Cirrhosis*: This occurs when the fibrosis has replaced functional liver tissue, and the damage cannot be reversed. Treatment at this stage will focus on preventing further worsening of the condition, and it may be possible to stop or slow the fibrosis.
- *Cancer*: Cirrhosis can lead to a number of complications, including liver cancer, the most common of which is when hepatocytes proliferate uncontrollably and become invasive (*hepatocarcinoma*).
- *Liver failure*: When sufficient tissue damage has resulted in almost complete loss of function. This becomes a life-threatening condition that demands urgent medical care and liver transplantation.

15.3.6 Application of Biomaterials

15.3.6.1 Intestinal Substitutes Unlike blood vessels that primarily function as a physical tube for guiding blood flow, the small intestine is where the vast majority of digestion and absorption of food takes place, rather than just a physical tube. To date, *no artificial polymers have been developed that can mimic this absorption function*. Some recent progress in artificial intestine development in animal models has been made, using a decellularized matrix [2], demonstrating the combined benefits of applications in biomaterials and stem cell approaches. Artificial sphincters have also been used to replace muscular sphincters, employing inflatable polymer cuff (Figure 15.8). A successful case of anal sphincter replacement has been reported [3].

15.3.6.2 Artificial Esophagus A similar concept to tracheal bioengineering in the respiratory system, an artificial esophagus, has been patented (US Patent 6241774) and applied clinically (Figure 15.9) [4], which is described as follows: "Disclosed is an artificial esophagus suitable for human use that includes a fine fibrous collagen layer and a tubular outer surface. The invention generally provides a degradable artificial structure that helps maintain an existing esophagus or forms a new esophagus. The invention has many important uses including improving esophageal reconstruction techniques."

Like the trachea, bioengineering of the esophagus represents an approach to creating synthetic artificial replacement of physical tubes that function mostly as transport conduits. At present, a tissue engineered esophagus remains experimental, with surgical replacement using skin grafts formed into a tube-like structure.

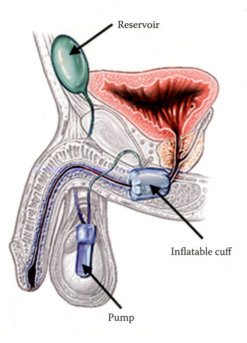

Reservoir

Inflatable cuff

Pump

Figure 15.8
Artificial sphincters employing inflatable polymer cuff. (From Benoist, S. et al., Dis. Colon Rectum, 48, 1978, 2005.)

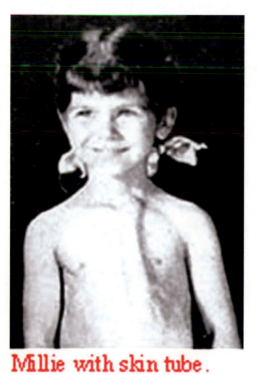

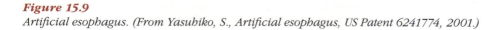

Figure 15.9
Artificial esophagus. (From Yasuhiko, S., Artificial esophagus, US Patent 6241774, 2001.)

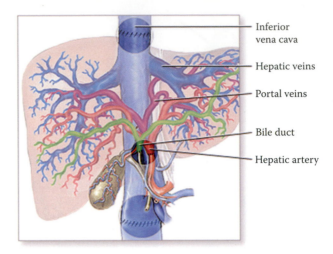

Inferior
vena cava

Hepatic veins

Portal veins

Bile duct

Hepatic artery

Figure 15.10
Extensive vascular network in the liver tissue.

15.3.6.3   Liver Tissue Engineering   Liver tissue engineering aims at the regeneration of liver at the late stages of liver diseases.

Liver tissue is populated with an extensive vascular network (Figure 15.10). The key issue to engineering survivable liver tissue is to develop vessels in the engineered liver tissue to replace those that have been lost due to fibrosis. *Revascularization is absolutely fundamental in tissue engineering of almost all tissue types, since every tissue (an exception is cartilage) has a blood supply.*

Currently, there is no artificial organ or device capable of emulating all the functions of the liver. Some functions can be emulated by liver dialysis, an experimental treatment for liver failure. The liver is thought to be responsible for up to 500 separate functions, usually in combination with other systems and organs. The bioartificial liver (BAL, Figure 15.11) is a support device similar to a portable dialysis machine, which uses live hepatocytes in a hollow-fiber bioreactor. The device is mostly only capable of filtration functions, and requires significant maintenance. Some progress has been made in miniaturizing the functional microduct units of the liver using polymer nano-surfacing and cell printing (the so-called liver on a chip; Figure 15.12) [5].

15.4   URINARY SYSTEM

15.4.1   Gross Anatomy of the Urinary System

The human urinary system is made up of the urinary organs, which produce the fluid called urine (Figure 15.13). The main anatomical features include the following:

- Kidneys
- Ureters
- Urinary bladder
- Urethra

In general, the main role of the urinary system is to maintain fluid and salt balance in the body, by removal of waste water and interstitial fluid, and retention of some of

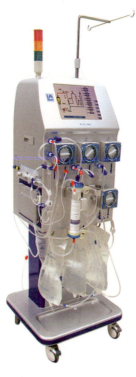

Figure 15.11
Bioartifical liver (artificial liver support system).

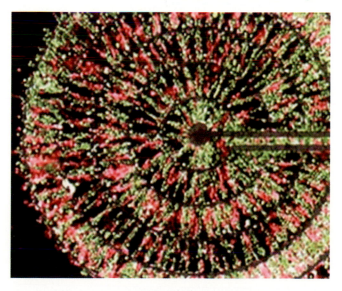

Figure 15.12
Liver on chip. (From Ho, C.T. et al., Lab Chip, 6, 724, 2006.)

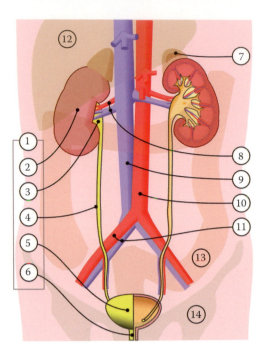

Figure 15.13

Gross anatomy of urinary systems. 1, Urinary system; 2, kidney; 3, renal pelvis; 4, ureter; 5, urinary bladder; 6, urethra (left side with frontal section); 7, adrenal gland; 8, renal artery and vein; 9, inferior vena cava; 10, abdominal aorta; 11, common iliac artery and vein; 12, liver; 13, large intestine; 14, pelvis. (From http://commons.wikimedia.org/produced by Jmarchn.)

the leftover water and salts. The adrenal gland, attached to the kidney, is also critical in blood pressure maintenance, by regulating systemic blood vessels, heart rate, and blood composition, to adapt to changes in metabolic demands and activity of the tissues. Food and water intake also have a major role in this balance, which is mainly controlled by endocrine signaling between the brain and the adrenal gland. Excess water intake can induce a dehydration reflex, which causes acute urine production.

After blood filtration in the kidneys, urine is drained from each one by its own collecting duct (ureter), which enters directly into the bladder, where urine is stored until it is evacuated (urination). Retention of urine is maintained by a sphincter, which is opened by conscious muscular control, but regulated automatically by sensing of hydrostatic pressure. The bladder itself is basically like an elastic balloon, which expands as it fills, and retracts as it empties through the urethra.

15.4.2 Kidney

The main role of the kidney is to remove waste from the blood and return the cleaned blood back to the body (Figure 15.14). The kidney is basically a very compact filtration device that maintains the body's electrolytes, acid base, and water balance. About 20% of the blood flowing from the heart enters the kidneys, where it passes through billions of microscopic arterioles and venules. Alongside these are similar sized microtubules called *nephrons*, across which ions are exchanged, resulting in net export of waste ions (NH_3^+, H^+) and solutes, and reabsorption of other ions (Na^+, Cl^+, HCO_3^-) back into the blood. This is essentially performed by an osmotic gradient across the membranes, like

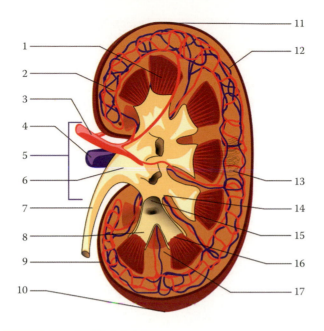

Figure 15.14
Gross structure and function of kidney. 1, Renal pyramid; 2, interlobular artery; 3, renal artery; 4, renal vein; 5, renal hilum; 6, renal pelvis; 7, ureter; 8, minor calyx; 9, renal capsule; 10, inferior renal capsule; 11, superior renal capsule; 12, interlobular vein; 13, nephron; 14, minor calyx; 15, major calyx; 16, renal papilla; 17, renal column. (From http://commons.wikimedia. org/produced by Piom.)

an ultrafilter, which occurs between the blood vessels and the nephrons at thousands of *glomeruli*, the functional filtration units of the kidney. These delicate structures are bit like the alveoli in the lungs, interfacing between the blood and the waste ducts over an extremely large surface area.

15.4.3   Regeneration of Kidney (Living with One Kidney)

The kidneys form a vital organ of the body, and the curative management of life-threatening conditions such as renal cell carcinoma (RCC) remains the surgical removal of one kidney, that is, *radical nephrectomy*. It is possible to survive with a single kidney; however, compensatory function of the remaining kidney results only from an increase in the size of nephrons, rather than their number (i.e., no cellular proliferation), so the kidney has no clinically relevant regenerative capacity. Supplementation of the patient functions is often with artificial dialysis, a long-term therapy where a patient's blood is fed through an automated filtration unit.

15.4.4   Kidney Failure and Diabetes

Kidney failure means the kidneys are no longer able to remove waste and maintain the level of fluid and salts that the body needs. *The most common single cause of kidney failure is diabetes*, due to complications associated with pathology of the microvessels that occurs in diabetics. In patients who do not manage their condition with insulin treatment, the high levels of glucose in the blood damage the millions of glomeruli within each kidney, eventually leading to kidney failure.

Around 20%–30% of people with diabetes develop kidney disease. More than 500,000 Australians a year see doctors for kidney disease. One in seven Australian adults has chronic kidney disease (CKD).

Current standard treatments for kidney failure include (1) hemodialysis (artificial blood filtration) (Figure 15.15), which is lifesaving but poorly tolerable, and (2) kidney transplantation, which is well-established, but usually suffers from a lack of donor organs.

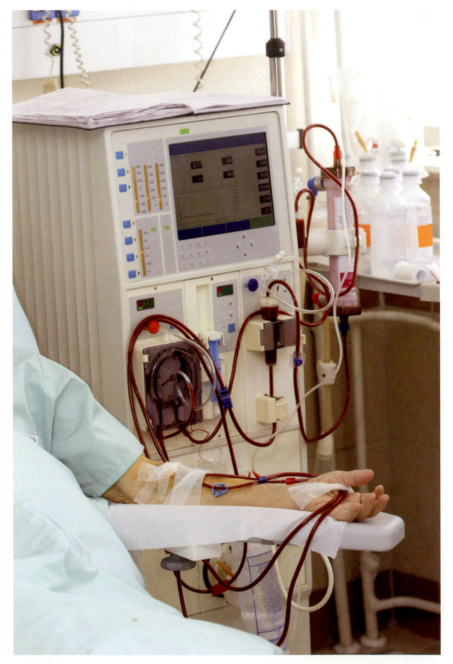

Figure 15.15
Hemodialysis (artificial kidney filter).

15.4.5   Application of Biomaterials

Like the small intestine and pancreas, the kidney is where a vast majority of biological activities (filtering) takes place. No solid biomaterials have the kidney-filtering function. Currently, artificial kidney-filtering equipment represents the application of biomaterials. Bioartificial kidneys have also been manufactured using 3D printing of cells, resulting in organs that look like kidneys, but have no specific vascular functions. Like the liver, some efforts have been made in miniaturizing the filtration process using microfabricated filtration devices (kidney on a chip) using PDMS.

Bladder replacement also represents a successful step toward the development of bioartificial organs using tissue engineering approaches. An artificial bladder was first developed in Boston in 1999, with the first successful clinical implantation published in 2006 [6]. The bladder itself was made from a biodegradable polymer scaffold, but no cellularization was used.

15.5   REPRODUCTIVE SYSTEM

The human male and female each has a system of organs, closely associated with the urinary system, specifically evolved for the production of new life. These systems are known as the reproductive or genital system. Since there are different systems for males and females, the genital systems are an example of sexual dimorphism (Figure 15.16).

Morph = form, shape
Di = two
Sexual = according to sex (gender)
Sexual Dimorphism = having two different forms according to sex

15.5.1   Gross Anatomy of the Human Reproductive System

Components of the genital systems may be considered in the following categories:

1. *Primary sex organs (Gonads)*: Primary sex organs produce sex cells (gametes). Male and female gametes fuse to form the one-cell embryo, which is the first stage after the process of fertilization that takes place in the oviduct. Primary sex organs also produce sex hormones.
2. *Secondary sex organs:* Secondary sex organs provide a support role for the products of the primary sex organs.
3. *Secondary sexual characteristics:* Secondary sexual characteristics are those traits that tend to make males and females more attractive to each other. Secondary sexual characteristics help to ensure mating. These characteristics first appear during puberty (10–15 years of age), under the influence of gonadal steroid hormones (a process also called sexual maturity). This involves complete anatomical maturation of the gonads and accessory tissues, which originally formed under the influence of the same hormones during late pregnancy.

The organs of the human female and male productive systems are listed in Table 15.1.

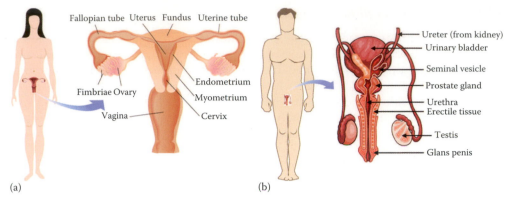

Figure 15.16
Gross anatomy of the (a) female and (b) male reproductive systems.

Table 15.1

The Human Female and Male Reproductive Systems

	Female	Male
Primary sex organs	Ovaries	Testes
Secondary sex organs	Uterine tubes (fallopian tubes, oviducts)	Epididymis Ductus (Vas) deferens Seminal vesicles Ejaculatory duct Prostate gland Penis
Secondary sexual characteristics	Growth of pubic hair, development of mammary glands, development of the pelvic girdle, and deposition of fat in the mons pubis and labia majora	Growth of facial, pubic, and chest hair; growth of the larynx to deepening of the voice; and deposition of protein to increase muscularity and general body size

15.5.1.1 Fertilization and Embryo Formation The female gametes (oocytes) are produced from the ovary by the process of ovulation which occurs in a monthly cycle. The oocyte contains all of the genetic programming unique to a female, and the processes necessary for the first 3–5 days of life. In the male, gametes (spermatozoa or *sperm*) are produced continuously, and expelled from the body during a process called ejaculation, a reflex occurring during copulation, when sperm passes from the epididymis to the prostate gland, where secondary proteins are added. The final ejaculated fluid exits from the urethra of the penis, which during sexual intercourse, is inside the vaginal canal. The sperm in the fluid then begin to migrate from the vaginal canal, across the cervix, through the uterine fluid to the oviduct, where they fertilize the ovulated oocyte. Of several million sperm, only a few hundred will survive the migration process, and ultimately only one sperm will undergo fertilization to form a new embryo. The embryo then spends the next 5 days developing into a blastocyst, which is a colony of embryonic stem cells that implants into the uterine wall, resulting in a pregnancy.

15.5.2 Diseases of the Reproductive System

15.5.2.1 Infections of the Reproductive System There are three mains types of reproductive tract infections (RTIs) that can develop in either males or females. These include endogenous infections, iatrogenic infections, and the more commonly known sexually transmitted infections. Some infections are easily treatable and can be cured, while some are more difficult, and *some conditions such as AIDS and herpes are not yet curable*. Many RTIs can result in secondary infection in other organs. In females, infections can spread from the vagina to the oviducts, causing oviduct blockages and infertility. This can also lead to inflammation of uterine lining (endometriosis), which causes tissue debris to exit from the oviducts into the pelvic cavity, causing pelvic inflammatory disease (PID). In the male, infections can also enter the urethra, causing painful urination, as well as secondary bladder and kidney problems.

15.5.2.2 Congenital Abnormalities Examples of congenital abnormalities of the reproductive system include the following:

- Kallmann syndrome—Genetic disorder causing decreased functioning of the sex-hormone-producing glands caused by a deficiency or both testes from the scrotum
- Androgen insensitivity syndrome—A genetic disorder causing people who are genetically male (i.e., XY chromosome pair) to develop sexually as a female due to an inability to utilize androgen
- Intersexuality—A person who has genitalia and/or other sexual traits which are not clearly male or female

Congenital abnormalities (L. con = with, genital = inherited) are occur usually during the formation of the fetus in utero, and many of these conditions are extremely rare. They are very well known to have a strong genetic cause, and can include conditions such as *polydactyly* (Gk. Poly = many, dactyl = digit), where children are born with extra fingers or toes.

15.5.2.3 Cancers Examples of cancers of the reproductive system include the following:

- Prostate cancer—cancer of the prostate gland
- Breast cancer—cancer of the mammary gland
- Ovarian cancer—cancer of the ovary
- Penile cancer—cancer of the penis
- Uterine cancer—cancer of the uterus
- Testicular cancer—cancer of the testicle (plural: testes)
- Cervical cancer—cancer of the cervix

Many cancers of the reproductive system remain can be caused by chemical toxicity, viral infection and radiation. This is often associated with endocrine and metabolic dysfunction. Common chemicals with known links to reproductive disorders include lead, chromium and other heavy metals, dioxins and dioxin-like compounds, styrene, toluene, and pesticides. The reproductive system, especially in the female, is particularly sensitive to such toxins, as illustrated by the acute increases in congenital malformations as a result of radiation exposure (e.g., due to nuclear fallout) or chemical warfare (e.g., defoliants).

15.5.3   Applications of Biomaterials

Anticancer drug delivery to treat cervical and prostate cancer is actively underway and may involve the use of biomaterials as drug delivery vehicles. Other applications include penile stents, for patients who suffer from blocked urethras due to congenital malformation or RTI. A bioartificial uterus has also been patented as early as 1955, but since then no progress has been made in the development of this complex idea using tissue engineering or biomaterial approaches. It is also questionable whether such an idea would have enough clinical relevance.

15.6   CHAPTER HIGHLIGHTS

1. Respiratory system includes the lungs and a system of tubes.
2. Two types of pneumocytes in alveoli:
   a. Type I pneumocytes (squamous alveolar) are responsible for gas exchange. No renewing ability.
   b. Type II pneumocytes (great alveolar, progenitor cells) secrete pulmonary surfactant. Renew and differentiate.
3. Emphysema begins with the destruction of air sacs (alveoli), a permanent damage in the lungs.
4. Application of biomaterials: medical glue in lung volume reduction surgery (LVRS).
5. Digestive system: The functions of stomach, small intestine, and large intestine (colon) cannot be replaced by biomaterials.

Biomaterials application: artificial esophagus

6. Liver
   a. Inflammation and fibrosis: curable.
   b. Cirrhosis, liver cancer and failure: not curable.
   c. Liver tissue engineering: vascularization is the key issue.
7. Kidney:
   a. The major function of kidney is to filter wastes.
   b. Kidney failure treatment: dialysis and organ transplantation.
8. Reproductive system: Anticancer drug delivery to treat cervical and prostate cancer.

ACTIVITIES

1. Read the article "liver on chips" http://www.rsc.org/Publishing/Journals/cb/Volume/2006/7/Liver_on_chip.asp.

SIMPLE QUESTIONS IN CLASS

1. *Air sac* is referred to as
   a. Pulmonary vein
   b. Pulmonary artery
   c. Alveolar duct
   d. Pulmonary alveolus
2. To regenerate lung tissue in vitro, you need to make a choice of cells. Which of the following cells is the best choice?
   a. Type I pneumocytes
   b. Fibroblasts
   c. Type II pneumocytes
   d. Macrophages
3. Lungs have a regenerative ability, but the major lung disease emphysema causes irreversible damage. The primary reason is
   a. The damage area is too large to be repaired
   b. The destruction of alveoli in the lung, where the progenitor type II pneumocytes reside, impedes repair
   c. The loss of blood vessels impedes repair
   d. The loss of macrophages impedes repair
4. The major component of current medical sealant is
   a. Collagen
   b. Fibrin
   c. Fibroblasts
   d. Platelets
5. Biomaterials (synthetic or natural) cannot be applied to compensate for the absence of the primary biological function of which organs?
   a. Bone
   b. Intestines
   c. Esophagus
   d. Blood vessels
6. Which of the following internal organs can not only repair the injured part but also regenerate the lost part?
   a. Pancreas
   b. Heart
   c. Liver
   d. Kidney
7. What is the major cause of kidney failure?
   a. High blood pressure
   b. High levels of sugar in the blood
   c. Bacterial infection
   d. Viral infection

PROBLEMS AND EXERCISES

1. What are the top three fatal diseases?
2. List six vital organs of the human body.

3. Discuss why the application of artificial tubes made of biomaterials is relatively more successful in the repair of blood vessels and the esophagus than in the repair of the large and small intestines.

4. There are many challenges associated with liver tissue engineering. According to the diagram Figure 15.10 of liver tissue, what is the major issue indicated?

5. What are the most threatening diseases for each of the following organs? What are the current standard treatments of these diseases? Discuss potentially alternative treatments using biomaterials.
   a. Lung
   b. Heart
   c. Liver
   d. Kidney

6. Discuss the regenerative ability of lungs, and the diseases of lungs that need a lung reduction surgery.

7. Discuss the major specialized cells of lungs. To regenerate lung tissues in vitro, what type of lung cells would you use? Explain your reason.

8. Discuss the regenerative ability and carcinogenicities of the following organs:
   a. Blood
   b. Heart
   c. Bone
   d. Lung
   e. Skin
   f. Cartilage
   g. Intestine
   h. Muscle
   i. Stomach
   j. Liver

9. Discuss the major diseases of the lymphatic system, correct standard treatments, and how biomaterials could be applied.

10. Discuss the major diseases of the kidneys, correct standard treatments, and how biomaterials have been applied.

BIBLIOGRAPHY

References

1. Macchiarini, P. et al., Clinical transplantation of a tissue-engineered airway. *Lancet*, 2008;**372**(9655):2023–2030. doi:10.1016/S0140-6736(08)61598-6.

2. Kajbafzadeh, A.M. et al., Sheep colon acellular matrix: Immunohistologic, biomechanical, scanning electron microscopic evaluation and collagen quantification. *Journal of Bioscience and Bioengineering*, 2013. doi:10.1016/j.jbiosc.2013.07.006.

3. Benoist, S. et al., Artificial sphincter with colonic reservoir for severe anal incontinence because of imperforate anus and short-bowel syndrome: report of a case. *Diseases of the Colon and Rectum*, 2005;**48**(10):1978–1982.

4. Yasuhiko, S., Artificial esophagus, United States Patent 6241774, 2001.

5. Ho, C.T., R.Z. Lin, W.Y. Chang, H.Y. Chang, and C.H. Liu, Rapid heterogeneous liver-cell on-chip patterning via the enhanced field-induced dielectrophoresis trap. *Lab on a Chip*, 2006;**6**:724–734. doi: 10.1039/b602036d.

6. Anthony, A. et al., Tissue-engineered autologous bladders for patients needing cystoplasty. *The Lancet*, 2006;**367**:9518:1241–1246. doi:10.1016/S0140-6736(06) 68438-9.

Websites

http://www.bartleby.com/107/.
http://www.healthline.com/human-body-maps.
http://www.innerbody.com/.
http://www.nhlbi.nih.gov/health/health-topics/topics/hlw/system.html.
http://hes.ucfsd.org/gclaypo/repiratorysys.html.
http://www.visiblebody.com/index.html.

Further Readings

Martini, F.H., M.J. Timmons, and R.B. Tallitsch, Human Anatomy, 5th edn. San Francisco, CA: Pearson/Benjamin Cummings, 2006. Related chapters.

Tate, S.S., Anatomy and Physiology, 8th edn. New York: McGraw Hill, 2008. Related chapters.

CHAPTER 16

CELLS AND BIOMOLECULES

LEARNING OBJECTIVES

After a careful study of this chapter, you should be able to do the following:

1. Describe the four types of biomacromolecules
2. Describe the structure of the cell membrane
3. Describe the major components of cells
4. Describe the phagocytosis process
5. Gain ability to communicate with cell biologists in laboratory, understanding some essential terms: phenotype, confluence, apoptosis, necrosis, lag phase, log phase, plateau stage
6. Describe how cells attach to a substrate (biomaterial) and proliferate
7. Describe characteristics of stem cells
8. Describe potency of stem cells: totipotency, pluripotency, and multipotency
9. Describe embryonic stem (somatic) cells
10. Name and describe adult (somatic) stem cells

16.1   INTRODUCTION

All organisms are made up of one or more cells, which are fused to each other in groups (tissues) and bound to the extracellular matrix. The cell is the most basic structural and functional unit of living organisms, and nothing less than the cell can live and reproduce individually.

Cells come with an immense diversity, in terms of size, shape, structure, and function, but can be divided into one of two types [1]: (1) *prokaryotic* cells, which exist as bacteria, around 1–5 μm long (Figure 16.1a) and characterized by its cell wall, rather than a lipid membrane; and (2) *eukaryotic* cells, which are larger, distinguished by a nucleus that contains the genetic material surrounded by a membranous envelope, and a lipid membrane instead of cell wall (Figure 16.1b).

Prokaryotes are considered an organism on their own, able to divide and form large colonies of independent cells. Eukaryotes are believed to have evolved from the former

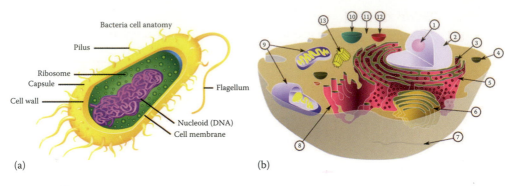

Figure 16.1
Two types of cells: (a) prokaryote (bacterial) and (b) eukaryote. (From the http://commons.wiki-media.org/.)

and still host cooperative colonies with the former (symbiosis, e.g., digestive system bacteria). The most important difference is that eukaryotes have evolved to exist as large collectives, where they are joined together to form tissues.

16.2   CELL BIOCHEMISTRY AND BIOSYNTHESIS

Every living organism is a complex chemical and physical system. There is nothing in a living organism that does not obey basic chemical and physical laws; however, the chemistry of life (biochemistry) is indeed of a special kind. The cell is based over-whelmingly on carbon compounds, which are the study subject of organic chemistry. However, cellular biochemistry and molecular biology are enormously complex.

16.2.1   Chemical Components of a Cell: Biomacromolecules

Of the 92 naturally occurring elements, living organisms are made up of only a small selection of these elements, mostly C, H, O, and N (96.5% of an organism's weight) with the remainder being either minor nutrients (<2 wt.%) or trace elements (<0.01 wt.%) (see Chapter 2). Water is the most abundant compound in cells, accounting for about 70 wt.% of a cell, and life depends almost exclusively on chemical reactions that take place in aqueous solution. Besides water, cells contain four major families of biomacro-molecules, made up of organic monomers (i.e., small organic molecules) [1]:

- Carbohydrates (polysaccharides), with sugar being the monomer
- Lipids (fats and oils), with fatty acids being their components
- Proteins, with amino acids being the monomer
- DNA and RNA, with nucleotides (five carbon sugar phosphates) being the monomer

Actually, all biomacromolecules, either inside or outside cells, fall into one of the afore-mentioned four types. Except for lipids, which are hydrophobic or polar, biomacromol-ecules are generally hydrophilic. The chemical compositions of a typical bacterium and mammalian cell are given in Table 16.1.

16.2.1.1   Polysaccharides (Sugar and Starch)   Polysaccharides are polymeric car-bohydrate structures, having a general formula of $C_x(H_2O)_y$ (Figure 16.2). *Sugars*

Table 16.1

Approximate Chemical Compositions of a Typical Bacterium and Mammalian (Eukaryotic) Cell

Component	Wt.%	
	E. Coli	Mammalian
Water	70	70
Inorganic ions (Na$^+$, K$^+$, Mg^{2+}, Ca^{2+}, Cl$^-$, etc.)	1	1
Miscellaneous small metabolites	3	3
Proteins	15	18
RNA	6	1.1
DNA	2	0.25
Phospholipids	1	3
Other lipids	—	2
Polysaccharides	2	2

Source: Alberts, B. et al., *Molecular Biology of the Cell.*

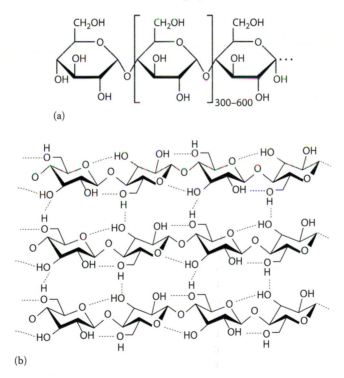

(a)

(b)

Figure 16.2

Two unit structures of polysaccharides (amylose), as (a) a linear backbone and (b) as a network cross-linked by hydrogen bonds. (From the http://commons.wikimedia.org/.)

provide an energy source for cells and are subunits of polysaccharides, but can also exist as oligosaccharides (e.g., di- or trisaccharides). Large polysaccharides can also form the basis of structures in cells, such as DNA and the surface coats of lipid membranes. Sugars are linked together through *condensation* to form polymers. The bonds created by condensation reactions can be broken by *hydrolysis*. Furthermore, in the same way as the polymers described in Chapter 8, sugars can exist as linear chains or branched chains.

16.2.1.2 Lipids (Fats and Oily Substances)

Lipids are essentially long-chain hydrocarbons, but not more than about 20 carbons long, although they can be either aliphatic or aromatic. Lipids can contain a variety of structural types of compounds, including alcohols, carboxylic acids, and esters (Figure 10.5). Generally defined by their physical properties, lipids can contain varying amounts of the following:

- Saturated and unsaturated aliphatic fatty acids
- Triacylglycerols (Figure 10.5b)
- Phospholipids (and related sphingolipids)
- Steroids/sterols
- Eicosanoids
- Hydrophobic vitamins

Lipids play various important roles in the processes of cell structure and function. In adipose tissue, lipids act as metabolic storage molecules, which can be oxidized in the mitochondria of all cells (e.g., bone marrow, liver). Lipids also form the raw materials for the biosynthesis of vitamins, hormones, pulmonary surfactant, molecular signaling molecules, and pigments. The most important lipid-based structures of cells are the phospholipid membrane bilayers (hydrophobic tails facing inward) that make up the cell and nuclear membranes in all cells, and other subcellular structures. The best example of this is in the multilayered insulation (myelin sheaths) in neurons that form the white matter of the brain. Lipids are transported in the blood as emulsified nanoparticles but can build up in arteries over time, causing cardiovascular disease, and increased lipid vesicles in adipocytes (fat cells) contribute to obesity.

16.2.1.3 Proteins

Proteins (also known as *polypeptides,* in the case of smaller proteins) (Figure 16.3a) are organic compounds made of *amino acids* (Figure 16.3b) arranged as a linear chain of amino acid monomers, and perhaps the most important biomolecules of living organisms. Proteins also have secondary sugar residues.

In the field of materials science, materials can be classified as structural and functional materials according to their roles in a construct. The bricks, steels, and concrete that form the walls of our houses are *structural materials*. The window glass that brings sunshine into the house (optical function) is a *functional material*. Likewise, proteins can also be categorized into structural and functional proteins.

Cells themselves are held in shape internally by long tubular proteins, microtubules and microfilaments, which anchor the cell membranes together, and give epithelial sheets their characteristic morphology (see more details in Section 16.3.2). These microtubules and microfilaments are structural proteins inside cells. Collagens are the main proteins of the extracellular matrix, which are the structural materials of the body. *Structural proteins* have more regular chain and sheet secondary structures, in long repeats.

Within cells, there are hundreds of different families of *functional proteins*. Most of the more functional proteins are globular, having more compact structures, depending on how specific amino acids are cross-linked. *Enzymes*, for example, are mostly globular proteins, with a specific catalytic region that binds and reacts

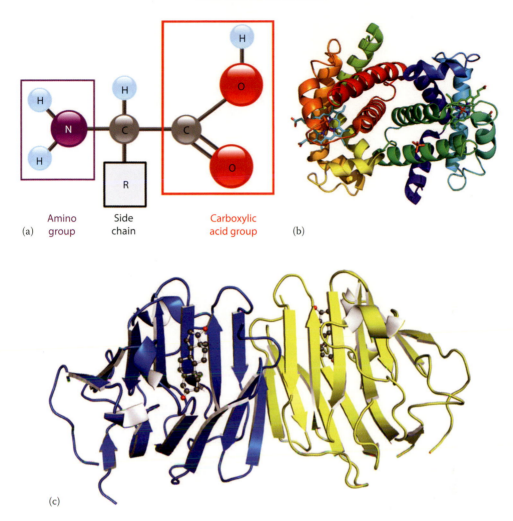

(a) Amino group Side chain Carboxylic acid group (b)

(c)

Figure 16.3
(a) The molecular structure of an amino acid (From the http://commons.wikimedia.org/produced by YassineMrabet.); (b) molecular structure of an alpha-helix structured protein: human oxyhemoglobin, enclosing two heme groups (left and right); and (c) a beta-sheet structured protein: testosterone-binding globulin, which is a glycoprotein that binds to the sex hormone testosterone, thereby regulating its activity and ability to enter a cell and activate its receptor.

with simpler compounds, to perform biochemical reactions in metabolism and biosynthesis. They are the major proteins inside the cells. Other proteins include *membrane proteins*, which can have adhesion and/or cell signaling roles (e.g., *receptors*). A good example of globular proteins that work outside cells is *hormones*, which travel through the bloodstream from a distant gland, to bind to receptors in other tissues.

The general structure of proteins is often described in terms of four levels (Figures 16.3 and 16.4):

- Primary structure: covalent bonding
- Secondary structure: hydrogen bonding

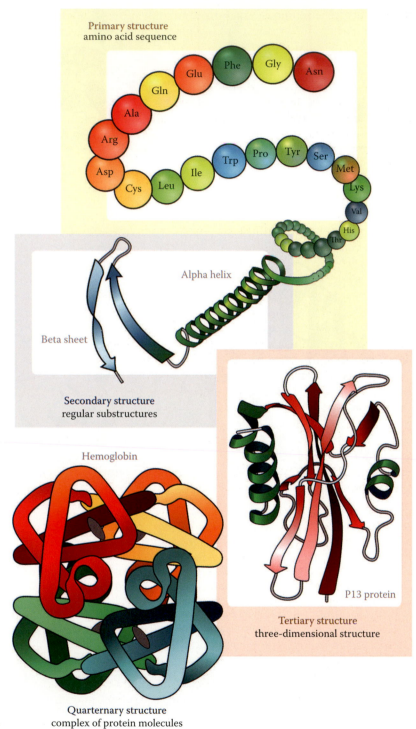

Figure 16.4
*Primary, secondary, tertiary, and quaternary structure of proteins. (From the http://commons.
wikimedia.org/)*

- Tertiary structure: encompasses all the noncovalent interactions
- Quaternary structure: usually not covalently connected, but might be connected by a disulfide bond

Proteins first twist into their *secondary structure* (Figure 16.4) when neighboring amino acids in the polypeptide sequence (*primary structure*) of the proteins form hydrogen bonds. Alpha-helix (Figure 16.3b) and beta-sheet (Figure 16.3c) are two major forms of secondary structure. The proteins' three-dimensional *tertiary structures* result from the interaction between amino acids at different points in the coiled secondary structure. When two or more polypeptide chains intertwine to form one molecule, the protein has a *quaternary structure* (Figure 16.4). [1]

16.2.1.4 DNA and RNA Nucleotides (Figure 16.5) make up the structural units of DNA (deoxyribonucleic acid) and RNA (ribonucleic acid), with DNA existing mostly as very long linear polymers, and RNAs as mostly compact globular or short chained molecules. Short-chain nucleotides (e.g., di- and trinucleotides) also act as short-range electron carriers and are readily oxidized or dephosphorylated to produce energy.

DNA polymer is probably the most widely studied biomacromolecule, mainly because it forms the basis of the so-called genetic *code*. Very long single chains, made of tens of thousands of nucleotides, form the information template used to assemble amino acids into whole proteins, within the nucleus. They form the basic structure of chromatin, a highly ordered protein complex that is packaged into individual chromosomes during cell division. Even though there are only five nucleotides (Figure 16.5) (with several different new forms of cytosine, for example, 5-methyl cytosine, 5-hydroxy-methyl cytosine), the complexity of DNA comes from its amazing diversity of combinations. First, DNA is normally assembled in a double-helical backbone, adenines bonded to thymines or uracils and guanines to cytosines in opposition. Second, these nucleotide pairs (base pairs) are grouped adjacently, converted to RNA, and then used to position a single amino acid in a sequence. Third, very large expanses of uniquely coded sequences form the basis of *genes*, for which there are about 20,000 in the human *genome*, each representing a specific protein. In scale, the sequence of human DNA contains more than three billion base pairs.

16.2.2 Types of Biomolecular Bonding

The chemistry of cells is dominated by the aforementioned four macromolecules. On a weight basis, carbon-based macromolecules are the most abundant in a living cell. Although covalent bonds bind atoms to form molecules, much of biology depends on the relatively weak binding of different molecules to each other. These weak bonds take less energy to bond or break upon demand, and in the case of very large polymers such as DNA, millions of weaker bonds in geometrically stable conformations lead to a relatively stable association. Also, such bonds under aqueous conditions have evolved to be ideal under physiological conditions (e.g., low temperatures, low ionic strength).

The four types of noncovalent interactions that help bring molecules together and to associate with each other in cells are as follows [1]:

- Ionic bonds
- Hydrogen bonds
- van der Waals attractions
- Hydrophobic forces

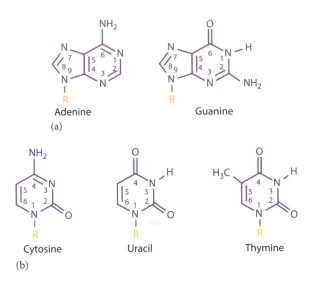

Figure 16.5
Five nucleotides: (a) purines and (b) pyrimidines. (From the http://commons.wikimedia.org/.)

The binding strength values of these bonds in aqueous environments are given in Table 7.5. Noncovalent bonds specify both the precise shape of a macromolecule and its binding to other molecules.

16.2.3 Biosynthesis and Metabolism: The Energy Balance of Cells

16.2.3.1 Cell Metabolism Each cell can be considered as a microscale bioreactor or a chemical processing factory. Two opposing streams of biochemical reactions occur in cells [1]:

1. The *catabolic pathways,* which break down food stuffs into smaller molecules, thereby generating high-energy molecules (usually in the form of dinucleotide phosphates) for cellular functions (e.g., cell division) and other small molecules that the cell uses as building blocks for synthesizing proteins and other macromolecules (for replicating chromatin, membranes, etc.).
2. The *anabolic (or biosynthetic) pathways* use the energy harnessed by catabolism to drive the synthesis of the many other molecules that form the cell.

Together these two sets of reactions constitute the *metabolism* of the cell (Figure 16.6), with the metabolic rate often associated with the particular cell type. For example, cardiomyocytes have a constant need for energy substrates, due to their periodic contractions, and neurons have high oxygen consumption due to their constant generation of rapid ion gradients. Cells have a net metabolic turnover, which is basically the balance between consumption and substrates and production of energy, to meet the demand. When there is low demand, there is more energy storage; when demand is high, stores are often exhausted, so supply must remain constant.

16.2.3.2 Why Is a Constant Input of Energy Needed to Sustain Living Organisms? According to the law of entropy, the universal tendency of things is to become disordered, which is a process of energy lowering. Therefore, to maintain an

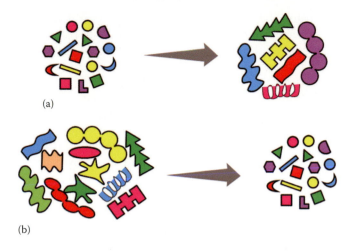

(a)

(b)

Figure 16.6
(a) Anabolic (or biosynthetic) pathways and (b) catabolic pathways.

order, the system needs constant input of energy. Biological order is made possible by the release of heat energy from cells to the living body (system). The synthesis of biological polymers (i.e., biological ordering processes) requires an energy input. However, the ability of cells to use and release energy is highly efficient, via the use of enzymes to catalyze multiple steps in what might be a single reaction in a cell-free system.

16.2.3.3 How Do Cells Obtain Energy?

Eukaryotic cells oxidize organic molecules in stepwise, enzyme-catalyzed reactions in a process called *cell respiration*, which produces carbon dioxide (CO_2) and water (H_2O) from carbohydrates (predominantly glucose and pyruvic acid). Carbons from this overall reaction are stored as *adenosine triphosphate (ATP)*, which is the universal high-energy metabolite for all cellular reactions. ATP is dephosphorylated by kinase enzymes, which liberates free energy stored in the covalent bonds.

16.2.3.4 How Do Enzymes Find Their Substrates?

The function of enzymes is to lower the barriers that block chemical reactions. How do enzymes find their substrates so fast? Rapid binding is possible because the motions caused by heat energy are enormously fast at the molecular level, via diffusion mechanisms. These molecular motions include translational motion, vibration, and rotation.

Cells are also equipped with proteins that assist transport of hydrophilic substrates across hydrophobic membranes, such as channel proteins, which act as shuttles, and which establish charge and proton gradients. These drive *facilitated diffusion*, to improve the efficiency of transport and availability of substrates within the cell. Furthermore, substrates often exist in excess, or in pools, so that a concentration gradient is established, which also helps the diffusion process [1].

- For sequential reactions, ΔG is additive:

$$X \xrightarrow{\text{+8 kcal/mol}} Z \text{ and } Y \xrightarrow{\text{+8 kcal/mol}} Z$$

Since ΔGs are additive in a series of sequential reactions, the unfavorable reaction $X \rightarrow Y$, which will not occur spontaneously, can be driven by the favorable reaction $Y \rightarrow Z$, provided that the second reaction follows the first. Cells can therefore cause the energetically unfavorable transition X → Y to occur if an enzyme that catalyzes the first reaction X → Y is supplemented by a second enzyme that catalyzes the energetically favorable reaction Y → Z.

- Activated carrier molecules are essential for biosynthesis. The most important of the energy carrier molecules are ATP, nicotinamide adenine dinucleotide (NADH), nicotinamide adenine dinucleotide phosphate (NADPH), and flavine adenine dinucleotide ($FADH_2$).
- The formation of energy carriers is coupled to an energetically favorable reaction. A part of the heat energy released by the oxidation reaction is stored in the energy-rich covalent bonds of the activated carrier molecules.
- ATP is the most widely used activated carrier molecule.
- NADH and NADPH are important activated electron carrier molecules.

16.2.3.5 How Do Cells Obtain Energy from Food?
Cells require a constant supply of energy to generate and maintain the biological order that keeps them alive. Energy is derived from chemical bond energy in food molecules, most importantly sugars. These are oxidized in a sequence of enzyme-catalyzed steps to ATP, with the by-products CO_2 and H_2O:

1. *Stage 1 digestion*: Enzymes break down polysaccharides to oligosaccharides to glucose.
2. *Stage 2 glycolysis*: This involves the generation of two molecules of pyruvate (a tricarboxylic acid) from glucose (a hexose).
3. *Stage 3*: The citric acid cycle forms citrate (6C) from pyruvate (3C) and acetate (3C), which can also be derived from amino acids and fatty acids after oxidation by their respective pathways. In a cyclic series of eight enzyme-catalyzed steps, citrate is decarboxylated twice (generating two molecules of CO_2) and dehydrogenated four times, generating four protons and four electrons to NADH. The protons are later used to establish a charge gradient in the mitochondria, which powers oxygen-dependent ATP synthesis.

In most complex sequential biochemical reactions such as this, each step is catalyzed by a single enzyme, which causes a slight conformational change in a molecule. Some key enzymes act as rate-limiting steps, by binding of reaction products or reaction cofactors, (if they are overproduced), and other mechanisms. Hence, energy usage can be effectively matched to demand, by feedback loops that activate these rate-limiting enzymes, like a braking system, to conserve energy. Rate-limiting enzymes can undergo structural changes, which inhibit their binding sites, or can also undergo competitive inhibition by more than one specific substrate, which also changes the reaction rate.

All cells need to maintain a high ATP/ADP ratio. Periodic access to food and decreases in demand during times of low activity, have led to the evolution of energy storage, the form of carbohydrate and fat stores. To compensate for long periods of fasting, for example, fatty acids can be stored as membrane-bound droplets composed of triacylglycerols, largely in specialized fat cells (adipocytes). For shorter-term storage, sugar is stored as glucose subunits in the large branched polysaccharides called glycogen, which is present as small granules in the cytoplasm of many cells, including liver and muscles. Both fatty acids and glycogen are very efficient as they can yield many ATP molecules on demand. Once stores have been depleted and substrates are also no longer available, cells begin to consume their own proteins (*autophagy*).

16.3   CELL STRUCTURE

All cells are bound by a lipid membrane called the *plasma membrane*, which serves as a dynamic interface between the internal environment of the cell and external environments [1]. The cell membrane is selectively permeable to ions and organic molecules and controls the movement of substances in and out of cells, using channel proteins, as described earlier. Cells favor water environments and tend to anchor on hydrophilic substrates. This is an important characteristic that should be considered in designing the surfaces of biomaterials. Plasma membranes also have a *net negative charge* and adherent surface proteins that are involved in adhesion, cell signaling, immune defense, and steric hindrance.

16.3.1   Structure of Cell Membrane

16.3.1.1   Phospholipid Bilayer   The cell membrane consists of the *phospholipid bilayer* with embedded proteins (Figure 16.7). The lipid bilayer is composed of two layers of amphiphilic phospholipid molecules, each of which has a hydrophilic head and two hydrophobic tails. The head is structured with polar groups, phosphate and glycerol, and the two tails are single-chain aliphatic fatty acids (Figure 16.8). The cell membrane is arranged such that the hydrophobic *tail* regions are shielded from the surrounding polar fluid, letting the more hydrophilic *head* regions to associate with water environments. The two (inner and outer) surfaces of cell membranes are hydrophilic, which ensures that cells can associate well with aqueous, ionic environments. The strongly hydrophobic middle layer in between the two phospholipid layer provides a protective wall to effectively prevent unwanted polar substances from entering the cell.

The embedded protein molecules, which are referred to as *protein complexes*, make up almost 50% of the total mass of the membrane, representing a so-called *mosaic model* of membrane structure. Proteins include channels, enzymes, receptors, and adhesion molecules, which all have specific parts of their amino acid sequence anchored into the hydrophobic region.

16.3.1.2   Receptors   On the external surface of the plasma membranes, many of the membrane proteins and lipids are conjugated with short chains of polysaccharide, in combinations called *glycoprotein* and *glycolipids* (Figure 16.7). Many of these glycoproteins and glycolipids are called receptors, because of their specific binding role. They participate in important interactions such as cell adhesion, recognition, and response to signaling proteins (e.g., hormones, cytokines, and antigens). Receptors have multiple domains in their protein structure. Membrane-binding domains do just that, enabling the protein to integrate into the membrane, usually containing hydrophobic amino acids to do this. Receptor-binding domains face the outside of the cell, being involved in binding to signaling molecules. Inside the cells, catalytic domains are involved in transducing the signal generated by a binding event to other metabolic or signaling pathways inside the cell.

16.3.2   Nucleus, Cytoplasm, and Cytoskeleton

The interior of eukaryotic cells is composed of two basic compartments, the *nucleus* and the *cytoplasm*. The nucleus is bound by its own lipid membrane, the nuclear membrane, and the cytoplasm refers to the space between this and the inner surface of

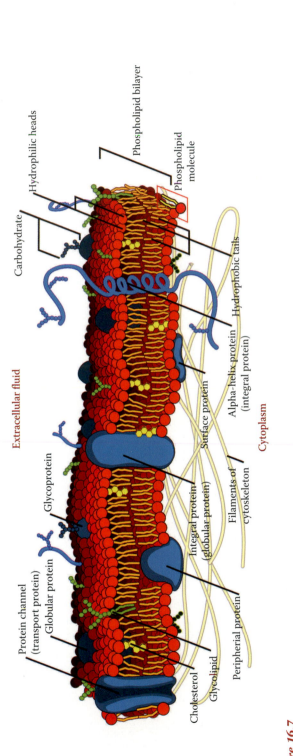

Figure 16.7

The membrane structure of cells. Lipid bilayer; protein complex (mosaic model), and carbohydrate receptors attached to proteins or lipids. (From http://commons.wikimedia.org/ produced by Mariana Ruiz Villarreal.)

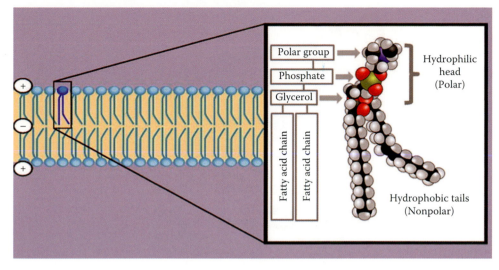

Figure 16.8
Molecular structure of amphiphile phospholipids.

the cell membrane. The *cytoskeleton* is the fibrous protein network that infiltrates the whole cytoplasm and anchors it to the cell membrane (Figure 16.1b). The cytoplasm contains other membrane-bound compartments that have very precisely specialized roles, called cytoplasmic *organelles*.

16.3.2.1 Nucleus The nucleus is the largest organelle and its substance is called *nucleoplasm*, bound by a membrane system called the *nuclear envelope* (Figure 16.9). Overall, the nucleoplasm is comprised of chromatin and other support proteins. The

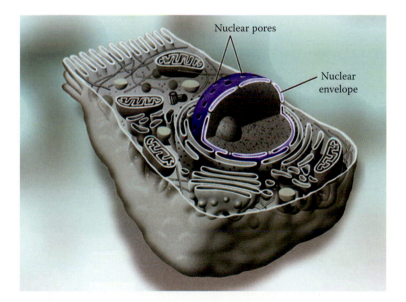

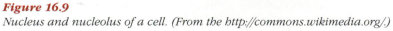

Figure 16.9
Nucleus and nucleolus of a cell. (From the http://commons.wikimedia.org/.)

531

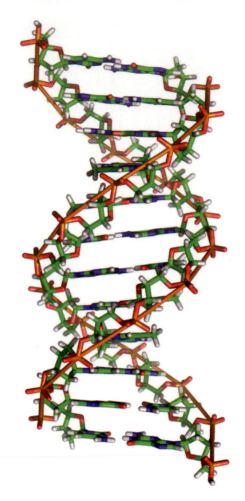

Figure 16.10
Double helix structure of DNA. (From the http://commons.wikimedia.org/.)

proteins form a large family that regulates the structure and access to specific genes belonging to all 23 human chromosomes.

As described earlier, individual nucleotide bases are bound to each other adjacently, via hydrogen bonds. These are then linked in antiparallel backbones by their phosphate groups, forming the famous double-helix arrangement (Figure 16.10). When DNA is in an open (decondensed) format in the chromatin, RNAs and other proteins can access the genes encoded in the DNA molecules, except during cell division, when chromatin is first replicated, then supercoiled tightly in individual chromosomes, using some of the support proteins in the nucleoplasm. During cell division, the chromosomes are pulled in opposite directions by cytoskeletal proteins into each new cell.

Gene transcription occurs in the nucleus. In the resting state, the DNA bases are *read* by some varieties of RNA, which then systematically convert the base sequences into other RNA molecules called messenger RNA (mRNA), which shuttle through the nuclear pores. These are then converted into amino acid sequences in the cytoplasm, as a kind of genetic template.

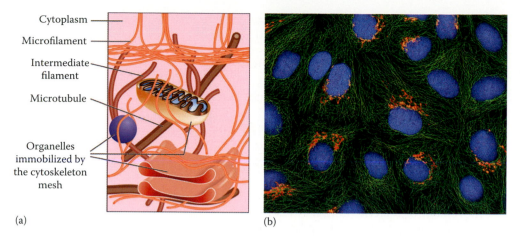

Cytoplasm

Microfilament

Intermediate filament

Microtubule

Organelles immobilized by the cytoskeleton mesh

(a)

(b)

Figure 16.11
(a) Schematic illustration and (b) microscopic images of cytoskeleton of hela cells. (From National Institute of Health Science, licensed via Science Photo Library.)

16.3.2.2 Cytoplasm The cytoplasm has three major elements, the cytosol, organelles, and inclusions. The cytoplasm itself is composed of a fluid medium (matrix) called the *cytosol*. In the cytosol are suspended (or embedded) a variety of *organelles*, and *inclusions* (e.g., carbohydrates and lipid droplets). In another words, the cytoplasm contains a viscous cytosol (containing water, ions, and macromolecules) and organelles (e.g., endoplasmic reticulum, Golgi apparatus, mitochondria, and secretory vesicles (or secretary granules). The endoplasmic reticulum (used for protein synthesis) and mitochondrial networks (used for ATP production and the citric acid cycle) are highly complex and fibrous, extending to all parts of the cell. Some specialized cell types have more specifically organized cytoplasms, such as muscle cells, which have fibrous, parallel endoplasmic reticulum, which provides a constant calcium supply for muscle contraction. Glandular cells, with more specific secretory roles, often have a top and bottom (apical and basal) side, where the apical side has many secretary vesicles, whereas the nucleus is near the bottom, with extensive endoplasmic reticulum in between.

16.3.2.3 Cytoskeleton The fibrous network known as the cytoskeleton is basically a kind of self-assembling and modifying scaffold system (Figure 16.11). The major function of cytoskeleton proteins is to provide a physical support to organelles, enabling them to relocate within the cytoplasm. The cytoskeleton is also involved in migration and changing cell shape, depending on its function. The cytoskeleton is very active during cellular division, allowing two newly copied daughter cells to move apart from each other and recompartmentalize, without becoming detached from the tissue network. The cytoskeleton also anchors intercellular adhesions that give tissues shape, and affect how they interact with the extracellular matrix.

16.4   TRANSPORT ACROSS PLASMA MEMBRANES

While the cell has a very well-defined structural morphology, it is important to realize that cells are highly dynamic, undergoing continuous remodeling, vesicle trafficking, gene expression, protein production, signaling, metabolism, and energy generation.

The plasma membrane, therefore, has several protein systems for exchange and interaction with the extracellular environment [1].

Transport of materials across the plasma membrane occurs by four principal mechanisms:

1. Passive diffusion
2. Facilitated diffusion
3. Active transport (against gradients)
4. Bulk transport

16.4.1   Passive Diffusion

Net movement of material from an area of high concentration to an area with lower concentration is said to move by passive diffusion, either across a membrane or from one region to another (e.g., between two adjacent tissues). It is driven by the difference in concentration between the two areas, called a concentration gradient. In short, passive diffusion moves materials down the concentration gradient, without the need to be driven by an external energy source. An example of this is passive oxygen diffusion from an arteriole, where oxygen moves from oxygenated red blood cells to deoxygenated tissues (e.g., brain arterioles).

Biological systems also employ a process called *osmosis*, where high concentrations of one type of solute (e.g., albumin, ions) accumulate on one side of a membrane, creating a water deficit (i.e., a concentration gradient). So water tries to equalize the pressure by moving across the membrane.

16.4.2   Facilitated Diffusion

Facilitated diffusion is also called carrier-mediated diffusion. It is the movement of molecules across a semipermeable membrane via microscale channel proteins embedded within the membrane, which function as gates or pores to aqueous dissolved molecules. Without these proteins, a hydrophobic phospholipid bilayer prevents strongly polarized solutes (e.g., amino acids, nucleic acids, carbohydrates, proteins, and ions, except for water) from diffusing across the membrane, but generally allows for the diffusion of hydrophobic (nonpolar) solutes (e.g., lipids, sterols).

To overcome this barrier, single polar molecules bind with their specific carrier proteins, triggering them to open and allowing them cross the channel, one molecule at a time. While this may seem slow, the presence of thousands of these channel proteins actually assists diffusion, by making the membrane semipermeable. This affords the cell the ability to control the bulk movement of substances, which has several advantages. First, it allows the membrane to be selectively permeable to only one variety of solute (e.g., glucose transporters for glucose). Second, the process is more controllable in speed, allowing for more efficient uptake than by diffusion alone, but also enabling uptake to slow down if there has been a reduction in the demand for the molecule inside the cell, or if supply has decreased externally. The third important advantage is that there is no net energy expenditure, like passive diffusion.

16.4.3   Active Transport (against a Gradient)

Active transport involves the movement of materials from an area of low concentration to higher concentration, against the spontaneous flow or concentration gradient. This may seem unnatural, but serves several important purposes. The shunting of molecules against a flow or against a concentration gradient requires energy in the form of ATP. Many proteins act as simple pumps by using energy to drive movement of solute molecules against a spontaneous flow. For example, in mitochondria, the NADH produced from the citric acid cycle establishes an internal charge and proton gradient, which drives oxidative respiration. Also in the endoplasmic reticulum, calcium pumps use ATP to remove calcium from the cytosol, to maintain low concentrations needed for control of signaling events.

16.4.4   Bulk Transport across Plasma Membranes

Transport of large or small particles into the cell occurs by a range of mechanisms collectively known as *endocytosis* (Figure 16.12). This generally occurs by changes in the conformation of the membrane at the side of uptake, and results in the formation of a membrane-bound vesicle.

16.4.4.1   Pinocytosis and Receptor-Mediated Endocytosis   Eukaryotic cells rely mainly on pinocytosis for the bulk uptake of substances nonspecifically, which includes molecules that are not able to pass through the plasma membrane, but have already been digested or broken down substantially. Pinocytosis occurs when membranes involute to take up extracellular fluid containing dissolved molecules, then merge again to form a spherical vesicle. Once inside, the vesicles merge with other vesicle traffic, such as lysosomes, which further digest food molecules. This process requires ATP, to drive cytoskeletal proteins, which reshape the membrane from underneath. Pinocytosis does not require binding of receptors to trigger the event, which occurs continuously, unlike *receptor-mediated uptake,* which requires solutes to bind to their matching receptors before being consumed by the cells. This mechanism also requires ATP, and examples include hormone-mediated binding and transport of iron by transferrin.

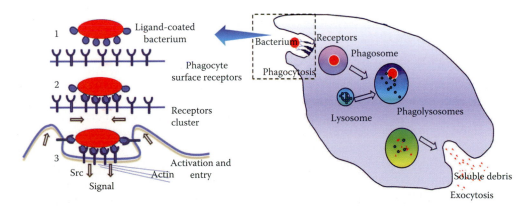

Figure 16.12
Schematic illustration of phagocytosis. (From the http://commons.wikimedia.org/.)

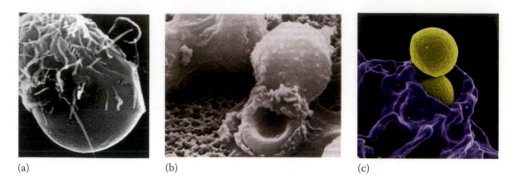

(a)   (b)   (c)

Figure 16.13

Phagocytosis of (a) a particle and (b) a dead red blood cell. (c) Colored scanning electron micrograph (SEM) of a neutrophil white blood cell (purple) engulfing methicillin-resistant Staphylococcus aureus bacteria (MRSA, yellow). This process is called phagocytosis. MRSA is a round (coccus) Gram-positive bacterium that is resistant to many commonly prescribed antibiotics. Neutrophils are the most abundant white blood cells and are part of the body's immune system. (From NIAID/National Institutes of Health/SCIENCE Photo Library.)

16.4.4.2 Phagocytosis   This process is used by some cells types (e.g., macrophages, which are a kind of white blood cell) to engulf solid particles using the cell membrane (Figure 16.12). Substances such as bacteria, dead cells, and small mineral and polymer particles may be phagocytosed (Figure 16.13), as opposed to dissolved compounds (Gk. *phago-* = "eat," *pino-* = "drink"). The ingested material is fused by the lysosome inside cells, leading to further decomposition of the particle.

16.4.4.3 Phagocytes: Cells of the Cellular Defense System   Nontoxic biomaterials are typically safely cleared from the body by phagocytosis. This job is done by specific *white blood cells*, which are collectively referred to as *phagocytes*, as listed in Table 16.2. These phagocytes are circulatory cells, which localize to areas such as infection sites, where removal of foreign bodies is required before tissue can begin to self-repair.

16.5   CELL PROLIFERATION

Eukaryotic cell survival is anchorage-dependent. A population of cells in a growing tissue occupies a localized environment, where cells are adherent to each other and an underlying substrate. Population renewal is referred to as *cell proliferation*, a controlled process of cell division, whereby cells make copies of themselves to increase the cell population and replace dead cells. This is especially necessary in *busy* tissues such as intestinal and dermal epithelium, where peripheral cells are shed every few hours. In any case, cell populations have been established from early development, and adult tissues are said to be maintained by base-line levels of cell proliferation.

In tissue engineering, the first and foremost function of most biomaterials (except for artificial vessels) is their role as substrates for cell attachment, which is critical in maintaining the environment that proliferating cells require. An exception is blood and sperm cells, which are no longer capable of dividing because they are the end-product of progenitor cell proliferation in a continually renewing tissue system (bone marrow,

Table 16.2
The Cells of the Defense System

White Blood Cells	Main Targets	Phenotype
Neutrophil[a]	Bacteria, fungi.	
Eosinophil	Parasites, allergic reactions.	
Basophil	Allergic reactions.	
Mast cells[a]	Allergic reactions.	
Lymphocyte	B-cells: pathogens (virus, bacteria, fungi…) T-cells: virus-infected and tumor cells.	
Monocyte[a]	They migrate from blood to other tissues and differentiate into tissue-resident *macrophages* or *dendritic cells*.	
Macrophage[a]	Engulf (eat) cellular debris and pathogens (e.g., osteoclast and fibroclast). These cells are dedicated to perform local phagocytosis.	
Dendritic cell[a]	Activate T-cells, help to engulf.	

[a] *Phagocytes.*

testis tubules). Cardiac and brain tissue have very low rates of cell proliferation, containing highly active cells that renew their composition and cell–cell interactions, rather than themselves.

16.5.1 Cell Attachment

Cells attach to each other and substrates via specific integral membrane proteins called *cell adhesion molecules*, including cell–matrix adhesion molecules (e.g., integrins, proteoglycans) and cell–cell adhesion molecules (e.g., cadherins) (Figure 16.14). Each of these adhesion molecules has a different function and recognizes different

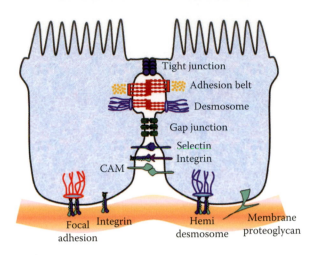

Figure 16.14
Schematic illustration of cell attachment to a substrate and between them.

binding sites of biomolecules. Knowledge of cell–matrix adhesion molecules provides us critical guides in surface chemical modification of biomaterials of implants.

Cell–cell adhesion is important in understanding the specific dynamics of the tissue itself, including its proliferation rate and transport processes, which have a major bearing on the healing rate. Cell proliferation in adherent colonies is highly regulated, compared to migratory cell types formed during early development (e.g., mesenchymal cells). In the adult, cells only reside and divide within tissues for their entire life span, although they can produce migratory cells, which are usually nonproliferative.

16.5.2   Mitosis and the Cell Cycle

Cell proliferation in adherent populations is very carefully controlled at the level of the *cell cycle*, a highly ordered sequence of intracellular protein signaling events that regulate cell replication and division. The first step in this process is the replication of the genetic material by *mitosis*. This is the most critical event, involving synthesis of new DNA and packaging of the chromatin into chromosomes, to ensuring that both daughter cells will inherit equal and exact copies of all genes (Figure 16.15). Of course, not all cells divide at once, or in the same location. For example, skin cells divide in the deeper dermal layers, before gradually moving toward the surface of the tissue. And only a small proportion of cells will divide, in balance with the rate of cell loss. If cell loss increases, then the cell cycle can be sped up to more rapidly regenerate tissues.

16.5.3   Regeneration versus Cancer

While upregulation of cell division is important in wound healing, the same process can become severely dysregulated, due to a defect in one or more proteins in the cell cycle or metabolic signaling systems, due to DNA damage. This can happen under a number of circumstances, including when cells have been exposed to chemical toxins (carcinogens), ionizing radiation, or viral attack, causing DNA mutations. Thus, cells can undergo a process called *transformation* into *cancer cells*.

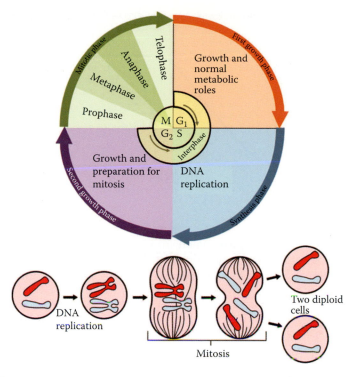

Figure 16.15
Cell division (mitosis).

Proliferative cell types (e.g., skin and glandular tissues) are particularly susceptible to cancer, resulting in cells that become *immortal* (able to divide indefinitely) and move to other tissues at a rapid rate (e.g., melanoma, adenoma, which are cancers of skin and gland, respectively). It is important to note that *migratory cancer cells are* anchorage-independent, reverting back to a mesenchyme-like state. Unlike normal cells, cancer cells can also survive without attachment to other cells of their own kind, so that even a single migratory cancer cell can establish a secondary colony in another tissue.

16.5.4   Cell Growth Curve

Cell proliferation has been observed to occur in three phases, called *lag, log,* and *plateau* phase (Figure 16.16). The *doubling time* is the period required for a population of cells to double in number. These growth dynamics occur under controlled growth conditions in vitro, in an excess of nutrients, with the lag phase an artifact of the recovery of cells from cryostorage. However, it is likely that similar proliferation dynamics occur in vivo as well. Routinely proliferating tissues are likely to be maintained with most cells being in the late-log to early plateau phase, unless an injury occurs. In that case, cells will then enter exponential log-phase growth for a short time, until healed. It is important to remember that cell division is an energy-dependent process.

16.5.5   Cell Aging (Senescence)

Normal tissue-specific cells have a limited number of cell cycles (typically 20–80). Natural aging and death of cells is genetically preprogrammed, which in the human

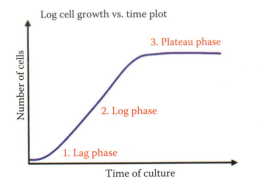

Log cell growth vs. time plot

Number of cells

Time of culture

1. Lag phase

2. Log phase

3. Plateau phase

Figure 16.16
A typical cell proliferation curve.

correlates with a life span of approximately 70 years. Many tissue types already begin to show morphological signs of senescence in middle age, including skin tissue. Cell cycles also slow down, so that the regenerative capacity of tissues gradually declines with age as well.

16.5.6   Phenotype of Proliferating Cells

A *phenotype* is any observable characteristic of a living cell, either dividing or produced from a proliferative tissue. Originally, this term was used to describe the visible signs of change in other organisms, in response to mutations is a specific gene (e.g., insects) under laboratory conditions. Today, the word can also describe the different types of cells according to their observable biological characteristics, such as extracellular and organelle morphology, proliferation rate, biomolecular properties, or behavior (Figure 16.17). In medical sciences, phenotype is more likely to be called tissue type, in relation to the basic cell types (see Chapter 17).

16.5.7   Cell Death

The natural process of gene-programmed cell death is called *apoptosis*. Apoptosis is important for body functions and health, in maintaining population size in balance with the innate proliferation rate of a specific tissue. For example, gut tissue is likely to have a higher apoptotic rate than brain tissue, due to more rapid cell turnover. During early embryo development, apoptosis is actually used in maintaining

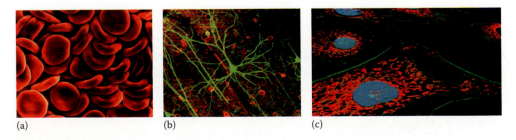

(a)   (b)   (c)

Figure 16.17
Diverse phenotypes of cells: (a) red blood cells; (b) nerve cells; and (c) fibroblasts.

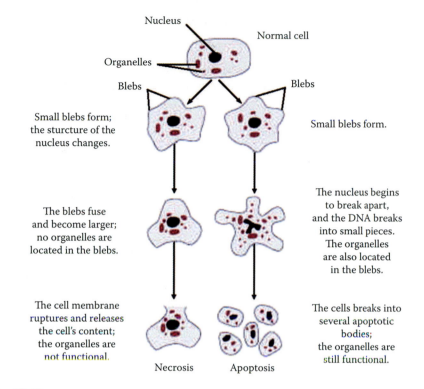

Figure 16.18
Morphological identification of cell death, necroses, or apoptosis. (From http://commons. wikimedia.org/.)

optimum population sizes and directs the removal of cells (e.g., removal of cells between digits in early limb plates). In the adult, uncontrolled cell proliferation leads to cancer (e.g., cancer cells can replicate without anchorage), where cells become unable to apoptose. On the other hand, uncontrolled cell death often occurs when cells have been deprived of nutrients or due to infections, leading to *necrosis*. Either apoptosis or necrosis can be identified morphologically using histological techniques (Figure 16.18).

16.6   CELL DIFFERENTIATION AND STEM CELLS

Specific *phenotypes* of adult cells have an autonomous and specialized physiological role in a proliferating tissue. A mature bone cell is very unlikely to function as a mature neuron, for example. However, in many tissues, small colonies of less mature (less specialized) cells exist, having maintained an immature phenotype from earlier in development. These include fibroblasts, hemopoietic progenitors, and tissue-specific progenitor cells (e.g., endometrial stromal cells). *Cellular differentiation* is the process by which a less specialized cell becomes a more specialized cell type. A cell that is able to differentiate into more than one cell type is referred to as a *stem cell*. Like branches of a tree, different cell types are thought of as *stemming* from a common progenitor cell type.

16.6.1 Common Characteristics of Stem Cells

Stem cells are characterized by the following:

1. The ability to self-renew almost indefinitely, through mitotic cell division. This characteristic is also *shared by cancer cells*. Stem cells, if not induced properly, can develop cancers, and in fact some of the earlier described experimental stem cell lines were derived from carcinoma-like cells.
2. The ability to differentiate into a diverse range of specialized cell types. *This is not possessed by cancer cells*. However, migratory cancer cells can induce blood vessel formation to obtain their own blood supply, very much like mesenchymal cells. The ability of stem cells to differentiate is also called *stem-ness*, a process that is still not very well understood. It does, however, involve reprogramming of developmentally important genes that are normally dormant in specialized cell types.

16.6.2 Embryonic Stem Cells

As described earlier in the section about the reproductive system, all humans have developed from a single cell, the oocyte. This is eventually fertilized to become a zygote (the first stem cell) from which the implantation-competent *blastocyst* develops. After implantation, the *inner cell mass (ICM)* (also called *embryoblast*) contains immature cells that ultimately develop into all the tissues in the body (Figure 16.19).

During development, these embryoblasts (from which *embryonic stem cells* have been derived in the laboratory) gradually form some of the first progenitor phenotypes in the developing embryo. These layers include the first two germ layers (ectoderm and endoderm), which are actually epithelial layers. Migratory mesoderm is formed when ectoderm cells break free of their cell–cell adhesions and move to populate other tissues, forming new blood supply and muscle (hence, all somatic tissues contain a blood supply and some muscle).

16.6.3 Potency of Stem Cells

Zygotes and embryonic stages before the blastocyst are characterized as *totipotent*, because they can differentiate into all embryonic tissues, including the extraembryonic (future placental) tissue (Figure 16.20). It is also possible to form an entirely new embryo from several cells of a cleavage stage embryo (e.g., 8-cell).

Embryoblasts are described as *pluripotent*, because these inner cells can differentiate into any tissue, but not extraembryonic tissues. In 1981, embryoblasts were isolated from mouse blastocysts and successfully used to generate the first pluripotent embryonic stem cell (ESC) lines, as proven by their ability to differentiate into each of the three germ layers (Figure 16.20) when implanted into immunodeficient mice.

The stem cells of any of these lineages are celled *multipotent*, as they can differentiate into specialized cells of more than one tissue, but are restricted to certain groups of tissues (e.g., mesoderm can only form muscle and vascular tissue, but not nerves). *Progenitor* cells are also a kind of stem cell, because they do renew and differentiate, although only toward one specialized cell type. For example, osteoblasts develop into osteocytes. Hemopoietic progenitor cells differentiate into the different blood cell types, for example.

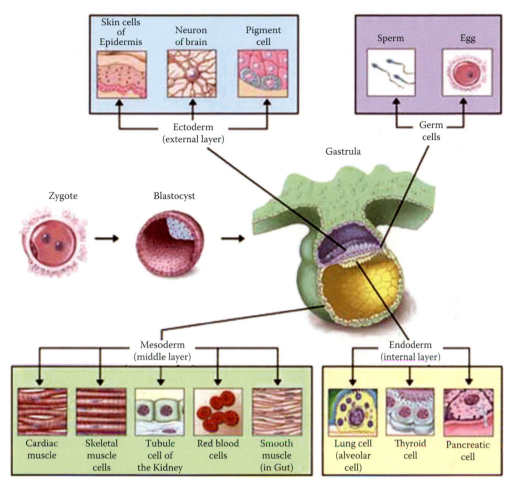

Figure 16.19
Cell differentiation during embryonic stages. (From National Centre for Biotechnology Information (NCBI), John Wetzel, an author at wikipremed.com.http://www.wikipremed.com/image.php?img=040601_68zzzz334000_Cell_differentiation_68.jpg&image_id=334000.)

16.6.4 Adult (Somatic) Stem Cells

As the fetus develops, it will form tissues derived from each of the multipotent cell types. These tissues are initially clusters of cells, eventually becoming organs that increase in size and complexity. Some stem cell types (so-called *fetal-derived stem cells*) have been derived from fetal blood progenitors present in the umbilical cord (e.g., cord blood stem cells).

Stem cells found throughout the body after most of the organism has developed are referred to as *adult (somatic) stem cells*. Focus on the derivation of these cells became more prevalent following legal and ethical issues that arose in association with experimental and medical trials of embryonic stem cells during the early 2000's. Adult stem cells divide and differentiate into tissue-specific cells during normal cell turnover, as well as during tissue repair. The regenerative ability of a tissue or organ is determined

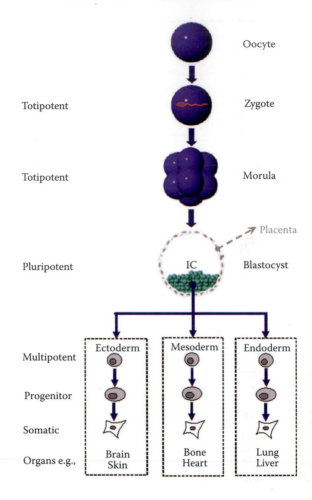

Oocyte

Totipotent — Zygote

Totipotent — Morula

Placenta

Pluripotent — IC — Blastocyst

Multipotent — Ectoderm — Mesoderm — Endoderm

Progenitor

Somatic

Organs e.g., — Brain Skin — Bone Heart — Lung Liver

Figure 16.20
Potency of stem cells.

by the amount of stem/progenitor cells that reside in small colonies within that tissue (e.g., tissues of the gastrointestinal tract).

Isolation and expansion of a patient's own stem cells (*autologous* stem cells) is also seen as advantageous in avoiding the immunological issues associated with implanting cells from another donor. *Bone marrow stem cells* have already been clinically trialled for this purpose, as an alternative to bone marrow transplantation. Adipose tissue also provides an abundant and accessible source of adult stem cells (*adipocyte progenitors*), which exist as undifferentiated fibroblasts that can be stimulated to form multiple types of cells.

In some instances, mature fibroblasts have been genetically modified in the laboratory to form new varieties of stem cells, called *induced pluripotent stem cells (iPSCs)*, although this represents a form of genetic modification. These types of stem cells have similarities to stem cells, but are still regarded as experimental as they are not fully defined. Nevertheless, they showed for the first time that pluripotency is indeed genetically programmed, and the differentiation process can be reversed, suggesting that any mature cell type could be used to generate stem cells.

16.7   CHAPTER HIGHLIGHTS

1. Four types of biomolecules:
   a. Carbohydrates (polysaccharides), with sugar being the monomer
   b. Lipids (fats and oils), with fatty acids being their components
   c. Proteins, with amino acids being the monomer
   d. DNA and RNA, with nucleotides (five carbon sugar phosphates) being the monomer
2. Cell membrane structure:
   a. Lipid bilayer membrane
   b. Mosaic model of membrane proteins
   c. Carbohydrate receptors
3. Cellular components inside membrane:
   a. Cytoplasm + Cytoskeleton + Nucleus
   b. Cytoplasm = Cytosol + Organelles
4. Four principal mechanisms to transport materials across the plasma membrane:
   a. Passive diffusion
   b. Facilitated diffusion: the transportation of polarized (hydrophilic) molecules
   c. Active transport (against gradients)
   d. Bulk transport, that is, phagocytosis: cellular engulf of solid foreign bodies
5. Most cells (an exception is blood cells) need to attach and spread out on a substrate before proliferation. Hence, the surface of most tissue engineering biomaterials (except vascular implants) must encourage cell attachment.
6. Cells do not attach directly to any substrates; rather they bind by *cell adhesion molecules.*
7. Apoptosis and necrosis: The natural process of gene-programmed cell death is called *apoptosis.* Cell death when cells have been deprived of nutrients or due to infections is called *necrosis.*
8. Stem cells are characterized by the following:
   a. The ability to self-renew almost indefinitely, through mitotic cell division
   b. The ability to differentiate into a diverse range of specialized cell types
9. Potency of stem cells:
   a. *Totipotent* stem cells can differentiate into all embryonic tissues, including the extraembryonic (future placental) tissue.
   b. *Pluripotent* stem cells cells can differentiate into any tissue, but not extra-embryonic tissues.
   c. *Multipotent*, as they can differentiate into specialized cells of more than one tissue, but are restricted to certain groups of tissues.
   d. *Progenitor* cells are also a kind of stem cell, because they do renew and differentiate, although only toward one specialized cell type.
10. Somatic (adult) stem cell sources:
   a. Umbilical cord
   b. Bone marrow
   c. Adipose tissue
   d. Induced pluripotent stem cells (iPSCs)

ACTIVITIES

Animation of passive facilitated diffusion

1. http://highered.mcgraw-hill.com/sites/0072495855/student_view0/chapter2/
   animation__how_the_sodium_potassium_pump_works.html
2. http://highered.mcgraw-hill.com/sites/0072495855/student_view0/chapter2/
   animation__how_osmosis_works.html

ADVANCED TOPIC: CELL THERAPY TO TREAT CARDIAC DISEASE

As early as 1978, Bader and Oberpriller demonstrated the regenerative capacity of amphibian hearts after autologous implantation of minced ventricular tissue samples (i.e., nonisolated cells) into injured newt hearts [1]. In this study, a partial regeneration of injured newt ventricles was observed. However, grafted tissue fragments remained morphologically and functionally separated from the native myocardium. True tissue engineering approaches emerged in the early 1990s when efforts to regenerate functional myocardial tissue were invested in grafting of isolated cells [2,3]. Since then, several early-stage clinical trials have been carried out using a variety of cell types with the hope of improving myocardial function. So far, a variety of cell models have been under intensive investigation. They can be categorized into three groups (Table 16.3): (1) somatic muscle cells, such as fetal or neonatal cardiomyocytes [4–13] and skeletal myoblasts [14–18]; (2) myocardium-generating cells, such as embryonic stem cells [19–23], (possibly) bone-marrow-derived mesenchymal stem cells [24–32], and adipose stem cells [33]; and (3) angiogenesis-stimulating cells, including fibroblasts [34] and endothelial progenitor cells.

Somatic Muscle Cells

Fetal or Neonatal Cardiomyocyte Early cell transplantation studies focused on using fetal or neonatal rodent (rat or mouse) cardiomyocytes, as these cells have the inherent electrophysiological, structural, and contractile properties of cardiomyocytes and still retain some proliferating capacity [3,4,13]. In their pioneering study, Soonpaa et al. [3] established the principles of cardiac cell implantation in the heart. They demonstrated that fetal cardiomyocytes could be transplanted and integrated within the healthy myocardium of mice, and that the surviving donor cells were aligned with recipient cells and formed cell-to-cell contacts [3]. This group also reported the same fetal cardiomyocyte grafting procedure in the myocardium of dystrophic mice and dogs [13].

More studies have demonstrated that cardiac myocytes from neonatal, embryonic, or adult models can also be engrafted into diseased (infarcted, cryoinjured, or cardiomyopathic) hearts [2,4–8,10–12,35]. These results also indicate that early-stage cardiomyocytes (fetal and neonatal) were better candidates than more mature cardiac cells due to their superior in vivo survival [11].

Time course studies for the survival of grafted cardiomyocytes in the healthy heart were carried out by Muller-Ehmsen et al. [36]. They isolated and injected male donor

Table 16.3
Potential Cell Sources for Myocardial Regeneration in Humans and Their Advantages and Disadvantages for Myocardial Repair

Cell Source	Autologous	Easily Obtainable	Highly Expandable	Cardiac Myogenesis	Clinical Trial	Safety
Somatic cells						
Fetal cardiomyocytes	No	No	No	Yes	No	No
Skeletal myoblasts	Yes	Yes	Depend on age	Debated	Yes	Yes, arrhythmias
Smooth muscle cells	Yes	Yes	Yes	No	No	No
Fibroblasts	Yes	Yes	Yes	No	No	No
Stem cells						
Somatic stem cells						
Mesenchymal stem cells	Yes	No	Depend on age	Yes	No	Yes, fibrosis calcification
Endothelial progenitor cells	Yes	Yes	Depend on age	Debated	No	Yes, calcification
Crude bone marrow	Yes	Yes	Depend on age	Debated	Yes	Yes, calcification
Umbilical cord cells (hemetopoietic stem cells)	No	Yes	Yes	Debated	No	No
Adipose stem cells	Yes	Yes	Yes	Yes	No	Yes
Embryonic stem cells						
Human embryonic stem cells	No	No	Yes	Yes	No	Yes, potential teratoma if cells escape differentiation

Source: Leor.J. et al., Pharmacol. Ther., 105(2), 151, 2005.

neonatal rat cardiomyocytes into the left ventricular (LV) wall of adult female inbred rats. They demonstrated that these cells could survive and improve cardiac function for up to 6 months in a rat model of chronic myocardial infarction [37]. Murry's group [38] showed, using syngeneic rats with cryoinjury, that cell graft survival after 7 days could be up to 33%.

Cardiomyocyte transplantation, which was applied to smaller infarcts [7], has been proven effective in the prevention of cardiac dilation and remodeling following infarction [40] and the improvement of the ventricular function [8,10]. Several mechanisms have been proposed for improved heart function following cardiac myocyte transplantation [40–43]:

1. Direct contribution of the transplanted myocytes to contractility
2. Attenuation of infarct expansion by virtue of the elastic properties of cardiomyocytes
3. Angiogenesis induced by growth factors secreted from the fetal cells resulting in improved collateral flow
4. Paracrine effects via the release of beneficial growth factors from the transplanted cells, which support the cardiomyocytes under strain in the failing heart, and may possibly recruit residential cardiac progenitor cells

However, the transplanted tissue decreased in size several months after transplantation [7,11]. An electron microscopy study revealed dead cells with necrotic and apoptic phenotypes. Based on the most recent experiments, it is apparent that cell death is rapid and extensive after cardiomyocyte grafting, with most cell death occurring during the first 2 days. However, after 1 week the graft is relatively stable [36,38]. Although this is important proof-of-concept work, there is no realistic possibility of human or rat neonatal cardiomyocytes coming to clinical application [38,44,45]. As a result, several alternative approaches have been developed to overcome the limitations of fetal cardiomyocyte transplantation and to obviate the need for immunosuppressants.

Skeletal Myoblast   Theoretically, skeletal muscle progenitor cells may be superior to cardiomyocytes for infarct repair, because skeletal myoblasts have almost all the properties of the ideal donor cell type except their noncardiac origin. Skeletal myoblast satellite cells can be harvested from autologous sources, which obviate the need for immune suppression. Satellite cells are mononuclear progenitor cells found in mature muscle. In undamaged muscle, the majority of satellite cells are quiescent. Upon muscle damage, satellite cells become activated and are able to differentiate and fuse to augment existing muscle fibers and to form new fibers. They can be rapidly expanded in an undifferentiated state in vitro to clinically applicable numbers of myoblasts without a risk for tumorigenicity, and they have the capabilities to withstand ischemia better than many other cell types. Continued proliferation in vivo may be an advantage when engrafting into an injured heart, since the input of a smaller number of cells might give rise to a large graft [43,46].

Although it was originally hoped that skeletal myoblasts would adapt a cardiac phenotype, it is now clear that within heart tissue the skeletal myoblasts remain committed to form only mature skeletal muscle cells that possess completely different electromechanical properties than those of heart cells. Moreover, given the inability of myoblasts to form electromechanical connections with host cardiomyocytes (due to lack of expression of adhesion and gap junction proteins), it is not surprising that physiological studies failed to demonstrate synchronous beating of the grafted cells within the host tissue [47].

However, studies in small and large animal models of infarction demonstrated beneficial effects of grafting of these cells on ventricular performance [48,49]. The mechanisms underlying the beneficial effects of skeletal myoblasts remain to be elucidated. The improvement in heart wall motion could be achieved by contraction of the transplanted cells, a local effect on scar remodeling by mechanical support and/or paracrine influences on the remodeling process.

Nevertheless, given their autologous origin, the capacity to amplify primary myoblasts from human muscle biopsies, and the encouraging preclinical results, skeletal myoblasts were the first cell type to reach clinical application [18,50–57]. The pioneering phase I clinical trials were performed either using a direct surgery approach (during coronary artery bypass graft surgery) or using a percutaneous endocardial catheter-delivery approach and have demonstrated both the feasibility of the procedure and the ability of the cells to engraft in the infarcted myocardium [18,50–52,54–59].

The clinical application of autologous skeletal myoblasts is currently limited by several concerns [46,60,61].

1. *Lack of myocardial phenotype*: This has been blamed for the disturbingly high incidence of life-threatening ventricular arrhythmias noted in the initial post-transplantation phase in these trials [50,51].
2. *Low recovery of satellite cells*. The recovery of satellite cells from muscle biopsies of elderly patients is low.
3. *Efficiency*: Grafting methods need be developed to improve the efficiency of cell engraftment and survival.
4. *Questionable beneficial effects*: The efficacy of skeletal myoblast therapy is still uncertain because of the following facts. Firstly, the phase I clinical trials were not randomized, and might be placebo controlled. Secondly, widely different cell transplantation protocols were used in a relatively small number of patients. Finally, the trials were associated with other confounding factors such as concomitant LVAD implantation or revascularization. Ongoing phase II clinical trials will hopefully address these concerns and thoroughly evaluate the safety and efficacy of myoblast transplantation.

Angiogenic Cells

Fibroblasts   Vascularization is a key step in tissue repair. At sites of injury, fibroblast-like cells are responsible for fibrous tissue formation. These cells are termed myofibroblasts because they contain alpha-smooth muscle actin microfilaments and are contractile. In vivo studies of injured rat cardiac tissues and in vitro cell culture studies [62] have shown that such fibroblast-like cells contain requisite components for angiotensin peptide generation and angiotensin II receptors. Such locally generated angiotensin II acts in an autocrine/paracrine manner to regulate collagen turnover and thereby tissue homeostasis in injured tissue.

Human dermal fibroblasts have been applied for myocardial regeneration to stimulate revascularization and preserve function of the infarcted LV in mice [63]. It has been shown that dermal fibroblasts functioned to attenuate further loss of LV function accompanying acute myocardial infarct and that this might be related in part to myocardial revascularization.

Endothelial Progenitor Cells   Endothelial progenitor cells (EPCs) are present in the bone marrow and the peripheral blood and exhibit phenotypical markers of mature endothelial cells [64]. It has been found that rats with inflammatory-mediated cardiomyopathy exhibited a significant mobilization of EPCs from the bone marrow to the periphery and their ability to adhere to fibronectin, mature endothelial cells, and cultured cardiomyocytes was significantly reduced when compared to healthy rats [65]. This result prompted studies in the application of EPCs in attenuating remodeling followed by acute myocardial infarction. Transfer of EPCs resulted in a functional improvement in cardiac performance. EPC transfer is effective in attenuating myocardial damage in a model of nonischemic dilated cardiomyopathy [65], probably exerting its beneficial effects via new vessel growth and improved blood supply to the failing heart.

Stem-Cell-Derived Myocytes

Basics of Stem Cells   Stem cells are undifferentiated, and thus unspecialized, cells that retain the ability to differentiate into multiple cell lineages [66]. In principle, stem cells are the optimal cell source for tissue regeneration, including myocardium. Firstly, they are capable of self-replication throughout life such that an unlimited number of stem cells of similar properties can be produced via expansion in vitro. Secondly, the stem cells are clonogenic, and thus each cell can form a colony in which all the cells are derived from a particular cell colony and have identical genetic constitution. Thirdly, they are able to differentiate into one or more specialized cell types. Hence, after expansion stem cells can be directed to differentiate into a cardiomyogenic lineage [20,67–69]. For these reasons, stem-cell-based therapy for cardiac muscle regeneration has been under intensive research during the last decade.

In this section, we focus on the applications of four types of stem cells in myocardial disease: bone-marrow-derived stem cells, adipose stem cells, native cardiac progenitor cells, and embryonic stem cells.

Bone-Marrow-Derived Stem Cells   Bone marrow stem cells are the most primitive cells in the marrow. These cells can be classified into: (1) bone-marrow-derived mesenchymal stem cell (MSC), and (2) hematopoietic stem cell (HSC).

Bone-Marrow-Derived Mesenchymal Stem Cells   Bone-marrow-derived mesenchymal stem cells are a subset of bone marrow stromal cells (the term "mesenchymal stem cell" is now used to include multipotent cells that are derived from either bone marrow or other tissues, such as adult muscle or the Wharton's jelly present in the umbilical cord). This multipotent cell type is derived from the stromal compartment of the bone marrow, and when induced artificially, can give rise to cells other than those of blood cell lineages, such as bone, cartilage, tendon, adipose, and endothelial cells [72].

A number of studies suggested that bone-marrow-derived MSCs could differentiate into cardiomyocytes both in vitro and in vivo [67,68,73–78]. Makino et al. [68] treated murine mesenchymal stem cells with 5-azacytidine and isolated a cardiomyogenic cell line after repeated screening of spontaneous beating cells. This result was confirmed by Tomita et al. [79]. Later, Orlic et al. [75] reported that a subpopulation of bone marrow stem cells was capable of generating myocardium in vivo in mice. More recently, it was reported that transplantation of mesenchymal stem cells into the infarcted myocardium of rats and pigs resulted in improved myocardial performance [77,80].

One possible advantage of mesenchymal stem cells is their ability to be either auto-transplanted or allotransplanted, as some reports suggested that they may be relatively privileged in terms of immune compatibility [81].

Hemopoietic Stem Cells   In addition to the initial hypothesis that bone marrow stem cells might be able to differentiate into myocardium in vivo, another major rationale behind the research of bone marrow stem cells for cardiac muscle regeneration was the essential roles of vascularization and angiogenesis in tissue regeneration. Studies in the animal models of ischemia and phase I and II clinical trials suggested that delivery of hemopoietic stem cells and circulating endothelial progenitor cells, both originating from bone marrow stem cells, may result in improvement in the ventricular function in ischemic heart disease patients [46]. Furthermore, since bone marrow stem cells reside in the bone marrow of all patients, they can be obtained by a relatively simple procedure of bone marrow aspiration, expanded in vitro with or without differentiation, and retransplanted into the patient, thus eliminating the need for immunosuppressants [43].

The initial assumption, regarding the capability of bone-marrow-derived stem cells to regenerate the heart by differentiation into cardiomyocytes, has been challenged by a number of recent studies. Balsam et al. [82,83] and Murry et al. [84] demonstrated that the hemopoietic stem cells continued to differentiate along the hemopoietic lineage, suggesting that the functional improvement observed may not be related to differentiation into the cardiac lineage, but rather from indirect mechanisms. A considerable body of data indicates that a specific subset of bone-marrow-derived angioblasts, expressing endothelial precursor markers, is responsible for neovascularization and angiogenesis [25,85–90]. Kocher et al. [25], for example, demonstrated that an intravenous injection of human bone marrow donor cells to the infarcted myocardium of rats resulted in a significant increase in neovascularization of postinfarction myocardial tissue, attenuation of cardiomyocyte apoptosis, and left-ventricular remodeling. The potential of bone marrow stem cells to heal a damaged heart by inducing vasculogenesis in the injured myocardium, thereby increasing heart viability and restoring cardiac function has rapidly promoted translation from animal studies to human clinical trial [46,91].

At present, the results of three medium-size clinical trials (100–200 patients) show a variable and modest effect of autologous bone marrow sstem cells in restoring cardiac function [92–94]. The application of bone marrow cells for cardiac disease is still in its preliminary phase, as determination of the correct cell source, delivery route, dose, and timing require further optimization. The application of bone-marrow-derived stem cells is also limited by a safety issue: obtaining adequate autologous cells from a patient with myocardial infarction in time to prevent postinfraction remodeling may be difficult. In addition, the presence of stem cells for cardiomyocytes in other parts of the body, including bone marrow, has not been widely accepted yet. Capsi and Gepstein [46] have given an excellently tabulated overview on the clinical trial results of using bone marrow stem cells in the treatment of acute and chronic heart diseases.

Adipose-Derived Stem Cells   Human adipose tissue provides a uniquely abundant and accessible source of adult stem cells for applications in tissue engineering and regenerative medicine [95–98]. Adipose-derived stem cells have the ability to differentiate along multiple lineage pathways. The cardiomyocyte phenotype from adipose-derived cells has been reported [33,99]. One study using rats showed that adipose-tissue-derived regenerative cells improved heart function following myocardial infarction [100].

Native Cardiac Progenitor Cells It had long been believed that the adult mammalian heart, a terminally differentiated organ, had no self-renewal potential. This notion about the adult heart, however, has been challenged by accumulated evidence that myocardium itself contains a resident progenitor cell population capable of giving rise to new cardiomyocytes [101–105]. There are scientists who have hypothesized that cardiac progenitor stem cells reside in the hearts of neonatal animals, and that these progenitor stem cells (if any) could eventually serve as the basis for cardiac cell lineage formation and thus its application in the treatment of cardiac disease in humans. Recently, cardiac progenitor cells were found in the hearts of neonatal humans, rats, and mice by a multi-institution group of United States and German researchers [105].

Nonetheless, given the limited regeneration ability of the adult heart, it is apparent that the existence of the aforementioned cells within the adult heart does not translate to a functionally significant cardiac differentiation following myocardial infarction [46]. The role of these cells in the normal adult heart is still to be elucidated. They may represent an intrinsic repair system capable of replacing cells lost in the normal process of ageing, or may simply reflect remnant cells from organ development in early life. The existence of these progenitor cells will no doubt open new opportunities for myocardial repair, though many issues still need to be addressed.

Embryonic Stem Cells Embryonic stem cells are thought to have much greater clinical value than other stem cell types, because of their specific advantages, in addition to the common features shared by all stem cells as mentioned earlier. First, they are pluripotent, which means they have a broader multilineage expressing profile. Unlike adult stem cells, which can differentiate to a relatively limited number of cell types, embryonic stem cells have the potential to contribute to all adult tissues. Second, they are robust. They have the long-term proliferation ability with a normal karyotype, and can be cryopreserved. Third, they can be genetically manipulated [106]. Hence, research using embryonic stem cells remains at the leading edge of progress in stem cell science. In 1981, the inner embryoblasts were isolated from mouse blastocysts and were successfully used to generate pluripotent stem cell lines, which were termed embryonic stem cells (ESC) [107,108]. However it was not until 1998 that two independent teams, Thomson et al. [20] and Shamblott et al. [109], described the generation of human embryonic stem cell lines from human blastocysts.

The embryonic stem cell is capable of continuous proliferation and self-renewal in vitro but also retains the ability to differentiate into derivatives of all three germ layers both in vitro and in vivo. Thus, following cultivation in suspension, the ESCs tend to spontaneously create three-dimensional aggregates of differentiating tissue known as embryoid bodies (EBs) [110]. Upon aggregation, differentiation is initiated and the cells begin to a limited extent to recapitulate embryonic development. Though they cannot form trophectodermal tissue (which includes the placenta), cells of virtually every other type present in the organism can develop. The aggregate at first appears as a simple ball of cells and then grows into an increasingly more complex appearance. After a few days a hollow ball (cystic embryoid body) forms, followed by the appearance of internal structures, such as a yolk sac and heart muscle cells (i.e., cardiomyocytes), which beat in a rhythmic pattern to circulate nutrients within the increasingly larger embryoid body.

The availability of the embryonic stem cell system has boosted the hope of heart regeneration. The first study using embryonic stem cell as a source for cell transplantation into the myocardium was reported by Klug et al. in 1996 [19]. By using genetically selected mouse embryonic stem-cell-derived cardiomyocytes, the study showed that the differentiated cells developed myofibrils and gap junctions between adjacent cells and performed synchronous contractile activity in vitro for up to 7 weeks. This study proved the feasibility to guide an unlimited number of embryonic stem cells into a cardiomyogenic cell linage and to utilize them for myocardial regeneration. Later studies [111–114], utilizing the infarcted rat heart model, demonstrated that transplantation of differentiated mouse embryonic stem-cell-derived cardiomyocytes can result in short- and long-term improvement of myocardial performance.

Theoretically, the undifferentiated ESCs, which might be able to differentiate in vivo into cardiomyocytes in the host microenvironment containing cardiac-specific differentiation signaling, could improve the heart function. However, controversial results have been reported, regarding the in vivo differentiation and outcome of the transplantation of undifferentiated ESCs. Puceat's group [115,116] showed that in infarcted myocardium, grafted stem cells differentiated into functional cardiomyocytes and integrated with surrounding tissue, improving contractile performance. However, Murry et al. [117] discovered that undifferentiated mouse ESCs consistently formed cardiac teratomas in nude or immunocompetent syngeneic mice, and that cardiac teratomas contained no more cardiomyocytes than hind-limb teratomas, suggesting lack of guided differentiation. Hence, the authors concluded that undifferentiated ESCs did not differentiate toward a cardiomyocyte fate in either normal or infarcted hearts [117].

As regards immunogenicity of the transplantation of undifferentiated ESCs, Menards et al. [118,119] reported that cardiac-committed mouse ESCs, which were transplanted to the infarcted sheep heart following incubation with BMP-2, differentiated to mature cardiomyocytes, and that cell transplantation resulted in a significant improvement in cardiac function independent of whether the sheep were immunosuppressed or not. However, another group [120] reported the increased immunogenicity (i.e., rejection) of mouse ESCs upon in vivo differentiation after transplantation into ischemic myocardium of allogeneic animals, implying that clinical transplantation of allogeneic ESCs or ESC derivatives for treatment of cardiac failure might require immunosuppressive therapy. This result was confirmed by Murry's group [117], who found no evidence for allogeneic immune tolerance of cell derivatives. Hence, successful cardiac repair strategies involving ESCs will need to control cardiac differentiation, avoid introducing undifferentiated cells, and will likely require immune modulation to avoid rejection.

Human Embryonic Stem Cells   The vast biomedical potential of human ESCs has stirred enthusiasm in the field of tissue engineering. From human ESCs, scientists hope to grow replacement tissues for people with various diseases, including bone marrow for cancer patients, neurons for people with Alzheimer's disease, pancreatic cells for people with diabetes, and cardiomyocytes for patients with heart damage. Furthermore, establishment of a tissue-specific differentiation system may have significant impact on the study of early human tissue differentiation, functional genomics, pharmacological testing, and cell therapy. Given these reasons, we think that the utilization of human ESCs in cardiac tissue engineering is worthy of a separate section. An overview of the relevant reports is given in Table 16.4. After the establishment of human ESC lines in 1998 [20,109], other research groups have been able to develop a reproducible cardiomyocyte differentiation system from the human ESCs [69,121–124]. The detailed protocols can be found in these reports.

It has been demonstrated that the human ESC-derived cardiomyocytes displayed structural properties of early-stage cardiomyocytes [69,121,122,125]. The presence

Table 16.4

Differentiation of Human ESCs toward Cardiomyocytes

Method of hESC Differentiation	Major Results	Ref
In vitro: via EBs in suspension	ESCs differentiated into cardiomyocytes, even after long-term culture. Upon differentiation, beating cells were observed after 1 week, increased in numbers with time, and retained contractility for >70 days. The beating cells expressed markers of cardiomyocytes.	[121]
In vitro: via EBs in suspension	ESCs showed consistency in phenotype with early-stage cardiomyocytes, and expression of several cardiac-specific genes and transcription factors.	[69]
In vitro: via EBs in suspension	ESCs showed a progressive ultrastructural development from an irregular myofibrillar distribution to an organized sarcomeric pattern at late stages.	[126]
In vitro: via EBs in suspension	ESC-derived myocytes at midstage development demonstrated the stable presences of functional receptors and signaling pathways, and the presence of cardiac-specific action potentials and ionic currents.	[128]
In vitro: coculture of differentiated rat cardiomyocyte and hESC-derived cardiomyocytes. In vivo: transplantation of hESC-derived cardiomyocytes into swine.	Tight electrophysiological coupling between the engrafted hESC-derived cardiomyocytes and rat cardiomyocytes was observed. The transplanted hES-cell-derived cardiomyocytes paced the hearts of swine.	[129]
In vitro: coculture of undifferentiated hESC with mouse endoderm-like cells	ESCs differentiated to beating muscle. Sarcomeric marker proteins, chronotropic responses, and ion channel expression and function were typical of cardiomyocytes. Electrophysiology demonstrated that most cells resembled human fetal ventricular cells.	[122]
In vitro: via EBs in suspension	ES cells differentiated into cardiomyocytes. Upon differentiation, beating cells were observed after 9 days, and retained contractility for longer than 6 months.	[139]
In vitro: coculture of hESC-derived cardiomyocytes with rat myocytes	Electrically active, hESC-derived cardiomyocytes are capable of actively pacing quiescent, recipient, ventricular cardiomyocytes in vitro and ventricular myocardium in vivo.	[130]
In vivo: differentiated hESC-derived cardiomyocytes transplanted into guinea pig		
In vivo: differentiated cardiac-enriched hESC progeny	hESCs can form human myocardium in the rat heart, permitting studies of human myocardial development and physiology and supporting the feasibility of their use in myocardial repair.	[125]

of cardiac-specific proteins and the absence of skeletal muscle markers have also been confirmed [125,126]. These studies also demonstrated the progressive maturation from an irregular myofilament distribution to a more mature (i.e., organized) sarcomeric pattern [69,125,126]. The human ESC-derived cardiomyocytes were also shown to display functional properties, consistent with an early-stage cardiac phenotype [69,122,123,127,128]. Functional improvement of heart following cell transplantation would require structural, electrophysiological, and mechanical coupling of donor cells to the existing network of host cardiomyocytes [46]. Hence, it is important to investigate whether cells derived from human ESCs can restore myocardial electromechanical properties. A study of the Gepstein group [129,130] demonstrated tight electrophysiological coupling between the engrafted human ESCs and host rat (or swine) cardiomyocytes both in vitro and in vivo.

In spite of the exciting potential of human ESCs, the cells are also giving rise to daunting legal and ethical concerns. ESCs are controversial because they are obtained from the destruction of a potential human embryo. Technologies for therapeutic and, especially, reproductive cloning add further ethical problems. In addition, a number of technical issues need to be addressed prior to clinical application [46], as discussed in the following.

1. *Scale-up*: One of the drawbacks of cell therapy is the difficulty in scaling up to meet larger production needs in clinical applications.
2. *Purification* of the differentiating cardiomyocyte population is necessary.
3. *In vivo delivery and efficiency of grafting*: Cell-delivery techniques should be developed to enable proper alignment of the grafted tissue, high seeding rate of the transplanted cells, and minimal damage to the host tissue.
4. *Immune rejection*: Human ESCs are derived from cell lines genetically distinct from the potential human recipient. Therefore, the potential for immune rejection following hESC transplantation into an immunocompetent adult recipient exists, as is observed with conventional solid organ transplantation. As hESCs are therefore allogenic, there is the potential requirement for coadministration of immunosuppression [131–136]. Encouragingly, there is some evidence that hESCs have an immunoprivileged status. Under certain conditions, both in vitro and in vivo, they display limited immunogenicity and are tolerated in cross-species (xeno-) transplantation without immunosuppression [137,138]. Reduced cell surface expression of both major histocompatibility complex and accessory proteins is believed to underlie this immunopriviledged status. However, this is mainly observed in undifferentiated hESCs, and with differentiation into specialized tissues such as cardiomyocytes, hESCs may acquire a greater immunogenic phenotype. Strategies aimed at preventing immunological rejection of the cells, such as genetic modification or graft-recipient tissue-type matching, should be explored.

STRATEGIES TO ADDRESS IMMUNE REJECTION IN CELLS

As mention earlier, the major limitation of cell therapy is immune rejection associated with most used cell types. Successful application of tissue engineering in the human will depend on the utilization of an autologous or nonimmunogeneic cell source, as well as synthetic scaffold materials, to avoid lifelong immunosuppression. Several strategies aimed at achieving immunological tolerance are being developed. These strategies include [46] the following:

1. Establishing banks of major histocompatibility complex (MHC) antigen-typed human ESC lines
2. Genetically altering the human ESC to suppress the immune response (e.g., by knocking out the major histocompatibility complexes)
3. The concept of hematopoietic chimerism
4. Generating immune-compatible ESC-derived cardiomyocytes with the patient's own genetic information, known as somatic cell nuclear transplantation or therapeutic cloning

The successful application of nuclear transfer techniques to a range of mammalian species has brought the possibility of human therapeutic cloning significantly closer. The objective of therapeutic cloning is to produce pluripotent stem cells that carry the nuclear genome of the patient and then induce them to differentiate into replacement cells, such as cardiomyocytes to replace damaged heart tissue. In the process, a somatic cell nucleus from a patient is transferred into an enucleated oocyte (i.e., its nucleus has been removed), as described in the cloning of Dolly the sheep [140]. The oocyte containing the new nucleus carries the genetic information of the patient. Using a tiny pulse of electricity to cause the new nucleus to fuse with the enucleated oocyte's cytoplasm, this manipulated oocyte can develop in vitro into a blastocyst. From this blastocyst, embryonic stem cells with the genetics of the patient can be isolated and expanded in vitro and then differentiated in vitro into genetically matched cardiomyocytes for transplantation. Obviously, cloning would eliminate the critical problem of immune incompatibility.

Strategies of Cell Delivery

In cell-based therapy, isolated cell suspensions are directly injected into injured heart via the pericardium, coronary arteries, or endocardium. Direct injection of isolated cells obviates an open-heart surgery. However, it is difficult to control the location of the grafted cells in the transplantation. To address these problems, 2D and 3D cell delivery vehicles have been under development using biomaterials.

SUMMARY OF CELL-BASED THERAPIES AND THEIR LIMITATIONS

Cell-based cardiac therapy represents an exciting strategy in, heart tissue regeneration and heart tissue engineering. Huge efforts have been invested in the development of cell sources for myocardial regeneration, including fetal cardiomyocytes, skeletal myoblasts, bone marrow stem cells, adipose stem cells, endothelial progenitors, native cardiac progenitor cells, and embryonic stem cells (ESC). A large number of studies has also been carried out to assess the roles of these potential cell types in the regeneration of myocardial tissue, both in vitro and in vivo. The translation of these basic scientific studies from bench to bedside has been progressing. Among these cell sources, embryonic stem cells possess the greatest promise because of their intrinsic pluripotency. These pluripotent cells can self-replicate tirelessly in the undifferentiated state in vitro and be induced to differentiate into cell derivatives of all three germ layers, including cardiomyocytes. The ability to generate human cardiac tissue in vitro using embryonic stem cells, therefore, provides the most exciting approach in the field of cardiac tissue regenerative medicine and tissue engineering.

Despite the enormous potential of cell-based therapy, a number of technical issues need to be addressed prior to clinical application. These include (1) scaling up of cells, (2) cell delivery, (3) efficiency of grafting, (4) suppression of alternative unwanted cell phenotypes when ES cells are applied, and (5) immune rejection. Improvements in the efficiency of cell delivery and grafting, in particular, could benefit immensely from advances in biomaterials, such as new developments in biodegradable materials.

SIMPLE QUESTIONS IN CLASS

1. The chemical bonding that helps bring molecules together in cells can be
   a. Metallic bonds
   b. Covalent bonds
   c. Ionic bonds
   d. Hydrogen bonds
2. Which of the following biomolecules is hydrophobic?
   a. Lipids (fats and oils)
   b. Carbohydrates (polysaccharides)
   c. Proteins
   d. Nucleotides (DNA and RNA)
3. Cells are
   a. Hydrophobic
   b. Hydrophilic
4. How many glycolipid receptors are on this cell membrane?

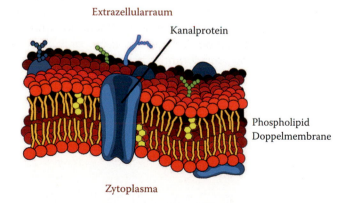

5. Which of following molecules and ions could passively diffuse across lipid bilayer membrane without facilitation?
   a. Amino acids
   b. Ca^{2+}, salt
   c. Lipids
   d. Sugar, carbohydrates

6. Which of the following descriptions about cells are incorrect?
    a. Most cells must attach to a surface before they start division.
    b. Blood cells can proliferate while in suspension.
    c. Cells tend to anchor on a hydrophobic substrate.
    d. Cells attach to a substrate through adhesion molecules.
7. "Cell necrosis" means
    a. Cell death caused by toxic chemicals
    b. Cellular phagocytosis
    c. Natural cell death due to aging
    d. Cellular mitosis
8. "Apoptosis" means
    a. Cell death caused by toxic chemicals
    b. Cellular phagocytosis
    c. Natural cell death due to aging
    d. Cell death caused by immune rejection
9. "Confluency" means
    a. The coverage of the dish or the flask by the cells
    b. The concentration of cells in suspension
    c. The flow ability of cells
    d. The components of a cell
10. "Phagocytosis" means
    a. Phenotype of cells
    b. Cellular pathology
    c. Necrosis of cells
    d. Cellular engulfing of solid particles
11. "Phenotype" means
    a. Functions of a cell
    b. Physiology of the cell
    c. Morphology of a cell
    d. Any observable characteristics or traits of a cell
12. Macrophages clean debris of biomaterials through which of the following mechanisms?
    a. Passive diffusion
    b. Facilitated diffusion
    c. Active transport
    d. Phagocytosis
13. Which of the following cells are not anchorage-dependent?
    a. Fibroblasts
    b. Osteoblasts
    c. Pneumocytes
    d. Blood cells
14. In which of the following applications should the biomaterials be designed to NOT encourage cell attachment onto the surface of materials?
    a. Liver tissue engineering
    b. Artificial blood vessel
    c. Bone filler for the repair of bone
    d. Total knee replacement

PROBLEMS AND EXERCISES

1. What are the four types of biomolecules? Give two examples for each type.
2. Describe the major structural features of a cell membrane and their functions.
3. Briefly explain why the diffusion of Ca^{2+} ions down a concentration gradient still needs protein-facilitation across a cell membrane.
4. What is cell apoptosis? What is cell necrosis? To evaluate the cytocompatibility of a biomaterial, will you assess the cell death on terms of apoptosis or necrosis?
5. Discuss the strategies to enhance cell attachment onto a biomaterial surface.
6. Discuss the strategies to modify the surface of a biomaterial used as artificial blood vessel.
7. Describe potency (totipotency, pluripotency, and multipotency) of the following stem (or progenitor) cells:
   1. Mesenchymal stem cells
   2. Embryonic stem cells
   3. Type II pneumonia cells
   4. Osteoblasts
   5. Adipose stem cells
8. To regenerate bone tissue in vitro, discuss how you will choose a cell of the following cell types:
   1. Osteoblast
   2. Progenitor osteoblast
   3. Mesenchymal stem cell
   4. Osteoclast
   5. Osteocyte
9. Discuss potential cell sources for the cell therapy of the treatment of the following diseases:
   1. Heart attack
   2. Emphysema
   3. Large bone defects
   4. Cirrhosis
   5. Full skin burn
   6. Articular cartilage damage
10. Discuss the advantages and risks of the cell therapy from embryonic stem cells.

BIBLIOGRAPHY

Reference for Text

1. Alberts, B., A. Johnson, J. Lewis, M. Raff, K. Roberts, and P. Walter, *Molecular Biology of the Cell.* Garland Science, New York, NY.

Websites

The Inner life of a Cell
http://ocw.mit.edu/courses/biology/
http://sparkleberrysprings.com/innerlifeofcell.html

http://www.cell-biology.org/
http://www.cellsalive.com/quiz.htm
http://www.studiodaily.com/main/searchlist/6850.html
http://www.youtube.com/watch?v=BtZEqQ1cpmk

References for Advanced Topic

1. Bader, D. and J.O. Oberpriller, Repair and reorganization of minced cardiac-muscle in adult newt (*Notophthalmus-Viridescens*). *Journal of Morphology*, 1978;**155**(3):349–357.
2. Koh, G.Y. et al., Long-term survival of at-1 cardiomyocyte grafts in syngeneic myocardium. *American Journal of Physiology*, 1993;**264**(5):H1727–H1733.
3. Soonpaa, M.H. et al., Formation of nascent intercalated disks between grafted fetal cardio-myocytes and host myocardium. *Science*, 1994;**264**(5155):98–101.
4. Leor, J. et al., Transplantation of fetal myocardial tissue into the infarcted myocar-dium of rat—A potential method for repair of infarcted myocardium? *Circulation*, 1996;**94**(9):332–336.
5. Li, R.K. et al., Cardiomyocyte transplantation improves heart function. *Annals of Thoracic Surgery*, 1996;**62**(3):654–660.
6. Li, R.K. et al., In vivo survival and function of transplanted rat cardiomyocytes. *Circulation Research*, 1996;**78**(2):283–288.
7. Li, R.K. et al., Natural history of fetal rat cardiomyocytes transplanted into adult rat myocar-dial scar tissue. *Circulation*, 1997;**96**(9):179–186.
8. Scorsin, M. et al., Does transplantation of cardiomyocytes improve function of infarcted myocardium? *Circulation*, 1997;**96**(9):188–193.
9. Scorsin, M. et al., Can grafted cardiomyocytes colonize peri-infarct myocardial areas? *Circulation*, 1997;**95**(1):A9 and 1996;**94**:337.
10. Scorsin, M. et al., Can cellular transplantation improve function in doxorubicin-induced heart failure? *Circulation*, 1998;**98**(19):II151–II155.
11. Reinecke, H. et al., Survival, integration, and differentiation of cardiomyocyte grafts—A study in normal and injured rat hearts. *Circulation*, 1999;**100**(2):193–202.
12. Murry, C.E. et al., Cellular therapies for myocardial infarct repair. *Cold Spring Harbor Symposia on Quantitative Biology*, 2002;**67**:519–526.
13. Koh, G.Y. et al., Stable fetal cardiomyocyte grafts in the hearts of dystrophic mice and dogs. *Journal of Clinical Investigation*, 1995;**96**(4):2034–2042.
14. Chiu, R.C., Cardiac cell transplantation: the autologous skeletal myoblast implantation for myocardial regeneration. *Advanced Cardiac Surgery*, 1999;**11**:69–98.
15. Dorfman, J. et al., Myocardial tissue engineering with autologous myoblast implantation. *Journal of Thoracic and Cardiovascular Surgery*, 1998;**116**(5):744–751.
16. Pouzet, B. et al., Intramyocardial transplantation of autologous myoblasts—Can tissue pro-cessing be optimized? *Circulation*, 2000;**102**(19):210–215.
17. Murry, C.E. et al., Skeletal myoblast transplantation for repair of myocardial necrosis. *Journal of Clinical Investigation*, 1996;**98**(11):2512–2523.
18. Menasche, P., Skeletal myoblast for cell therapy. *Coronary Artery Disease*, 2005;**16**(2):105–110.
19. Klug, M.G. et al., Genetically selected cardiomyocytes from differentiating embry-onic stem cells form stable intracardiac grafts. *Journal of Clinical Investigation*, 1996;**98**(1):216–224.
20. Thomson, J.A. et al., Embryonic stem cell lines derived from human blastocysts. *Science*, 1998;**282**(5391):1145–1147.
21. McLachlan, C.S. et al., Transfer of mouse embryonic stem cells to sheep myocardium. *Lancet*, 2006;**367**(9507):301–302.
22. Singla, D.K. et al., Transplantation of embryonic stem cells into the infarcted mouse heart: Formation of multiple cell types. *Journal of Molecular and Cellular Cardiology*, 2006;**40**(1):195–200.

23. Heng, B.C., H. Liu, and T. Cao, Transplanted human embryonic stem cells as biological 'catalysts' for tissue repair and regeneration. *Medical Hypotheses*, 2005;**64**(6):1085–1088.

24. Bittner, R.E. et al., Recruitment of bone-marrow-derived cells by skeletal and cardiac muscle in adult dystrophic mdx mice. *Anatomy and Embryology*, 1999;**199**(5):391–396.

25. Kocher, A.A. et al., Neovascularization of ischemic myocardium by human bone-marrow-derived angioblasts prevents cardiomyocyte apoptosis, reduces remodeling and improves cardiac function. *Nature Medicine*, 2001;**7**(4):430–436.

26. Itescu, S., M.D. Schuster, and A.A. Kocher, Myocardial neovascularization by adult bone marrow-derived angioblasts: Strategies for improvement of cardiomyocyte function. *International Journal of Artificial Organs*, 2002;**25**(7):647–653.

27. Bartunek, J. et al., Ex vivo cardiac specification of adult bone marrow-derived mesenchymal stem cells is feasible using biological growth factors and facilitates cardiac repair of the chronically infarcted myocardium. *Circulation*, 2004;**110**(17):69–69.

28. Noiseux, N. et al., Transplantation of bone marrow-derived mesenchymal stem cells expressing Akt into infarcted murine heart produces dramatic improvement in cardiac function despite infrequent cellular fusion. *Circulation*, 2004;**110**(17):68–68.

29. Yoon, J. et al. Cardiac differentiation of bone marrow-derived mesenchymal stem cells by microenvironment factors. *Circulation*, 2003;**107**(19):E146–E146.

30. Beeres, S.L. et al., Human adult bone marrow-derived mesenchymal stem cells repair experimental conduction block in cardiomyocyte cultures in contrast to skeletal myoblasts and cardiac fibroblasts. *Circulation*, 2005;**112**(17):U147–U147.

31. Yoon, Y.S., N. Lee, and H. Scadova, Myocardial regeneration with bone-marrow-derived stem cells. *Biology of the Cell*, 2005;**97**(4):253–263.

32. Haider, H.K. and M. Ashraf, Bone marrow stem cell transplantation for cardiac repair. *American Journal of Physiology—Heart and Circulatory Physiology*, 2005;**288**(6):H2557–H2567.

33. Planat-Benard, V. et al., Spontaneous cardiomyocyte differentiation from adipose tissue stroma cells. *Circulation Research*, 2004;**94**(2):223–229.

34. Leor, J. et al., Genetically modified fibroblasts obtained from the infarcted myocardium as donor cells for transplantation. *European Heart Journal*, 2001;**22**:489–489.

35. Scorsin, M. et al., Can transplantation of skeletal myoblasts improve function of infarcted myocardium? *Circulation*, 1998;**98**(17):200–200.

36. Muller-Ehmsen, J. et al., Survival and development of neonatal rat cardiomyocytes transplanted into adult myocardium. *Journal of Molecular and Cellular Cardiology*, 2002;**34**(2):107–116.

37. Muller-Ehmsen, J. et al., Rebuilding a damaged heart—Long-term survival of transplanted neonatal rat cardiomyocytes after myocardial infarction and effect on cardiac function. *Circulation*, 2002;**105**(14):1720–1726.

38. Zhang, M. et al., Cardiomyocyte grafting for cardiac repair: Graft cell death and anti-death strategies. *Journal of Molecular and Cellular Cardiology*, 2001;**33**(5):907–921.

39. Leor, J., Y. Amsalem, and S. Cohen, Cells, scaffolds, and molecules for myocardial tissue engineering. *Pharmacology and Therapeutics*, 2005;**105**(2):151–163.

40. Etzion, S. et al., Influence of embryonic cardiomyocyte transplantation on the progression of heart failure in a rat model of extensive myocardial infarction. *Journal of Molecular and Cellular Cardiology*, 2001;**33**(7):1321–1330.

41. Reinlib, L. and L. Field, Cell transplantation as future therapy for cardiovascular disease? A workshop of the National Heart, Lung, and Blood Institute. *Circulation*, 2000;**101**(18):E182–E187.

42. Kessler, P.D. and B.J. Byrne, Myoblast cell grafting into heart muscle: Cellular biology and potential applications. *Annual Review of Physiology*, 1999;**61**:219–242.

43. Etzion, S. et al., Myocardial regeneration: Present and future trends. *American Journal of Cardiovascular Drugs*, 2001;**1**(4):233–244.

44. Varda-Bloom, N. et al., Cytotoxic T lymphocytes are activated following myocardial infarction and can recognize and kill healthy myocytes in vitro. *Journal of Molecular and Cellular Cardiology*, 2000;**32**(12):2141–2149.

45. Hosenpud, J.D. et al., The registry of the international society for heart and lung transplantation: Sixteenth official report—1999. *Journal of Heart and Lung Transplantation*, 1999;**18**(7):611–626.

46. Caspi, O. and L. Gepstein, Stem cells for myocardial repair. *European Heart Journal Supplements*, 2006;**8**(Supplement E):E43–E54.

47. Rubart, M. et al., Spontaneous and evoked intracellular calcium transients in donor-derived myocytes following intracardiac myoblast transplantation. *Journal of Clinical Investigation*, 2004;**114**(6):775–783.

48. Taylor, D.A. et al., Regenerating functional myocardium: Improved performance after skeletal myoblast transplantation. *Nature Medicine*, 1998;**4**(8):929–933.

49. Scorsin, M. et al., Comparison of the effects of fetal cardiomyocyte and skeletal myoblast transplantation on postinfarction left ventricular function. *Journal of Thoracic and Cardiovascular Surgery*, 2000;**119**(6):1169–1175.

50. Menasche, P. et al., Autologous skeletal myoblast transplantation for severe postinfarction left ventricular dysfunction. *Journal of the American College of Cardiology*, 2003;**41**(7):1078–1083.

51. Smits, P.C. et al., Catheter-based intramyocardial injection of autologous skeletal myoblasts as a primary treatment of ischemic heart failure—Clinical experience with six-month follow-up. *Journal of the American College of Cardiology*, 2003;**42**(12):2063–2069.

52. Herreros, J. et al., Autologous intramyocardial injection of cultured skeletal muscle-derived stem cells in patients with non-acute myocardial infarction. *European Heart Journal*, 2003;**24**(22):2012–2020.

53. Pagani, F.D. et al., Autologous skeletal myoblasts transplanted to ischemia-damaged myocardium in humans—Histological analysis of cell survival and differentiation. *Journal of the American College of Cardiology*, 2003;**41**(5):879–888.

54. Siminiak, T. et al., Autologous skeletal myoblast transplantation for the treatment of postinfarction myocardial injury: Phase I clinical study with 12 months of follow-up. *American Heart Journal*, 2004;**148**(3):531–537.

55. Siminiak, T. et al., Percutaneous trans-coronary-venous transplantation of autologous skeletal myoblasts in the treatment of post-infarction myocardial contractility impairment: The POZNAN trials. *European Heart Journal*, 2005;**26**(12):1188–1195.

56. Siminiak, T. et al., Percutaneous transvenous transplantation of autologous myoblasts in the treatment of postinfarction heart failure—One year follow-up of the POZNAN trial series. *Journal of the American College of Cardiology*, 2005;**45**(3):57A.

57. Dib, N. et al., Safety and feasibility of autologous myoblast transplantation in patients with ischemic cardiomyopathy—Four-year follow-up. *Circulation*, 2005;**112**(12):1748–1755.

58. Pagani, F.D. et al., Autologous skeletal myoblasts transplanted in ischemia damaged myocardium in humans: Histological analysis of cell survival and differentiation. *Circulation*, 2002;**106**(19):463–463.

59. Hagege, A.A. et al., Skeletal myoblast transplantation in ischemic heart failure—Long-term follow-up of the first phase I cohort of patients. *Circulation*, 2006;**114**:I108–I113.

60. Laflamme, M.A. and C.E. Murry, Regenerating the heart. *Nature Biotechnology*, 2005;**23**(7):845–856.

61. Murry, C.E., L.J. Field, and P. Menasche, Cell-based cardiac repair—Reflections at the 10-year point. *Circulation*, 2005;**112**(20):3174–3183.

62. Weber, K.T., Y. Sun, and L.C. Katwa, Myofibroblasts and local angiotensin II in rat cardiac tissue repair. *International Journal of Biochemistry and Cell Biology*, 1997;**29**(1):31–42.

63. Kellar, R.S. et al., Cardiac patch constructed from human fibroblasts attenuates reduction in cardiac function after acute infarct. *Tissue Engineering*, 2005;**11**(11–12):1678–1687.

64. Urbich, C. and S. Dimmeler, Endothelial progenitor cells—Characterization and role in vascular biology. *Circulation Research*, 2004;**95**(4):343–353.

65. Werner, L. et al., Transfer of endothelial progenitor cells improves myocardial performance in rats with dilated cardiomyopathy induced following experimental myocarditis. *Journal of Molecular and Cellular Cardiology*, 2005;**39**(4):691–697.

66. Alison, M.R. et al., An introduction to stem cells. *Journal of Pathology*, 2002;**197**(4):419–423.
67. Wakitani, S., T. Saito, and A.I. Caplan, Myogenic cells derived from rat bone-marrow mesenchymal stem-cells exposed to 5-azacytidine. *Muscle and Nerve*, 1995;**18**(12):1417–1426.
68. Makino, S. et al., Cardiomyocytes can be generated from marrow stromal cells in vitro. *Journal of Clinical Investigation*, 1999;**103**(5):697–705.
69. Kehat, I. et al., Human embryonic stem cells can differentiate into myocytes with structural and functional properties of cardiomyocytes. *Journal of Clinical Investigation*, 2001;**108**(3):407–414.
70. Vats, A. et al., Stem cells: Sources and applications. *Clinical Otolaryngology*, 2002;**27**(4):227–232.
71. Wobus, A.M. and K.R. Boheler, Embryonic stem cells: Prospects for developmental biology and cell therapy. *Physiological Reviews*, 2005;**85**(2):635–678.
72. Pittenger, M.F. et al., Multilineage potential of adult human mesenchymal stem cells. *Science*, 1999;**284**(5411):143–147.
73. Tomita, S. et al., Autologous transplantation of bone marrow cells improves damaged heart function. *Circulation*, 1999;**100**(19):247–256.
74. Orlic, D. et al., Transplanted adult bone marrow cells repair myocardial infarcts in mice. In *Hematopoietic Stem Cells 2000 Basic and Clinical Sciences* 2001. New York: New York *Acad. Sciences*, 938, pp. 221–230.
75. Orlic, D. et al., Bone marrow cells regenerate infarcted myocardium. *Nature*, 2001;**410**(6829):701–705.
76. Toma, C. et al., Human mesenchymal stem cells differentiate to a cardiomyocyte phenotype in the adult murine heart. *Circulation*, 2002;**105**(1):93–98.
77. Mangi, A.A. et al., Mesenchymal stem cells modified with Akt prevent remodeling and restore performance of infarcted hearts. *Nature Medicine*, 2003;**9**(9):1195–1201.
78. Pittenger, M.F. and B.J. Martin, Mesenchymal stem cells and their potential as cardiac therapeutics. *Circulation Research*, 2004;**95**(1):9–20.
79. Tomita, S. et al., Bone marrow cells transplanted in a cardiac scar induced cardiomyogenesis and angiogenesis and improved damaged heart function. *Circulation*, 1999;**100**(18):91–92.
80. Amado, L.C. et al., Cardiac repair with intramyocardial injection of allogeneic mesenchymal stem cells after myocardial infarction. *Proceedings of the National Academy of Sciences of the United States of America*, 2005;**102**(32):11474–11479.
81. Le Blanc, K., Immunomodulatory effects of fetal and adult mesenchymal stem cells. *Cytotherapy*, 2003;**5**(6):485–489.
82. Balsam, L.B. et al., Functional benefits after transplantation of hematopoietic stem cell enriched bone marrow into ischemic myocardium are not due to transdifferentiation. *American Journal of Transplantation*, 2004;**4**:469–469.
83. Balsam, L.B. et al., Haematopoietic stem cells adopt mature haematopoietic fates in ischaemic myocardium. *Nature*, 2004;**428**(6983):668–673.
84. Murry, C.E. et al., Haematopoietic stem cells do not transdifferentiate into cardiac myocytes in myocardial infarcts. *Nature*, 2004;**428**(6983):664–668.
85. Asahara, T. et al., Isolation of putative progenitor endothelial cells for angiogenesis. *Science*, 1997;**275**(5302):964–967.
86. Takahashi, T. et al., Ischemia- and cytokine-induced mobilization of bone marrow-derived endothelial progenitor cells for neovascularization. *Nature Medicine*, 1999;**5**(4):434–438.
87. Shintani, S. et al., Augmentation of postnatal neovascularization with autologous bone marrow transplantation. *Circulation*, 2001;**103**(6):897–903.
88. Kamihata, H. et al., Implantation of bone marrow mononuclear cells into ischemic myocardium enhances collateral perfusion and regional function via side supply of angioblasts, angiogenic ligands, and cytokines. *Circulation*, 2001;**104**(9):1046–1052.
89. Kawamoto, A. et al., Autologous, percutaneous, intramyocardial transplantation of endothelial progenitor cells enhances neovascularization and attenuates chronic myocardial ischemia in swine. *Circulation*, 2001;**104**(17):443–443.

90. Kawamoto, A. et al., Transplantation of ex vivo expanded endothelial progenitor cells for myocardial neovascularization. *Circulation*, 2000;**102**(18):5–5.

91. Dimmeler, S., A.M. Zeiher, and M.D. Schneider, Unchain my heart: The scientific foundations of cardiac repair. *Journal of Clinical Investigation*, 2005;**115**(3):572–583.

92. Assmus, B. et al., Transcoronary transplantation of progenitor cells after myocardial infarction. *New England Journal of Medicine*, 2006;**355**(12):1222–1232.

93. Schachinger, V. et al., Intracoronary bone marrow-derived progenitor cells in acute myocardial infarction. *New England Journal of Medicine*, 2006;**355**(12):1210–1221.

94. Lunde, K. et al., Intracoronary injection of mononuclear bone marrow cells in acute myocardial infarction. *New England Journal of Medicine*, 2006;**355**(12):1199–1209.

95. Gimble, J.M., Adipose tissue-derived therapeutics. *Expert Opinion on Biological Therapy*, 2003;**3**(5):705–713.

96. Gimble, J.M. and F. Guilak, Differentiation potential of adipose derived adult stem (ADAS) cells. In *Current Topics in Developmental Biology*, Vol. 58, 2003. San Diego, CA: Academic Press Inc., pp. 137–160.

97. Rodriguez, A.M. et al., The human adipose tissue is a source of multipotent stem cells. *Biochimie*, 2005;**87**(1):125–128.

98. Gimble, J.M., A.J. Katz, and B.A. Bunnell, Adipose-derived stem cells for regenerative medicine. *Circulation Research*, 2007;**100**(9):1249–1260.

99. Liu, J.B. et al., Autologous stem cell transplantation for myocardial repair. *American Journal of Physiology—Heart and Circulatory Physiology*, 2004;**287**(2):H501–H511.

100. Wang, L. et al., Adipose-derived stem cells significantly improve cardiac function of the infarct rat hearts. *Journal of Molecular and Cellular Cardiology*, 2007;**42**:S97–S97.

101. Beltrami, A.P. et al., Adult cardiac stem cells are multipotent and support myocardial regeneration. *Cell*, 2003;**114**(6):763–776.

102. Oh, H. et al., Cardiac progenitor cells from adult myocardium: Homing, differentiation, and fusion after infarction. *Proceedings of the National Academy of Sciences of the United States of America*, 2003;**100**(21):12313–12318.

103. Pfister, O. et al., CD31(-) but not CD31(+) cardiac side population cells exhibit functional cardiomyogenic differentiation. *Circulation Research*, 2005;**97**(1):52–61.

104. Messina, E. et al., Isolation and expansion of adult cardiac stem cells from human and murine heart. *Circulation Research*, 2004;**95**(9):911–921.

105. Laugwitz, K.L. et al., Postnatal isl1+cardioblasts enter fully differentiated cardiomyocyte lineages. *Nature*, 2005;**433**(7026):647–653.

106. Shamblott, M.J. et al., Human embryonic germ cell derivatives express a broad range of developmentally distinct markers and proliferate extensively in vitro. *Proceedings of the National Academy of Sciences of the United States of America*, 2001;**98**(1):113–118.

107. Evans, M.J. and M.H. Kaufman, Establishment in culture of pluripotential cells from mouse embryos. *Nature*, 1981;**292**(5819):154–156.

108. Martin, G.R., Isolation of a pluripotent cell-line from early mouse embryos cultured in medium conditioned by teratocarcinoma stem-cells. *Proceedings of the National Academy of Sciences of the United States of America—Biological Sciences*, 1981;**78**(12):7634–7638.

109. Shamblott, M.J. et al., Derivation of pluripotent stem cells horn cultured human primordial germ cells. *Proceedings of the National Academy of Sciences of the United States of America*, 1998;**95**(23):13726–13731.

110. Doetschman, T.C. et al., The invitro development of blastocyst-derived embryonic stem-cell lines—Formation of visceral yolk-sac, blood islands and myocardium. *Journal of Embryology and Experimental Morphology*, 1985;**87**(June):27.

111. Min, J.Y. et al., Transplantation of embryonic stem cells improves cardiac function in postinfarcted rats. *Journal of Applied Physiology*, 2002;**92**(1):288–296.

112. Min, J.Y. et al., Long-term improvement of cardiac function in rats after infarction by transplantation of embryonic stem cells. *Journal of Thoracic and Cardiovascular Surgery*, 2003;**125**(2):361–369.

113. Min, J.Y. et al., Stem cell therapy in the aging hearts of Fisher 344 rats: Synergistic effects on myogenesis and angiogenesis. *Journal of Thoracic and Cardiovascular Surgery*, 2005;**130**(2):547–553.

114. Min, J.Y. et al., Homing of intravenously infused embryonic stem cell-derived cells to injured hearts after myocardial infarction. *Journal of Thoracic and Cardiovascular Surgery*, 2006;**131**(4):889–897.

115. Behfar, A. et al., Stem cell differentiation requires a paracrine pathway in the heart. *FASEB Journal*, 2002;**16**(12):1558–1566.

116. Behfar, A. et al., Administration of allogenic stem cells dosed to secure cardiogenesis and sustained infarct repair. In *Stem Cell Biology: Development and Plasticity*. New York: New York Acad. Sciences, 2005, 1049, pp. 189–198.

117. Nussbaum, J. et al., Transplantation of undifferentiated murine embryonic stem cells in the heart: Teratoma formation and immune response. *FASEB Journal*, 2007;**21**:1345–1357.

118. Menard, C. et al., Transplantation of cardiac-committed mouse embryonic stem cells to infarcted sheep myocardium: A preclinical study. *Lancet*, 2005;**366**(9490):1005–1012.

119. Menard, C. et al., Cardiac specification of embryonic stem cells. *Journal of Cellular Biochemistry*, 2004;**93**(4):681–687.

120. Swijnenburg, R.J. et al., Embryonic stem cell immunogenicity increases upon differentiation after transplantation into ischemic myocardium. *Circulation*, 2005;**112**(9):I166–I172.

121. Xu, C.H. et al., Characterization and enrichment of cardiomyocytes derived from human embryonic stem cells. *Circulation Research*, 2002;**91**(6):501–508.

122. Mummery, C. et al., Differentiation of human embryonic stem cells to cardiomyocytes—Role of coculture with visceral endoderm-like cells. *Circulation*, 2003;**107**(21):2733–2740.

123. Kehat, I. and L. Gepstein, Human embryonic stem cells for myocardial regeneration. *Heart Failure Reviews*, 2003;**8**(3):229–236.

124. Xu, C.H. et al., Basic fibroblast growth factor supports undifferentiated human embryonic stem cell growth without conditioned medium. *Stem Cells*, 2005;**23**(3):315–323.

125. Laflamme, M.A. et al., Formation of human myocardium in the rat heart from human embryonic stem cells. *American Journal of Pathology*, 2005;**167**(3):663–671.

126. Snir, M. et al., Assessment of the ultrastructural and proliferative properties of human embryonic stem cell-derived cardiomyocytes. *American Journal of Physiology—Heart and Circulatory Physiology*, 2003;**285**(6):H2355–H2363.

127. Kehat, L. et al., High-resolution electrophysiological assessment of human embryonic stem cell-derived cardiomyocytes—A novel in vitro model for the study of conduction. *Circulation Research*, 2002;**91**(8):659–661.

128. Satin, J. et al., Mechanism of spontaneous excitability in human embryonic stem cell derived cardiomyocytes. *Journal of Physiology—London*, 2004;**559**(2):479–496.

129. Kehat, I. et al., Electromechanical integration of cardiomyocytes derived from human embryonic stem cells. *Nature Biotechnology*, 2004;**22**(10):1282–1289.

130. Xue, T. et al., Functional integration of electrically active cardiac derivatives from genetically engineered human embryonic stem cells with quiescent recipient ventricular cardiomyocytes—Insights into the development of cell-based pacemakers. *Circulation*, 2005;**111**(1):11–20.

131. Hassink, R.J. et al., Stem cell therapy for ischemic heart disease. *Trends in Molecular Medicine*, 2003;**9**(10):436–441.

132. Dowell, J.D. et al., Myocyte and myogenic stem cell transplantation in the heart. *Cardiovascular Research*, 2003;**58**(2):336–350.

133. Reffelmann, T. and R.A. Kloner, Cellular cardiomyoplasty—Cardiomyocytes, skeletal myoblasts, or stem cells for regenerating myocardium and treatment of heart failure? *Cardiovascular Research*, 2003;**58**(2):358–368.

134. Reffelmann, T. et al., Cardiomyocyte transplantation into the failing heart—New therapeutic approach for heart failure? *Heart Failure Reviews*, 2003;**8**(3):201–211.

135. Leor, J. and I.M. Barbash, Cell transplantation and genetic engineering: New approaches to cardiac pathology. *Expert Opinion on Biological Therapy*, 2003;**3**(7):1023–1039.

136. Bradley, J.A., E.M. Bolton, and R.A. Pedersen, Stem cell medicine encounters the immune system. *Nature Reviews Immunology*, 2002;**2**(11):859–871.
137. Drukker, M. et al., Characterization of the expression of MHC proteins in human embryonic stem cells. *Proceedings of the National Academy of Sciences of the United States of America*, 2002;**99**(15):9864–9869.
138. Drukkera, M. et al., Human embryonic stem cells and their differentiated derivatives are less susceptible to immune rejection than adult cells. *Stem Cells*, 2006;**24**:221–229.
139. Harding, S.E. et al., The human embryonic stem cell-derived cardiomyocyte as a pharmacological model. *Pharmacology and Therapeutics*, 2006;**113**(2):341–353.
140. Wilmut, I. et al., Viable offspring derived from fetal and adult mammalian cells. *Nature*, 1997;**386**(6621):200 and 1997;**385**:810.

Further Readings

Alberts, B., A. Johnson, J. Lewis, M. Raff, K. Roberts, and P. Walter. *Molecular Biology of the Cell*. New York: Garland Science.
Walter, P., B. Alberts, D. Bray, K. Hopkin, J. Lewis, M. Raff, K. Roberts, and A.D. Johnson, *Essential Cell Biology*. Garland Publishing, New York, NY.

CHAPTER 17

HISTOLOGY AND TISSUE PROPERTIES I
Epithelial, Neuronal, and Muscle Tissue

LEARNING OBJECTIVES

After a careful study of this chapter, you should be able to do the following:

1. Describe the structure and function of the four basic types of tissues:
   a. Epithelium
   b. Nerve tissue
   c. Muscle tissue
   d. Connective tissue
2. Describe active and passive mechanical performance
3. Explain the passive J-shaped stress–strain curve of biological tissues
4. Describe passive stiffness–stress, stress–strain relationships
5. Define stiffness constant

17.1   INTRODUCTION

Histology is a branch of medical science that focuses on the microstructure of tissues and their cellular composition. It is basically anatomy at the microscopic level, based on the morphology of tissue after it has been chemically preserved, mounted in a solid (usually wax), and serially cut using a mechanical bladed tool called a microtome. The end result of this process is a 5–10 µm slice of tissue, where the 3D structure has been kept intact. Once prepared, the slices can be imaged using various types of microscopy.

From histological studies, we learn about the spatial arrangements (microstructures) of the basic tissues, which provide the key to understanding the functions of each tissue and the organs they populate. This is also complementary to understanding the studies of organ and system physiology. For example, understanding the histology of neural tissue enables us to learn about neural connectivity and local differences in brain structure, which complements live brain imaging using magnetic resonance imaging (MRI).

If we want to mimic a tissue, we must first understand its structure and basic functions. This also provides clues about the physical and mechanical nature of tissues and organs, which is central to tissue engineering.

17.1.1 Four Types of Tissues

Despite its complexity, the human body is composed of only four basic types of tissues as mentioned in Chapter 13 (Figure 17.1):

1. Epithelium (epithelial cells)
2. Muscle (myocytes)
3. Nerve tissue (neurons)
4. Connective tissue (fibroblasts, blood)

As discussed, organs are composed of each of these tissue types, in different proportions and locations. For example, skin is a multilayered sheet of epithelium, but it also contains blood and nerve supply, smooth muscle, and glandular tissue.

It is also important to note that one basic tissue type will vary slightly in morphology, between different tissues, depending on its function. For example, compared to skin epithelium, digestive tract epithelium is more specialized toward transport functions (e.g., cilia, high surface area of membranes, transport vesicles, etc.).

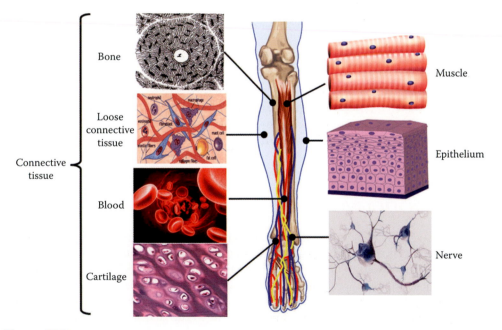

Figure 17.1
Four types of tissues.

17.1.2 Tissue Composition and Basic Structure

In gcncral, tissues are composed of cell populations in highly ordered, three-dimensional (3D) arrangements. Cells are held together by adherent biomolecules and produce their own fibrous matrix (*extracellular matrix* (ECM)), which forms part of the interstitial space, acting as a structural scaffold to support the cells in 3D. The ECM in connective tissues is composed of the following:

- Protein fibers (structural molecules), the dominant component of the ECM
- Glycosaminoglycans (GAGs), which are structural proteins with some signaling molecules (i.e., functional molecules)
- Glycoproteins, which are smaller proteins, usually with adhesion and signaling roles
- Interstitial fluid, produced by the cells themselves and free to exchange with the blood plasma

17.1.3 Regeneration and Carcinogenic Susceptibility of Tissues

In general, the cells of epithelial and connective tissues are highly renewable, while muscular and nervous cells have very limited capacity to reproduce and regenerate. Gene mutation mostly occurs during mitosis (Section 16.5.2), and as a consequence, cancer rates are highest in epithelial tissue, where frequent stem cell divisions keep pace with the regeneration of damaged or lost tissue, and relatively low in neural and muscle tissues, where stem cell divisions do not normally occur. There is also a strong association between cancer and endocrine control of highly metabolic and dividing tissues (e.g., breast, gastrointestinal tract, liver, and pancreas), so these tissues tend to have a higher susceptibility to cancer formation.

17.2 EPITHELIUM

The epithelia are a diverse group of tissues that line all of the continuous surfaces of the body, as well as cavities and tubes. Note that epithelium lines both the outer surface and internal cavities of the body (Figure 17.2), as described earlier in relation to the integumentary and digestive systems. Epithelial layers function as interfaces between different biological compartments, acting mostly as a physical barrier, with selective transport and secretory functions. They form an effective barrier to fluids and prevent the entry of pathogens (e.g., microbes) and toxins.

17.2.1 Epithelial Cells

Cells that form epithelial sheets are closely bound to one another at their peripheral sides by tight junction proteins (see Section 16.5.1) while supported on their basal sides by a *basement membrane*, a type of ECM that they produce. As a result, epithelial cells form either a monolayer or a multilayered (stratified) sheet. The forms and dimensions of epithelial cells also vary, ranging from high columnar to cuboidal to low squamous cells and including all intermediate forms (Figure 17.3). Skin is well known as being stratified squamous type, whereas digestive tract epithelium is columnar, with extensive tight junctions and much higher cell density.

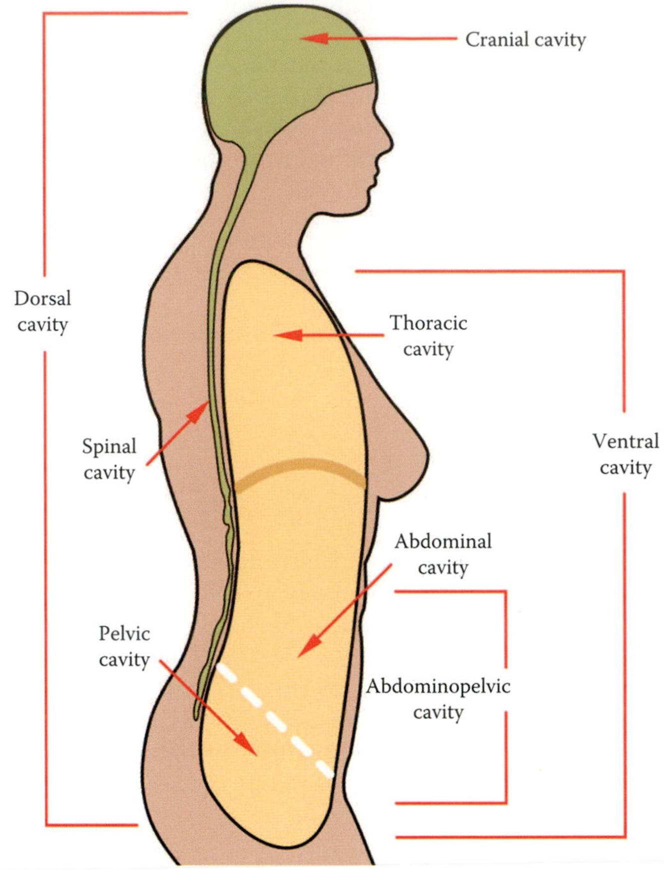

Figure 17.2
Epithelial tissues. (From http://training.seer.cancer.gov/module_anatomy/unit1_3_terminology3_cavities.html., C/-wikipemedia.)

17.2.2 Examples of Epithelia

As shown in Figure 17.3, epithelia are traditionally classified according to three morphological characteristics:

1. The spatial arrangement of cells: simple or stratified
2. The shape of the component cells: columnar, cuboidal, or squamous
3. The presence of surface specializations and other structural features (e.g., cilia, surface proteins, types of cell–cell junctions, and density of vesicles and granules).

The formation of these different types is genetically determined during early development of the fetus. It is regulated by the different compositions of cytoskeletal and junctional proteins that are unique to an epithelial cell type in a specific location.

Epithelia can also be grouped into two broad classifications, according to their structure and function:

1. *Covering epithelia*: Tissues in which the cells are organized in layers that cover the external surface or line the cavities of the body.

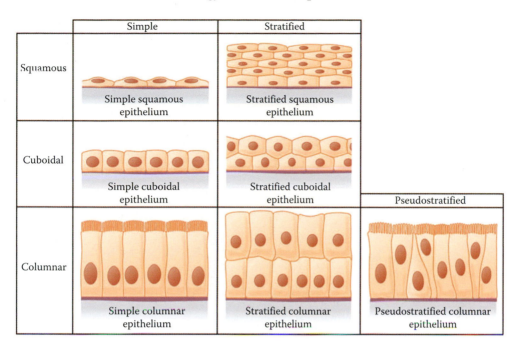

Figure 17.3
Spatial arrangements of epithelial cells. (From OpenStax College—Anatomy & Physiology, Connexions web site. http://cnx.org/content/col11496/1.6/, June 19, 2013.)

2. *Glandular epithelia*: Tissues formed by epithelial cells specialized to produce a fluid secretion that differs in composition from blood or extracellular fluid. The term *gland* is usually used to designate large, complex aggregates of glandular epithelial cells, often in larger organs (e.g., pancreas, which is the largest gland).

3. *Covering epithelia with dispersed glands*: Many epithelia also contain small exocrine glands, such as the epidermis (sebaceous and sweat glands), and ear epidermis (secretes wax). Another example is the ependymal cells that line the brain cavity, responsible for secreting some of the cerebral spinal fluid.

The epidermis is a stratified squamous epithelium, composed of four or five layers, depending on the anatomic position of skin. These layers in descending order are cornified, clear/translucent, granular, spinous, and basal/germinal cells (Figure 17.4). The epidermis is avascular, nourished by nutrients that diffuse into the interstitial spaces from deeper dermal and hypodermal vessels. The avascular structure is the major reason why epidermal tissue engineering is relatively successful compared to other vascularized tissues.

17.2.3 Endothelium

Epithelial cells lining the inner surface of blood and lymphatic vessels, and the serous body cavities are termed *endothelium* and *mesothelium*, respectively. Mesothelium lines the lung, heart, brain, and peritoneal cavities, producing a fluid that assists in lubrication or hydrostatic support (e.g., lowering pericardial friction). In the case of blood vessels, Figure 17.5 schematically illustrates the intima, media, and adventitia layers of blood vessels, where the intima comprises an elastic basement membrane that supports the internal endothelial layer.

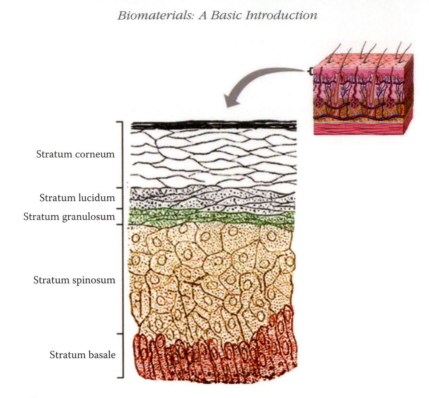

Stratum corneum

Stratum lucidum

Stratum granulosum

Stratum spinosum

Stratum basale

Figure 17.4
Avascular epidermis structure. (From http://en.wikipedia.org/wiki/Image:Gray941.png.)

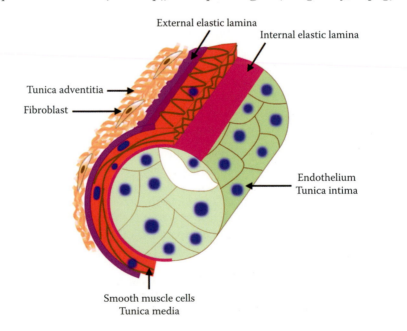

External elastic lamina

Internal elastic lamina

Tunica adventitia

Fibroblast

Endothelium
Tunica intima

Smooth muscle cells
Tunica media

Figure 17.5
Three major layers (tunicae) of an artery wall shown in cross-section. The tunica intima is endothelium with an elastic basement membrane. Over this, the tunica media is attached, represented by smooth muscle, also encased in an external elastic membrane. Thirdly, the tunica adventitia is outer connective tissue.

17.2.3.1 Endothelium and Vascular Tissue Engineering Vascular endothelial cells have the intrinsic ability to form tubes, as depicted in Figure 17.6. In addition to epithelium, blood vessels also include the other three types of tissues, that is, nerve, muscle, and connective tissues, as depicted in Figure 17.7. Therefore, to engineer blood vessels, it is critical to use endothelial cells to form the basic vascular tube. To stabilize the tube, we also need specialized cells to regenerate muscular and connective tissues, or

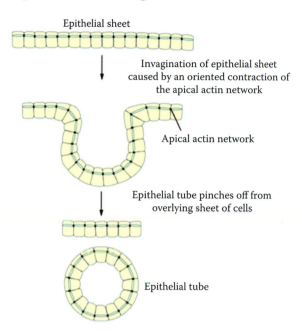

Figure 17.6
Tubing of vascular epithelial cells. (http://commons.wikimedia.org/wiki/File:Folding_of_epithelial_sheet.svg).

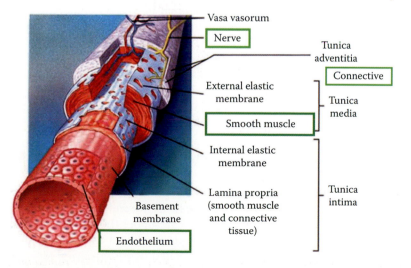

Figure 17.7
Blood vessel structure and four types of tissues in it. (From Seeley, R. et al., Anatomy and Physiology, 2002, with permission of McGraw-Hill Education.)

stem cells that are possibly able to form both, as well as interact with the peripheral nerves, such as in larger arteries.

Mechanically, vascular endothelium is also unique from other epithelia, in its response to shear stress. Endothelial cells form elongated squamous layers, where the cells become orientated lengthways, in the direction of blood flow. This is an example of mechanosensory function of tissues, which is also an important consideration in vascular tissue engineering. A much studied alternative cell type for vascular grafting purposes is human umbilical vein endothelial cells (HUVECs), having similar properties.

17.3   MUSCULAR TISSUE

17.3.1   *Microanatomy of Muscle*

As described in Section 13.3, there are three types of muscular tissues with their associated cell types:

1. Skeletal (voluntary, striated) muscle
2. Cardiac (involuntary, striated) muscle
3. Smooth (involuntary, nonstriated) muscle

17.3.1.1   Skeletal Muscle   The structure of skeletal muscle is highly hierarchical (Figure 17.8). Each skeletal muscle can be regarded as an independent organ, organized in bundles of fibers called fascicles, embedded with vascular and nerve networks. A fascicle consists of muscle fibers, each of which is a muscle cell containing contractile proteins (Figure 17.9). Hence, muscular tissue is primarily composed of muscle cells, which are connected to one another by endomysium (a connective tissue). Muscle cells are terminally differentiated. Collagen constitutes 1%–2% of soft muscle tissue, and accounts for 6% of strong, tendinous muscles.

Functionally, this compartmentalization of muscle serves several purposes. Firstly, it allows fibers to be aligned in parallel for maximal power generation when leveraging a joint. Secondly, since only one nerve activates a muscle, specific fibers are contracted in a coordinated manner by specific nerve branches consecutively, as a joint is lifted, which gradually controls lifting. This occurs at the level of groups of fibers (called *muscle recruitment*). Thirdly, connective tissue interspersed in the muscle allows for additional support to fibers, with additional leverage between compartments.

Figure 17.9 schematically shows a skeletal muscle fiber, that is, a muscle cell. Each muscle cell is constituted of myofibrils, which in turn are made up of filaments. In short,

$$\text{Filaments} \xrightarrow{\text{form}} \text{Fibrils} \xrightarrow{\text{form}} \text{Fibers}$$

17.3.1.2   Cardiac Muscle (Also Called Myocardium)   Heart muscle is a type of involuntary striated muscle, forming the walls of the heart. *Involuntary* means that we cannot consciously control this muscle. These muscles are under the control of the autonomic nervous system. This system controls many systems without us being aware of them.

The cells that constitute cardiac muscle are called *cardiomyocytes*. Most of these cell has a single nucleus, although some are uniquely multinucleated, relates to their integrated function and size. Cardiomyocytes are joined end to end to form fibers, which are branched and interconnected in networks (Figure 17.10a). At its end, where one cell

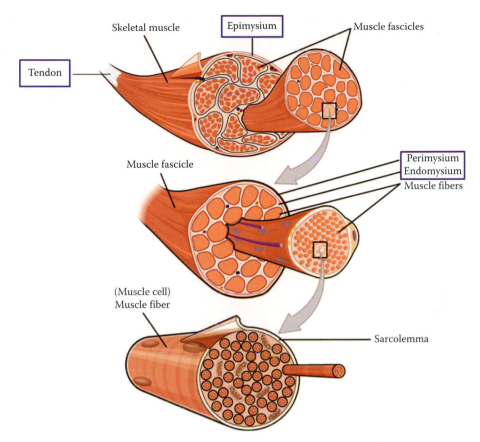

Figure 17.8
Structure of skeletal muscular tissue. (From http://cnx.org/content/col11496/1.6/, June 19, 2013.)

touches another, there is a specialized intercellular junction called an *intercalated disc*, which occurs only in cardiac tissue. It is this specialized junction that enables adjacent cells to beat in unison (Figure 17.10b). A more detailed description of heart muscle contraction is provided in Section 17.3.2.

17.3.1.3 Smooth Muscle Smooth muscles are found within the walls of hollow organs, such as blood vessels, the gastrointestinal tract, the bladder, or the uterus. In blood vessels, smooth muscles occur as the tunica media layer of the aorta and smaller arteries, wihere they are arranged concentrically, allowing vessels to contract lengthwise.

Smooth muscles are responsible for the contractility of hollow organs. They are arranged in layers with the fibers in each layer running in various directions (Figure 17.11). This makes the muscle contract in different directions. For example, there are three independent layers in the stomach wall, allowing longtitudinal, oblique and concentric contractions.

17.3.2 Proteins in Muscle Cells and Muscle Contraction

17.3.2.1 Skeletal Muscle Each tubular myocyte is made up of chains of myofibrils, rod-like units of highly organized proteins that contain *sarcomeres*. Proteins within

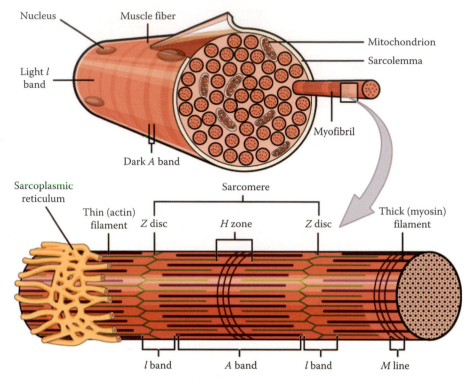

Figure 17.9
A muscle cell forms a muscle fiber. (From http://cnx.org/content/col11496/1.6/, June 19, 2013.)

the sarcomere sections include *actin, myosin,* and *titin,* as illustrated in Figure 17.12. Both actin and myosin are dynamic proteins, requiring energy to contract, and occur in regular repeated units (striations, hence skeletal muscle is also called *striated* muscle). Titin is the main structural protein element.

During a single contraction, nerve stimulation causes local calcium release into the sarcomeres, triggering the activation of regulatory proteins, which in turn activate myosin. The heads of the activated myosin proteins make contact with the actin filaments, beating cooperatively in the same direction, and move the actin filament relative to the myosin filament toward the center of each sarcomere. This essentially shortens the sarcomere, resulting in compression of the elastic protein titin. At the end of contraction, the myosin chain heads then stop beating, and lie down, allowing the actin filaments to be released, moved back by the compressed titin to their original position.

Titin is the largest protein known,its structure and function are very similar to those of an elastic spring (Figure 17.13), it comprises over 200 folded domains forming the secondary structure of the protein chain. The elastic deformation and reshaping mechanism lies in these secondary and tertiary structures, which are like a molecular spring. Unwinding of titin is basically caused by unfolding of the folded chains sections in series.

The mechanism of elastic properties of titin is determined by the general structures of protein. As described in Section 16.2.1 (Figure 16.4), structure of proteins is often described in terms of four levels: (1) primary structure: covalent bonding; (2) secondary structure: hydrogen bonding; (3) tertiary structure: encompasses all the non-covalent interactions; and (4) quaternary structure: usually not covalently connected, but might be connected by a disulfide bond.

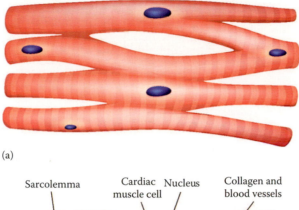

(a)

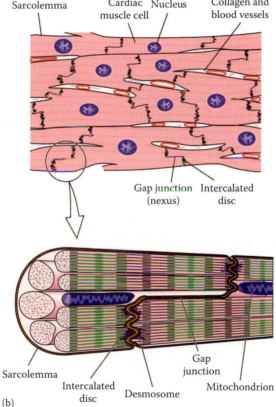

(b)

Figure 17.10
Cardiac muscle: (a) cardiac muscle anatomy; (b) cardiac muscle histology.

17.3.2.2 Cardiac Muscle and Cardiomyocytes Cardiac muscle operates using the same protein mechanisms as skeletal muscle, although it has a thicker myosin, and shorter sarcomeres, which favor short, sharp contractions. The ends of the cardiac sarcomeres are also unique, compared to skeletal muscle, because they contain microscopic structures called *intercalated discs*. These are specialized junctional proteins between two adjacent ends of cardiomyocytes. Here, the membranes are highly convoluted, enabling cells to be very strongly bound together, both at the membrane and at the cytoskeletal level. This provides strength, but also flexibility, and also enables adjacent cells to beat in unison. Furthermore, the higher branching between multiple cardiomyocytes also enables them

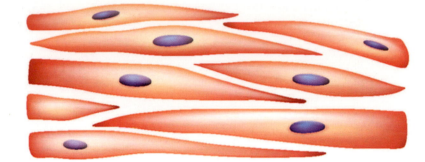

Figure 17.11
Smooth muscle.

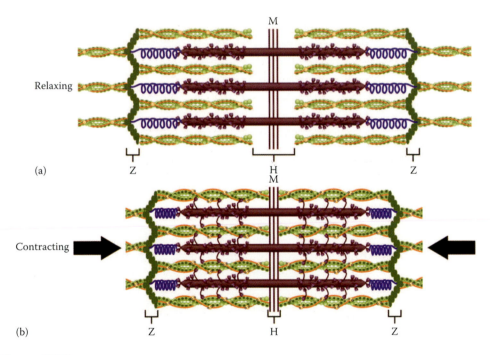

Figure 17.12
(a) Relaxing sarcomeres and (b) mechanism of contraction. (From http://cnx.org/content/col11496/1.6/, June 19, 2013.)

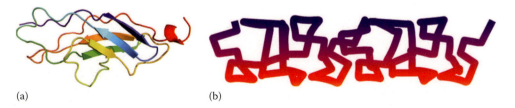

Figure 17.13
(a) Tertiary structure of titin and (b) a schematic biological spring. (From http://en.wikipedia.org/wiki/Titin#mediaviewer/File:1BPV.png).

to beat in unison, rather than sequentially. Both of these modifications allow the entire heart wall to beat at once, then relax at once. This occurs with a regular frequency under autonomic nerve stimulation via *pacemaker* neurons and a small number of cardiomyo-cytes, forming the functional basis of the mechanical performance of the heart.

17.3.3 Mechanical Performance of Muscular Tissue

There are two types of mechanical behaviors in muscle:

1. Active mechanical properties
   The mechanical behavior of stimulated muscle (e.g., the systole process) is referred to as active. Mechanical measurement is carried out inside the body, such as via pressure transducers or dynamic imaging.
2. Passive mechanical properties
   The mechanical behavior of unstimulated muscle (e.g., during the diastole pro-cess) is referred to as passive. Mechanical testing in a controlled laboratory set-ting provides information about the passive mechanical properties of the muscle.

17.3.4 Stress–Strain Relationships of Muscular Tissues

Passive mechanical properties of heart muscle (human and mouse) have been exten-sively studied. Figure 17.14a shows a few typical stress–strain curves of heart muscles of humans and rats, as well as stress–strain curves of a number of soft tissues, which all exhibit the following features:

1. *Nonlinear elasticity*: stress–strain curves are J-shaped (Figure 17.14a)
2. *Hysteresis*: stress–strain curves differ during loading (imposition of an external force) and unloading (Figure 17.14b)
3. *Viscoelasticity*: stress–strain curves have time-dependent characteristics (Figure 17.14c)

For a nonlinear stress–strain curve, the stiffness (i.e., Young's modulus) is not a constant but varies with stress (or strain). Hence, it is difficult to compare the elastic strength properties of different tissues based on stiffness alone. It has been discovered in many experimental reports that the stiffness value of a J-shaped (passive) stress–strain curve of many tissues is linearly proportional to stress (Figure 17.15), that is,

$$\frac{d\sigma}{d\varepsilon} = k\sigma + \alpha \tag{17.1}$$

After the following mathematical processes:

$$\frac{d\sigma}{d\varepsilon} = k\sigma + \alpha = k\left(\sigma + \frac{\alpha}{k}\right)$$

$$\frac{d\sigma}{\sigma + \frac{\alpha}{k}} = k\,d\varepsilon$$

$$d\ln\left(\sigma + \frac{\alpha}{k}\right) = d(k\varepsilon)$$

$$\ln\left(\sigma + \frac{\alpha}{k}\right) = k\varepsilon + \text{cons.}$$

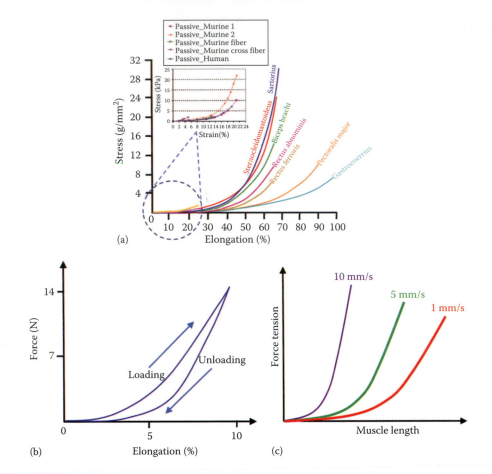

(a)

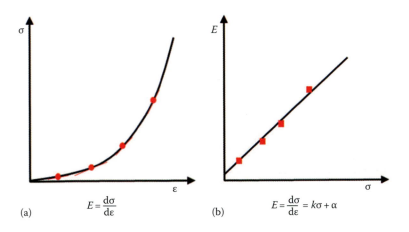

(b)

(c)

Figure 17.14

Stress–strain curves of heart muscle tissues. (a) Nonlinear elasticity: J-shaped stress -strain curves of human and mouse heart, (b) hysteresis reflected by stress-strain curves, and (c) viscoelasticity reflected by stress-strain curves.

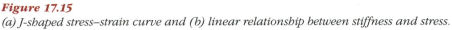

(a)

$$E = \frac{d\sigma}{d\varepsilon}$$

(b)

$$E = \frac{d\sigma}{d\varepsilon} = k\sigma + \alpha$$

Figure 17.15

(a) J-shaped stress–strain curve and (b) linear relationship between stiffness and stress.

We have

$$\sigma = Ae^{k\varepsilon} - \frac{\alpha}{k} \tag{17.2}$$

The boundary condition is $\sigma = 0$, $\varepsilon = 0$, which derives

$$A = \alpha/k$$

Hence,

$$\sigma = \frac{\alpha}{k}\left(e^{k\varepsilon} - 1\right) \tag{17.3}$$

where k is defined as the *stiffness constant*, can be used to describe the stiffness level of different tissues. Typical mechanical properties of heart muscle are listed in Table 17.1.

The k value of heart muscle is in the middle of the range of most skeletal muscles (10–15), which itself varies depending on the species, age, anatomical positions, and health conditions. Similar variation occurs in other tissues, for example, the stiffness of skin increases with age (Figure 17.16), which indicates a decrease in softness and stretchability with age.

Table 17.1

Mechanical Properties of Heart Muscle

Mechanical Properties	Value
Stiffness E	0.01–0.5 MPa
Strain at rupture	20%–25%
Strain at the end of diastole	12%–15%
Stiffness constant k	10–15

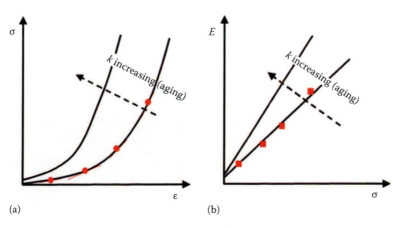

(a) (b)

Figure 17.16
Stiffness constant of your skin increases with aging, as indicated by (a) stress-strain curves and (b) stiffness-stress lines.

581

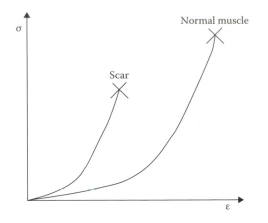

Figure 17.17
Stress–strain curves of normal heart muscle and its scarred tissue.

   In all tissue types at any age, the stiffness of fibrous scar tissue at an injury sight is always significantly higher than that of original tissue, being less stretchable compared with the original tissue. Thus a heart (which is already likely to be aged) that has suffered from myocardial infarction will show a significant shift leftward and downward in the stress–strain curve (Figure 17.17).

17.3.5   Reproducing J-Shaped Mechanical Properties in Synthetic Materials

As discussed in Chapter 10, the fibrous structure of biological tissues renders them with J-shaped, nonlinearly elastic deformation behavior. Hence, textiles offer a readily manufacturable technique to produce J-shaped stress–strain curves with nonbiological materials. In addition to J-shaped stress–strain curves, knitted structures also behave elastically (Figure 17.18). The popular game facility, trampoline, is the application of good elasticity (softer and more stretchable) of knitted steel wire, compared with bulk steel materials.

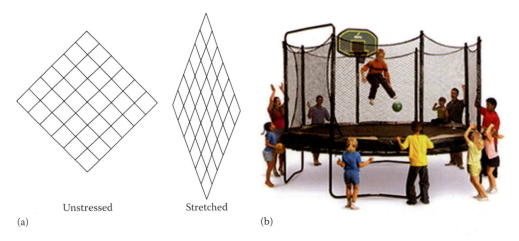

(a)   (b)

Figure 17.18
(a) Deformation of textile showing J-shaped stress–strain curve. (b) A trampoline is an application that takes advantage of the elastic behavior of textile materials.

17.4   NERVOUS TISSUE

Nerve cells (neurons) respond to environmental changes (stimuli) by altering electric potentials that exist between the inner and outer surfaces of their membranes. In the case of peripheral nerves, these stimuli can be transmitted over long distances, where a stimulus at one end (e.g., brain) results in a response at the other end (e.g., where nerve cells terminate at a muscle). Within the brain, neurons are much shorter, denser, and very highly interconnected. In all cases, Nerve tissue is mechanically less durable than other tissue types.

17.4.1   Cellular Organization and Histology of Nerve Tissue

Nerve tissue consists of two basic cell types, the neurons and the supporting glial cells (Lat. *glia* = glue), which account for more than 98% of Nerve tissue. In the central nervous system, neurons and glia coexist in densely packed three-dimensional populations. In the peripheral Nerve system, neurons exist as elongated cable-like structures, which run in parallel with the blood and lymph supply of all tissues.

17.4.1.1   Neurons   Histologically, a typical neuron consists of three parts:

1. Dendrite
2. The cell body (soma)
3. Axon

The cell body of neurons contains the nucleus and surrounding cytoplasm. Emanating from the cell body are branches (dendrite), comprising of neuronal membrane. One dendrite is larger and longer than the others (the *axon*), and contains a high abundance of microtubules on the inside of the neural membrane, while (for most type of neurons) being insulated outside by concentric membranes of *Schwann cells* (Figure 17.19), which contain high concentrations of myelin (the *myelin sheath*). At the end of the axon, plasma membranes terminate into microscopic structures called *synapses*, which join other neuron cells bodies, or muscles (*neuromuscular junctions*).

Neurons are highly specialized for transmission and processing of cellular signals, in the form of ion mediated depolarization across their membranes. In this respect, the most important feature of neurons is their directionality. A stimulus arrives at the cell body via a dendrite, is always transmitted directionally down the axon, and results in secretion of biochemicals at the synapses. Here, microvesicles containing bioactive amines (neurotransmitters) are released from the membranes, then recycled back. This forms the basis of a nerve impulse. Propagation of the impulse along the axon is maintained by the myelin sheath, which acts as an insulator, preventing loss of the signal.

There are different kinds of neurons, defined by their specific function. *Sensory neurons* respond to external stimuli, such as pressure and temperature changes, resulting in signal transduction back to the brain. These neurons are usually associated with the sensory organs (eyes, ears, nose, tongue, and touch-sensitive areas). *Motor neurons* are typically muscle stimulators, which run from the brain to the various muscles of the body, initiating movement. Both types of neurons are characterized by having extremely long axons (e.g., sciatic nerve axon ~ 1 m), and vary both in diameter (0.2–20 μm) and speed of signal conduction (0.5–120 m/s). The cerebral cortex contains about 10 different types of *cortical neurons*, which are very short, and characterized by their high dendrite density and differences in axon polarity, which dramatically increases their speed

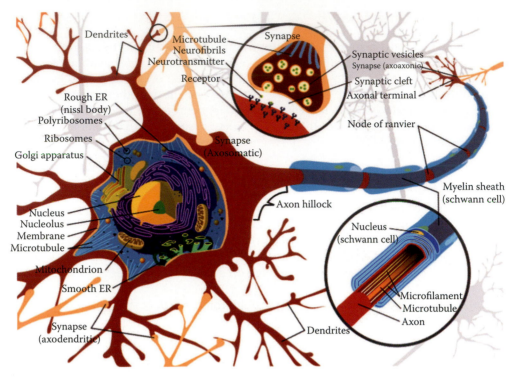

Figure 17.19
Structure of a typical myelinated neuron. (From http://commons.wikimedia.org/wiki/User:LadyofHats/gallery2#mediaviewer/File:Complete_neuron_cell_diagram_en.svg.)

of signaling and level of connectivity. Hence these neurons act like a living circuit, able to rapidly process complex signals and integrate signals from all over the body.

17.4.1.2   Glial Cells   The neurons are both physically and biochemically supported by the glial cells within the nervous system (Figure 17.20), especially in the brain and spinal cord. Glial cell types include:

- Oligodendrocytes (produce myelin sheaths in the brain)
- Schwann cells (produce myelin sheaths in peripheral nerves)
- Astrocytes (signal integration, biochemical support, blood supply interface, repair of scar tissue)
- Ependymal cells (lining of brain cavity, secretion of cerebrospinal fluid (CSF))
- Microglia (immune cells of the brain, like macrophages)

In general, glial cells have some capacity for cell division, whereas neurons do not typically divide. In the peripheral nervous system, the most important glial cells are Schwann cells, which are able to renew and render the axon with an ability to regenerate by a mechanism of new dendrite formation. In the brain, the most abundant and critical cells are the astrocytes. These are highly branched (star-like) in structure, which relates to their very dense system of dendrites, which is involved in signal integration and maintaining tissue shape. In terms of repair, they are involved in the remodeling of scar tissue, and have a host of other maintenance functions including regulating blood flow, stimulating oligodendrocytes to produce myelin, and supply of glucose to neurons.

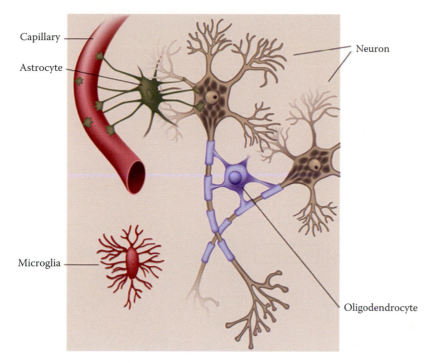

Figure 17.20
Neuron cells of the central nervous system with glial cells glued on them.

17.4.2 Anatomy of Peripheral Nerve Fibers

Neurons in the peripheral nervous system are connected in a head-to-end style, forming a single nerve filament (Figure 17.21). Each fiber is sealed by endoneurium, a connective tissue. A bundle of nerve fibers is held together by perineurium, another connective tissue type, which forms a fibril. Finally several fibrils are sealed by epineurium to form a complete nerve fiber. Blood vessels are embedded between nerve fibers (Figure 17.22).

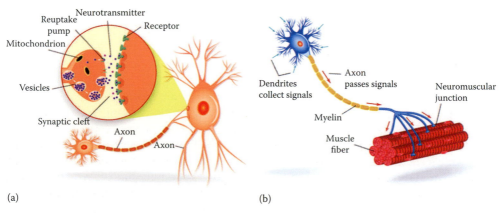

Figure 17.21
(a) Synapse of neurons and (b) synapse of neuron to muscle.

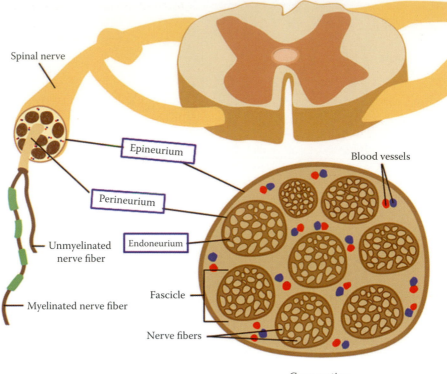

Spinal nerve

Epineurium

Blood vessels

Perineurium

Unmyelinated
nerve fiber

Endoneurium

Fascicle

Myelinated nerve fiber

Nerve fibers

Cross section

Figure 17.22
Nerve fiber structure. Framed items are connective tissues.

17.5 CHAPTER HIGHLIGHTS

1. Four basic types of tissues:
   - Epithelial (epithelium)
   - Muscular (myocytes)
   - Nervous (neurons)
   - Connective tissue

   Most organs (e.g., blood vessels) contain all four types of tissues.

2. In general, tissues are composed of
   - Cells
   - ECM

   However, epithelial, muscular, and nerve tissues are primarily composed of their cells, which account for more than 98% of the tissue. Only in connective tissues is ECM the primary component.

3. Epithelial tissues are a diverse group of tissues which cover or line all body surfaces, cavities, and tubes.

4. Active and passive mechanical performance of muscle tissue
   - Active: Stimulated muscle. Active deformation (i.e., contraction) is caused by internal chemical energy.
   - Passive: Unstimulated muscle. Passive deformation is caused by *external* force, and restored by the elastic protein, titin.

5. Passive J-shaped stress–strain curve of biological tissues
   Mechanism: progressive recruitment of strain-resistant fibers
   Passive stiffness: linear relationship between stiffness and stress
   Stiffness constant, k
6. Nerve tissue consists of two cell types:
   Neurons (also known as nerve cells) and supporting Glial cells (*glia* means glue).
   Neuron consists of dendrites, the cell body, and axon.
   The most important glial cells are Schwann cells, which have renew ability, and render the axon an ability to regenerate by a sprouting mechanism.
7. Connective tissue: Support structures, loose vs. dense, reticular structure are examples. Different amounts of elastin vs. collagen, varying vascularity.

ACTIVITIES

Watch video on YouTube of the muscle contraction process.

ADVANCED TOPIC: PROPERTIES OF PROTEINS IN MAMMALIAN TISSUES

Structural Elastic Proteins

As in the field of materials science where materials are classified into structural and functional materials, proteins can be grouped into these two general categories as well. Functional proteins include enzymes, ligands and receptors, antibodies, and adhesion proteins, which have specialized amino acid domains for binding and catalysis. Amongst the structural ones are the elastic proteins that fulfill specific biological roles, such as maintaining tissue integrity and 3D morphology [1]. The best-known elastic proteins include collagen, elastin, titin, and fibrillin in vertebrate muscle and connective tissue. Other biological examples include byssus and abductin from molluscs, resilin and silk proteins from arthropods, and gluten from plants [1]. They are widely distributed and exhibit unique elastic characteristics; however, only a few have been well characterized in detail [1].

Polypeptide-based biomaterials are increasingly being investigated for their application in tissue engineering. This interest is fuelled by the remarkable properties of structural proteins, such as elasticity and intrinsic biocompatibility, as well as their ability to self-assemble. Just as the development of any material requires a fundamental knowledge of structure–function relationship, to develop protein-based biomaterials it is essential to understand their basic biological attributes, including biochemistry (primary, secondary, tertiary, quaternary structure, and related biochemical activities) and physiological function. This knowledge has been well documented in a large amount of literature elsewhere, including *Handbook of Proteins: Structure, Function and Methods* [2], *Proteins: Structures and Molecular Properties* [3], *Proteins: Biochemistry and Biotechnology* [4].

In this section, we review the protein attributes relevant to biomedical engineering, including biodegradability and elastic properties, focusing on four of the best studied elastic proteins in mammalian tissues: collagen, elastin, fibrin, and titin. Since these proteins cause little or no foreign body reaction, their biocompatibility is not a major concern and thus will not be discussed. The mechanical properties of proteins are greatly influenced by the testing conditions, especially temperature and hydration states. In this review, all mechanical data were collected from mechanical testing that was carried out at temperature and hydration states that correspond to in vivo conditions for the proteins. For example, tendon collagen and elastin were tested in water or physiological saline [5].

COLLAGEN

Collagens in Biological Tissues

Collagen is the most abundant protein present in the human body, providing tensile strength and structural integrity for connective tissue such as dermis, bone, cartilage, tendon, ligament, and structural parts of internal organs [6]. Although collagen is ubiquitous in the mammalian body, it is generally extracted from those tissues rich in fibrous collagen such as skin and tendons. There are more than 22 different types of collagen identified so far in the human body, with collagens I–V being the five major types [6,7]. Collagens typically form a triple helix, cross-linked at glycine and proline residues by hydrogen bonding. These fibers often occur in parallel as highly organized fibrillar tracts with complex structure, which imparts variable strength in tissues.

Mechanical Properties

Collagen fibers, as seen in tendons, are often described as inelastic in terms of stretchiness, because their extensibility, ε_{max}, is between 10% and 20%, typically 13%–15% [8–11]. Collagen is also relatively less soft than other elastic proteins such as elastin), with an exceptionally wide range of Young's modulus from several MPa to one GPa. However, collagen is a truly elastic protein. Figure 17.23 shows a typical stress–strain curve of tendon collagen, with a high resilience of 90%, similar to that of elastin at the cardiac frequency (1–3 Hz) [5,12]. Collagen has consistently been shown to be capable of reversible deformation. It is this aspect of collagen that established it as an elastic protein [5].

Biodegradability

Collagen undergoes enzymatic degradation, depending on the types of collagen and the sites it is implanted to. In normal connective tissue, collagen degrades at a very slow and controlled rate while extensive degradation occurs during rapid tissue growth and in diseased states such as arthritis, cancer, and chronic non-healing ulcers [6]. Different forms of collagen are also transiently deposited during different phases of tissue healing and remodeling, which imparts different levels of rigidity.

Applications of Collagen in Tissue Engineering

Due to its good solubility in acidic aqueous solutions, collagen can be processed into different forms, including sheets, tubes, sponges, foams, nanofibrous matrices, powders, fleeces, and injectable viscous solutions and dispersions [7]. Besides, as a major component of the ECM, collagen can serve as a natural substrate for cell attachment, proliferation, and differentiation, which makes collagen a good matrix material for tissue engineering and wound dressing applications. For example, collagen-based bilayer dressings with or without seeded cells for the treatment of exuding diabetic ulcers (Integra®, TransCyte®, Orcel®, Apligraf®) have been approved by the FDA and

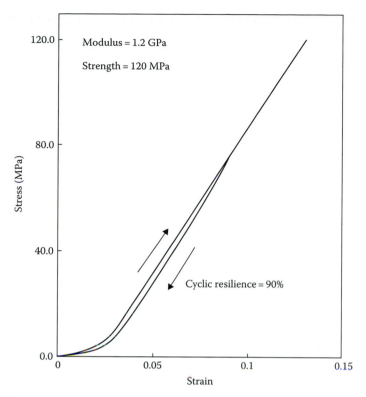

Figure 17.23
A typical stress–strain curve of tendon collagen. (From Gosline, J. et al., Philos. Trans. R. Soc. Lond. B Biol. Sci., 357(1418), 121, 2002. With permission of The Royal Society.)

are commercially available [13,14]; an absorbable, 3D collagen matrix graft (Duragen®) has been developed for spinal dural repair and regeneration [15]; an FDA approved product, Collagraft®, is a composite made of collagen, hydroxyapatite, and tricalcium phosphate, and is applied as a bone graft substitute; and many other forms of collagen have been developed as scaffolds in cardiovascular, musculoskeletal, and neuronal tissue engineering [16]. In addition, collagen can be cross-linked to produce collagen gels or made into collagen/polymer hybrid materials for use as carriers to deliver drugs, proteins, and even genomic and plasmid DNA for targeted therapies [17,18].

In summary, although collagen possesses several advantages such as its inherently good biocompatibility and natural biodegradability, its poor mechanical properties and variable physical properties with different sources of the protein matrices have hampered progress with these approaches. Concerns have arisen regarding immunogenic problems associated with the introduction of nonhuman collagen or recombinant versions [19], a common issue with materials of biological origin that have potential immunogenic properties.

ELASTIN

Biological Function of Elastin

Elastin is an important component in tissues that are subjected to repetitive strain such as skin, lung alveoli, arterial walls, mucous membranes, gut lining, and elastic cartilage [20]. In these tissues, elastin is responsible for their reversible extensibility and provides the initial low modulus region of the stress–strain curve while collagen offers the rigid constraint that limits the deformation of the elastic element [21]. Elastin is an especially important component of arteries (Figure 17.7), where the elasticity (including large extensibility and good resilience) allows arteries to efficiently transfer pulsatile waves of bulk blood flow from the heart, lowering peak blood pressure and mechanical work of the heart, and maintaining a relatively steady flow of oxygen through tissues [5].

Mechanical Properties of Elastin

Compared to collagen, elastin is more flexible and stable. Natural elastin has Young's modulus of 300–1000 kPa and elongation at a break of 100%–150% [5,22]. Figure 17.24 provides data for the mechanical behavior of elastin under a number of conditions, including varying strain rate, hydration level, and temperature, where storage modulus (E') is the stiffness associated with the storage of elastic energy, and loss modulus (E'') is the stiffness associated with molecular friction and energy dissipation.

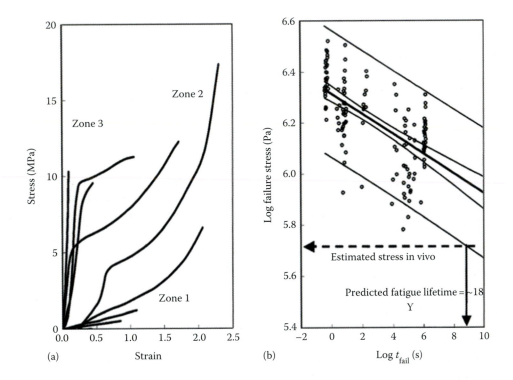

Figure 17.24

Static-fatigue lifetime estimates for purified, pig-arterial elastin. (a) Sample stress–strain curves for constant strain rate tests. Samples tested under full hydration at low strain rates show typical rubber-like behavior (zone 1), but as the strain rate is increased elastin passes through its glass transition, first becoming tough (zone 2) and then becoming a brittle polymeric glass (zone 3). (b) Correlation of failure stress and failure time for fully hydrated elastin at a broad range of strain rates. Extrapolation of this failure envelope to long times provides an estimate of static-fatigue lifetime at in vivo stress. (From Gosline, J. et al., Philos. Trans. R. Soc. Lond. B Biol. Sci., 357(1418), 121, 2002. With permission of The Royal Society.)

Resilience of Fully Hydrated Elastin

At cardiac frequencies (typically 1–3 Hz), E' is about two orders of magnitude greater than E''. This indicates high resilience for elastin at rates of deformation that occur in the cardiovascular system [5]. Resilience, R, can be calculated from the following equation:

$$R = e^{-2\pi\delta}, \qquad (17.4)$$

where $\delta = E''/E'$ is the damping factor. At 1 Hz, the resilience for fully hydrated elastin is about 90%. However, as frequency rises above 1 Hz, E' rises slowly and E'' rises quite rapidly, indicating glass transition in elastin. By 100 Hz, δ has risen to such a level that reliance is only 50% [5].

Resilience of Partially Hydrated Elastin

When water content is reduced in elastin, the mobility of molecules decreases, which in turn causes a dramatic change in its elastic properties. For instance, when water content is reduced by about 50%, the efficient elastic behavior only occurs at frequencies below 10^{-2} Hz; and at cardiac frequencies, the resilience is below 50%. Hence, increasing frequency or reducing water content both reduces resilience of elastin and limits the utility of elastin in strain energy storage devices [5].

Cyclic (Fatigue) Lifetime of Elastin

Elastin remains in place throughout the full life span of the organism, which for humans is ~80 years, suggesting that elastin is an extremely durable material [5]. However, a baseline level of turnover occurs regularly, depending on the tissue, and elasticity declines with tissue age. Figure 17.24 shows the fatigue properties of elastin and depicts how failure stress and strain of elastin are strongly influenced by test conditions. At low strain rates and high temperatures, the fully hydrated elastin behaves as a typical rubber (Zone 1 in Figure 17.24a). Under these test conditions, the failure stresses are low, while the extensions and times to break are high. Conversely, at high strain rates and low temperatures, low hydration gives elastin the properties of a rigid polymeric glass, with very high stiffness and low extensibility (Zone 3). Failure stresses here are high, but the extensions and times to break are extremely low. At intermediate test conditions, elastin is in the middle of its glass transition, where it is a tough, semi-rigid polymer that fails at high stress and high strain (Zone 2) [5]. It has been estimated from Figure 17.24b that the fatigue lifetime of porcine arterial elastin is 18 years, which is consistent with the lifetime of the animal species from which this elastin was isolated [5].

It is interesting to compare the mechanical properties of collagen and elastin with those of an engineering material, elastic steel (Table 17.2). It is striking that the soft, weak elastin has the same elastic energy storage capacity as the spring steel, which indicates that elastin is indeed a highly efficient spring material. Moreover, the spring energy storage capacity of collagen is about 10 times greater than that of both elastin and steel [5].

Table 17.2

Mechanical Properties of Elastin, Collagen, and Spring Steel

Protein	Modulus (MPa)	Stress-in-Use (MPa)	Density (g/cm³)	Resilience (%)	Energy Storage Capacity (J/kg)
Elastin	1.1	0.55	1.3	90	95
Collagen	120	60	1.3	90	1000
Spring steel	200,000	600	7.8	99	115

Source: Gosline, J. et al., *Philos. Trans. R. Soc. Lond. B Biol. Sci., 357(1418), 121, 2002.*

Biostability of Elastin

Elastin is remarkably stable in healthy tissue, with an associated half-life of up to 70 years due to its resistance to enzymatic, chemical, and physical degradation [23]. In vivo biocompatibility tests have showed that elastins have no cytotoxicity problems, and are supportive to cell adhesion and proliferation [24].

Self-Assembling Characteristics of Elastin

One of the remarkable properties of elastin is the ability of its precursor protein tropo-elastin to self-assemble under physiological conditions. This is the basis of the coacervation process, which leads to alignment of tropoelastin molecules prior to intermolecular cross-linking into a spherical droplet arrangement [25,26]. The temperature above which coacervation occurs is referred to as an inverse transition temperature (T_t) or lower critical solution temperature (LCST), meaning that the protein forms ordered structures as temperature increases. The coacervation behavior can be affected by many factors, including protein concentration, salt concentration, temperature, pH, and the presence of other molecules such as GAGs [26–28]. This self-assembling behavior of elastin is especially useful in preparing various elastin-based biomaterials, such as hydrogels [29], sheets [21], sponge-like isotropic networks [30], and nanoscale materials [31]. It is also because of this self-assembling property that elastin has a potential in the development of novel applications in the areas of bio-actuators, implantable sensors, and drug delivery vehicles [20].

Applications of Elastin in Tissue Engineering

There is an increasing number of research studies on elastin and elastin-based bio-materials investigated for their application in tissue engineering, specialized mechanical properties, ability to self-assemble, and their long-term stability [32]. Elastin can be used in its natural state (i.e., insoluble elastin occurring in autografts, allografts, and xenografts), processed into different forms prior to applications (e.g., decellularized ECM, purified elastin or hydrolyzed soluble elastin), or synthesized with other molecules to form biomaterial blends (e.g., elastin–fibronectin, silk–elastin, and elastin–synthetic polymer). Excellent reviews have been recently provided on the processing and synthesis of elastin-based biomaterials, and readers can refer to Reference [32] for details. These biomaterials have been applied to the construction of skin substitutes [33], vascular grafts [34], heart valves [35], and elastic cartilage [36] (Tables 17.3 and 17.4).

Table 17.3

Applications of Elastin-Related Biomaterials in Skin Tissue Engineering

Materials	Model	Major Results	Refs.
Decellularized collagen/elastin membrane	Rat-excised wound	A histologically satisfactory result was obtained. Due to wound contraction, the membrane formed pleats within the layer of elastic fibers.	[37]
Chemically cross-linked collagen/elastin membrane by a carbodiimide	Rat-excised wound	The collagen/elastin membrane caused activation of macrophages and the formation of inflammatory tissue, which indicated potentially undesirable chronic processes in the healing wound.	[38]
Collagen coated with 3% α-elastin	Porcine-excised wound	When combined with meshed split skin grafts, the collagen–elastin matrix was shown to reduce wound contraction and improve tissue regeneration, compared with the epidermal transplantation control group. Matrix remodeling and elastin regeneration occurred both in the superficial and deep dermal layers.	[39]
	Human clinical trials	Short-term follow-up revealed that skin elasticity was considerably improved by the collagen/elastin dermal substitute.	[40]
		The long-term evaluation showed improved elasticity, but the difference with controls is insignificant after 1 year.	[41,42]
	In 46 patients, 69 pairs 12 year follow-up	This is the first long-term and objective follow-up of this dermal substitution. Scar parameters were found to be improved in both reconstructed wounds treated with the collagen–elastin substitute, indicating a long-lasting improvement in scar integrity.	[43]
Collagen coated with 3% α-elastin	Ten patients with severe burn injuries of the hand	Showed full range of hand motion after 3 months.	[44]
Elastin–laminin peptide	In vitro	The hybrid material promoted attachment and proliferation of normal human dermal fibroblasts in culture.	[45]
	Rabbit ear skin	Alginate dressings lined with elastin–laminin peptides re-epithelialized faster than controls.	

Skin Tissue Engineering

Currently autologous skin grafting remains the gold standard in skin repair. Collagen or mixed ECM–based scaffolds such as Dermograft® and Alloderm® have also been intensively investigated and applied clinically. However, the use of elastin-containing biomaterials as skin substitutes has not been extensively applied. Some examples include

Table 17.4

Applications of Elastin-Related Biomaterials in Vascular Tissue Engineering

Approach to Obtain Tubular Constructs	Major Results	Refs.
Decellularized blood vessels from rat aorta	In vivo, decellularized rat aorta showed inflammation-resistant properties and inhibited smooth muscle cell proliferation compared to collagen-containing matrices, while endothelial cell migration was maintained.	[56]
Decellularized blood vessels from porcine carotid arteries	In an acute thrombogenicity model, the decellularized blood vessels had a longer patency time than synthetic tubing.	[24,53–55]
	Elastin–aSIS–fibrin conduits also occluded, but the thrombus appeared to be associated with the suture line, not the vessel wall itself.	
	Calcification was observed upon subcutaneous implantation of decellularized porcine arteries.	
	In a preliminary rabbit carotid bypass model, platelet adhesion was much lower than the positive control.	[57]
Tubing from collagen–elastin acid solution	In vitro culture, smooth muscle cells were able to adhere to and proliferate in these porous 3D collagen–elastin tubes for up to 14 days, while maintaining their contractile phenotype as evidenced from smooth muscle actin staining.	[58–63]
Electrospinning	Fibroblasts, smooth muscle cells, and endothelial cells were successfully seeded onto the scaffolds.	[34]

mixed materials such as decellularized porcine membrane comprising approximately 70% collagen and 30% insoluble elastin, with minor amounts of GAGs [37]. Synthetic scaffolds of type I collagen coated with 3% α-elastin [46], hybrid peptides of elastin [45], and injectable α-elastin [47] have also been used.

In a porcine excised wound model, a combination of collagen/3% α-elastin dermal matrix and meshed split skin grafts was shown to reduce wound contraction and improve tissue regeneration, compared with the epidermal transplantation control group, and no myofibroblasts were observed. Matrix remodeling and elastin regeneration occurred both in the upper and lower dermis [39]. The same collagen/3% α-elastin dermal matrix has also been applied in a clinical trial [40]. Short-term follow-up revealed that skin elasticity was considerably improved by the collagen/elastin dermal substitute as analyzed by Cutometer measurements [40]. Long-term evaluations with respect to elasticity are consistent with the former findings, but the difference between controls was not significant after 1 year [41,42]. In the study of another group, the same collagen/3% α-elastin dermal matrix was used in 10 patients as a dermal substitute in severe burn injuries of the hand. The result was encouraging, showing full range of hand motion after 3 months [44].

Vascular Tissue Engineering

The reason why elastin becomes promising for vascular tissue engineering is twofold. First, biocompatibility requires that the tissue-engineered grafts can encourage remodeling of the internal blood vessel cell wall (endothelium) which is confluent, and adherent throughout the interior of the vessel, but resistant to thrombosis. This is especially important to coronary artery bypass surgery, in which small-diameter vascular graft with long-term patency and non-thrombogenicity are required. Elastin coatings applied to synthetic tubular, elastin-like polypeptides have been reported to reduce thrombogenicity in animal models [48,49]. Second, the mechanical properties of vascular grafts should be similar to the native vessel [50]. As described, elastin is an important component of vascular tissue and plays a critical role in the elastic properties of blood vessels, especially arteries. Hence, it is biologically relevant to apply elastin in engineering vascular tissues; however, there are few examples of where elastin has been incorporated in most tissue-engineered blood vessels [51].

There are generally three approaches to obtain tubular constructs: (1) preparation of decellularized blood vessels, which have retained the intrinsic ECM organization but have reduced immunogenic potential by removal of smooth muscle, fibroblasts, and endothelial cells; (2) preparation of tubular scaffolds from individual matrix components (with or without seeded cells), and (3) encouraging cells to produce the ECM [32,52]. In general, the decellularized blood vessels have a longer patency time than synthetic tubing. However, calcification has been observed upon subcutaneous implantation of decellularized arteries [24,53–55]. Calcification is a serious concern here, as it may cause failure of the vascular graft.

In relation to the use of elastin for tubular structures, some have been prepared from elastin-based materials synthetically. Starting from purified components, one can prepare grafts substrates that are more defined at the molecular level than decellularized natural material. This can be done by: (1) pouring a diluted acetic acid suspension of purified type I collagen fibrils and elastin fibers in a tubular mold, freezing, and lyophilizing [59,63]; (2) winding of a sheet or (3) electrospinning. Electrospinning is a widely used method for vascular reconstruction by scaffold construction, and future research is needed to better define its use in in vivo applications.

Elastin and elastin-based biomaterials are promising candidates in the field of tissue engineering, particularly for dermal and vascular areas. They have desired properties, especially biomechanical behavior, which may promise to go a long way toward the successful clinical applications. However, there are issues with native elastin biomaterials, among which the number one drawbacks such as the tendency to calcify when implanted subdermally [64]. This problem is still a poorly understood phenomenon in biomaterial science, often occurring in cardiovascular prosthetic implants (e.g., bioprosthetic heart valves and aortic homografts) [64].

FIBRIN

Fibrin in Blood Clotting

Fibrin is a biopolymer involved in the natural blood clotting process, derived from the preprotein fibrinogen. During the process of the fibrin clot formation, a number of factors such as the ratio of thrombin to fibrinogen, the ionic strength and divalent cation concentration of the medium, or the presence of very specific types of plasma proteins (e.g., serum albumin and so-called clotting adhesion proteins), regulate the rate of fibrin polymerization, structure, and composition [65]. Mechanically, fibrins form the structural framework of extracellular microfibrils in connective tissues that endow dynamic connective tissues with long-range elasticity.

Mechanical Properties of Fibrin

Although fibrin is a well-defined protein structurally, much less is known about how it forms heterogeneous mesh-like secondary structures in vivo. Fibrin forms complex ultrastructure, essentially like a random meshwork of linear microfibrils with large pores. It has proved a major challenge both to define their structural organization and to relate it to their biological and mechanical function, although the clot structure is remarkably good at trapping platelets and conforming to any lesion size. The fibrin clot structure and composition, concentration of fibrinogen and protein factor XIII (which mediates cross-linking) considerably influence the elastic modulus and tensile strength of fibrin clots [66–69]. The modulus of fibrin was reported to be ~50 Pa [70], and insufficient mechanical support was reported to be the main drawback of fibrin for its application in articular cartilage repair strategies tested in animal models [71].

Biodegradation of Fibrin

Fibrin is subject to enzyme-mediated hydrolytic degradation, known as fibrinolysis both in vivo and in vitro. The degradation rate of fibrin can vary from 4 to 26 weeks [71,72]. Also, depending on where fibrin clots occur (e.g., in skin or within larger vessels), the mechanical stability of these structures will vary, which will likely accelerate degradation rates.

Applications of Fibrin in Tissue Engineering

Due to the excellent biocompatibility, biodegradability, injectability, and the presence of several ECM proteins (e.g., fibronectins that favorably affect cell adhesion and proliferation), fibrin was one of the earliest biopolymers used as a biomaterial [7]. One of the first products was a fibrin sealant (Fibrinkleber Human Immuno®), which is currently approved for use in surgical procedures to achieve rapid hemostasis and to seal tissue surfaces [73]. This fibrin-based bioresorbable adhesive coating is especially useful for soft tissues and organs such as cardiovascular and thoracic tissues.

Another important application of fibrin is as a carrier vehicle of tissue-specific cells. Horch and colleagues found that a keratinocyte/fibrin matrix suspension, after injection to skin lesion sites, resulted in the regeneration of epidermal tissue, which assisted in the wound-healing process [74]. In addition to skin wound-healing, fibrin-based biomaterials have been demonstrated to be effective for urinary system repair. Urothelial cell/fibrin matrix suspensions successfully transplant to lesion sites and help to regenerate multilayered urothelium in urethral reconstruction procedures [75,76]. Other cells including tracheal epithelial cells, preadipocytes [77], chondrocytes [78], human myofibroblasts [79], and osteoprogenitor cells [80] have also been applied in fibrin gels and tested for tissue regeneration applications.

Furthermore, the combination of fibrin-based biomaterials and other biomaterials (for example, fibrin blends with inorganic bone ceramics) to add additional biological activity while improving the biomechanical properties of the composite matrix provides several viable possibilities for tissue regeneration [7]. Lastly, fibrin has been applied as coatings to functionalize a range of biomaterial surfaces [81–89].

Fibrillin-rich microfibrils of the ECM have been shown to play an essential role in the provision of long-range extensibility to many dynamic connective tissues. Their complex ultrastructure has hindered our understanding of the biological and mechanical roles of these proteins. The major application of these extremely soft elastic proteins is as injectible scaffold materials and surgical sealants.

TITIN

Titin in Muscles

Titin, also known as connectin, is a protein found in human and other mammalian muscle tissue. Titin is a giant protein, the largest known single polypeptide [90], which functions as a molecular spring responsible for the passive elasticity of muscle (Figure 17.10). It is composed of folded protein domains, which can unfold when the protein is stretched and refold when the tension is removed [91]. It is necessary to mention the concepts associated with the *active* and *passive* mechanics of muscle. Active mechanical properties refer to the mechanical behaviors of muscle triggered by metabolic energy that causes proteins to move in fast, ratchet-like actions, under direct nerve stimulation or externally applied stimulation. Passive mechanical properties refer to mechanical behaviors of unstimulated muscle under an external force. Uniquely, functional muscle also undergoes active responses to passive stimulation.

Titin is important in the contraction of striated muscle tissues, where it connects the *Z* line to the *M* line in the sarcomere, the functional unit of all muscle fibers. The *A*-band part of the molecule is functionally stiff [92,93] while the *I*-band section of titin is elastic along most of its length, except near the *Z*-line [92,94,95].

Mechanical Properties of Titin

The entropic-chain characteristics of titin result in a nonlinear force response to stretching (Figure 17.25). The elastic modulus of titin is 350 kPa, a value similar to

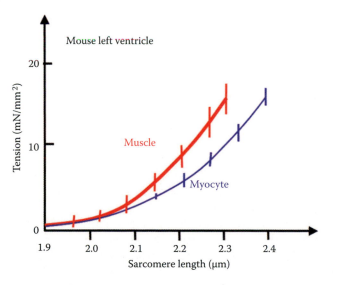

Figure 17.25
Sensitive tension levels of cardiac muscle (red line) and single cardiac myocytes (blue line). (From Wu, Y. et al., J. Mol. Cell. Cardiol., 32(12), 2151, 2000.)

that reported for elastin. The maximum active isometric tension in a single myofibril at a sarcomere length of 2.1–2.3 µm is about 150 kPa [96]. Titin is highly resilient at low strain and shock absorbent at high strains. The shock absorbance at high strains comes from the ability of titin to unravel and dissipate energy. The stretching of titin prevents the strain from damaging other tissues, such as tendon and ligaments [97].

Need for Titin Modification in Titin-Related Diseases

Certain genetic diseases result in mutant forms of titin being produced in the individual. This has led to cardiomyopathy [99] and various forms of dystrophy, including tibial muscular dystrophy [100], Duchenne muscular dystrophy (DMD)—where it was degraded extensively after 5 years, Becker muscular dystrophy (mild degradation), and myotonic and limb girdle dystrophy (minimal degradation) [101]. In certain autoimmune diseases, such as scleroderma [102] and myasthenia gravis [103], titin is attacked by antibodies. Amyotrophic lateral sclerosis and Charcot–Marie–Tooth disease also led to minimal degradation of titin [101]. The use of a replacement or tissue engineering strategy using titin may be a worthwhile option to treat some of these problems; however, genetic problems have undefined causes, and the treatment may not be a permanent cure.

Titin in Tissue Engineering

Artificial elastomeric proteins have been synthesized in an attempt to mimic the mechanical properties of titin [97]. Since the natural protein is made of regions with different mechanical properties, artificial titin has been made by cross-linking protein domains with resilin (see the following text). The resulting biomaterials have high resilience at low strain and shock absorbance at high strain, similar to the passive elastic properties of muscle. This new muscle-mimetic biomaterial is anticipated to have important applications as scaffolds and the matrix for the engineering of artificial muscles [97].

SUMMARY OF NATURAL ELASTIC PROTEINS

Theoretically, naturally occurring polymers, such as collagen, fibrin, and titin should not cause a foreign materials response when implanted in humans, unless there are residual immunogenic factors. They provide a natural substrate for cellular attachment, proliferation, and differentiation in their native state, with several inherent advantages, including bioactivity, the ability to present receptor-binding ligands to cells, susceptibility to cell-triggered proteolytic degradation and natural remodeling [7]. For these reasons, naturally occurring polymers could be a favorite substrate for tissue engineering [104].

The mechanical properties of naturally occurring elastic proteins are summarized in Table 17.5. The structural proteins are exceptionally diverse in terms of material properties. Each elastic protein is biologically adapted to be a good match to the environmental conditions and biological role. Elastin and resilin work well as strain-energy storage devices at low frequencies, body temperature, and aqueous media, and they have material properties that could probably be equaled by commonly available synthetic materials. Collagen fibers and spider silks, on the other hand, represent truly exceptional

Table 17.5
Mechanical Properties and Biodegradability of Elastic Proteins

Protein	Young's Modulus	UTS	Elongation at Break (%)	Resilience (%)	Toughness (MJ/m³)	Degradability	Refs.
Collagen (skin)	2–46 MPa		<50	90–95		Generally fast	[5,8–11]
Collagen (human tendon)	1.2 GPa	120 MPa	13	90	6		[5]
Elastin	300–1000 kPa	2 MPa	60–150	90–92	1.6	Remarkably stable, half-life being up to 70 years	[5,22]
Fibrin	50 Pa					Completely absorbed in 4–26 weeks	[70,79,80]
Titin	350 kPa						[96]
Resilin (dragonfly tendon)	2 MPa	4 MPa	200–300	92	4	Readily digested by proteolytic enzymes, fast enzymatic degradation rate	[5,106,107]
Mussel byssus, distal	870 MPa	75 MPa	109	28	45		[5]
Mussel byssus, proximal	16 MPa	35 MPa	200	53	35		[5]
Dragline silk	10 GPa	1.1 GPa	30	30–40	160		[5]
Viscid silk	3 MPa	500 MPa	270	30–40	150		[5]

materials that challenge the elastomeric material limits. Collagen has unmatched capacity for the storage of elastic-strain energy and spider silks have unmatched toughness [5].

In addition, when the natural elastic proteins were tested under environmental conditions beyond those seen in their normal function, a much broader range of material properties have been discovered. For example, dragline silk becomes rubber-like when hydrated, but it retains essentially all of its remarkable strength, making it a candidate for a high-performance elastomeric material for biomedical implantation. Mussel byssal fibers normally function in seawater, but when plasticized by other solvents, they may achieve greater strength with little compromise in extensibility. Natural proteins have a number of downsides, such as costly purification (depending on the source), strong immunogenic response, degradation reliant on enzyme activity and concentration that varies from individual to individual and even site to site, possible calcification in vivo, complexities in processing due to thermal instability and denaturation in organic solvent, and possibility of disease transmission [7,105]. Further studies are needed to understand the molecular mechanisms in elastic proteins. The resultant knowledge could have tremendous impact on the design of novel synthetic elastomeric materials.

SIMPLE QUESTIONS IN CLASS

1. Which of the following tissues is *not* connective tissue?
   a. Epidermis
   b. Dermis
   c. Blood
   d. Cartilage
2. Which of following tissues is not epithelial tissue?
   a. Epidermis
   b. Endothelium of blood vessels
   c. Endothelium of intestine
   d. Smooth muscle of blood vessels
3. A muscle cell is a muscle
   a. Fibril
   b. Filament
   c. Fiber
   d. Protein
4. Which of the following tissues contains less than 2% ECM?
   a. Bone
   b. Skin
   c. Cartilage
   d. Nerve
5. In a pressure-volume loop of heart (**Figure 14.12**), which stage is largely a passive mechanical process?
   a. Relaxation
   b. Filling
   c. Contraction
   d. Ejection
6. Which of the stress-strain curves has a stiffness constant k larger than k_1?
   a. Curve A
   b. Curve B

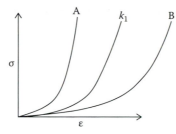

7. In the following diagram, which cell is a neuron?
   a. Cell in the frame A
   b. Cell in the frame B
   c. Cell in the frame C
   d. Cell in the frame D

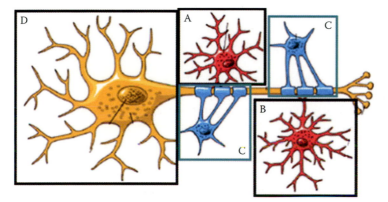

8. List the four basic types of tissues. In the following vessel structure, give tissue generic names of adventitia, media, and intima.

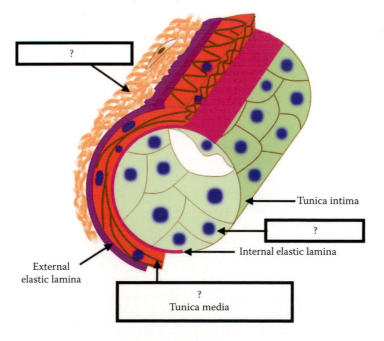

9. During the active muscle contraction and subsequent passive relaxation, which protein(s) change(s) in length?
   a. Actin
   b. Titin
   c. Myosin
   d. All of them

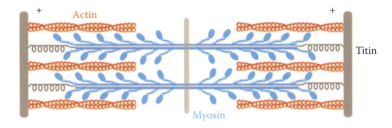

PROBLEMS AND EXERCISES

1. Briefly describe the histological structure of epithelial tissue. Illustrate anatomic positions of five organs where epithelial tissue is present.
2. Briefly describe the histological structure of skeletal muscular tissue.
3. What is passive mechanical behavior of muscle? What is active mechanical behavior of muscle?
4. If the stress–strain ($\sigma - \varepsilon$) relation of a tissue is $\sigma = A(ek^\varepsilon - 1)$, derive the relation of its Young's modulus E and stress σ.
5. What is the stiffness constant? Explain how scar is always harder and less elastic than natural skin? The formation of a scar is a protective mechanism of our defense system. Explain why this mechanism eventually leads to heart failure after heart attack.
6. What are the shapes of the stress–strain curves of synthetic elastomers and human elastin? Explain the reason for the difference.
7. Discuss the regenerative ability of the following three types of tissues:
   a. Nerve
   b. Muscle
   c. Epithelium
8. What is the major difference in the mechanical behavior of muscle and synthetic elastomeric polymers? Discuss possible strategies to produce the mechanical performance of biological elastin with synthetic elastomers.
9. Briefly describe the histological structure of a nerve organ.
10. Schematically demonstrate the histological structure of a neuron, and discuss the regeneration ability of the neuron.

BIBLIOGRAPHY

References for Text

1. Junqueira, L.C., J. Carneiro, and R.O. Kelley, *Basic Histology*, 9th edn. New York: McGraw-Hill, 1995.

2. Young, B. and J.W. Heath, *Functional Histology, A Text and Colour Atlas*, 4th edn. London, U.K.: Churchill Living Stone, 2000.
3. Fawcett, D.W. and E. Raviola, *A Textbook of Histology*, 12th edn. Chapman and Hall, New York, NY, 1993.

Websites

http://cueflash.com/Decks/M1-C2-L19_—%26gt%3B_Cell_to_Cell_Communication/.
http://droualb.faculty.mjc.edu/Lecture%20Notes/Unit%203/chapter_9__skeletal_muscle_tiss%20with%20figures.htm.
http://histology-online.com/.
http://intranet.tdmu.edu.ua/data/kafedra/internal/histolog/classes_stud/en/stomat/ptn/1/09%20Nerve%20tissue.%20Nerve%20cells.%20Glial%20cells.%20Nerve%20fibers.%20Nerve%20endings.htm.
http://www.histology-world.com/.
http://www.med.umich.edu/histology/dmindex.html.
http://www.wikispaces.com/.
https://histo.life.illinois.edu/histo/atlas/slides.php.

References for Advanced Topic

1. Shewry, P.R. et al., *Elastomeric Proteins Structures, Biomechanical Properties, and Biological Roles*, 2003, Cambridge, U.K.: Cambridge University Press.
2. Cox, M.M. and G.N. Phillips (eds.), *Handbook of Proteins: Structure, Function and Methods*, New York: Wiley, 2008.
3. Creighton, T.E., *Proteins: Structures and Molecular Properties*, 2edn. New York : W.H. Freeman & Co Ltd, 1993.
4. Walsh, G., *Proteins: Biochemistry and Biotechnology*. New York: John Wiley & Sons, 2002.
5. Gosline, J. et al., Elastic proteins: Biological roles and mechanical properties. *Philosophical Transactions of the Royal Society of London Series B-Biological Sciences*, 2002;**357**(1418):121–132.
6. Beckman, M.J., K.J. Shields, and R.F. Diegelmann, Collagen. In *Encyclopedia of Biomaterials and Biomedical Engineering*, 2nd edn., G.E. Wnek and G.L. Bowlin, eds. London, U.K.: Informa Healthcare, 2004, pp. 324–334.
7. Nair, L.S. and C.T. Laurencin, Biodegradable polymers as biomaterials. *Progress in Polymer Science*, 2007;**32**(8–9):762–798.
8. Chandran, K.B., *Cardiovascular Biomechanics*. New York: New York University Press, 1992.
9. Mark, J.E., *Polymer Data Handbook*. New York: Oxford University Press. 1999, xi, 1018pp.
10. Misof, K. et al., Collagen from the osteogenesis imperfecta mouse model (oim) shows reduced resistance against tensile stress. *Journal of Clinical Investigation*, 1997;**100**(1):40–45.
11. Webb, A.R., J. Yang, and G.A. Ameer, Biodegradable polyester elastomers in tissue engineering. *Expert Opinion on Biological Therapy*, 2004;**4**(6):801–812.
12. Nyman, J.S. et al., Age-related effect on the concentration of collagen crosslinks in human osteonal and interstitial bone tissue. *Bone*, 2006;**39**(6):1210–1217.
13. Thornton, J.F. and R.J. Rohrich, Dermal substitute (Integra) for open nasal wounds. *Plastic and Reconstructive Surgery*, 2005;**116**(2):677.
14. Purna, S.K. and M. Babu, Collagen based dressings—A review. *Burns*, 2000;**26**(1):54–62.
15. Narotam, P.K. et al., Collagen matrix (DuraGen) in dural repair: Analysis of a new modified technique. *Spine*, 2004;**29**(24):2861–2867; discussion 2868–2869.
16. Duan, X. et al., Biofunctionalization of collagen for improved biological response: Scaffolds for corneal tissue engineering. *Biomaterials*, 2007;**28**(1):78–88.

17. Jeckle, J. et al., Novel natural polymer-based material with improved properties for use in human and veterinary medicine and the method of manufacturing such. Patent WO 2001066159 A1, filed 2000.

18. Sano, A. et al., Atelocollagen for protein and gene delivery. *Advanced Drug Delivery Reviews*, 2003;**55**(12):1651–1677.

19. Vacanti, C.A., L.J. Bonassar, and J.P. Vacanti, Structure tissue engineering. In *Principles of Tissue Engineering*, R.P. Lanza, R. Langer, and J.P. Vacanti, eds. San Diego, CA: Academic Press, 2000, pp. 671–682.

20. Brinkman, W.T., K. Nagapudi, and E.L. Chaikof, Elastin. In *Encyclopedia of Biomaterials and Biomedical Engineering*, 2nd edn., G.E. Wnek and G.L. Bowlin, eds. London, U.K.: Informa Healthcare, 2008, Chapter 85.

21. Mithieux, S.M., J.E.J. Rasko, and A.S.A.S. Weiss, Synthetic elastin hydrogels derived from massive elastic assemblies of self-organized human protein monomers. *Biomaterials*, 2004;**25**(20):4921–4927.

22. Fung, Y.C., *Biomechanics: Mechanical Properties of Living Tissues*, 2nd edn. New York: Springer-Verlag, 1993, xviii, 568pp.

23. Petersen, E., F. Wågberg, and K.A. Ängquist, Serum concentrations of elastin-derived peptides in patients with specific manifestations of atherosclerotic disease. *European Journal of Vascular and Endovascular Surgery: The Official Journal of the European Society for Vascular Surgery*, 2002;**24**(5):440–444.

24. Lu, Q. et al., Novel porous aortic elastin and collagen scaffolds for tissue engineering. *Biomaterials*, 2004;**25**(22):5227–5237.

25. Cox, B.A., B.C. Starcher, and D.W. Urry, Communication: Coacervation of tropoelastin results in fiber formation. *Journal of Biological Chemistry*, 1974;**249**(3):997–998.

26. Wu, W.J., B. Vrhovski, and A.S. Weiss, Glycosaminoglycans mediate the coacervation of human tropoelastin through dominant charge interactions involving lysine side chains. *Journal of Biological Chemistry*, 1999;**274**(31):21719–21724.

27. Mecham, R.P. and G. Lange, Antigenicity of elastin: Characterization of major antigenic determinants on purified insoluble elastin. *Biochemistry*, 1982;**21**(4):669–673.

28. Vrhovski, B., S. Jensen, and A.S. Weiss, Coacervation characteristics of recombinant human tropoelastin. *European Journal of Biochemistry*, 1997;**250**(1):92–98.

29. Wright, E.R. et al., Thermoplastic elastomer hydrogels via self-assembly of an elastin-mimetic triblock polypeptide. *Advanced Functional Materials*, 2002;**12**(2):149–154.

30. Bellingham, C.M. et al., Recombinant human elastin polypeptides self-assemble into biomaterials with elastin-like properties. *Biopolymers*, 2003;**70**(4):445–455.

31. Zhang, S., Fabrication of novel biomaterials through molecular self-assembly. *Nature Biotechnology*, 2003;**21**(10):1171–1178.

32. Daamen, W.F. et al., Elastin as a biomaterial for tissue engineering. *Biomaterials*, 2007;**28**(30):4378–4398.

33. Lamme, E.N. et al., Living skin substitutes: Survival and function of fibroblasts seeded in a dermal substitute in experimental wounds. *Journal of Investigative Dermatology*, 1998;**111**(6):989–995.

34. Boland, E.D. et al., Electrospinning collagen and elastin: Preliminary vascular tissue engineering. *Frontiers in Bioscience*, 2004;**9**:1422–1432.

35. Neuenschwander, S. and S.P. Hoerstrup, Heart valve tissue engineering. *Transplant Immunology*, 2004;**12**(3–4):359–365.

36. Xu, J.W. et al., Tissue-engineered flexible ear-shaped cartilage. *Plastic and Reconstructive Surgery*, 2005;**115**(6):1633–1641.

37. Hafemann, B. et al., Use of a collagen/elastin-membrane for the tissue engineering of dermis. *Burns*, 1999;**25**(5):373–384.

38. Klein, B. et al., Inflammatory response to a porcine membrane composed of fibrous collagen and elastin as dermal substitute. *Journal of Materials Science-Materials in Medicine*, 2001;**12**(5):419–424.

39. Lamme, E.N. et al., Extracellular matrix characterization during healing of full-thickness wounds treated with a collagen/elastin dermal substitute shows improved skin regeneration in pigs. *Journal of Histochemistry and Cytochemistry*, 1996;**44**(11):1311–1322.

40. van Zuijlen, P.P.M. et al., Graft survival and effectiveness of dermal substitution in burns and reconstructive surgery in a one-stage grafting model. *Plastic and Reconstructive Surgery*, 2000;**106**(3):615–623.

41. van Zuijlen, P.P.M. et al., Dermal substitution in acute burns and reconstructive surgery: A subjective and objective long-term follow-up. *Plastic and Reconstructive Surgery*, 2001;**108**(7):1938–1946.

42. van Zuijlen, P.P.M. et al., Long-term results of a clinical trial on dermal substitution. A light microscopy and Fourier analysis based evaluation. *Burns*, 2002;**28**(2):151–160.

43. Bloemen, M.C.T. et al., Dermal substitution in acute burns and reconstructive surgery: A 12-year follow-up. *Plastic and Reconstructive Surgery*, 2010;**125**(5):1450–1459.

44. Haslik, W. et al., First experiences with the collagen-elastin matrix Matriderm((R)) as a dermal substitute in severe burn injuries of the hand. *Burns*, 2007;**33**(3):364–368.

45. Hashimoto, T. et al., Development of alginate wound dressings linked with hybrid peptides derived from laminin and elastin. *Biomaterials*, 2004;**25**(7–8):1407–1414.

46. Devries, H.J.C. et al., Reduced wound contraction and scar formation in punch biopsy wounds—Native collagen dermal substitutes: A clinical-study. *British Journal of Dermatology*, 1995;**132**(5):690–697.

47. de Chalain, T., J.H. Phillips, and A. Hinek, Bioengineering of elastic cartilage with aggregated porcine and human auricular chondrocytes and hydrogels containing alginate, collagen, and kappa-elastin. *Journal of Biomedical Materials Research*, 1999;**44**(3):280–288.

48. Woodhouse, K.A. et al., Investigation of recombinant human elastin polypeptides as non-thrombogenic coatings. *Biomaterials*, 2004;**25**(19):4543–4553.

49. Jordan, S.W. et al., The effect of a recombinant elastin-mimetic coating of an ePTFE prosthesis on acute thrombogenicity in a baboon arteriovenous shunt. *Biomaterials*, 2007;**28**(6):1191–1197.

50. Mitchell, S.L. and L.E. Niklason, Requirements for growing tissue-engineered vascular grafts. *Cardiovascular Pathology*, 2003;**12**(2):59–64.

51. Patel, A. et al., Elastin biosynthesis: The missing link in tissue-engineered blood vessels. *Cardiovascular Research*, 2006;**71**(1):40–49.

52. L'Heureux, N. et al., A completely biological tissue-engineered human blood vessel. *FASEB Journal*, 1998;**12**(1):47–56.

53. Karnik, S.K. et al., A critical role for elastin signaling in vascular morphogenesis and disease. *Development*, 2003;**130**(2):411–423.

54. Hinds, M.T. et al., Biocompatibility of a xenogenic elastin-based biomaterial in a murine implantation model: The role of aluminum chloride pretreatment. *Journal of Biomedical Materials Research Part A*, 2004;**69A**(1):55–64.

55. Hinds, M.T. et al., Development of a reinforced porcine elastin composite vascular scaffold. *Journal of Biomedical Materials Research Part A*, 2006;**77A**(3):458–469.

56. Liu, S.Q., C. Tieche, and P.K. Alkema, Neointima formation on vascular elastic laminae and collagen matrices scaffolds implanted in the rat aortae. *Biomaterials*, 2004;**25**(10):1869–1882.

57. Simionescua, D.T. et al., Biocompatibility and remodeling potential of pure arterial elastin and collagen scaffolds. *Biomaterials*, 2006;**27**(5):702–713.

58. Buijtenhuijs, P. et al., Tissue engineering of blood vessels: Characterization of smooth-muscle cells for culturing on collagen-and-elastin-based scaffolds. *Biotechnology and Applied Biochemistry*, 2004;**39**:141–149.

59. Engbers-Buijtenhuijs, P. et al., Biological characterisation of vascular grafts cultured in a bioreactor. *Biomaterials*, 2006;**27**(11):2390–2397.

60. Buttafoco, L. et al., Electrospinning of collagen and elastin for tissue engineering applications. *Biomaterials*, 2006;**27**(5):724–734.

61. Buttafoco, L. et al., First steps towards tissue engineering of small-diameter blood vessels: Preparation of flat scaffolds of collagen and elastin by means of freeze drying. *Journal of Biomedical Materials Research Part B-Applied Biomaterials*, 2006;**77B**(2):357–368.

62. Buttafoco, L. et al., Porous hybrid structures based on P(DLLA-co-TMC) and collagen for tissue engineering of small-diameter blood vessels. *Journal of Biomedical Materials Research Part B—Applied Biomaterials*, 2006;**79B**(2):425–434.

63. Buttafoco, L. et al., Physical characterization of vascular grafts cultured in a bioreactor. *Biomaterials*, 2006;**27**(11):2380–2389.

64. Vyavahare, N. et al., Elastin calcification and its prevention with aluminum chloride pretreatment. *American Journal of Pathology*, 1999;**155**(3):973–982.

65. Helgerson, S.L. et al., Fibrin. In *Encyclopedia of Biomaterials and Biomedical Engineering*, 2nd edn., G.E. Wnek and G.L. Bowlin, eds. London, U.K.: Informa Healthcare, 2008, Chapter 103.

66. Mosesson, M.W., K.R. Siebenlist, and D.A. Meh, The structure and biological features of fibrinogen and fibrin. *Annals of the New York Academy of Sciences*, 2001;**936**:11–30.

67. Blomback, B., Fibrinogen and fibrin—Proteins with complex roles in hemostasis and thrombosis. *Thrombosis Research*, 1996;**83**(1):1–75.

68. Mosesson, M.W. et al., Studies on the ultrastructure of fibrin lacking fibrinopeptide B (beta-fibrin). *Blood*, 1987;**69**(4):1073–1081.

69. Ferry, J.D. and P.R. Morrison, Preparation and properties of serum and plasma proteins. VIII. The conversion of human fibrinogen to fibrin under various conditions1,2. *Journal of the American Chemical Society*, 1947;**69**(2):388–400.

70. Urech, L. et al., Mechanical properties, proteolytic degradability and biological modifications affect angiogenic process extension into native and modified fibrin matrices in vitro. *Biomaterials*, 2005;**26**(12):1369–1379.

71. Van Susante, J.L.C. et al., Chondrocyte-seeded hydroxyapatite for repair of large articular cartilage defects. A pilot study in the goat. *Biomaterials*, 1998;**19**(24):2367–2374.

72. Meinhart, J., M. Fussenegger, and W. Hobling, Stabilization of fibrin-chondrocyte constructs for cartilage reconstruction. *Annals of Plastic Surgery*, 1999;**42**(6):673–678.

73. Sierra, D.H., Fibrin sealant adhesive systems: A review of their chemistry, material properties and clinical applications. *Journal of Biomaterials Applications*, 1993;**7**(4):309–352.

74. Horch, R.E. et al., Single-cell suspensions of cultured human keratinocytes in fibrin-glue reconstitute the epidermis. *Cell Transplantation*, 1998;**7**(3):309–317.

75. Wechselberger, G. et al., Fibrin glue as a delivery vehicle for autologous urothelial cell transplantation onto a prefabricated pouch. *Journal of Urology*, 1998;**160**(2):583–586.

76. Bach, A.D. et al., Fibrin glue as matrix for cultured autologous urothelial cells in urethral reconstruction. *Tissue Engineering*, 2001;**7**(1):45–53.

77. Wechselberger, G. et al., Successful transplantation of three tissue-engineered cell types using capsule induction technique and fibrin glue as a delivery vehicle. *Plastic and Reconstructive Surgery*, 2002;**110**(1):123–129.

78. van Susante, J.L.C. et al., Resurfacing potential of heterologous chondrocytes suspended in fibrin glue in large full-thickness defects of femoral articular cartilage: An experimental study in the goat. *Biomaterials*, 1999;**20**(13):1167–1175.

79. Ye, Q. et al., Fibrin gel as a three dimensional matrix in cardiovascular tissue engineering. *European Journal of Cardio-Thoracic Surgery*, 2000;**17**(5):587–591.

80. Tholpady, S.S. et al., Repair of an osseous facial critical-size defect using augmented fibrin sealant. *Laryngoscope*, 1999;**109**(10):1585–1588.

81. Fei, X. et al., Effect of fibrin glue coating on the formation of new cartilage. *Transplantation Proceedings*, 2000;**32**(1):210–217.

82. Samii, M. and C. Matthies, Protective coating of cranial nerves with fibrin glue (Tissucol) during cranial base surgery: Technical note—Comment. *Neurosurgery*, 1998;**43**(5):1246.

83. Kobayashi, S., Protective coating of cranial nerves with fibrin glue (Tissucol) during cranial base surgery: Technical note—Comment. *Neurosurgery*, 1998;**43**(5):1246.

84. de Vries, J. et al., Protective coating of cranial nerves with fibrin glue (Tissucol) during cranial base surgery: Technical note. *Neurosurgery*, 1998;**43**(5):1242.

85. Al-Mefty, O., Protective coating of cranial nerves with fibrin glue (Tissucol) during cranial base surgery: Technical note—Comment. *Neurosurgery*, 1998;**43**(5):1246.

86. Carr, M.E., S.A. Sajer, and A. Spaulding, Fibrin coating of bladder-tumor cells (t24) is not protective against lak cell cytotoxicity. *Journal of Laboratory and Clinical Medicine*, 1992;**119**(2):132–138.

87. Schrenk, P. et al., Fibrin glue coating of E-Ptfe prostheses enhances seeding of human-endothelial cells. *Thoracic and Cardiovascular Surgeon*, 1987;**35**(1):6–10.

88. Schuenemann, B. et al., Fibrin coating of the peritoneal catheter as a cause of recurrent peritonitis. *Artificial Organs*, 1981;**5**(4):454.

89. Adachi, M., M. Suzuki, and J.H. Kennedy, Preoperative coating of velour-lined circulatory assist devices with a fibrin coagulum membrane (FCM). *Transactions American Society for Artificial Internal Organs*, 1970;**16**:7–11.

90. Trinick, J., Elastic filaments and giant proteins in muscle. *Current Opinion in Cell Biology*, 1991;**3**(1):112–119.

91. Chaikof, E.L., Materials science: Muscle mimic. *Nature*, 2010;**465**(7294):44–45.

92. Furst, D.O. et al., The organization of titin filaments in the half-sarcomere revealed by monoclonal antibodies in immunoelectron microscopy: A map of ten nonrepetitive epitopes starting at the Z line extends close to the M line. *The Journal of Cell Biology*, 1988;**106**(5):1563–1572.

93. Trombitas, K. et al., Nature and origin of gap filaments in striated muscle. *Journal of Cell Science*, 1991;**100**(Pt 4):809–814.

94. Trombitas, K. et al., Elastic properties of titin filaments demonstrated using a "freeze-break" technique. *Cell Motility and the Cytoskeleton*, 1993;**24**(4):274–283.

95. Trombitas, K., J.-P. Jin, and H. Granzier, The mechanically active domain of titin in cardiac muscle. *Circulation Research*, 1995;**77**(4):856–861.

96. Linke, W.A., V.I. Popov, and G.H. Pollack, Passive and active tension in single cardiac myofibrils. *Biophysical Journal*, 1994;**67**(2):782–792.

97. Lv, S. et al., Designed biomaterials to mimic the mechanical properties of muscles. *Nature*, 2010;**465**(7294):69–73.

98. Wu, Y. et al., Changes in titin and collagen underlie diastolic stiffness diversity of cardiac muscle. *Journal of Molecular and Cellular Cardiology*, 2000;**32**(12):2151–2162.

99. Satoh, M. et al., Structural analysis of the titin gene in hypertrophic cardiomyopathy: Identification of a novel disease gene. *Biochemical and Biophysical Research Communications*, 1999;**262**(2):411–417.

100. Hackman, P. et al., Tibial muscular dystrophy is a titinopathy caused by mutations in TTN, the gene encoding the giant skeletal-muscle protein titin. *American Journal of Human Genetics*, 2002;**71**(3):492–500.

101. Matsumura, K. et al., Immunochemical study of connectin (titin) in neuromuscular diseases using a monoclonal antibody: Connectin is degraded extensively in Duchenne muscular dystrophy. *Journal of the Neurological Sciences*, 1989;**93**(2–3):147–156.

102. Machado, C., C.E. Sunkel, and D.J. Andrew, Human autoantibodies reveal titin as a chromosomal protein. *The Journal of Cell Biology*, 1998;**141**(2):321–333.

103. Greve, B. et al., The autoimmunity-related polymorphism PTPN22 1858C/T is associated with anti-titin antibody-positive myasthenia gravis. *Human Immunology*, 2009;**70**(7):540–542.

104. Seal, B.L., T.C. Otero, and A. Panitch, Polymeric biomaterials for tissue and organ regeneration. *Materials Science and Engineering R—Reports*, 2001;**34**(4–5):147–230.

105. Stankus, J.J., J. Guan, and W.R. Wagner, Elastomers, biodegradable. In *Encyclopedia of Biomaterials and Biomedical Engineering*, 2nd edn., G.E. Wnek and G.L. Bowlin, eds. London, U.K.: Informa Healthcare, 2008, Chapter 86, pp. 484–494.

106. Weis-Fogh, T., A rubber-like protein in insect cuticle. *Journal of Experimental Biology*, 1960;**37**(4):889–907.
107. Charati, M.B. et al., Hydrophilic elastomeric biomaterials based on resilin-like polypeptides. *Soft Matter*, 2009;**5**(18):3412–3416.

Further Readings

Relevant chapters of

Fawcett, D.W. and E. Raviola, *A Textbook of Histology*, 12th edn.

Junqueira, L.C., J. Carneiro, and R.O. Kelley, *Basic Histology*, 9th edn. New York: McGraw-Hill, 1995.

Park, J. and R.S. Lakes, *Biomaterials: An Introduction*, 3rd edn. New York: Springer, 2007.

Young, B. and J.W. Heath, *Functional Histology, a Text and Colour Atlas*, 4th edn. London, U.K.: Churchill Living Stone, 2000.

CHAPTER 18

HISTOLOGY AND TISSUE PROPERTIES II
Connective Tissues

LEARNING OBJECTIVES

After a careful study of this chapter, you should be able to do the following:

1. Describe the constituents of connective tissue
2. Recognize which tissues are connective tissues
3. Describe elasticity of collagen and elastin
4. Understand the difference between synthetic and biological elastomers
5. Discuss potential strategies to reproduce the elasticity of biological tissue from synthetic polymers
6. Understand why cartilage has a poor regenerative ability, while cartilage tissue engineering is most successful
7. Describe bone histology

18.1 OVERVIEW OF CONNECTIVE TISSUES

As briefly described in the previous chapter, connective tissue is a form of support tissue, containing varying amounts of fibrous proteins (collagen, elastin, and proteoglycans) and cells. The matrix structure of connective tissue provides varying degrees of mechanical support to all tissues, depending on the function of the tissue, particularly variable elasticity, fluid content, and porosity. Hence, biomaterials play a major role as a connective tissue substitute. Unlike epithelial, muscular, or nervous tissue, the major constituent of connective tissue is the extracellular matrix (ECM), with the cells that produce this matrix embedded within it. The ECM of connective tissues is what a biomaterial is aimed to replace.

As well as physical support, connective tissue also has a barrier function, which together with resident phagocytic and immunologically active cells contributes to the immune defense of the organism. During infection (foreign bodies) or inflammation (tissue irritation), porous connective tissue (e.g., subdermal layers) is actively infiltrated by leukocytes, which causes local fluid production and short-term swelling. Variable elasticity of connective tissue helps to contain and moderate fluid accumulation. For more serious or larger lesions, fibrous connective tissue is less elastic but is able to regenerate with the formation of *granulation tissue*, which is basically new connective tissue with a regenerated blood supply. This forms in deeper wounds and fills them from the bottom upward.

Most connective tissues originate from the mesoderm, the middle germ layer of the embryo (Figure 16.18). Mesoderm cells differentiate to become the mesenchymal cells, and the tissue they form is called mesenchyme. In developing organs before birth, mesenchyme is also regarded as a connective tissue on its own. In adult tissues, some mesenchyme remains in the undifferentiated state as mesenchymal stem cell populations (e.g., bone marrow stromal cells, BMSCs). These assist in the formation of new connective tissue, where there has been significant loss or dying of the tissue.

18.2 TYPES OF CONNECTIVE TISSUE

The conventional groupings of connective tissue are based on the structure of connective tissue. However, some connective tissues have specialized properties (similar to functional materials), and some have supporting connective tissues (similar to structural materials). In addition, embryonic connective tissues (in embryo) are grouped as a separate type of connective tissue.

18.2.1 Connective Tissue Proper

There are two subclasses of connective tissue proper:

1. Loose connective tissue
   a. Areolar tissue (e.g., subdermal layers)
   b. Mucous tissue (gel-like or fluid-producing tissue, some with high hyaluronic acid content)
   c. Adipose tissue (loose, vascularized tissue with high fat content)
2. Dense connective tissue
   a. Ligament
   b. Tendon

18.2.2 Connective Tissue with Specialized Properties

• Hematopoietic (lymphatic and myeloid) tissue, also called reticular tissue. Specialized loose connective tissue providing mechanical support for bone marrow tissue, spleen, and lymph nodes)
• Blood
• Adipose tissue (also considered a specialized tissue, owing to its functional ability to store fat, a mobilizable energy store)

18.2.3 Supporting Connective Tissue

• Cartilage
• Bone

18.2.4 *Embryonic Connective Tissue*

This type of connective tissue includes two subtypes:

1. Mesenchymal connective tissue
2. Mucous connective tissue

Regardless of how connective tissue is grouped, it is important to remember that connective tissues are highly integrated with all of the other tissue types. Ultimately they *connect* tissue together, allowing a very high degree organization and integration at a structural and functional level. In this respect, all connective tissues can be regarded as having a support role, some with more functional than simply structural support roles.

18.3 CONNECTIVE TISSUE PROPER (SKIN, TENDON, LIGAMENT)

The skin is a good example of a tissue that relies on a connective tissue. Beneath epithelial layers and basement membranes of the skin is a loose connective tissue (Figure 18.1) consisting of

- Epidermal and stromal cells
- ECM:
  - Proteoglycans (nonfibrous gel)
  - Protein fibers
  - Extracellular fluid (aqueous fluid, containing ions and other solutes)

18.3.1 *Cells Present in Connective Tissue*

Connective tissue contains various types of cells, each of which performs specific functions, as summarized in Table 18.1. Those residing within connective tissue include blast cells, plasma cells, adipocytes, and macrophages, whereas the remainder are leukocytes that infiltrate the tissue by crossing over the blood vessels from the blood stream.

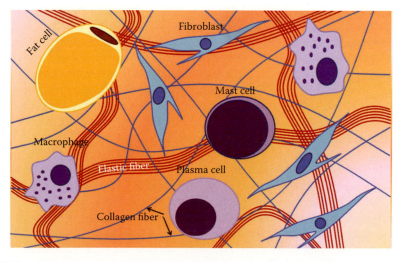

Figure 18.1
Diagrammatic representation of histology of dermis, a loose connective tissue.

Table 18.1

Functions of Connective Tissue Cells

Cell Type	Main Product or Activity	Main Function	Origin
Fibroblasts (e.g., chondroblasts, osteoblasts, odontoblasts)	Production of fibers and nonfibrous gel substance	Structural	Tissue itself
Plasma cells	Production of antibodies	Immunological	Blood
Lymphocytes	Production of immunocompetent cells	Immunological	Blood
Eosinophils	Phagocytosis of antigen–antibody complex	Immunological	Blood
Macrophages, neutrophils	Phagocytosis of foreign substances, bacteria	Immunological	Blood, some resident in tissues
Mast cells, basophils	Liberation of pharmacologically active substances	Immunological	Blood
Adipocytes	Storage of neutral fats, heat production	Energy reservoir, heat production	Tissue itself

18.3.1.1 Fibroblasts and Fibrocytes Fibroblasts (*blast* means *to generate*, fiber-generating cells) are responsible for the synthesis of fibers and nonfibrous gel substances. Fibroblasts are generally in nondividing resting (*quiescent*) state, where they are involved in routine support of fiber integrity and renewal. However, they can begin to undergo a more highly synthetic (*active*) state, where their production of fibrous connective tissue is upregulated. This happens especially during acute tissue damage, where repair processes depend on the production of new connective tissue (e.g., rupture of connective tissue). The term *fibroblast* is also considered to be the more active form of this cell type, with the *fibrocyte* defined as the quiescent form (e.g., osteoblast vs. osteocyte).

Histologically, fibrocytes have less protein synthetic organelles (e.g., rough endoplasmic reticulum) than fibroblasts. Fibrocytes are spindle-shaped cells, randomly embedded within the matrix they have synthesized. When it is adequately stimulated, such as during wound healing, the fibrocyte reverts to the fibroblast state and its synthetic activities are reactivated. In such instances the cell reassumes the phenotype of a fibroblast. Fibroblasts synthesize collagen, reticulin, and elastin, and the glycosaminoglycans (GAGs) and glycoproteins of the intercellular ground substance. Fibrocytes rarely undergo division (mitosis). Mitosis is observed only when additional fibroblasts are required, such as during connective tissue repair.

18.3.1.2 Macrophages As described earlier in relation to the immune system, macrophages are resident to specific tissues, and function to engulf and accumulate foreign substances and bacteria in their cytoplasm in the form of granules or vacuoles. Tissue macrophages can proliferate locally, increasing in number, depending on the degree of infection or inflammation. In specific regions, macrophages have special names (Table 18.2).

Macrophages are long-lived cells and may survive for several months in tissues. When adequately stimulated, these cells may increase in size, or several may fuse to form multinuclear *giant cells, which are usually found under pathological conditions.*

Table 18.2

Macrophages in Specific Tissues

Cell Type	Location	Main Function
Monocytes	Blood	Circulating precursor of macrophages
Macrophages	Connective tissue, lymphoid organs, lungs	Production of cytokines, chemotactic factors, and several other molecules that participate in inflammation (defense); antigen presentation
Kupffer cells	Liver	As per macrophages
Microglial cells	Central nervous system	As per macrophages
Langerhans cells	Skin	Antigen presentation
Osteoclasts	Bone (fusion of several macrophages)	Digestion of old bone during new bone formation
Multinuclear giant cell	Connective tissue (fusion of several macrophages)	Digestion and segregation of foreign bodies

The currently accepted hypothesis regarding the mechanism of phagocytosis is summarized in Figure 16.12b.

18.3.1.3   Mast Cells   Mast cells are oval or round, 20–30 μm in diameter, whose cytoplasm is filled with basophilic granules. The rather small and spherical nucleus is centrally situated. The principal function of mast cells is the storage of chemical mediators of the inflammatory response.

18.3.1.4   Plasma Cells   There are few plasma cells in most connective tissues. They are numerous in pathologic sites.

Plasma cells are large, ovoid cells. The nucleus of the plasma cell is spherical and eccentrically placed. Plasma cells seldom divide; their average life is 10–20 days.

18.3.1.5   Adipose Cells   Adipose cells are connective tissue cells that have become specialized for storage of neutral fats or for the production of heat. Fat stores act as a reserve source of metabolizable hydrocarbons, in the event of dietary deprivation, for example. When glucose and other carbohydrates are in excess of routine metabolism, they are polymerized to form fatty acids, and stored in vesicles inside the adipocytes. This explains why adipose tissue is commonly located near the digestive system. The bone marrow also has a high content of adipose tissue, used to supply energy for the acute regeneration of blood during hemorrhage.

18.3.1.6   Leukocytes   These have been described earlier with respect to cells of the circulatory system. Leukocytes of all different varieties are able to occupy connective tissues from blood, especially areolar and adipose tissue (Table 18.1). Leukocytes cross the endothelial layer of blood vessels by squeezing between the endothelial cells. A specific low-abundance type of leukocyte are plasma cells (derived from B lymphocytes), which circulate in the plasma and are numerous at pathological sites. These cells have a spherical nucleus that is eccentrically placed, and seldom divide, with an average life-span of 10-20 days. When active, plasma cells are known to produce very large amounts of antibody protein, but of a limited type, depending on the foreign particles they encounter.

18.3.2 *Acellular Components of Connective Tissue*

18.3.2.1 Nonfibrous Gel-Like Substance This component of ECM (also called ground substance in histological and electron microscopy tissue sections) is a flexible, amorphous, colorless, transparent material, which has the properties of a semi-fluid gel (a low cross-linked polymer network infiltrated by water). Chemically, it is a complex mixture of proteoglycans (Figure 18.2a) and glycoproteins (Figure 18.2b) that participates in binding cells to the fibers of connective tissues.

Proteoglycans are very high molecular weight fibrous proteins that are heavily glycosylated. The basic proteoglycan unit consists of a *core protein* with covalently attached *glycosaminoglycan* (GAG) chains, a polysaccharide. Figure 18.2c shows eight sugars commonly found in human glycoproteins. GAG chains are electrostatically linked to one another and water molecules to form a hydrogel. The size of the spaces between the GAG molecules and the nature of electrostatic changes determines the permeability characteristics of the support tissue they occupy. This is particularly significant in the structure of basement membranes, which passively filter

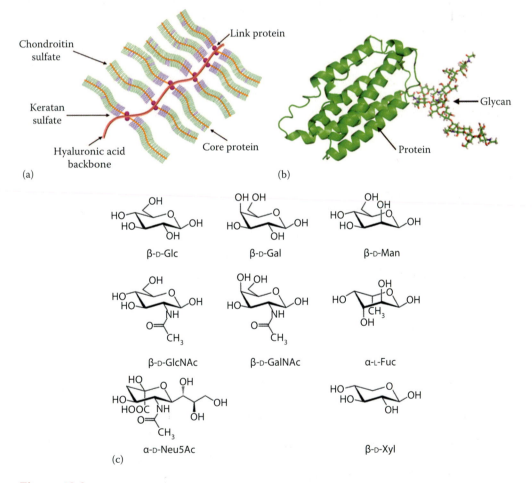

Figure 18.2
Schematic illustrations of (a) proteoglycans, attached to the large cartilage protein, aggrecan. (b) fibrillin glycoprotein. (c) Eight sugars commonly found in human glycoproteins.

diffusible metabolites and ions between blood vessels and specific tissue, such as epithelia. This hydrated state also gives cartilage its compressive properties, owing to its high levels of aggrecan (Figure 18.2(a)), which contains very high densities of GAG chains.

Structural glycoproteins contain oligosaccharide chains (*glycans*) covalently attached to residues on the polypeptide chain. These glycoproteins play an important role not only in the interaction between neighboring cells but also in the adhesion of cells to their substrate. Two most important glycoproteins are fibronectin and laminin:

1. Fibronectin is synthesized by fibroblasts and some epithelial cells. This molecule has binding sites for cells, collagen, and GAGs. Interactions at these sites help to mediate normal cell adhesion and migration.
2. Laminin is a large glycoprotein that participates in the adhesion of epithelial cells to the basal lamina, a structure rich in laminin.

18.3.2.2   Tissue Fluid (Interstitial Fluid)   Connective tissue consists of a small quantity of fluid called *tissue fluid* (interstitial fluid), residing both in the spaces between fibers, and in the hydrated GAGs of the nonfibrous gel. This fluid is similar to blood plasma in its content of ions and low molecular weight diffusible molecules. Like adipose tissue for fatty acid storage, hydrogels of proteoglycans and structural glycoproteins can also act as a water store, conserving water when the dietary supply is limited. This is also as a result of water retention in the venous circulation at these times. The degree of hydration also has a structural effect on the degree of elasticity and compressibility of the connective tissue.

18.3.3   Structural Protein Fibers

Connective tissue fibers are long, slender protein filaments. The three types of connective tissue fibers include collagen, reticulin, and elastin. Collagen is also grouped together with reticulin, because it is basically a cross-linked form of collagen. Both collagen and elastin are the two critical components of connective tissue.

18.3.3.1   Collagen   Among the 28 different types of collagens which are defined according to their specific molecular characteristics and biological roles, there are basically five types:

1. *Collagen I*: skin, tendon, vessels, organs, bone (main component of the organic part of bone). This comprises about 90% of all connective tissue collagen.
2. *Collagen II*: main component of cartilage.
3. *Collagen III*: main component of reticular fibers, found alongside type I.
4. *Collagen IV*: forms basement membrane.
5. *Collagen V*: cell surfaces, hair, placenta.

Collagens can also be broken into the following functional groups:

- Fibril-forming collagens
- Fibril-associated collagens
- Network-forming collagens
- Anchoring collagens

The mechanical properties of collagen will be described in more detail in Section 18.4.

18.3.3.2 Reticular Fibers (Reticulin) Reticular fibers are extremely thin collagen III fibers, with diameters between 0.5 and 2 μm. They form an extensive network in certain organs, for example, smooth muscle, endoneurium, and within the framework of hemopoietic organs, with random alignment and cross-linkages of collagen. They are also found in skin, dentin, and bone.

18.3.3.3 Elastic Fiber System The elastic fiber system is considered separate from collagen and elastin fibers, and a more complex system of variable diameter and orientation fibers present in connective tissues of very specific areas of the body. In general, elastic fiber is composed of the protein fibrillin and elastin. The three types of fibers of this system include the following [1]:

1. *Oxytalan*—short fibers—are a component of the ECM in the periodontal ligaments of teeth. These fibers are elastic-like fibers that run parallel to the tooth surface and bend to attach to cementum. Fibrillin builds the oxytalan fibers, which causes the elastic behavior. They can also be found on the surface of smooth muscles, and are mainly associated with blood vessels. According to the observations under electron microscopy, oxytalan is composed of microfibrillar units, 7–20 nm in diameter with a periodicity of 12–17 nm. These fibers are considered to be an immature form of elastic tissue.
2. *Elaunin*—as a word, elaunin is derived from the Greek verb ἐλαύνω, meaning *I steer*—is another component of the ECM in the periodontal ligament and in the connective tissue of the dermis, particularly in association with sweat glands. They are elastic fibers formed from a deposition of elastin between oxytalan fibers.
3. *Elastin* is a protein of the ECM in connective tissue that is elastic and helps many organs and their tissues (e.g., skin, lungs, bladder, blood vessels, and elastic cartilage) in the body to resume their shape after stretching or contracting [2]. Elastin allows skin to return to its original position when it is poked or pinched. Elastin is also an important component of cartilage in load-bearing organs, such as joints and vertebra, where mechanical energy

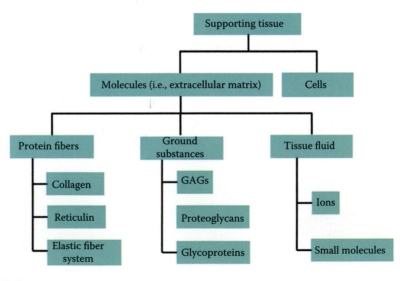

Figure 18.3
Constituents of connective tissues.

is required to be stored. Elastin forms the major component of elastic fibers from the arterial walls and plays an important role in elastic properties of large blood vessels (e.g., aorta). Elastin is made up of simple amino acids, such as glycine, valine, alanine, and proline [2].

Figure 18.3 summarizes the main structural organization of connective tissue.

18.4 MECHANICAL PROPERTIES OF STRUCTURAL PROTEINS

18.4.1 Elasticity of Biological Tissues

Long-term good elasticity is an intrinsic nature of most biological tissues, such as skin, heart, lungs, and bladder. In Section 3.4, the concepts of stretchability and elasticity of materials were described. Generally speaking, a full description of elasticity of any material should include both its measured resilience and rupture elongation values. Resilience is the property of the material to absorb energy after elastic deformation, with partial energy recovery upon unloading.

Since biological tissues have virtually no yield point, quantitative resilience is better described by the *coefficient of restitution*, *R*, which is represented by the ratio of the two areas under the loading and recovering curves in the elastic region of the stress–strain curve (Figure 3.4 and Equation 3.3).

18.4.2 Mechanical Properties of Collagen

Collagen is the main protein of connective tissue, making up about 25%–35% of the total protein in the body. Because of their molecular configuration (Figure 18.4), collagen fibers have a high tensile strength. Consequently, collagen imparts a unique combination of flexibility and strength to the tissues it supports.

Figure 18.5 demonstrates a typical stress–strain curve of tendon, ~86 wt.% of which (in the dried condition) is type I collagen. The reported properties of collagen are mostly in the following ranges:

- Young's modulus (linear region): 1–1.5 GPa
- Ultimate tensile strength (UTS): 100–150 MPa
- Strain at rupture: 10%–20%.

18.4.2.1 Elasticity of Collagen Much literature (including medical textbooks) incorrectly describes collagen as inelastic because it has a smaller elastic strain range (10%–20%), compared with elastin (150%). Collagen is however truly elastic within its rupture strain (10%–20%). Figure 18.6 shows loading–unloading curves of tendon (collagens).

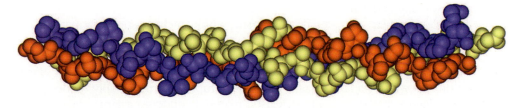

Figure 18.4
Molecular configuration of collagen.

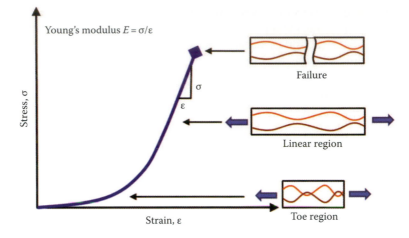

Figure 18.5
Stress–strain curves of collagen.

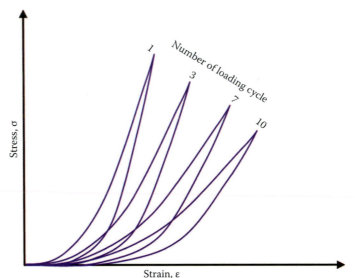

Figure 18.6
Cyclic stress–strain curves of tendon. The stress–strain curves gradually slide to the right, and the peak load reduces. Usually, after 10 cycles, the curves become quite repeatable and steady.

Although the cyclic curves shift down with the increase in the number of cycles, during each cycle the tested sample is completely reshaped to its original length, leaving little residual plastic deformation.

As described earlier, all materials are elastic within their elastic deformation limits. In materials science, *elastic deformation* is defined as a reversible change in the dimensions of a material sample. A *plastic deformation* is a permanent and irreversible change in shape (Figure 18.7). A plastic material, which undergoes a small elastic deformation followed by a large plastic one before rupture, can arguably be described as *inelastic* (Figure 18.8a). In contrast, elastic materials undergo a large elastic deformation, and experience little plastic deformation before rupture (Figure 18.8b and c). Hence, it is appropriate to describe collagen as elastic.

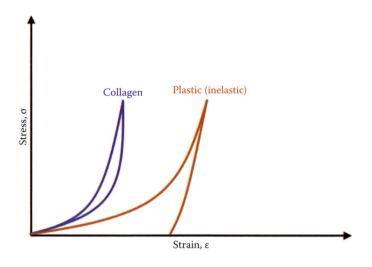

Figure 18.7
Elastic vs. plastic (inelastic).

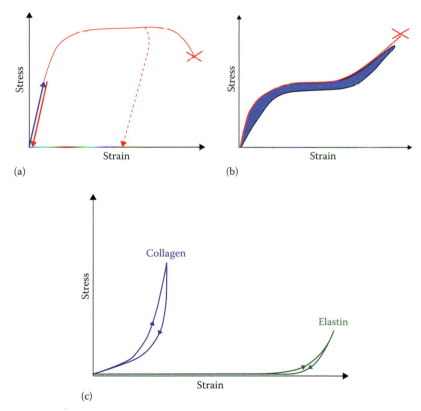

Figure 18.8
Inelastic versus elastic deformation performance of biomaterials. (a) Elastic strain range of metallic materials: <0.2%; thermoplastics: <5%; these experience a large plastic deformation before rupture. (b) Elastic strain range of synthetic elastomer: >100%; these experience little plastic deformation before rupture. (c) Elastic strain range of collagen: 10%–20%; elastin: 150%; these experience little plastic deformation before rupture.

18.4.3 Mechanical Properties of Elastin

Elastin is abundant in large elastic blood vessels such as the aorta, and plays an important role in the elastic properties of connective tissue in the lungs, ligaments, skin, bladder, elastic cartilage, and intervertebral disc. Elastin has an irregular, randomly coiled conformation (Figure 18.9a), formed by the linkage of many hydrophilic molecules of a protein called tropoelastin, to form a massive insoluble, cross-linked array. It is interesting to compare the conformation of elastin to a synthetic elastomer (Figure 18.9b), which is randomly tangled.

Elastin fibers are much softer and more stretchable than collagen, exhibiting a large toe-region in their J-shaped stress–strain curves (Figure 18.8c). As in synthetic elastomers, elastin fiber arrays show a time-dependent elastic behavior (viscoelasticity) and hysteresis.

In Chapter 10, it was discussed that the randomness in molecular conformation contributes to the initial segment of S-shaped stress–strain curves of synthetic elastomers (Figure 10.15), and that an aligned conformation produces J-shaped stress–strain curves. A question that should be asked here is, why is the stress–strain curve of elastin not S-shaped, even though it has an irregular, random conformation? The difference is that in synthetic elastomers, the long polymer chains are tangled together, while elastin is composed of short, cross-linked molecules that are coiled individually. Elastin fibers are also coiled in living tissue, much like titin. During the uncoiling of the short elastin chains, the process does not involve any friction between molecules. In a synthetic elastomer network, it is friction between the linear polymer chains that requires extra stress during the early stage of deformation. Without the friction, the uncoiling of individual elastin molecules can occur easily with little force. Hence elastin is extremely soft in the toe region (Figure 18.8c). Table 18.3 provides typical ranges of mechanical properties of collagen, elastin, and some synthetic materials.

18.4.4 Resilience of Proteins

Table 18.4 provides the resilience values of some proteins. Collagen has a resilience of more than 90%, within its typical 15% stretchability, again indicating that collagen is elastic.

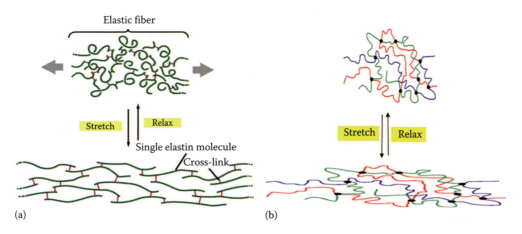

(a) (b)

Figure 18.9

Molecular conformation of elastic fibres made from (a) cross-linked elastin (From Molecular biology of the cell 5/e (© Garland science 2008)) and (b) a randomly arranged synthetic elastomer.

Table 18.3
Mechanical Properties of Collagen and Elastin

Proteins/Polymers	Stiffness *E* (GPa)	Ultimate Tensile Strength (UTS) (GPa)	Strain at Rupture (%)	Toughness (MJ/m³)
Type I collagen	1–1.5	*E*/10	10–20	7.5
Elastin	0.001	0.002	150	1.6
Synthetic rubber	0.001–1	0.002–2	100–1000	100
Nylon	5	0.95	18	80
Carbon fiber	300	4	1.3	25

Table 18.4
Coefficient of Restitution (Resilience)

Proteins	Sources	Resilience (%)
Resilin	Found in the wing hinges of insects	97
Collagen	**Found in tendons, ligaments, skin, etc.**	**90–95**
Elastin	**The main elastic protein of vertebrates**	**90–92**
Spider silk	Capture threads	35
Extreme case	**Perfectly elastic (no hysteresis, no plastic)**	**100**
Extreme case	**Completely plastic**	**0**

18.5   CARTILAGE

18.5.1   General Aspects of Anatomy and Function

Cartilage is a specialized form of connective tissue, usually associated with bone. Cartilage is characterized by an ECM enriched with GAGs and proteoglycans that interact with collagen and elastin fibers. The *firm, gel-like* consistency of cartilage allows the tissue to bear mechanical stresses without permanent distortion. Another function of cartilage is to support soft tissues. Because of its smooth surface and resilience, cartilage acts as a shock-absorber and frictionless sliding area for joints, facilitating bone movements (e.g., knee, hip, and ankle joints). Cartilage is also essential for the development and growth of long bones both before and after birth, during endochondrial ossification, where cartilage centers are converted to bone.

Embedded within cartilage (Figure 18.10) are *chondrocytes*, derived from mesenchymal stem cells (MSCs), which secrete the main protein component of the extensive ECM. The cells are located in cavities within the gel matrix called *lacunae*, and obtain nutrients via passive diffusion. Unlike the other tissue types, cartilage does not have its own blood or nerve supply, so can truly be considered an avascular tissue. There are three types of cartilage:

1. Hyaline cartilage
2. Elastic cartilage
3. Fibrocartilage

18.5.1.1   Hyaline Cartilage   In the unborn fetus, hyaline cartilage serves as a temporary skeleton, which is gradually ossified into bone during the first few years of life.

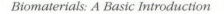

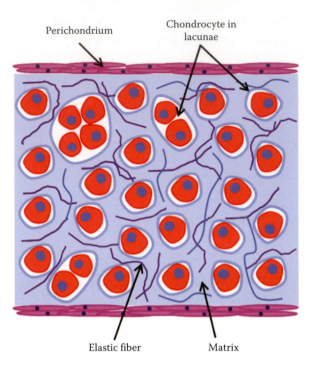

Figure 18.10
Diagrammatic representation of cartilage histology.

In adults, hyaline cartilage is located on the articulating surfaces of the moving joints, in the ventral ends of ribs, where they articulate with the sternum. Hyaline cartilage also forms the epiphyseal plate, where it is responsible for the longitudinal growth of bone, and supports soft tissues of the nose, trachea, bronchi, and large vessels.

A unique type of hyaline cartilage occurs in the central region of the spongy discs between vertebrae of the spinal column. These are also load-bearing joints, with a spongy, inner area (*nucleus pulposus*) of hyaline cartilage, surrounded by a capsule. The main difference is that the ratio of proteoglycan to collagen is 10-fold higher in the nucleus (~30:1) compared to joint cartilage (~3:1), which makes it almost fluid-like.

Except in articulating surfaces of joints, hyaline cartilage is covered by another layer of fibrous connective tissue called the *perichondrium*, which is vascular and can supply some nutrients to the chondrocytes. Hyaline cartilage is also often encased in a fibrous membrane called the *synovial membrane*, which contains fibroblasts that secrete a fluid that lubricates these joints (e.g., knee and interdigital joints). The synovial membrane encases hyaline cartilage in a fibrous compartment called the *joint capsule*.

18.5.1.2 Elastic Cartilage   Elastic cartilage is essentially identical to hyaline cartilage except that it contains an abundant network of fine elastic fibers in addition to collagen type II fibrils. Chondrocytes are embedded in between the elastin fibrils. The most common location for elastic cartilage is in auricle of the ear, Eustachian tube, and the epiglottis (opening of the trachea). Elastic cartilage is highly resistant to repeated deformations.

18.5.1.3 Fibrocartilage Fibrocartilage is a much denser connective tissue than hyaline cartilage, due to its much higher collagen content, and regularly aligned fibers. Thus, fibrocartilage is located where there is a need for tensile support, with limited elasticity. While this type of cartilage contains chondrocytes, they are very often arranged in long rows, interspersed with dense bundles of collagen fibrils, usually spanning short distances. Fibrocartilage forms the outer capsule of spinal discs, and joints between the pubic bones, knee cartilages, and jaw bone to the skull. Interestingly, the spinal disc fibrocartilage fibers are arranged obliquely, rather than perpendicularly, which improves joint mobility and elasticity, especially during torsional movements.

18.5.2 Histology and Structural Aspects of Cartilage

18.5.2.1 Extracellular Matrix of Cartilage Approximately 40% of the dry weight of hyaline cartilage consists of collagen embedded in a firm, hydrated gel of proteoglycans and structural glycoproteins. Hyaline cartilage contains primarily type II collagen. The proteoglycans are noncovalently associated with long molecules of hyaluronic acid, forming proteoglycan aggregates that interact with collagen (Figure 18.10).

In addition to type II collagen and proteoglycans, an important component of cartilage matrix is the structural glycoprotein *chondronectin*, a macromolecule that binds specifically to GAGs and collagen type II, mediating the adherence of chondrocytes to the ECM. The cartilage surrounding each chondrocyte is rich in GAG and poor in collagen, as indicated by its more purple hematoxylin staining, when observed in histological sections. The peripheral zone is called the territorial, or capsular matrix, with intervening areas called the interterritorial matrix.

18.5.2.2 Perichondrium Except in the regions of joint cartilage directly involved in articulation, all hyaline cartilage is covered by a layer of dense connective tissue called perichondrium, as described previously. Perichondrium is rich in type I collagen fibers and contains numerous fibroblasts, as well as a blood supply.

18.5.2.3 Chondrocyte Growth in Cartilage Chondrocytes are usually present as single cells within each lacuna, however they are frequently found in groups of up to 8–10 cells when they are actively proliferating. These groups are called isogenous nests and are typically derived from the one cell, produced from chondroblasts with mesenchymal origins. The growth of cartilage is attributable to two processes:

1. *Interstitial growth*: resulting from the mitotic division of preexisting chondrocytes
2. *Appositional growth*: resulting from the differentiation of some cells residing in the perichondrium (most of these cells are osteoblastic)

In epiphyseal growth plates, proliferating chondrocytes begin to enlarge (hypertrophy) as they move toward the ends of the plates, later becoming osteoblasts.

18.5.3 Repair of Diseased or Damaged Cartilage

Except in young children, damaged cartilage regenerates with difficulty and often incompletely, because it is avascular compared to other connective tissues. *Mesenchymal stem cells* (MSCs, also known as bone marrow stromal cells [BMSCs]) can migrate to sites of bone and cartilage damage, able to differentiate into either chondroblasts or osteoblasts, depending on the specific cellular signals received, at specific locations in joints and cartilage centers. There are also resident osteo- and chondroblasts in these tissues, although these are less effective. In general,

- Differentiation of MSCs in vascularized areas (e.g., bone) yields an osteoblast
- Differentiation of MSCs in a nonvascularized area yields chondroblast and, ultimately, cartilage

18.5.3.1 Articular Cartilage Damage   Cartilage damage can result from a variety of causes, including sudden impact (a bad fall or traumatic sport-accident) or gradual damage (wear over time). Painful inflammatory disease caused by this type of long-term damage to the cartilage is known as *osteoarthritis*. The risk of developing osteoarthritis is increased in patients who are overweight (obesity) or who have had previous surgical intervention of joints, resulting in altered joint mechanics. According to the arthroscopic grading system set up by The International Cartilage Repair Society, cartilage defects are ranked as

- Grade 0: (normal) healthy cartilage
- Grade 1: the cartilage has a soft spot or blisters
- Grade 2: minor tears visible in the cartilage
- Grade 3: lesions have deep crevices (more than 50% of cartilage layer)
- Grade 4: the cartilage tear exposes the underlying (subchondral) bone

Articular cartilage has a very limited capacity to regenerate after injury or disease, leading to loss of tissue and formation of a defect. Low level damage does not repair itself and can often get worse over time. As cartilage is aneural and avascular (lack of nerve and blood supply, respectively), shallow damage (grade 1) often does not trigger pain. However, the small articular cartilage defect could potentially progress to reach the subchondral bone (grade 4). Although articular cartilage damage is not life threatening, it does strongly affect one's quality of life. Articular cartilage damage is often the cause of severe pain, knee swelling, substantial reduction in mobility, and severe restrictions to one's activities.

18.5.3.2 Current Clinical Treatments of Cartilage [3]   The aim of an articular cartilage repair treatment is to restore the surface of an articular joint's hyaline cartilage.

- Nonsurgical treatment
  A number of nonsurgical treatments can help to relieve symptoms of damaged articular cartilage, including physiotherapy, painkillers, supportive devices, and lifestyle changes.
- Surgical treatment
  Surgical treatment for damaged articular cartilage includes the following procedures:
  - Arthroscopic lavage/debridement: is a technique used to flush out pieces of cartilage have become loose in the joint, causing the joint to lock.
  - Arthroscopic chondroplasty: This is an outpatient procedure, which is used to repair a small area of damaged cartilage in the knee. The damaged tissue is removed, allowing healthy cartilage to grow in its place. It is performed through small incisions on the sides of the knee with the aid of a small video camera called an arthroscope.

- Marrow stimulation: involves making tiny holes (microfractures) into the bone beneath the damaged cartilage. This releases the bone marrow from inside the bone and leads to a blood clot forming within the damaged cartilage. The marrow cells then begin to stimulate production of new cartilage. The drawback to marrow stimulation is that the newly generated cartilage is fibrocartilage rather than hyaline cartilage. As fibrocartilage is not as supple as hyaline cartilage, there is a risk that after a few years it will wear away and further surgery may be needed. There is also a risk of osteogenesis rather than chondrogenesis.
- Mosaicplasty: is a technique where small rods of healthy cartilage from the non-weight-bearing areas of a joint, such as the side of the knee, are removed and used to replace the damaged cartilage.
- Autologous or allograft osteochondral transplantation
  - Meniscal transplant surgery

A meniscal transplant replaces the damaged meniscus with donor cartilage.

18.5.3.3 Total Joint Replacement   In cases of severe cartilage damage caused by underlying osteoarthritis, an artificial joint replacement may be recommended to replace the damaged one. Total joint replacement (also called arthroplasty) is the ultimate treatment, including total knee (Figure 4.14) and total ankle arthroplasty (Figure 4.15).

18.5.3.4 Success of Cartilage Tissue Engineering   Over the last decades, research has focused on regenerating damaged joints in vitro. These regenerative procedures are believed to delay osteoarthritis of injuries on the articular cartilage of the knee, by slowing down the degeneration of the joint compared to untreated damage. According to Mithoefer et al. (2006), these articular cartilage repair procedures offer the best results when the intervention takes place in the early stages of the cartilage damage.

Tissue-engineered cartilage in vitro refers to the use of biomaterial scaffolds to direct the differentiation of MSCs into chondrocytes to regenerate cartilage. Because of the avascular nature, cartilage tissue engineering is one of two most successful applications of tissue engineering (already applied clinically). Nonetheless, up to now none of the short- or mid-term clinical results of tissue-engineering techniques with scaffolds have been reported to be better than *conventional* autologous chondrocyte implantation (ACI) [4].

18.6   BONE

Bone is a specialized connective tissue composed of intercellular calcified material (i.e., the bone matrix) and four cell types (~2 wt.% of the total weight of bone):

1. Osteoblasts
2. Osteoclasts
3. Osteocytes
4. Osteoprogenitor cells

18.6.1   Bone Matrix

Inorganic matrix (carbonated apatite, see Chapter 11) represents about ~50 vol.% (~65 wt.%) of the dry weight of bone matrix. Calcium and phosphorus are especially abundant, but bicarbonate, citrate, magnesium, potassium, and sodium are also found. Crystalline HA is the major phase, although significant quantities of amorphous (noncrystalline) calcium phosphate are also present. HA crystals of bone appear as plates that lie alongside the collagen fibrils but are surrounded by ground substance. The surface ions of HA are hydrated, and a layer of water and ions forms around the crystal. This layer, the hydration shell, facilitates the exchange of ions between the crystal and the body fluids.

The organic matter (~35 dry-wt.%) in bone matrix is type I collagen and ground substance. Bone collagen differs slightly from soft-tissue collagen of the same type in *having a great number of intermolecular cross-links*. Ground substance contains proteoglycan aggregates and several specific structural glycoproteins. Some of the glycoproteins are produced by osteoblasts and demonstrate affinity for both HA and the cell membrane; they might be involved in binding osteoblasts or osteoclasts to bone matrix. Bone glycoproteins may also be responsible for promoting calcification of bone matrix. Other tissues containing type I collagen are not normally calcified and do not contain these glycoproteins.

The association of HA with collagen fibers is responsible for the hardness and resistance of bone tissue. After a bone is decalcified by acid treatment during histological processing, its shape is preserved, but it becomes as flexible as a tendon. Removal of the organic part of the matrix—which is mainly collagenous—also leaves the bone with its original shape; however, it becomes fragile, breaking and crumbling easily when handled.

18.6.1.1 Periosteum and Endosteum   External and internal surfaces of bone are covered by layers of bone-forming cells and connective tissue called *periosteum* and *endosteum* respectively. They supply new osteoblasts for repair or growth of bone. The Periosteum consists of an outer layer of collagen fibers and fibroblasts. The inner, more cellular layer is composed of fibroblast-like cells called *osteoprogenitor cells*, with the potential to divide by mitosis and differentiate into osteoblasts. Osteoprogenitor cells play a prominent role in bone growth and repair. The endosteum lines all internal cavities within the bone and is composed of a single layer of flattened osteoprogenitor cells and a very small amount of connective tissue.

18.6.1.2 Types of Bone   Macroscopically, bone tissue is composed of *compact* (dense, lamellar) bone, which occupies the outer cortical area of long bones. This surrounds the *cancellous* (spongy, woven, or trabecular) bone within the center of the bone (Figure 18.11), where the bone marrow can be found. Osteon lamellae within the compact bone (Figure 18.11) are organized in multiple layers, which are comprised of the following (Figure 18.11):

- Outer circumferential lamellae (or simplified as circumferential lamellae)
- Inner circumferential lamellae (or concentric lamellae)
- Interstitial circumferential lamellae (simplified as interstitial lamellae)

Cancellous bone has a porous structure, and thus has a high surface area to mass ratio. The greater surface area in comparison with cortical bone makes cancellous bone suitable for metabolic activity, for example, exchange of calcium ions. The primary anatomical and functional unit of cancellous bone is the trabecula. The surface of trabeculae is covered by a layer of osteoblasts with a few osteoclasts (Figure 18.12). As described in relation to the femoral head earlier on, trabeculae follow stress lines in

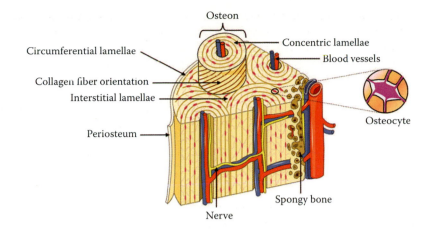

Figure 18.11
Diagrammatic 3D representation of the histology of cortical bone (also called compact, dense or lamellar bone).

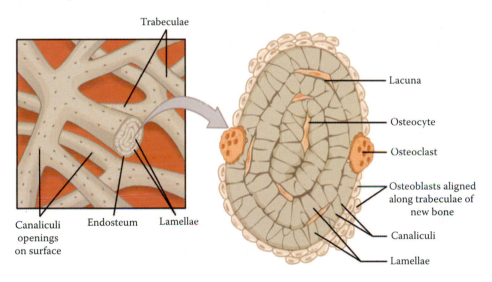

Figure 18.12
Diagrammatic representation of the histology of cancellous bone (also called spongy or trabelular bone).

this are, thus responding to mechanical stimuli. Hence, in people with osteoporosis, trabeculae are thinner and fewer. Cancellous bone is typically found at the ends of long bones, proximal to joints and within the interior of vertebrae (Figure 11.6a). Cancellous bone is highly vascular and frequently contains red bone marrow where hemopoiesis, the production of blood cells, occurs.

Both compact and cancellous bones are also further defined histologically as primary and secondary types.

- *Primary bone* is the first bone tissue to appear in embryonic development and in fracture repair. It is usually temporary and replaced in adults by secondary bone tissue. Primary bone is characterized by random deposition (or irregular

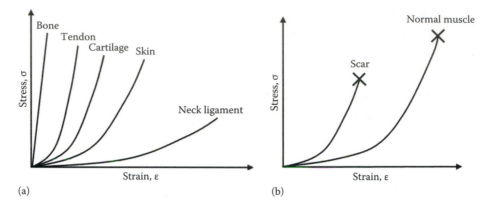

Figure 18.13
Comparison of different connective tissues and scar.

array) of fine collagen fibers. Other characteristics of primary bone tissue are a lower mineral content and a higher proportion of osteocytes than that in secondary bone tissue.

- *Secondary bone* shows collagen fibers and osteocytes arranged in lamellae (3–7 μm thick) that are parallel to each other and concentrically organized around canals (Haversian canals, forming a functional unit called an *osteon*) (Figure 18.13). Surrounding each osteon is a deposit of amorphous material called cementing substance that consists of mineralized matrix with few collagen fibers.

Bones are also classified based on their growth manner. Bones formed by endochondral ossification are called *cartilage bones*, whereas those formed by intramembranous ossification are called *membrane bones*.

18.6.2 Cells in Bone

18.6.2.1 Osteoblasts Osteoblasts are responsible for the synthesis of the organic components of bone matrix (type I collagen, proteoglycans, and glycoproteins) and inorganic components. Osteoblasts are exclusively located at the surface of bone tissue (Figure 18.12). A new bone matrix is secreted at the osteoblast interface with the older bone matrix, producing a layer of new (but not yet calcified) matrix called *osteoid*. This process is called bone apposition, and is completed by subsequent deposition of calcium salts.

18.6.2.2 Osteoclasts Osteoclasts are multinucleated cells, containing as many as 5–50 nuclei. They are derived from the fusion of bone marrow-derived cells of the mononuclear phagocyte lineage. Osteoclasts are responsible for resorbing bone matrix by acid secretion, controlling the production of new bone by osteoblasts.

18.6.2.3 Osteocytes Osteocytes are derived from osteoblasts, and compared to osteoblasts, are almond-shaped with reduced rough endoplasmic reticulum and Golgi complex and more condensed nuclear chromatin. These cells are actively involved in the maintenance of the bone matrix, and their death is followed by the resorption of this matrix. Like chondrocytes in cartilage, osteocytes are embedded within the bone matrix, except that their nutrient supply is derived directly from blood vessels.

Table 18.5
Mechanical Properties of Some Tissues

	Young's Modulus	Strength	Max. Strain (%)
Muscle	0.01–0.5 MPa	0.01–0.05 MPa	~20
Skin (connective)	0.7–16 MPa	~20 MPa	~60
Tendon (collagen)	~1.5 GPa	~0.15 GPa	~15
Bone	~20 GPa	~0.16 GPa	~3

18.6.2.4   Osteoprogenitor Cells   These bone lining cells are essentially inactive osteoblasts. They cover all of the available bone surface and function as a barrier for certain ions. Once the bone is injured, these cells are activated, proliferating and differentiating into osteoblasts.

18.6.3   Mechanical Properties of Bone

The mechanical properties of bone have been discussed in Chapter 11. Table 18.5 summarizes the properties of bone with three representative soft tissues including muscle, skin, and tendon. Figure 18.13 schematically demonstrates the rank of bone and other connective tissues in terms of stress–strain curves.

18.6.4   Bone Growth and Regeneration

In general, *bone growth* refers to the process of young bone ossification and elongation, whereas *bone remodeling* involves replacement and repair during maintenance of bone in adults. As described in Section 13.2.3, bone is formed by either *endochondral ossification* (mineralization of preexisting cartilage) or *intramembranous ossification* (the direct mineralization of the HA matrix secreted by osteoblasts). In both processes, the bone tissue appearing first is woven bone (hence the term *primary*), soon to be replaced by lamellar or secondary bone. Areas of primary bone deposition, resorption, and secondary bone deposition appear side by side, mediated by osteoblasts.

Cartilage formation precedes both forms of ossification, which involves an irregular collagenous network, in growing, remodeling, or repairing bone. Woven bone is then extensively remodeled by osteoclast resorption and appositional growth, gradually converting the cartilage to highly organized osteon structures that are characteristic of lamellar bone.

18.7   CHAPTER HIGHLIGHTS

1. Constituents of connective tissue:

       Cells + ECM (major constituent).

2. Be able to recognize what tissues are connective tissues:
    a.   Dermis (ECM is a soft fiber-reinforced gel)
    b.   Hypodermis (ECM is a soft fiber-reinforced gel)
    c.   Cartilage (ECM is a firm gel)
    d.   Bone (ECM is a hard solid)
    e.   Blood (ECM is liquid)

3. Appreciate elasticity of collagen and elastin:
   Collagen is elastic with a smaller strain range than elastin.
4. Understand the difference between synthetic and biological elastomers:
   Synthetic: long chains are tangled together.
   Biological: short molecules are coiled individually.
5. Understand why cartilage has a poor regenerative ability, while cartilage tissue engineering is most successful:
   a. The progenitor cells (MSCs) of cartilage are located in bone marrow, rather than in cartilage, and cartilage is avascular which means MSCs cannot migrate to cartilage.
   b. However, it is because the avascular nature of cartilage that eliminates, from cartilage tissue engineering, the challenge associated with the development of vascular network, which is essential to engineering of many other tissues.
6. Bone histology:
   a. Compact vs Cancellous
   b. Four types of cells: osteocytes, osteoblasts, osteoclasts, osteoprogenitor cells.

LABORATORY PRACTICE 6

Histological analysis of biomaterials (tri-calcium phosphate or hydroxyapatite) grafted bone defects.

SIMPLE QUESTIONS IN CLASS

1. Which of the following tissues have ECM as its major constituent?
   a. Nervous tissue
   b. Muscular tissue
   c. Connective tissue
   d. Epithelial tissue
2. The categorical relation between enzymes and collagens is similar to
   a. Ceramic and metallic materials
   b. Polymeric and metallic materials
   c. Metallic and composite materials
   d. Functional and structural materials
3. Type I Collagen is (choose the best description)
   a. Elastic with a large strain range
   b. Completely inelastic
   c. Elastic with a strain rage of 10%–20%
   d. Plastic
4. When biomedical researchers say, *Collagen is inelastic*, it actually means
   a. Collagen is plastic.
   b. Collagen has no elasticity at all.
   c. Collagen is less elastic than elastic proteins, having a smaller elastic strain range.
   d. Collagen cannot be elastically deformed.

5. Which of following tissues is avascular?
   a. Nerve tissue
   b. Bone tissue
   c. Cartilage tissue
   d. Heart muscle
6. Cartilage has a poor regenerative ability. The major reason is
   a. A lack of progenitor cells of chondrocytes in the body
   b. A lack of progenitor cells of chondrocytes in the cartilage
   c. Cartilage has no vessels to deliver nutrition
   d. Cartilage has no macrophages to clean the injured tissue
7. Cartilage tissue engineering is the most successful example of tissue engineering. The primary reason is
   a. Cartilage is the simplest tissue to engineer.
   b. The regeneration of cartilage does not need blood circulation.
   c. Cartilage tissue engineering has been investigated longer than any other tissue engineering.
   d. Cartilage disease affects a large population, and thus the research has been strongly supported by governments globally.
8. Which of the following cells are bone-forming cells?
   a. Osteoprogenitor cells
   b. Osteocytes
   c. Osteoblasts
   d. Osteoclasts
9. Which of the following cells are bone-specific macrophages?
   a. Osteoprogenitor cells
   b. Osteocytes
   c. Osteoblasts
   d. Osteoclasts
10. Which of the following cells are bone-maintaining cells in a healthy individual?
    a. Osteoprogenitor cells
    b. Osteocytes
    c. Osteoblasts
    d. Osteoclasts
11. Which of following cells are cells of the body's immune (defense) system?
    a. Chondrocytes
    b. Osteocytes
    c. Fibroblasts
    d. Macrophages
12. Which of the following terms is NOT a name for cells?
    a. Fibroblast
    b. Fibrin
    c. Fibroclast
    d. Fibrocyte
13. Which of the following terms is a name for cells?
    a. Myelin
    b. Fibrin
    c. Osteoclast
    d. Collagen

PROBLEMS AND EXERCISES

1. Describe the components of dermis and the functions of major cell types in dermis.
2. Describe the major histological structure of cartilage.
3. Discuss the reasons why cartilage has poor regenerative ability.
4. To regenerate cartilage, what cells would be ideal? Explain the reason.
5. Marrow stimulation is a treatment of cartilage damage. However, it has a major drawback. Discuss the reason.
6. Discuss why cartilage has a poor regenerative ability, while cartilage tissue engineering is most successful among all types of tissue engineering.
7. Discuss the regeneration capacity of the following connective tissues and the carcinogenicity of the related organs:
   a. Bone
   b. Blood
   c. Cartilage
   d. Dermis
   e. Tendon
   f. Ligament
8. Describe the major histological structures of compact bone and cancellous bone tissues.
9. Describe the four types of cells in bone, including their locations and functions.
10. To regenerate bone in vivo using cell therapy, which type of cells is your choice? Explain your reason.

BIBLIOGRAPHY

References

1. Cotta-Pereira, G., GuerraRodrigo, F., and S. Bittencourt-Sampaio, Oxytalan, elaunin, and elastic fibers in the human skin. *Journal of Investigative Dermatology*, 1976;**66**(3):143–148.
2. Keeley, F.W., Bellingham, C.M., and K.A. Woodhouse, Elastin as a self-organizing biomaterial: use of recombinantly expressed human elastin polypeptides as a model for investigations of structure and self-assembly of elastin. *Philosophical Transactions of the Royal Society of London Series B: Biological Sciences*, 2002;**357**(1418):185–189. doi:10.1098/rstb.2001.1027.
3. Dhinsa, B.S. and A.B. Adesida, Current clinical therapies for cartilage repair, their limitation and the role of stem cells. *Current Stem Cell Research & Therapy*, 2012;**7**(2):143–148.
4. Iwasa, J., Engebretsen, L., Shima, Y., and M. Ochi. Clinical application of scaffolds for cartilage tissue engineering. *Knee Surgery, Sports Traumatology, Arthroscopy*, 2009;**17**(6):561–577. doi: 10.1007/s00167-008-0663-2.

Websites

http://asavory.edublogs.org/2012/11/05/connective-tissues/.
http://classes.midlandstech.edu/carterp/Courses/bio210/chap06/lecture1.html.
http://en.wikipedia.org/wiki/Articular_cartilage_repair.
http://orthoinfo.aaos.org/menus/treatment.cfm.
http://themedicalbiochemistrypage.org/.
http://webanatomy.net/.

http://webanatomy.net/anatomy/histology_printer.htm.
http://www.nhs.uk/Conditions/Cartilage-damage/Pages/treatment.aspx.
http://www.rci.rutgers.edu/~uzwiak/AnatPhys/APFallLect8.html.
http://www.studyblue.com/notes/note/n/bones—cartilage/deck/5438189.

Further Reading

Park, J. and R.S. Lakes, Ceramic implant materials. In *Biomaterials: An Introduction*, 3rd edn. New York: Springer, 2007, Chapter 6.

CHAPTER 19

IMMUNE SYSTEM AND BODY RESPONSES TO BIOMATERIALS

LEARNING OBJECTIVES

After a careful study of this chapter, you should be able to do the following:

1. Describe the immune system, including the organs and cells of the immune system.
2. Describe two types of cells of immune system and their defense roles.
3. Describe wound healing processes of skin and bone.
4. Describe cellular activities of the inflammation phase.
5. Describe systemic reactions: Long-term responses to implants

19.1 IMMUNE SYSTEM

The immune and lymphatic systems are two closely related organ systems that share several organs and physiological functions (Figure 19.1). The immune system is the defense system against *infectious organisms* (such as bacteria and viruses) and *foreign materials*. Through a series of molecular binding and signaling events mediated by circulating blood cells, the immune system can recognize, attach to, and destroy these invasive factors (also called pathogens), preventing local or systemic infection and preventing disease. Hence, in order to understand the body response to an implanted material, it is essential to study the immune system of the body [1].

The immune system is broadly classified into two main subsystems:

1. *Innate immune response*: the first line of defense, based on a learned or pre-programmed, nonspecific reaction to foreign bodies.
2. *Adaptive* or *acquired immune response*: where a new foreign stimulus has been encountered, creating a molecular *memory*, which is stored in the case of a later repeated event.

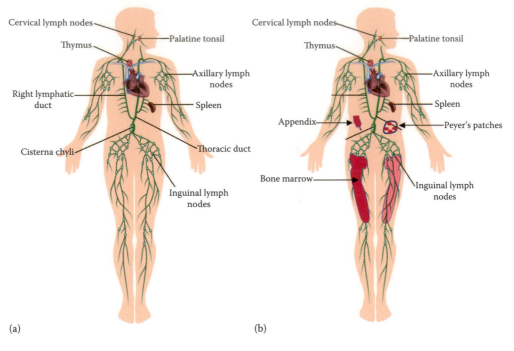

(a)   (b)

Figure 19.1
Comparison of the organs (a) lymphatic and (b) immune system.

Both systems involve highly complex families of soluble molecules that signal between cells and receptors that respond to these signals, presented by immune cells and circulating in the blood plasma. Binding receptors are also present on the surface of these cells, allowing recognition and tagging of pathogens, and binding of cells to these pathogens. All of these signaling events are in turn mediated by the immune cells themselves, which infiltrate tissues on demand [1].

19.1.1 Cells of the Immune System

The immune system is made up of a network of cells, tissues, and organs that work together to protect all other tissues in the body, linked via the blood and lymph vessels (Figure 19.1b). The cells involved are the *white blood cells* (*leukocytes*), which originate in the bone marrow, but are stored in many locations in the body, including the thymus, spleen, and lymph nodes, collectively called the lymphoid organs. Locally, the lymph nodes act as local centers for immune defense, becoming inflamed with excess lymph (interstitial fluid) during localized infections (e.g., swollen tonsils during tonsillitis). In adults, the thymus degenerates from its earlier role during childhood and adolescence, in presenting leukocytes with antibodies, to provide them molecular information about foreign bodies, as they develop a molecular memory [1].

Two basic types of leukocytes are *phagocytes*, cells that consume and digest invading organisms (i.e., phagocytosis, Figure 16.12), and *lymphocytes*, cells that remember and recognize previous invasive entities and destroy them (Figure 19.2). Both cell

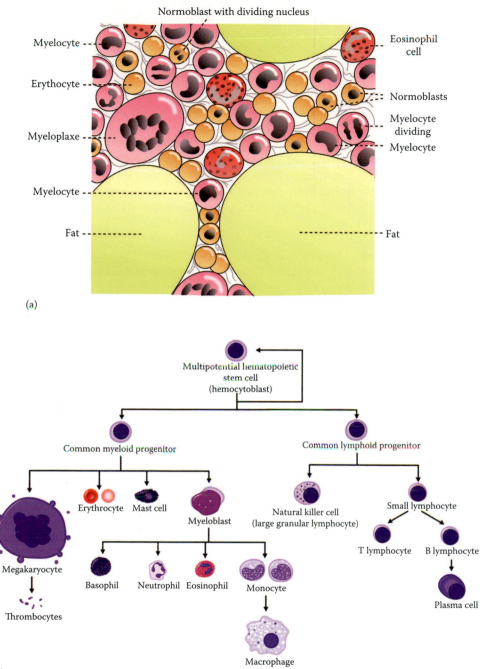

Figure 19.2

Cells of the immune system (a) in bone marrow (Gray's anatomy 72) (From http://commons. wikimedia.org/wiki/File:Gray72.png) and (b) their categorical illustration. (Image:Hematopoiesis_ (human)_diagram.png by A. Rad, linked to http://en.wikipedia.org/wiki/File:Hematopoiesis_ simple.svg.)

types are in the circulation and start to populate regions of infection or inflammation, in response to local signalling molecules that are produced by the affected tissue (e.g., cytokines). The immune cells then proliferate and produce more factors, which mobilize other types of immune cells to the site [1].

19.1.2 Phagocytes

Phagocytes are often described as either *professional* or *nonprofessional*, depending on how effective they are at phagocytosis. The key difference between professional and nonprofessional phagocytes is that the professional phagocytes have molecular receptors on their surfaces that can detect foreign or infectious substances. Phagocytes are crucial in fighting infections, as well as in maintaining healthy tissues by removing dead and dying cells that have reached the end of their lifespan. The professional phagocytes include neutrophils, monocytes, macrophages, dendritic cells, and mast cells (Figure 19.2).

19.1.2.1 Neutrophils Neutrophils are the most abundant type of phagocyte and are normally found in the blood stream. During the beginning (acute) phase of inflammation, particularly as a result of bacterial infection, environmental toxicity, and some cancers, neutrophils are one of the first-responders of inflammatory cells to migrate toward the site of inflammation. Neutrophils are recruited to the site of injury within minutes following trauma and are the hallmark of acute inflammation.

19.1.2.2 Macrophages Macrophages are multinucleated cells, also known as *giant cells*. The major function of macrophages is phagocytosis. They also function as antigen-presenting cells (APCs) (Figure 19.2) because they ingest foreign materials and present these antigens to other cells of the immune system, such as T-cells and B-cells. This is one of the important first steps in the initiation of an immunological response.

19.1.2.3 Dendritic Cells Dendritic cells are professional APCs that have long outgrowths called dendrites, which help to engulf microbes and other invaders. Dendritic cells are present in the tissues that are in contact with the external environment (such as the skin and the inner lining of the nose, lungs, stomach, and the intestines).

19.1.2.4 Mast Cells Mast cells play a key role in the inflammatory process. These cells have toll-like receptors and interact with dendritic cells, B-cells, and T-cells to help mediate responses such as hypersensitivity and allergic reactions. Mast cells can consume and kill certain (gram-negative) bacteria and process their antigens.

19.1.2.5 Eosinophils and Basopils Eosinophils are phagocytic cells that play a crucial role in the killing of parasites, though they have a limited ability to participate in phagocytosis. They are professional APCs and regulate other immune cell functions. Basophils are the rarest type of leukocyte, also involved in acute allergic reactions, mediated by the production of histamine. Eosinophils, basophils, and mast cells are important mediators of allergic responses. They are found in tissues where allergic reactions occur and contribute to the severity of these reactions, such as the integumentary and respiratory systems.

19.1.3   Lymphocytes

Lymphocytes are subdivided into B- and T-lymphocytes (B- and T-cells) according to their functions:

- *B-cells* act as the body's "military intelligence" system, homing to molecular targets and binding to them, via surface molecules
- *T-cells* act as "soldiers", destroying the "invaders", once B-cells have identified them and have been activated after binding and signaling

19.1.3.1   B-Cells (from Bone Marrow)

Foreign bodies (e.g., invading bacteria and cancer cells) contain surface molecules called *antigens*. Following stimulation by phagocytosis of the foreign body, B-cells develop into memory B-cells or antibody-secreting *plasma cells* (Figure 19.3a), as mentioned in Chapter 18. They produce a Y-shaped protein called an antibody (Ab), also known as an *immunoglobulin* (Ig) (Figure 19.3b). *Antibodies* are specialized to recognize and bind to the specific antigens, which act as a tag that other leukocytes can recognize.

19.1.3.2   T-Cells (Produced in the Thymus)

T-lymphocytes are usually divided into two major subsets that are functionally and phenotypically different. *T helper (Th) cells,*

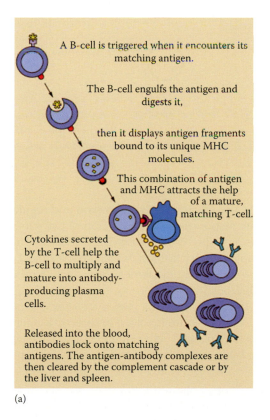

A B-cell is triggered when it encounters its matching antigen.

The B-cell engulfs the antigen and digests it,

then it displays antigen fragments bound to its unique MHC molecules.

This combination of antigen and MHC attracts the help of a mature, matching T-cell.

Cytokines secreted by the T-cell help the B-cell to multiply and mature into antibody-producing plasma cells.

Released into the blood, antibodies lock onto matching antigens. The antigen-antibody complexes are then cleared by the complement cascade or by the liver and spleen.

(a)

Figure 19.3
(a) B-cells label antigens with a Y-shaped protein called an antibody (Ab), which is also known as (b) immunoglobulin (Ig). *(Continued)*

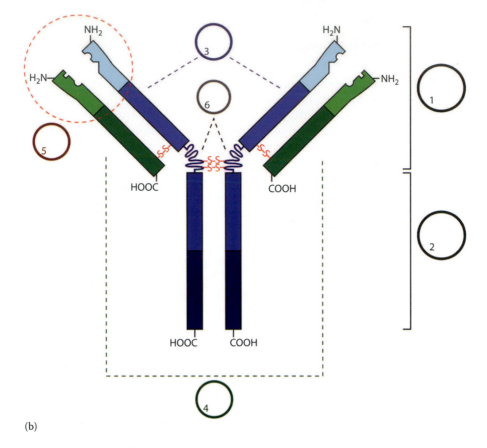

(b)

Figure 19.3 (Continued)
(a) B-cells label antigens with a Y-shaped protein called an antibody (Ab), which is also known as (b) immunoglobulin (Ig). (From http://en.wikipedia.org/wiki/B_cells#mediaviewer/File:B_cell_activation.png).

also called CD4+ T-cells, are involved in coordination and regulation of immunological responses. They mediate responses by the secretion of cytokines that stimulate B-cells to differentiate into plasma cells (Figure 19.4a). They also recognize residual B-cell antigens and bind in a complementary fashion, which enables the T-cells to bind to B-cells and remain localized to them. The cytokines then signal to the B-cells to proliferate and produce more antibodies [1].

The second subset type of T-lymphocytes is cytotoxic *T-lymphocytes (Tc cells or CTLs)* or CD8+ T-cells. These cells are involved in directly killing malignant tumor cells, virus-infected cells, and transplanted cells (Figure 19.4b). They basically treat these cells as not belonging to the body, and therefore the same as foreign bodies.

19.1.3.3 Natural Killer Cells Natural killer cells, known as NK cells, are similar to CTLs, able to directly and rapidly kill certain tumor cells such as those from melanomas, lymphomas, and virus-infected cells. However, unlike Tc cells, NK cells kill their target cells without need for recognition of antigens.

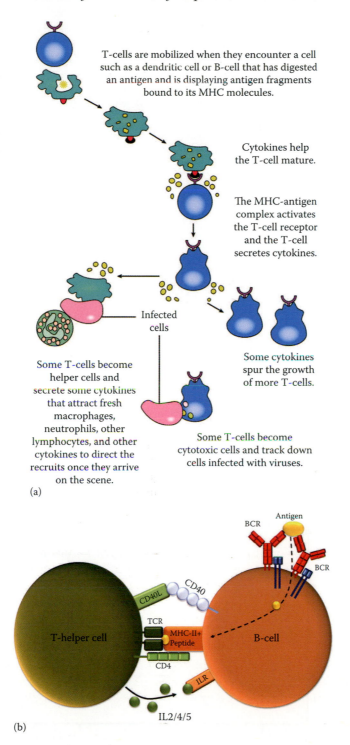

Figure 19.4

(a) T-helper-dependent B-cell activation (From http://en.wikipedia.org/wiki/T_lymphocytes#mediaviewer/File:T_cell_activation.svg) and (b) T-lymphocyte activation. (http://en.wikipedia.org/wiki/File:T-dependent_B_cell_activation.png).

19.2   TISSUE RESPONSE TO INJURIES

The implantation of a medical device always involves host tissue injury. The surgeon first cuts the tissue, and then removes injured or diseased tissues in the process. The knowledge of tissue responses to these injuries, the *normal wound healing processes* in the absence of implants, is fundamental for us to distinguish the normal body response to a tissue injury from a pathological response to an implant [2].

Normal wound healing process involves two distinct phases, the *acute inflammatory phase* and the *remodeling phase* of tissue repair. Depending on the size of injury and tissue type, the inflammatory response may vary. Also, repair of the wound may be prolonged if there is less original tissue. Other factors such as age and preexisting medical conditions can also affect the wound healing process, in terms of the repair rate and scar formation [2].

19.2.1   Inflammation

When tissues are injured, cells adjacent to the lesion respond to repair them. An immediate response to any injury, the *acute inflammation*, is a protective attempt by the organism to remove the injurious stimuli and to initiate the healing process. Where blood vessels have been ruptured, larger vessels will constrict by spasm of arterial smooth muscle, preventing excessive blood loss, while smaller lesions are plugged by fibrin clots during the reaction of circulating clotting factors in the plasma. This is followed by tissue dilation caused by increased permeability of blood vessels to allow more blood to enter the site, once blood loss has been stemmed. The increased permeability also allows plasma to enter the tissues, bringing with it antibodies, and flushes the stimulus from the area.

The classic signs of acute inflammation are pain, heat, redness, swelling, and loss of function. During inflammation, the immune system strongly responds to injury. Typically, neutrophil and macrophage cells appear at a wound site (Figure 19.5), attracted to the area along gradients of cytokines and other secreted soluble factors.

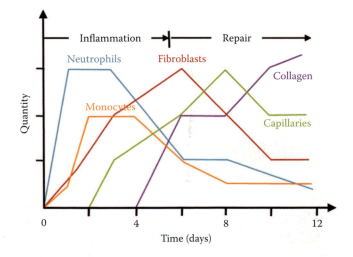

Figure 19.5
Cellular activity during the skin wound healing process.

Once the stimulus has been removed, the acute phase stops. This is partly due to the labile nature of the circulatory molecules that mediate the process. Hence, the acute phase must be sustained over the course of the stimulus/response, until it has been removed or deactivated [2].

19.2.2 Remodeling Phase: Soft Tissue

Following acute inflammation, the repair process mainly involves the restructuring of collagen by fibroblasts. The collagen restructuring process requires more than 6 months to complete, although the repaired tissue at the wound site is never the same as the original tissue, in terms of elasticity and appearance, mostly due to changes in the proportion of collagen relative to elastin and other matrix molecules. This is evident in focal skin scars, where the more strongly elastic collagen applies tension to the surrounding tissues, with radial lines. When the amount of collagen starts to increase, it marks the onset of the remodeling process (Figure 19.5). In deeper and wider lesions, granulation tissue is formed from resident fibroblasts, which fill the wound from the bottom up. In more simple wounds (e.g., cuts), apposed edges of an epithelium will fuse, without further evidence of a scar, depending on the orientation with respect to collagen fibers (i.e., scars after a cut run parallel to the fibers and are less visible than those across the fibers) [2].

19.2.3 Remodeling Phase: Hard Tissue

Bone remodeling is an extremely complicated process. Fibroblasts not only lay down new collagen fibers but differentiate into chondroblasts, which form hyaline cartilage (Figure 19.6). Spongy bone is formed from cartilage by calcification, and compact bone is formed from spongy bone by becoming dense (Figure 19.7). Compared with the formation of bone during development (Figure 19.8), the process of bone healing goes through a very similar chain of events. In brief, the major chain steps of bone remodeling are as follows:

- Collagen deposition and formation of granulation tissue
- Cartilage formation (a firm gel of collagen)
- Spongy (cancellous) bone formation
- Dense (compact) bone formation

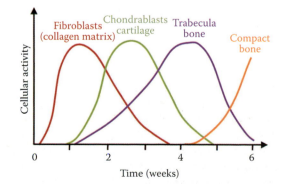

Figure 19.6
Bone remodeling process.

643

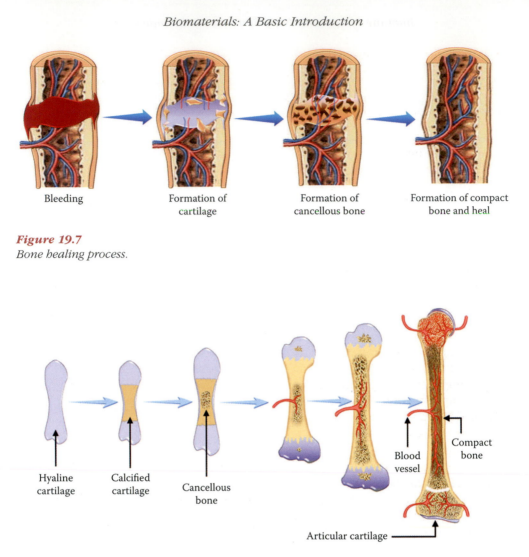

Bleeding   Formation of   Formation of   Formation of compact
                             cartilage   cancellous bone   bone and heal

Figure 19.7
Bone healing process.

Hyaline   Calcified   Blood   Compact
cartilage   cartilage   Cancellous   vessel   bone
                                 bone

Articular cartilage

Figure 19.8
Bone formation (developmental biology).

19.3   BODY RESPONSE TO IMPLANTS

The success of an implant depends on not only how tissues respond to the surgical procedure, but more importantly how on tissues and implants interact. Both the local and systemic responses of the tissues toward implants comprise the most important aspect of the biocompatibility of a medical device, both in the short and long term. Local effects can be both acute and prolonged. For example, implant rejection occurs rapidly, whereas mismatch between the modulus of a THR and the adjacent bone may not be evident for months after a procedure. Systemic impacts are generally more prolonged, often resulting from toxicity of a material that has arisen over time; however, acute toxicity may also occur due to allergic reactions to specific materials (e.g., acrylic monomers) [2].

19.3.1 Local Tissue Responses

The local response of a tissue to an implant varies with the chemical and physical properties of the materials, the physiological conditions (such as pH) of the specific tissue at the implantation site and the localized immune response.

A local tissue response typically falls in one of the following outcomes:

1. Complete biointegration (little or no toxicity or inflammation)
2. Encapsulation
3. Foreign body effect (immune response)
4. Necrosis (toxic effect, followed by tissue death)
5. Carcinogenicity (cancer-causing effects of a material)

19.3.1.1 Biointegration   Several excellent biomaterials are completely accepted by the body and are able to be integrated within host tissue. These materials include hydroxyapatite and related calcium phosphates, bioactive glasses and titanium alloys.

19.3.1.2 Encapsulation   More generally, the body reacts to foreign materials in order to remove them. The foreign material can be extruded from the body if it is movable (as in the case of a wood splinter in the surface layer of the skin). Otherwise, the material may be isolated in the event that it is difficult to dislodge.

If an implant is chemically and physically inert, only a thin layer of collagenous tissue encapsulates the implant. Most ceramic materials, such as TiO_2, Al_2O_3, ZrO_2, $CaO–Al_2O_3$, $CaO–ZrO_2$, and $CaO–TiO_2$, and some inert metals, such as Au, Zr, Ta, and Nb, show minimal local tissue reactions with a thin layer of encapsulation (Figure 6.3).

19.3.1.3 Foreign Body Effects   Many implants are either a chemical or physical irritant to the surrounding tissue, and prolonged inflammation occurs at the implant site. Prolonged inflammation involves the appearance of granulocytes (also known as *polymorphonuclear leukocytes*) (Figure 19.2) near the implant followed by the *macrophages (also called foreign body giant cells)*. As the implanted material becomes broken down into particulates (e.g., wearing debris) or fluids (decomposed polymers), it is subsequently phagocytosed and removed (Figure 16.12). Hence, the appearance of macrophages is a typical indicator of a foreign body effect. Most alloy implants (stainless steels, CoCrMo alloys, and Ti alloys) trigger this type of foreign body response, as do the particulate forms of even some of the more inert polymeric materials.

19.3.1.4 pH Change at Implantation Sites   Implants typically prolong the inflammation phase of wound healing. One mechanism for this is the production of acidic by-products, which can decrease the normal values of 7.2–7.4 to below 5.2 (even as low as to 3.5) at the implantation site. Depending on the type of tissue and wound healing time, this decrease in pH may actually be beneficial, as slightly acidic environments are believed to stimulate fibroblast activity and inhibit damaging proteases. Conversely, high levels of acidity can degrade the natural signaling proteins produced by the healing tissues. In any case, degradation product chemistry and kinetics should be complementary to the molecular process that regulates wound healing, for specific tissue types.

19.3.1.5 Necrosis Some implants may cause necrosis of tissues by chemical, mechanical, and thermal trauma. Alloys with poor corrosion and wear resistances and degradable and toxic polymers can induce tissue necrosis. In addition, incomplete revascularization or other causes of oxygen deficits to a cellularized tissue construct may also result in tissue death by necrosis, leading to implant failure.

19.3.1.6 Local Carcinogenicity It has been found that many polymers produce cancer when implanted in animals, and that the physical form of the implant is important. Sheets or films of many polymers produced cancer when implanted in rats. Fibers and fabrics produced fewer tumors than sheets of the same material, and powders produced almost no tumors. Nevertheless, there are few well-documented cases of tumors in humans directly related to implants. There is also evidence to support the conjecture that carcinogenesis is species-specific and that physical shape of an implant in human tissue does not necessarily influence tumor formation. However, it may be premature to conclude that the latency time for tumor formation in humans may be longer than 20–30 years. In any case, as long as a material may be carcinogenic in animal models, it is still considered carcinogenic in general, which will influence its approval for clinical use by regulatory bodies (see the next chapter).

19.3.2 Local Tissue Responses to Different Materials

The degree of the local tissue responses varies according to both the physical and chemical nature of an implant. Pure metals (except the noble metals) tend to evoke severe tissue reactions, due to their high-energy state or large free energy, which tends to readily oxidize and corrode, strongly reacting with tissue and resulting in rapid necrosis.

Corrosion-resistant metal alloys such as Ti, CoCrMo, and 316 stainless steel have an oxide layer once they are passivated, which is ceramic-like and very inert, showing minimal tissue reactions with only a thin layer of encapsulation or a direct bonding between implant and bone (e.g., Ti).

Most ceramic materials investigated for their tissue compatibility are oxides. These materials show minimal tissue reaction, again with only a thin layer of encapsulation. Carbon implants have similar reactions. Some glass-ceramics show a direct bonding between implant and tissue, in the case of bone repair.

Polymers are quite inert toward tissue if there are no additives such as antioxidants, filters, anti-discoloring agents, plasticizers, and other compounds. On the other hand, monomers and oligomers can evoke an adverse tissue reaction since they are readily reactive. Thus, the degree of polymerization is somewhat related to the tissue reaction. Since complete polymerization is almost impossible to achieve, a range of different sizes of polymer molecules exist, with smaller molecules (oligomers) able to be leached out of the polymer. In particulate form (e.g., powders and granules), very inert polymeric materials can cause severe tissue reactions, likely due to the increased surface area, which promotes increased release of oligomers and monomers, as well as free radical release.

19.3.3 Systemic Impact of Implants on the Body

There are concerns regarding the systemic effects of biodegradable implants such as absorbable sutures and surgical adhesives, and the large number of wear and corrosion particles released by the metallic implants. The latter fact is especially important in view of the fact that the period of implantation is becoming longer as materials are implanted in younger patients.

19.3.3.1   Metal and Trace Additive Allergy   The elevated ion concentration in various organs may interfere with normal physiological activities. Divalent metal ions may, for example, inhibit the activities of various enzymes. Release of Ni and Cr from CoCrMo or NiTi implants can have long-term adverse effects in some patients, including painful muscle fatigue and cramps, dyspnea, decline in cognitive function, memory difficulties, depression, severe headaches, anorexia, and weight loss. The psychological effects are possibly due to accumulation of metal ions in the peripheral and central nervous systems.

Polymeric materials contain additives that cause systemic reactions to a greater degree than the bulk polymer itself. Even the well-tolerated polymer dimethylsiloxane (PDMS) contains a filler, silica powder, to enhance its mechanical properties. Although the bulk material itself is generally nonreactive to most tissues, silica powder itself is an irritant when implanted in a concentrated area, and can induce a systemic immune reaction as shown recently [3].

19.3.3.2   Carcinogenicity in Other Tissues   A variety of chemical substances in implants are known to induce cancers in human tissues, via entry into the circulation, ingestion, inhalation, or direct tissue contact. Usually, the chemical nature of the compound causes it to either mutate DNA or interfere with signaling and metabolic pathways, which induces cancer phenotypes in normal cells. Some metals, notably Cr and Ni, can be carcinogenic systemically in this way. Materials are therefore considered carcinogenic if they contain components that are potentially carcinogenic. In these cases, the risk would be greater in proportion to the surface area exposed, which is greatest for fine powders.

19.3.4   Blood Compatibility

The most important requirement for *blood-interfacing implants* (e.g., artificial blood vessels) is blood compatibility, with blood coagulation (thrombogenicity) being the most important factor. The implant should not damage proteins, enzymes, or blood cells/platelets. However, there are several factors involved in the modulation of blood coagulation.

19.3.4.1   Thrombogenicity

1. *Surface roughness*: A rough surface promotes faster blood coagulation than a highly polished surface of glass, PMMA, polyethylene, and stainless steel, due to adhesions formed by fibrous clotting proteins. Sometimes, thrombogenic materials with rough surfaces are used to promote clotting in porous interstices to prevent initial leakage of blood, and to allow tissue ingrowth through the pores of vascular implants at later stages.
2. *Surface wettability*: Hydrophobicity has been postulated to be an important factor. However, the wettability parameter (indicated by contact angle with liquids) does not correlate consistently with the blood clotting time.
3. *Surface electrical nature*: Since blood cells have a net negative charge on their membrane surfaces, negatively charged surfaces have low thrombogenicity (thromboresistant).

4. *Surface chemical nature*: The chemical nature of a material surface interfacing with blood is closely related to the electrical nature of the surface. The type of functional groups of a polymer determines the net surface charge.

19.3.4.2   Thromboresistance

1. *Heparin and other biological coatings*: Implant materials with heparin coatings show a significant increase in thromboresistance compared with untreated materials, due to their net negative surface charge. Many polymers have been heparinized, including polyethylene and silicone rubber. This reduces the tendency of initial bleeding through the fabric, and a thin neointima is later formed. Some studies also describe the testing of cardiovascular implant surfaces with other biological molecules such as albumin and gelatin. Vascular grafts coated with inert materials such as carbon, by methods such as ultra-low-temperature isotropic (ULTI) pyrolytic deposition, show excellent compatibility, and are widely used for artificial hearts.

2. *Surfaces coated with anionic radicals*: Addition of a single electron to a neutral (uncharged) molecule generates a unique chemical species, called an *anion radical* (or *radical anion*) that simultaneously has a unit of negative charge and an unpaired electron. An example of a non-carbon radical anion is the superoxide anion, formed by transfer of one electron to an oxygen molecule. Anion radical is a type of antimicrobial agent. An *antimicrobial surface* contains an antimicrobial agent that inhibits or reduces the ability of microorganisms to grow on the surface of a material. The most common and most important use of antimicrobial coatings has been in the healthcare setting for sterilization of medical devices to prevent hospital-associated infections. (e.g. Au with charge amine groups, $AgNO_3^-$ nanoparticles etc.)

3. *Inert surfaces*: Hydrogels of both hydroxyethyl methacrylate and acrylamide are classified as inert materials since they contain neither anionic radicals nor negatively charged surfaces.

4. *Solution-perfused surfaces*: Perfusion of water (saline solution) through the interstices of a porous material that interfaces with blood is a new approach to preventing blood coagulation. This has the advantage of avoiding damage to blood cells; however, blood plasma is diluted locally and the treatment is only temporary.

19.4   CHAPTER HIGHLIGHTS

1. Two types of immune cells: phagocytes and lymphocytes.
2. Their defense roles:
   a. Phagocytes: consume pathogens
   b. Lymphocytes: B-cells: "intelligence"
       i. T-cells: kill or help to kill
3. The wound healing process of skin and bone.
   Two distinct phases:
   a. The inflammatory phase
   b. The repair (remodeling) phase

4. Skin healing: inflammation followed by the restructuring of collagen.
5. Bone healing: inflammation followed by the restructuring of collagen (the formation of cartilage), then the formation of spongy bone, and finally dense bone.
6. Cellular activity of inflammation phase.
   a. Dilatation of blood capillaries, the leakage of fluids from blood capillaries, and plug of the damaged lymphatics.
   b. Cells of the immune system (typically neutrophils and macrophages) appear at a wound site.
7. Body responses to implants: to reject them.
   a. The foreign material can be extruded from the tissue if it can be moved (as in the case of a wood splinter) or walled off it is immobile.
   b. If the material is particulate (e.g. from wearing debris) or fluid (e.g. polymer degraded polymers), it can be removed after ingestion by giant cells (macrophages).
8. Effects of implants on wound healing and body.
   a. Intensification of (acute) inflammation
   b. Prolonged inflammation (chronically)
   c. Severe tissue destruction
   d. pH change
   e. Systemic toxicity
   f. Carcinogenic

ACTIVITIES

Study the immune system online via http://www.innerbody.com/image/lympov.html.

SIMPLE QUESTIONS IN CLASS

1. Which of the following organs belongs to the immune system only?
   a. Spleen
   b. Heart
   c. Lymph vessels
   d. Tonsils
   e. Thymus
   f. Appendix
   g. Bone marrow
   h. Thoracic duct
2. Which of the following organs belongs to the lymphatic system only?
   a. Spleen
   b. Heart
   c. Tonsils
   d. Thymus
   e. Appendix
   f. Bone marrow
   g. Lymph nodes
   h. Thoracic duct

3. Which of the following organs belongs to both lymphatic and immune systems?
    a. Spleen
    b. Heart
    c. Tonsil
    d. Thymus
    e. Appendix
    f. Bone marrow
    g. Lymph nodes
    h. Thoracic duct
4. Which of the following cell types is the hallmark of acute inflammation?
    a. Macrophages
    b. Master cells
    c. Lymphocytes
    d. Neutrophils
    e. Eosinophils and basophils
5. Which of the following descriptions is incorrect for B-cells?
    a. They act as the body's *intelligence* system.
    b. They label the foreign invaders for T-cells to kill.
    c. They kill bacteria and fungi.
    d. They are produced in the bone marrow.
6. Which of the following descriptions is incorrect for T-cells?
    a. They act as soldiers of the defense system of the body.
    b. They label the foreign invaders so as to kill them.
    c. They kill bacteria and fungi.
    d. They are produced in the thymus.
7. Which of the following reactions are systemic impacts of implants?
    a. Necrosis
    b. Cancer development
    c. Encapsulation
    d. Allergy
8. Which of the following reactions are local impacts of implants?
    a. Biointegration
    b. Cancer development
    c. Allergy
    d. Encapsulation

PROBLEMS AND EXERCISES

1. Discuss the relationships between the immune and lymphatic systems.
2. Describe the major cellular activities during the wound healing process.
3. Describe the relationships between B- and T-cells in the lymphatic system.
4. Describe the major stages of the skin healing process.
5. Describe all the possible immune responses of the body to an inert implant.
6. Describe all the possible immune responses of the body to a degrading implant.
7. Describe the three stages of bone development.
8. Describe the three stages of the bone healing process.
9. Describe the major roles of B- and T-lymphocytes in the immune system.
10. Describe three major systematic reactions of a living body to a metallic implant.

BIBLIOGRAPHY

References

1. Sell, S., *Immunology, Immunopathology, and Immunity*, 4th edn. New York: Elsevier Science Ltd., 1987.
2. Park, J. and R.S. Lakes, Chapter 10: Tissue response to implants. In *Biomaterials: An Introduction*, 3rd edn. New York: Springer, 2007.
3. Hirai, T. et al., Amorphous silica nanoparticles size-dependently aggravate atopic dermatitis-like skin lesions following an intradermal injection. *Part Fibre Toxicology*, 2012 Feb 2;**9**:3. doi:10.1186/1743-8977-9-3.

Websites

http://www.innerbody.com/image/lympov.html.
http://www.niaid.nih.gov/topics/immuneSystem/Pages/structureImages.aspx.

Further Readings

Black, J. and G. Hastings, *Handbook and Biomaterials Properties*. London, U.K.: Chapman & Hall, 1998, Part III, Chapters 1–7.
Park, J. and R.S. Lakes, Chapter 10: Tissue response to implants. In *Biomaterials: An Introduction*, 3rd edn. New York: Springer, 2007.
Sell, S., *Immunology, Immunopathology, and Immunity*, 4th edn. New York: Elsevier Science Ltd., September 1987.

EVALUATION AND REGULATION OF MEDICAL DEVICES

CHAPTER 20

EVALUATION OF BIOMATERIALS

LEARNING OBJECTIVES

After a careful study of this chapter, you should be able to do the following:

1. Describe all aspects of evaluation.
2. Be familiar with the major systems of standards.
3. Know how to schedule testing of new biomaterials.
4. Understand what a control is and know how to choose a control.
5. Understand and conduct cytotoxicity testing.

20.1 OVERVIEW OF BIOMATERIALS EVALUATION

Evaluation of a biomaterial destined for medical uses involves validation of both the materials properties and biological effects. Characterization of structures and measurement of the material properties is established in the materials field, while biological assessment is performed in the laboratory (in vitro), in animal models (in vivo), in humans (clinical trials), and in postimplantation follow-up studies [1,2].

20.1.1 Evaluation in the Context of Materials Science and Engineering

The structure and properties of a material are generally different at the surface and within the material (Figure 20.1). The most frequently conducted characterization of bulk and surface properties of materials is listed in Table 20.1.

20.1.2 Evaluation of Biomaterials in the Context of Biotechnology

Biological validation of biomaterials starts with in vitro assessments, followed by animal studies and ultimately clinical trials in humans in that specific order, before they are suitable for clinical use, as summarized in Table 20.2. To save time, biological and materials-based evaluation can be performed in parallel in their respective wet laboratories.

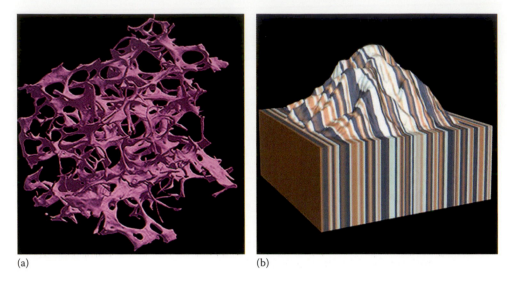

(a)   (b)

Figure 20.1
(a) Tomography and (b) topography.

Also, preliminary information from CAS numbers of individual components may provide some indication of whether there has been some previous testing of the raw materials used in products with probable processing.

20.2 STANDARDS

20.2.1 What Are Standards?

Standards are used in almost all aspects of our life, from the building of houses, production of foods and medicines, making of clothes, and manufacture of various implements and electronic devices to large industrial equipment and public facilities. Why do we need them? Rather than asking why we need standards, we might usefully ask ourselves what the world would be like without standards. Products might not work as expected. They may be of inferior quality and incompatible with other equipment; in fact they may not even connect with them, and in extreme cases, nonstandardized products may even be dangerous or fatal. Plugs and sockets (Figure 20.2) are a good example of the risks caused by lack of a uniform standard.

In industries, manufacturing to defined standards enables maintenance of the consistency of a mass-produced item, to avoid deviation from its original specifications. This involves not only strict quality control through product testing to within nominal ranges but also the maintenance of the standard testing procedures (e.g., calibration of equipment, diagnostics, etc.). For product development, standards are also necessary to enable effective comparisons between older and newer designs or formulations.

The same principles apply to biomaterials, although the product in this case is more difficult to manufacture and test, with multiple time-consuming steps in both processes. Material properties can also vary significantly with the testing conditions, so they can only be effectively compared under standardized testing procedures. As a result, standardized production and testing techniques are widely accepted, commonly

Table 20.1

Major Aspects of Characterization of Materials and Typical Techniques

Bulk characterization methods

Mechanical characterization

    Static testing: tensile, compression, bending, or torsion

    Dynamic testing: creep and fatigue

    Impact testing: impact strength and fracture toughness

    Hardness testing

    Wear/friction testing

Physical properties include

    Density

    Melting temperature (DSC)

    Glass transformation temperature (DSC)

    Molecular weight and distribution (GPC)

    Thermal properties

    Electric properties

    Magnetic properties

    Optical properties (color, opacity, etc.)

    Porosity

    Particle size and distribution (drug delivery)

Chemical characterization

    Chemical composition (x-ray, NMR, EDX, etc.)

    Corrosion kinetics

    Degradation kinetics

    Chemical bonding (FTIR, Raman, mass spectrum, etc.)

Structure characterization

    Macrostructure

    Tomography (of a 3D porous network, Figure 20.1a)

    Microstructure

    Crystalline structure

    Electronic structure

Surface characterization

Surface *topography* (surface shape and features, Figure 20.1b) (SEM, Zygos)

Surface atomic structure (AFM)

Surface composition (XPS, ESCA, AES, SIMIS)

Surface wettability (water contact angle)

trusted, and highly valued. There is far more stress on standards to ensure the safety of biomaterials developed for tissue engineering applications, with the degree of testing dependent on the class of device or implant.

Standards are documented agreements containing technical specifications and practices, or other precise criteria to be used consistently as rules, guidelines, or definitions of characteristics. They ensure that materials, products, processes, and services are fit for their end purpose.

Table 20.2
Biological Evaluations of Biomaterials and Medical Products

In vitro assessment
  1. Cytotoxicity
  2. Cell proliferation
  3. Histochemistry
  4. Cytochemistry
  5. Immunocytochemistry

In vivo evaluation
  1. Various imaging assessments
  2. Various biochemical assessments (histochemistry, cytochemistry, immunocytochemistry), physiological and pathological techniques monitoring organ functions
  3. Patient feedback postoperatively

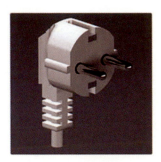
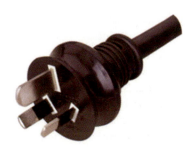
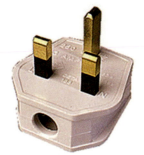
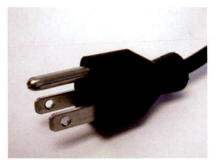

Figure 20.2
Plugs of different countries.

20.2.2 Major International Standardization Organizations

There are many international organizations associated with standardizing science and engineering, including

- International Organization for Standardization (ISO) (*Note:* not IOS)
- International Electrotechnical Commission (IEC)
- International Telecommunication Union (ITU)
- American Society for Testing and Materials (ASTM), an international organization that develops and publishes standards for materials.

Table 20.3

Standardization Organizations Related to Biomaterials Evaluation

Bulk characterization	}ASTM, ISO
Surface characterization	
In vitro biological assessment	}ISO
In vivo evaluation	

20.2.2.1 Standards of Biomaterials Evaluation   ASTM and ISO standards are both widely used in the evaluation of materials properties, with the former being more popular in the United States, and the latter dominant in Europe. Biological evaluation of biomaterials is primarily standardized by ISO (Table 20.3).

20.2.3 Reference Materials (Controls)

A convenient way to measure the quality of a new product is to compare it with an existing reference product with well-established parameter values. This reference material is typically called the *control*. The so-called *Standard reference materials (SRMs)* are thoroughly characterized and controlled for composition and reproducibility of processing. SRMs are available from authorities such as the National Institute of Standards and Technology (NIST), but are expensive and may not be available in sufficient quantities for many analyses or tested properties.

There are actually other options to obtaining controls, as long as a material satisfies some of the following criteria. In general, control materials must be

- Chemically and physically homogeneous
- Chemically stable or preservable
- Able to be made with reproducible properties
- Of similar physical features to tested samples (e.g., porous, fibrous, sheet, or gel)
- Present in sufficient quantities

Any material that satisfies the aforementioned criteria is a good candidate for a control sample. In practice, researchers often use reputable, clinically applied biomaterials as controls, such as titanium, HA, PLA, PGA, and PLGA.

20.2.3.1 Blood–Material Interaction Studies   SRMs selected by NHLBI (National Heart, Lung and Blood Institute) include

- Low-density polyethylene (LDPE)
- Polydimethylsiloxane (PDMS)
- Fluorinated ethylene propylene (FEP)

Other recommended reference materials for blood material interactions include:

- *Pyrolytic carbon*: This is low temperature isotropic (LTI) pure carbon, polished to a smooth surface finish with 0.25-micron diamond dust.
- *Metals*: A large number of metals could serve well as reference materials, for instance, the more corrosion-resistant stainless steels, the CoCr alloys, and titanium.
- *Ceramics*: Calcium hydroxylapatite (HA) is an obvious choice as a reference material.

- *Stabilized tissue*: Biological tissue materials currently used in medical devices would fill the need for reference materials. Stabilized tissue materials include
  - Pericardium
  - Porcine heart valves
  - Bovine heterografts
  - Human umbilical cord vein grafts marketed by cardiovascular devices companies.

20.2.4 Sterilization Practices

There are a variety of sterilization methods using physical and/or chemical agents which can be considered suitable for a particular device. Sterilization effects must be considered immediately after treatment, and for extended storage periods afterwards.

20.2.4.1 Choice of Sterilization Methods Design requirements of sterilization can be found outlined in the quality and sterilization standards of ISO, regulations published by the US Food and Drug Administration (FDA) regulations, and the guidelines of Good Manufacturing Practice (GMP). Here in Australia, there are also various standard procedures for sterilization of devices and materials used for medical and surgical procedures, published by Standards Australia.

Sterilization methods include the following treatments:

- Radiation (x-ray, UV)
- Heated steam, typically 121°C–133°C (autoclave)
- Dry heat (~180°C for specific times)
- Liquid chemical (70% alcohol–water solution)
- Plasma irradiation
- Gas treatment (ozone, H_2O_2, ClO_2, or EtO)

20.3 TOXICOLOGICAL EVALUATION

Toxicological testing may be referred to as either *toxicity tests* or *safety tests* based upon the specific approaches and goals, with the latter also including material processing, handling, storage and implantation procedures, beyond just the effects of the implanted material on the tissue. If consideration of the biocompatibility of a material is ignored in the early phases of planning or development, it could be very expensive to rectify the problem, resulting in considerable loss of time for the developer.

Toxicological evaluation of candidate biomaterials is an extremely important part of their development for biomedical applications. It is best to start by determining the toxicological profile of a new biomaterial or device, just as it would be for a new drug, in order to ensure compatibility of the biomaterials with the biological environment in which they are to be used.

When considering benefits versus risks for biomedical devices, it is not adequate simply to consider them in terms of whether the risks to the patient are greater if the device is used or not, but rather in terms of whether or not *the device produces the* maximum *benefit to the patient with a* minimum *of risk,* using existing treatment strategies. Note, however, that absolute safety cannot be guaranteed in any case.

20.3.1   Scheduling of Testing

To emphasize again, *biocompatibility is the first consideration in developing new bio-materials*. The following schedule is a basic stepwise guide to validation of a candidate biomaterial:

1. The material should be evaluated in an appropriate series of tests to obtain a multifactorial *toxicological profile*:
   a. *Outcome 1*: The material is toxic. Re-design or modify the existing material (e.g., processing conditions or surface treatment) to improve its biocompatibility.
   b. *Outcome 2*: The material is nontoxic within nominal values. Once evaluated to be suitable after redesign or modification, the fabrication of a biomedical item may proceed.
2. *Identify a probable application* for the nontoxic material. While a more logical approach would be to begin with the application and working backward to define which material would be suitable, the reverse is more common in tissue engineering, with a single material usually identified to be useful for many applications.
3. *Optimize the design and manufacturing* needs of the material for the application(s) identified. This may include fine-tuning the material properties, configuration for specific tissues, inclusion of cells or drugs, use of biological molecules, ECM, etc.
4. *In vitro and preclinical testing* of the material. The last preclinical phase involves preparing the material for its device configuration. Once the item is in its finished form, it should again be subjected to toxicological evaluation to ensure that the procedures involved in its fabrication, sterilization, etc., have not introduced substances or modified the material in such a way that the biocompatibility of the original material has been altered (e.g., sterilization treatment of the material may have caused changes in the surface chemistry or topography, which may result in surface erosion after implantation). The evaluation for toxicity and/or safety should always start with animal models that mimic, as much as possible, the clinical application of the device.

20.3.2   Causes of Toxicity Problems

Both chemical and physical factors, alone or in combination, may play a role in the toxicity of a material, with the usual causes for biological incompatibility being:

- Biologically active leachable substances (e.g., unreacted monomers in polymers)
- Biodegradation of the material (e.g., overdose of trace elements, excess acidity or alkalinity)
- Physical contact of the material (particularly with regard to thrombosis and cancer induction following direct tissue–material interactions)
- Physical damage of the material (fragments, surface erosion products, etc.)

Most cases of acute biological incompatibility appear to be due to the release of one or more substances (called leachates or *leachables*) into the biological system. Toxic leachables may also be due to sterilization residues or degradation products produced by excessive heat or radiation of some materials. Since toxic leachables are most often responsible for adverse effects noted in short-term screening tests, it may be possible to clean up the existing material to eliminate this aspect of its toxicity. This involves identifying the leachable and/or its source, so as to prevent its occurrence or remove it from the material. Depending upon the leachable and its source, *it may be necessary to alter the processing by*:

- Using more highly purified starting materials
- Modifying the formulation
- Employing better stoichiometric synthesis
- Preventing extraneous contamination during the manufacturing process

20.3.2.1 Leaching from Polymers The presence of biologically active leachables in a polymer is the most frequent cause for acute incompatibility of this type of material in biological systems, mainly because of their solubility in aqueous environments. Sources of leachables in polymers include

- *Intentional additives*: plasticizers, stabilizers, colorants, radiopaques, ultraviolet (UV) absorbants, residual monomers, incompletely polymerized molecules and polymerization initiators
- *Unintentional additives:* contaminants from impure starting materials, sterilant residues, and products of polymer degradation

20.3.2.2 Sterilization by-products Selection of an appropriate sterilization method is of prime importance. If an inappropriate method is used, or if it is simply not used properly, a biologically compatible device may become one that is physically and biologically unacceptable. This is one reason why a finished device should be evaluated for toxicity even if previous tests have indicated that all of its component materials were suitable. Details of the CAS numbers of each component of the material will provide further information of their specific short- and long-term chemical stability and biohazard information.

20.3.2.3 Drug–Plastic Interactions Permeation and sorption are often concurrent with polymer implants. Sorption tends to remove substrates from the contacting medium, either onto its contacting surface or into the matrix of the polymer. Permeation is the process of a substance migrating through the polymer.

Selective permeability of a polymer to specific molecular species may be a highly desirable characteristic and serve as the basis for certain biomedical applications, such as hemodialysis devices and oxygenators. On the other hand, permeation (and sorption) may have a detrimental effect upon a diagnostic or therapeutic product.

20.3.2.4 Biodegradation and/or Biotransformation of Materials Prolonged contact of a biomaterial with biological systems often results in alterations of the chemical and physical properties of the biomaterial. There are, of course, a few biomedical applications (such as absorbable sutures, or bioceramics used in some controlled drug release systems), for which biodegradation of the material is a desirable characteristic, but it is undesirable for most applications. Biodegradation and/or biotransformation may involve biological molecules attaching to (or penetrating into) a polymer, or biological reactions altering the structure of a polymeric material.

Because this type of problem involves an interaction between the biological environment and the material, in vitro tests are of little value in predicting a problem of this nature. Only in vivo testing can ensure that the original unchanged material will perform satisfactorily for the anticipated duration of its service during implantation.

20.3.2.5 Physical Contact Most biomaterials exhibit relatively good compatibility during short-term contact with tissues, excluding blood, unless toxic leachables are involved. However, after a biomaterial is implanted, the body's defense systems attack it in an attempt to destroy or isolate it. Most implanted biomaterials are biodegraded rather slowly, and thus, it is common for the body to enclose them in a fibrous capsule. Overall, long-term effects of a biomaterial in direct contact with tissues are still not well-understood.

20.3.3 Toxicity Test Methods

The industrial toxicology testing methods most often used to evaluate biocompatibility of materials and devices are discussed as follows.

20.3.3.1 Cytotoxicity Various methods are described in the literature [3], in the US Pharmacopeia [4], and in ISO 109993-5: Tests for Cytotoxicity: in vitro Methods [5]. One or two methods can be used to screen materials or to qualify materials initially. Cytotoxicity methods are known to be sensitive, economical, and relatively quick to conduct.

20.3.3.2 Sensitization There is always a likelihood that an implanted material can cause an allergic response following exposure to the patient, and this needs to be determined for the final product, especially if components of the biomaterial are previously documented as allergenic. This is especially critical for invasive or implantable devices because they cannot easily be retrieved. Some of the typical reactions noted in the literature are skin rashes to eyeglass frames containing nickel, patient and user reaction to rubber gloves, and anaphylactic reactions to latex balloons on barium enema catheters, for example. This is again related to the immune response of a biomaterial, which may not necessarily be obvious in animal models.

20.3.3.3 Tissue Reactivity after Irritation or Intracutaneous Injection Materials are tested in vivo by several methods, such as using more penetrative techniques to induce an immune reaction. The nature of device exposure to the body dictates the type of method used to show compatibility in vivo, as outlined in "ISO 10993 Part 10: Tests for Irritation and Sensitization." The investigator is responsible for selecting the appropriate method, according to the matrix outlined, and depending on contact duration, and the location of the implant. Irritation implies that the material is used to physically abrade the tissue, as opposed to an inflammatory response (reaction), whereas the intracutaneous injection requires placement of the material into the tissue.

The three main testing procedures, which are typically for validation of surface devices, but are required as a basic method for all materials, include

1. Primary skin irritation—where the material is used to physically abrade the tissue
2. Mucosal irritation—where the material is used to physically abrade mucosal tissue
3. Intracutaneous injection—where a tissue reaction is determined after placement via injection under the skin

20.3.3.4 Acute Systemic Toxicity Systemic toxicity of metal ions can be tested using one of the following methods, using animal models, typically rodents:

- Mouse injection test (e.g. sensitization)
- Oral and dermal tests (e.g. irritation/inflammation)
- Pyrogen test (e.g. fever response)

20.3.3.5 Subchronic Toxicity These tests determine the effects of constant tissue exposure or repeated treatment in to an animal model for a period of time up to 10% of the animal life span. Such a study would be necessary for any device in contact with the patient for more than 1 day and up to 30 days.

20.3.3.6 Genotoxicity Devices that contact the body for more than 30 days and are in contact with circulating blood or are implantable would require a mutagenicity screen. The most common test for this is the Ames *Salmonella* bacteria reverse mutation assay. In addition to the Ames test, which evaluates primarily gene mutations in a bacterial model, there is also a requirement to evaluate DNA and chromosomal effects on mammalian cells.

20.3.3.7 Implantation Virtually any implantable devices will require an evaluation following implantation in an animal model. The most relevant guidance may be found in ISO 10993 Part 6: Tests for Local Effects Following Implantation.

There are several issues to keep in mind. First, most reviewers and regulators are accustomed to seeing a simple muscle implant test on materials that have prolonged or permanent contact with mucosal tissue, blood, or bone, as well as subcutaneous, brain, or muscle tissue. Second, implant studies are essentially an examination of local reaction at the site of the implantation. Thirdly, for devices in contact with the body for more than 2 weeks, it is important to set the implant intervals to bracket the time of human exposure or to show that the reaction to the implant has stabilized.

20.3.3.8 Hemocompatibility Traditionally, toxicologists used red blood cell hemolysis and thrombogenicity as measures of blood compatibility. A more thorough evaluation of hemocompatibility has been left to those investigators actually doing efficacy-like studies in animal models or clinical trials. There are currently no standard methods for the assessment of blood compatibility study of materials and devices that can predict the performance in vivo. The guideline document for this type of testing is ISO 10993 part 4: Selection of Tests for Interactions with Blood.

20.3.3.9 Chronic Toxicity Ready-made protocols for systemic toxicity tests do not exist. Guidance can be found in ISO 10993 Part 11: Tests for Systemic Toxicity, but there are no protocols described or referenced. For doing systemic toxicity work, one needs to conduct studies similar to those described earlier, but for longer periods of time. Chronic evaluations, defined as greater than 10% of the animal lifespan, are required for all materials in contact with the body for more than 30 days, regardless of the exposure site. Common sense dictates that the length of the study need only slightly exaggerate the human exposure time.

20.3.3.10 Carcinogenicity/Reproductive Toxicity Biocompatibility studies that address the tumorigenic and teratogenic potential of implantable devices are rarely conducted, but would involve exposure of materials to gestational females, to determine if any systemic toxicity is transmitted to the fetal tissues during pregnancy. At this time, there is heavy reliance on a battery of genotoxicity studies to rule out potential carcinogenicity, as there is an evidence of a high correlation between these in vitro assays and lifetime tumorigenic studies in rodents.

In the event that carcinogenicity testing is required, there are some guidelines available. One such protocol is ASTM F-1439-92. The second is OECD Guidelines 451 that provides general information but does not address implantables.

20.4   CYTOTOXICITY TESTING

Cytotoxicity test methods are useful for screening materials that may be used in medical devices because they serve to separate reactive from nonreactive materials, providing predictive evidence of material biocompatibility. The ISO 10993-1 standard, "Guidance on the Selection of Tests," considers these tests so important that they are prescribed for every type of medical device, along with sensitization and irritation testing. Testing for cytotoxicity is a good first step toward ensuring the biocompatibility of a medical device.

A *negative* result indicates that a material is free of harmful leachables or has an insufficient quantity to cause acute effects under exaggerated conditions with isolated cells. A *positive* cytotoxicity test result can be taken as an early warning sign that a material contains one or more leachable or reactive substances that could be of clinical importance. In such cases, further investigation is required to determine the utility of the material.

Cytotoxicity testing is certainly not, on its own merit, evidence that a material can be considered biocompatible; it is simply a first step. Cytotoxicity testing is a rapid, standardized, sensitive, and inexpensive means to determine whether a material contains significant quantities of biologically harmful extractables. Results of cytotoxicity tests correlate reasonably well with short-term implant studies. However, they do not necessarily correlate well with other standard tests of biocompatibility that are designed to examine specific endpoints (such as sensitization).

20.4.1   Cytotoxicity Test Methods

In standard cytotoxicity test methods, cell *monolayers* are grown to near *confluence* (Figure 20.3) in flasks and are then exposed to test or control samples directly or indirectly

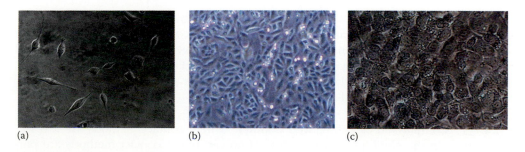

(a)   (b)   (c)

Figure 20.3
(a) Nonconfluent, (b) confluent, and (c) super-confluent cell layer.

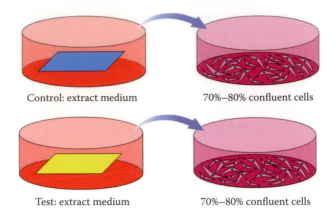

Figure 20.4
Cytotoxicity method I: extract.

by means of fluid extracts. A mammalian cell culture medium is the preferred extractant because it is a simulated physiological solution, capable of extracting a wide range of soluble chemical structures and trace amounts of hydrophobic species. Antibiotics can be added to the medium to eliminate potential interference from microbial contamination that may be present on the test material and control samples, as long as they do not affect the material chemically or otherwise. The choice of solution also depends on which cells are used.

20.4.1.1 Cytotoxicity Method I: Extract (Elution)   In the *elution test method* (Figure 20.4), which is widely used, extracts are obtained by placing the test and control materials in separate cell culture media under standard conditions (for example, 3 cm² or 0.2 g/mL of culture medium for 24 h at 37°C in a controlled gas atmosphere).

Each fluid extract obtained is then applied to a cultured-cell monolayer, replacing a portion of the medium that had supported the cells to the point of 70%–80% confluence. In this way, test cells are supplied with a medium containing extractables derived from the test or control material. The cultures are then returned to the 37°C incubator and periodically removed for microscopic examination at designated times for up to 3 days. Cells are observed for visible signs of toxicity (such as a change in the size or appearance of cellular components or a disruption in their configuration) in response to the test and control materials.

20.4.1.2 Cytotoxicity Method II: Contact   Alternatively, samples of test and control materials can be applied directly to monolayers of cells covered with nutrient medium or to a semisolid, such as an agar overlay that cushions the cells from any physical effects that may be caused by contact with the samples (Figure 20.5). After incubation, the monolayers are evaluated in terms of the presence or absence of a zone of cellular effects beneath and surrounding the sample.

20.4.1.3 Comparison of Extract and Contact   Direct contact methods are less rigorous than in the elution (extraction) test. However, direct contact methods are particularly relevant to many clinical scenarios, such as for materials destined for surface devices (e.g., patches).

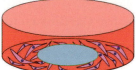
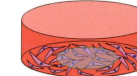

Control: Contact/*above* cells   Test: Contact/*above* cells

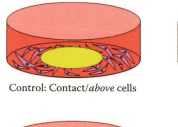
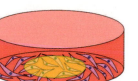

Control: Contact/*below* cells   Test: Contact/*below* cells

Figure 20.5
Cytotoxicity method II: contact.

20.5   EVALUATION IN ANIMALS

20.5.1   Ethical Issues

Evaluation of surgically implanted materials in animals represents a relatively recent concept in medicine. For centuries, new procedures were trialed immediately on patients, and therefore, willingly or not, intended or not, many of them became a sacrifice to the goal of medical progress.

While preclinical animal trials have been widely practiced, western society also evolved an increasing concern for the well-being of animals, such that today this is a legal requirement. There is considerable agreement in both the scientific community and the population at large regarding the duty to ensure laboratory animals are treated humanely. Most medical research centers and industry groups now have their own governing committees, operating in line with federal, state and institutional regulations, to implement and maintain approval for animal trials, without which the work is not permitted. There are also major documentation and data recording responsibilities involved.

The process of development and licensing of biomaterials or implantable devices will invariably involve research and/or testing in animals at some point. Even when research and development begins in vitro, animal studies are eventually required to assess safety, efficacy, and interactions with the intact tissue being repaired, in a living organism. The approval process for devices requires testing in animals prior to testing in humans. These requirements are designed to protect people from exposure to ineffective or dangerous agents, and this is a standard procedure in industry research and development.

20.5.2   Selection of Animal Models

The test design regarding which animal model to use for a specific material must be based on how the material and its endpoint device are intended to be applied in the human. Although as a model, direct comparison to the human is not completely possible owing to species differences, so human trials are still required. While there are major similarities between mammalian models and humans, in terms of specific physiological and biochemical nature of tissues and organ systems being investigated, there

Table 20.4
Animal Models for Cardiovascular Implants

Grafts	Animal Models
Arterial healing and vascular grafts	Goats
Thrombogenicity	Pigs and nonhuman primates
Hemodynamics	Dog and secondarily in nonhuman primates
Heart valves	Sheep
Artificial hearts and left ventricular assist devices	Calves, mice/rats

are still subtle differences. These include differences in immune responses, recovery rates, toxicity tolerance and level of vascularity, which can all influence the end result of a material implantation test. One of the lesser known factors is also the stress response to the actual procedure, which can have major hormonal effects on tissue and organ physiology. A *sham* control is therefore required, where all treatments on the animal are performed identically in the absence of the material.

20.5.2.1 Abdominal   The anatomy and physiology of the *canine* abdominal cavity is more similar than other animals to that of humans, making this species the ideal animal model for any experimental surgery involving the abdomen.

20.5.2.2 Cardiovascular   There are many considerations in cardiovascular research, and nearly all laboratory species have been used. The choice of the model depends upon the objective of the experiment (Table 20.4).

20.5.2.3 Neurology   Rat and nonhuman primates are the preferred models for testing of the effect of implant materials on the peripheral nervous system.

20.5.2.4 Ophthalmology   Rabbits, white domestic geese and cynomolgus monkeys are commonly used in testing procedures to determine effects of biomaterials on eyesight, and health of the eye itself.

20.5.2.5 Orthopedics   The healing of bone and its reaction to biomaterials in the sheep and goat has been shown to very closely resemble that seen in humans with regard to cell type, collagen structure, organization of both hard and soft tissue structures, and time of repair.

20.5.2.6 Dental Applications   Dogs, monkeys, baboons, and pigs are all recommended. Although the specific anatomy is quite different between these species and humans, the tissue response to periodontal disease and gingival recession is quite similar. These models are also mostly omnivorous, like humans, suggesting gross similarities in the influence of dietary factors on oral implant effectiveness.

20.5.2.7 Otology   The microscopic anatomy of the temporal bone and its contents (including bones of the inner ear) in the cat and chinchilla shows a remarkable resemblance to that of the human.

20.5.2.8 Respiratory System   Because of a similar anatomical size and healing characteristics, dogs and pigs are used for testing of biomaterials used for lung and thoracic tissue engineering.

20.5.2.9 Urogenital Tract Primarily because of the size of these structures, as well as similar anatomical and healing characteristics, dogs and pigs are used.

20.5.2.10 Wound Healing Young domestic pigs are used. This is because the skin of the young domestic pigs is nearly identical to that of humans (11 hair follicles/cm^2).

20.6 CHAPTER HIGHLIGHTS

1. The evaluation of biomaterials include
   a. Bulk characterization
   b. Surface characterization
   c. In vitro biological assessment
   d. In vivo evaluation.
2. ASTM and ISO are the two most frequently used systems for standardized evaluation of biomaterials.
3. Controls are Reference Materials that are thoroughly characterized and controlled as to composition and reproducibility. You can also use established biomaterials as a control.
4. Cytotoxicity test methods: extract and contact.
5. Animal model selection.

LABORATORY PRACTICE 5

Cytotoxicity evaluation of Ti64 alloys, hydroxyapatite, and polylactide

CASE STUDY: EVALUATION OF HEART PATCH IN RATS*

Introduction

Mortality and morbidity from heart failure following myocardial infarction remain high, despite the best currently available pharmacological therapies. This is because drugs cannot regenerate the tissue lost during infarction and endogenous tissue repair is not sufficient to prevent deleterious remodeling of cardiac morphology and reduced function. Currently two tissue engineering approaches are under intensive investigation: cell therapy [1] and passive left ventricular restraint [2]. These strategies aim to address the massive cell loss and negative remodeling associated with disease progression, respectively. Embryonic and adult stem cells have the potential to revolutionize treatment for heart-failure patients by differentiating into functional cardiomyocytes, smooth muscle, and endothelial cells, thereby regenerating heart tissue and restoring contractile function. However, current cell delivery methods are inefficient, with most cells rapidly lost after direct injection or intravenous infusion [3,4]. Another technical hurdle in cell delivery is caused by the increased size of predifferentiated cardiomyocytes compared with progenitor cells. Although predifferentiation may eliminate

---

* *Tissue Engineering*, 16:3395–3402, 2010.

tumorigenicity and provide authentic cardiac muscle [5], the increased cell size could lead to microinfarction following coronary cell infusion [6].

In vitro tissue engineering of a scaffold material seeded with cells prior to grafting into the infarcted heart may offer a method for improving the efficacy of cell delivery [7–10] while incorporating the added benefit of direct mechanical support offered by the scaffold material. This could reduce postinfarction wall stress, prevent excessive remodeling or aneurism, and augment systolic contraction [11,12]. Many different cell encapsulating biomaterials have been suggested for engineering of cardiac tissue constructs [11], including naturally occurring gels (Matrigel [13], fibrin glue [14], alginate [7,15] and collagen [16]) and synthetic thermoplastic polyester, for example, poly(lactic acid). These materials support cell growth and retention, but are either mechanically weak or nonelastic [17].

To quantitatively design the heart patch, it is necessary to introduce a concept, structural modulus Ω, which describes the capability of a sheet material to resist expansion under pressure. Structural modulus not only reflects the material's property (i.e., Young's modulus) but also the construct's geometry (i.e., thickness) [17]. In the application of a heart patch, the structural modulus Ω is

$$\Omega = Et, \tag{20.1}$$

where
  E is the Young's modulus of the material
  t is the thickness of the sheet

Therefore, mechanocompatibility requires

$$\Omega_{patch} \approx \Omega_{heart}, \tag{20.2}$$

that is,

$$E_{patch}t_{patch} \approx E_{heart}t_{heart}. \tag{20.3}$$

There is a hypothesis embedded in Equations 20.2 and 20.3; that is, the mechano-therapeutic effect is optimal when the injured area is free of stress and its contractile function is temporarily replaced by the elastic patch. The Young's modulus E_{heart} of heart muscle is 0.05 MPa and rat heart wall thickness at end diastole, t_{heart}, is 2 mm [18], giving a structural modulus of 0.1 N/mm. The heart patch thickness t_{patch} should be 0.2–0.5 mm to prevent tearing during attachment, and adhesion to or pressure on the chest wall [8]. Using Equation 20.3, a 0.33 mm thick patch should have a Young's modulus of 0.3 MPa to match the structural modulus of the myocardium. However, the mechanical function of a heart patch is complicated by material degradation and the healing profile of the diseased heart muscle. Further, true restraint of expansion may require a modulus significantly greater than one just matching the properties of the myocardium. This suggests that an initial structural modulus greater than 0.1 N/mm may be required. Hence, we tested three elastomeric biomaterials, PGS, PED, and PED–TiO$_2$ with a range of structural moduli, 0.117, 0.924, and 8.811 N/mm respectively.

To test the theory that an elastically compatible scaffold will reduce postinfarct remodeling and hypertrophy we used MRI to evaluate in vivo the mechanically-related therapeutic effect (mechano-therapeutics) of these three patch materials grafted onto the hearts of infarcted rats. The results will form the basis for a decision on which material might be taken forward to a combined stem cell/material patch therapy. A further goal was to develop MR imaging methods that gain information about the interaction between patch materials and the beating heart in vivo. MRI sets the gold standard for measuring in vivo cardiac function in both small animals and humans [19,20]. The use of MRI contrast agents gives information on myocardial viability [20] and has been used to track stem cell location in live animals [3], but its potential for studying material/cardiac interactions has not been fully realized.

Methods

Experimental Design

Ex vivo study: A pilot study was performed using the two stiffest materials to ensure that no immediate morbidity or mortality would be seen in the animals and to determine whether they could be detected by MRI under ideal conditions. PED ($n = 6$) and PED–TiO$_2$ ($n = 6$) scaffolds were grafted onto control rat hearts, which were excised after 1 week and imaged using 3D-MR-microscopy.

In vivo study: PED–TiO$_2$ ($n = 6$) and PGS ($n = 6$) scaffolds were grafted onto infarcted hearts. Infarcted hearts without scaffolds were used as controls (MI group, $n = 6$). In vivo MRI was performed 1 and 6 weeks after infarction; then hearts were fixed for histology.

Scaffold Material Synthesis
PGS was synthesized through polycondensation. Briefly, an equimolar mixture of glycerol (Sigma) and sebacate (Aldrich) was melted at 120°C under argon for 24 h. The prepolymer was dissolved into tetrahydrofuran (THF), cast on glass slides to produce sheets and incubated for 48 h at 120°C under a vacuum. After cooling at room temperature under vacuum, sheets were autoclaved for sterilization. PGS sheets had Young's modulus of 0.3 MPa and a thickness of 0.39 mm.

PED and PED–TiO$_2$ scaffolds were synthesized as described elsewhere [21]. Briefly, transesterification of dimethyl terephthalate (DMT, Poland) and ethylene glycol (Aldrich) was performed at elevated temperature in the presence of Zn(Ac)$_2$ (Aldrich) and Sb$_2$O$_3$ (Aldrich). A dimer fatty acid (Uniqema, The Netherlands; acid value 196 mg KOH/g) and TiO$_2$ nanoparticles of mean particle size 23 nm (Aeroxide® P25, Degussa, Germany) were added to the PED–TiO$_2$ scaffolds and polycondensation was carried out at 285°C–290°C and 0.5–0.6 mmHg of vacuum. The Young's moduli of PED and PED–0.2 wt%TiO$_2$ used in this work were 2.8 and 26.7 MPa, respectively. The thickness of sheets was 0.33 mm.

Myocardial Infarction and Scaffold Grafting
All procedures were conducted in accordance with The University of Oxford and Imperial College, London, Animal Ethics Review Committees and the Home Office, London. Myocardial infarction or sham surgery was performed in 30 male Wistar rats by ligation of the left anterior descending coronary artery as described [22]. Scaffolds were attached to the epicardial surface shortly after the induction of infarction using 12–16 continuous stitches.

3D-MR-Microscopy
Hearts were excised, fixed in paraformaldehyde and embedded in 1% agarose doped with gadolinium diethylenetriaminepentaacetic acid (Gd-DTPA). MRI was performed at 11.7 T using a 40-mm quadrature-driven birdcage coil (Rapid

Biomedical, Würzburg, Germany) and a 3D fast gradient echo sequence (TE/TR 1.8/15 ms; 15° pulse; field of view 32 × 32 × 64 mm; matrix size, 512 × 512 × 512; voxel size 32 × 32 × 64 µm; 6 averages) [22].

In Vivo MRI   Cardiac cine-MRI was performed as described [23]. Briefly, using an 11.7 T MR system with a Bruker console running Paravision 2.1.1 and 52 mm birdcage coil, a stack of contiguous 1.5 mm thick true short-axis ECG and respiration-gated cine images (TE/TR 1.43/4.6 ms; 17.5° pulse; field of view 51.2 × 51.2 mm; matrix size 256 × 256; voxel size 200 × 200 × 1500 µm; 25–35 frames per cardiac cycle) were acquired to cover the entire left ventricle (7–9 slices). Long-axis two-chamber and four-chamber images were also acquired. Delayed enhancement MRI (DE-MRI) was performed on slices containing scaffold material at 10–25 min after Gd-DTPA infusion using the same cine-MRI sequence, but with flip angle increased to 60° to induce saturation of signal in normal myocardium. The entire imaging protocol was performed in approximately 60 min.

MRI Data Analysis   Image analysis was performed using Image J (NIH Image, Bethesda, MD). Left ventricular volumes, ejection fractions, and scar sizes (defined as akinetic myocardium) were calculated as described [22]. DE-MR images were thresholded to two standard deviations above the mean signal intensity from normal tissue and qualitatively assessed for regions of tissue necrosis. To measure scaffold volumes, images were thresholded to enhance contrast between the myocardium and the scaffold, and semi-automated analysis of the scaffold area was performed in each MRI slice.

Histology   Hearts were excised, washed, and frozen. Serial 10 µm cryosections were cut in the short axis-orientation and stained with hematoxylin and eosin.

RESULTS AND DISCUSSION

Ex Vivo Detection of Grafted Patches

Ex vivo experiments aimed to test the mechanical integrity of the patch materials and the feasibility of visualizing the patch using MRI. Since the physical integrity of grafted PGS has been demonstrated [24,25], only PED or PED–TiO$_2$ scaffolds were grafted onto normal rat hearts. At 1 week, hearts were excised and MR microscopy was performed. Scaffolds were clearly identifiable as signal voids on the epicardial surface of the myocardium (Figure 20.6), indicating that MRI can be used to evaluate scaffold materials. The solid nature and very limited water permeability of the scaffold materials meant that they produced no MRI signal, which allowed their identification as signal voids in a proton rich, aqueous environment.

MR microscopy revealed that PED scaffolds had become fractured into 2–4 pieces by the stresses exerted during repeated cardiac contraction, while the PED–TiO$_2$ and PGS remained intact. There was no difference in patch volume between the PED and PED–TiO$_2$ scaffolds (46 ± 6 vs. 42 ± 4 mm³). The fracture of PED was likely caused by hydrolysis of ester links in the soft dimer fatty acid segments, leaving nondegradable polyethyleneterephthalate behind. This may occur faster in vivo owing to the catalytic function of enzymes, including esterase and oxidoreductase [26]. Hence, PED was excluded from further in vivo studies.

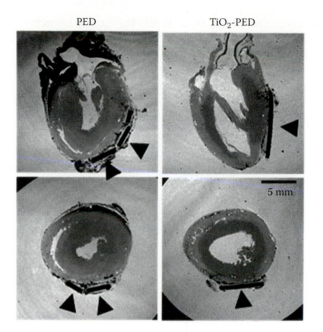

Figure 20.6
Ex vivo scaffold detection; MR microscopy images of PED and PED–TiO$_2$ scaffolds attached to the epicardium of control rat hearts. Images are in the long-axis (a) and short-axis (b) orientation. Arrows indicate scaffold location.

In Vivo Detection of Grafted Patches

PED–TiO$_2$ and PGS scaffolds were grafted onto infarcted rat hearts shortly after coronary occlusion. Implantation of the patch did not lead to excess mortality or obvious morbidity. In vivo MRI was performed 1 and 6 weeks after implantation. The grafted scaffolds were identifiable as signal voids on the epicardial surface of the myocardium and were visible throughout the cardiac cycle (Figures 20.7 and 20.8).

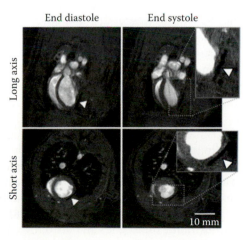

Figure 20.7
In vivo scaffold detection; long and short axis cine-MR images acquired at end diastole and end systole. Arrow heads show the location of the PED–TiO$_2$ scaffold.

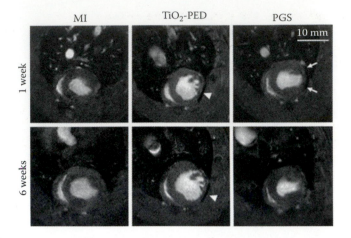

Figure 20.8
Serial cine-MRI: representative end systolic frames of cine images acquired at 1 and 6 weeks after infarction. Arrowheads show the location of the scaffolds. Note the larger end systolic volume of the PED–TiO$_2$ image at 6 weeks; the PGS scaffold has bowed with the curvature of the heart (white arrows); by 6 weeks, little PGS scaffold material is detectable. PGS, poly(glycerol sebacate).

The PED–TiO$_2$ scaffolds remained in a rigid flat sheet during systole, while PGS scaffolds were more compliant, bowing during cardiac contraction and matching the curvature of the heart.

In Vivo Measurement of Heart Patch Degradation

The high contrast between scaffold and surrounding tissue permitted accurate measurement of scaffold volume and quantification of degradation. The size of the scaffold-induced signal void within each MR image was measured at 1 and 6 weeks after implantation. At 1 week, the volumes of PED–TiO$_2$ and PGS scaffolds were similar (32 ± 7 vs. 36 ± 8 mm^3). At 6 weeks, the volumes of the PED–TiO$_2$ scaffolds had not changed, while PGS scaffolds had almost completely degraded (32 ± 7 vs. 3 ± 2 mm^3), with only small fragments remaining attached to the epicardium. These observations were confirmed by histology. This result was unexpected, as incubation of PGS material for 60 days in cell culture media at 37°C resulted in ~20% reduction in size [17]. The rapid in vivo degradation of PGS can be attributed to esterase and oxidoreductase mediated hydrolysis of the ester links.

In Vivo Measurement of Cardiac Morphology and Function

Myocardial infarction rapidly leads to tissue necrosis and reduced contractility within the territory of the occluded artery [27]. By 1 week after infarction a collagenous scar begins to form, ejection fraction, normally 72% in similar sized control rats [23], has decreased, and end systolic volume, normally 115 µL [23], has increased, as demonstrated by the control MI group of this study (Figure 20.8 and Table 20.5). From 1 to 6 weeks the surviving myocardium undergoes hypertrophy and dilation to maintain cardiac output, even with lower ejection fraction, as is evident from the increased LV mass and end diastolic volumes of the control MI group (Table 20.5). Although hypertrophy can initially compensate for the infarcted akinetic myocardium, the increased

Table 20.5

In Vivo Measurements of Cardiac Morphology and Function at 1 and 6 Weeks

	MI	TiO$_2$–PED	PGS
LV mass (mg)			
1 week	525 ± 37	537 ± 28	616 ± 18
6 weeks	834 ± 33	827 ± 27	750 ± 32
Change	309 ± 16	290 ± 19	132 ± 30[a]
LV mass/body mass (mg/g)			
1 week	2.13 ± 0.15	2.21 ± 0.08	2.31 ± 0.07
6 weeks	2.37 ± 0.11	2.38 ± 0.09	2.24 ± 0.08
Change	0.24 ± 0.06	0.19 ± 0.07	−0.07 ± 0.05[a]
End diastolic volume (μL)			
1 week	523 ± 42	487 ± 31	533 ± 49
6 weeks	726 ± 41	772 ± 27	670 ± 101
Change	202 ± 26	285 ± 33	137 ± 65
End systolic volume (μL)			
1 week	277 ± 34	285 ± 20	302 ± 39
6 weeks	369 ± 44	492 ± 13[a]	403 ± 99
Change	92 ± 20	207 ± 16[a]	100 ± 67
Stroke volume (μL)			
1 week	246 ± 17	202 ± 15	230 ± 16
6 weeks	357 ± 19	280 ± 20[a]	267 ± 8[a]
Change	111 ± 19	78 ± 24	37 ± 15[a]
Ejection fraction (%)			
1 week	48 ± 3	41 ± 2	44 ± 3
6 weeks	50 ± 3	36 ± 2[a]	44 ± 6
Change	2.2 ± 1.8	−5.4 ± 3.0[a]	0.1 ± 4
Heart rate (bpm)			
1 week	367 ± 12	359 ± 11	369 ± 13
6 weeks	363 ± 7	399 ± 16	365 ± 6
Change	−4 ± 16	41 ± 23	−4 ± 7
Cardiac output (μL/min)			
1 week	90 ± 6	74 ± 5	85 ± 5
6 weeks	129 ± 7	112 ± 9	94 ± 4[a]
Change	40 ± 7	39 ± 9	8 ± 6[a]
Body weight (g)			
1 week	247 ± 7	244 ± 7	271 ± 5
6 weeks	352 ± 7	348 ± 6	335 ± 4
Change	106 ± 6	104 ± 6	64 ± 3[a]
Absolute scar size (mm^2)			
1 week	52 ± 11	72 ± 5	59 ± 15
6 weeks	60 ± 12	101 ± 9[a]	62 ± 25
Change	8 ± 5	29 ± 9	3 ± 13
Relative scar size (% of LV)			
1 week	23 ± 3	32 ± 4	21 ± 5
6 weeks	19 ± 3	31 ± 2[a]	19 ± 6
Change	−4 ± 1	−1 ± 3	−2 ± 2

[a] $p < 0.05$ compared with MI group.

wall stress associated with chamber enlargement can lead to excessive dilation and eventually heart failure, where cardiac output is reduced to a level insufficient to perfuse the body.

At 1 week there were no significant differences in any of the measured parameters of cardiac morphology and function between the MI, PED–TiO$_2$, and PGS groups (Table 20.5). However, delayed enhancement MRI performed at 1 week identified extensive tissue necrosis adjacent to the sites of attachment of the PED–TiO$_2$ but not PGS scaffolds (Figure 20.9). This tissue damage probably resulted from the much higher Young's modulus of the PED–TiO$_2$ patch making it insufficiently compliant, leading to different extension profiles during contraction and thus sliding of the heart wall against the attached patch. Consequently, the heart, which is the softer of the two, was damaged. In a separate study we have confirmed that the TiO$_2$ nanoparticle component of PED–TiO$_2$ has little effect on adult cardiac myocytes, eliminating this as a possible source of the damage observed [28]. Opportunities to improve the PED–TiO$_2$ composite patch are being explored also by reducing TiO$_2$ nanoparticle content and by optimizing the patch design, adding porosity to reduce stiffness.

After 6 weeks severe remodeling occurred in the PED–TiO$_2$ group, with 33% higher end systolic volumes, 14% lower ejection fractions and 68% higher scar sizes compared with the MI group ($p < 0.05$, Table 20.5). Hence, the rigid PED–TiO$_2$ patch impeded contraction, induced necrosis, and exacerbated postinfarct remodeling and hypotrophy, resulting in increased end systolic volumes and scar sizes and reduced stroke volumes and ejection fractions.

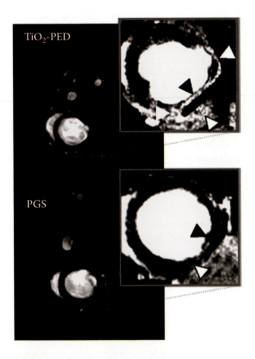

Figure 20.9
DE-MRI: images acquired at 1 week after scaffold attachment. The inset of the upper panel shows extensive hyperenhancement in the vicinity of the PED–TiO$_2$ scaffold attachment sites (white and black arrowheads), whereas in the lower panel enhancement is localized to the site of infarction and not adjacent to the PGS scaffold attachment sites. DE, delayed enhancement.

Hearts treated with the PGS scaffold showed similar ejection fractions and end diastolic and systolic volumes to the control MI group at 6 weeks. The increase in myocardial mass was 57% lower ($p < 0.0005$, Table 20.5) and the LV to body mass ratio was also significantly lower compared with control infarcts. This indicates that hypertrophy in the PGS group was reduced. However, this potential benefit was outweighed by a negative effect on stroke volumes and cardiac outputs, which increased from 1 to 6 weeks in the MI group, but remained unchanged in the PGS group (Table 20.5), suggesting that the scaffold mediated reduction in hypertrophy had compromised systolic function.

The grafted scaffold materials were designed to perform two functions; (1) limit excessive chamber dilation and (2) aid systolic contraction. Our MRI results indicate that the PED–TiO$_2$ patch was too rigid to perform these functions and that it damaged the myocardium. The PSG scaffold successfully reduced hypertrophy, giving it potential as a biomaterial for limiting excessive remodeling. PGS was unable to assist systolic contraction: cardiac remodeling is a strategy that initially allows cardiac output to be maintained and its prevention may have been counter-productive. Modification of the biodegradation properties to prevent the rapid breakdown in vivo could possibly enhance the support by PGS. We have shown that altering the curing temperature is able to reduce degradation rates [17]. However, if the goal is to use the patch to deliver cardiac stem/progenitor cells then these will provide the contractile component required for the heart patch to assisted systolic function. Embryonic stem cells can be cultured on the surface of elastomeric scaffold materials (Harding, Unpublished), whereas neonatal cardiac fibroblasts and myocytes can be seeded within porous PGS constructs [29]. The properties of PGS in terms of temporary support to reduce remodeling during the period of functional cellular integration, followed by rapid degradation to remove the material, may be advantageous.

Histology

No evidence of infarction was found after patch grafting onto control hearts. When hearts were removed from infarcted rats, PGS scaffolds were found to have few adhesions to the chest wall, whereas PED–TiO$_2$ scaffolds exhibited strong adhesions. Examination of histological sections stained with hematoxylin and eosin indicated that PED–TiO$_2$ scaffolds had remained intact and unchanged in shape. Moreover, fibrous tissue was found on the surface of PED–TiO$_2$ scaffolds, as well as some thinning of myocardium at the adjoining points (Figure 20.10), which forms further evidence that there was severe wearing or friction on the surface myocardium caused by PED–TiO$_2$. The majority of PGS scaffolds had degraded with only small strings remaining on the LV. Similarly, a previous study in which porous PGS scaffolds were attached to infarcted hearts found that 2 weeks after grafting, scaffolds had partially degraded and incorporated into the myocardium, with invasion of host cells and vessels [29].

Significance of Using MRI in Tissue Engineering

Tissue engineering has become a reality for bone regeneration [30], treatment of burns [31], cartilage replacement [32], and airway reconstruction [33]. Engineered heart tissue is also under development and has great potential for the treatment of myocardial infarction and prevention of heart failure. Development of engineered heart tissue requires the application of noninvasive and nondestructive in vivo imaging, which can

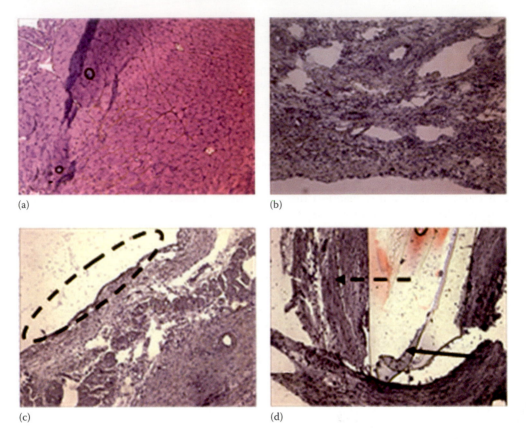

Figure 20.10

Histology: hematoxylin and eosin-stained sections from (a) normal myocardium; (b) fibrous scar tissue; (c) infarcted tissue after PED–TiO2 grafting—the PED–TiO2 scaffold (arrow) can be clearly seen with fibrous tissue on the surface (dashed arrow); (d) infarcted tissue after PGS grafting—the PGS scaffold was completely degraded (dashed line) from the left ventricle (LV) surface.

give scaffold location and degradation, and can assess the effect on cardiac function. Here we report the first noninvasive method for measurement of cardiac scaffold location and degradation in vivo.

The properties of scaffold materials implanted into animals have previously been studied by histology of material recovered after sacrifice, precluding serial measurements of the same sample and making temporal changes impossible to record [6]. Noninvasive techniques, including single photon computed tomography (SPECT) [34], bioluminescence imaging [35], and ultrasound [36], have been used to monitor drug [34] and cell [35] seeded materials implanted subcutaneously [35,36] or into bone [34] of mice and rats. Although these methods give valuable information, the ionizing radiation, poor spatial resolution, and/or requirement for genetic modification of donor cells make the techniques sub-optimal. MRI overcomes these limitations and produces high resolution three-dimensional images from naturally abundant protons within the sample. MRI has been used to characterize cell-seeded bioscaffolds in vitro [37,38] and in vivo [39,40] with bone formation serially monitored after subcutaneous implantation of demineralized bone matrix [39] and iron oxide labeled bone marrow cell seeded scaffolds located [40] in live rats. The present work showed for the first time that MRI can be used to locate cardiac scaffolds in vivo, characterize the integrity of scaffold materials grafted onto rat hearts, and make serial measurements of biomaterial degradation, in addition to accurate assessment of cardiac function.

SUMMARY

The present work explored the mechano-therapeutic effects of biomaterial heart patches using in vivo MRI. We show that a rigid PED–TiO$_2$ scaffold damaged heart muscle via surface friction, which increased tissue necrosis, scar size, adhesions to the chest and fibrosis, and reduced cardiac function compared with control infarcted rats. It may be possible to improve the PED–TiO$_2$ scaffolds by reducing TiO$_2$ nanoparticle content and by adding porosity, this being investigated separately.

The present results showed that mechanically compatible PGS patch effectively prevented postinfarction hypertrophy, but did not assist contractile function, resulting in lower stroke volumes and cardiac outputs. The properties of in vivo biocompatibility and limitation of remodeling, as well as the previously demonstrated tuning of biodegradation rates and support of human embryonic stem cell–derived cardiomyocytes, makes PGS a promising candidate for further development as a heart patch [24]. In addition, this work has shown for the first time that MRI can be used as a noninvasive method for the evaluation of tissue engineering scaffolds in vivo.

SIMPLE QUESTIONS IN CLASS

1. Which of the following materials is the best choice of a control for the evaluation of biocompatibility of a new metallic implant?
   a. Ti–6Fe–4Al
   b. Bioactive glass
   c. Ti–6Al–4V
   d. PMMA
2. Which of the following materials is the best choice of a control for the evaluation of biocompatibility of a new degradable polymer?
   a. Ti–6Al–4V
   b. PMMA
   c. Hydroxyapatite
   d. Poly(lactic acid-*co*-glycolic acid) (PLGA)
3. Which of following materials is the best choice of a control for the evaluation of biocompatibility of a new bioceramics?
   a. Hydroxyapatite
   b. Ti–6Al–4V
   c. Bioglass
   d. Poly(lactic acid-*co*-glycolic acid) (PLGA)
4. When should you evaluate the biocompatibility of a potential biomaterial?
   a. After achieving the desired mechanical properties
   b. After proceeding with design and development of the device
   c. When it is in the finished form (in the device)
   d. At an early stage in its consideration for a biomedical application

5. Which of the following statements is incorrect?
   a. Cytotoxicity test methods can provide predictive evidence of material biocompatibility.
   b. Cytotoxicity testing is a rapid, standardized, sensitive, and inexpensive means to assess the biocompatibility of a biomaterial.
   c. Cytotoxicity testing, on its own merit, provides evidence that a material can be considered biocompatible.
   d. Cytotoxicity testing is a rapid and inexpensive first step.
6. A negative result indicates that a material is _____ extractables or has _____ of them to cause acute effects under exaggerated conditions with isolated cells.
7. A positive cytotoxicity test result indicates that a material contains one or more extractable substances that could be _____.

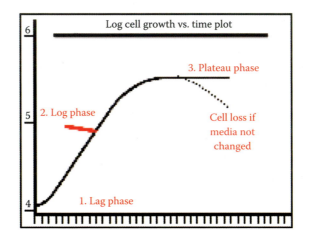

8. On the following cell growth curve, which stage indicates that confluence has been reached?
   1. Lag phase
   2. Log phase
   3. Plateau phase

PROBLEMS AND EXERCISES

1. Define the terms "confluency," "apoptosis," and "necrosis."
2. To evaluate an orthopedic implant used for aging people, should you evaluate the cell death in terms of apoptosis or necrosis? Explain your reason.
3. Discuss the importance of cytotoxicity evaluation. If a material shows to be cytotoxic in vitro, would it be toxic in vivo? Explain your reason.
4. Compare and discuss the advantages and disadvantages of the two cytotoxicity test methods: extract and contact.
5. Discuss your scheduling of testing during the development of an inert bioceramics.
6. Discuss your scheduling of testing during the development of a degrading polymer.
7. Discuss the choice of controls in the evaluation of new ceramic, metallic, and polymeric implant materials. Give examples.

8. Discuss the animal models for the evaluation of a new artificial blood vessel.
9. Discuss the animal models for the evaluation of a new orthopedic implant for the treatment of knee joint.
10. Discuss the benefits of using a rodent model for the evaluation of heart muscle patch.

BIBLIOGRAPHY

References for Text

1. Von Recum, A.F., *Handbook of Biomaterials Evaluation*. CRC Press, New York, NY, 1998.
2. Braybrook, J.H., *Biocompatibility Assessment of Medical Devices and Material*. Wiley, NY, 1997.
3. Wilsnack, R.E., F.J. Meyer, and J.G. Smith, Human cell culture toxicity testing of medical devices and correlation to animal tests. *Biomaterials, Medical Devices and Artificial Organs*, 1973;**1**(3):545–562.
4. US Pharmacopeia, Biological reactivity tests, in vitro. In *U.S. Pharmacopeia, 23*. Rockville, MD: United States Pharmacopeial Convention Inc., Rockville, MD, 1995, pp. 1697–1699.
5. Tests for cytotoxicity: In vitro methods. *Biological Evaluation of Medical Devices,* Part 5, ANSI/AAMI, 1993, pp. 10993–10995.

Websites

http://www.astm.org/.
http://www.iso.org/iso/home.html.
http://www.nist.gov/index.html.
http://www.usp.org/.

References for Case Study

1. Soonpaa, M.H., G.Y. Koh, M.G. Klug, and L.J. Field, Formation of nascent intercalated disks between grafted fetal cardiomyocytes and host myocardium. *Science*, 1994;**264**:98–101.
2. Mann, D.L. and J.T. Willerson, Left ventricular assist devices and the failing heart—A bridge to recovery, a permanent assist device, or a bridge too far? *Circulation*, 1998;**98**:2367–2369.
3. Stuckey, D.J. et al., Iron particles for noninvasive monitoring of bone marrow stromal cell engraftment into, and isolation of viable engrafted donor cells from, the heart. *Stem Cells*, 2006;**24**:1968–1975.
4. Sheikh, A.Y., S.A. Lin, F. Cao, Y. Cao, K.E. van der Bogt, P. Chu, C.P. Chang, C.H. Contag, R.C. Robbins, and J.C. Wu, Molecular imaging of bone marrow mononuclear cell homing and engraftment in ischemic myocardium. *Stem Cells*, 2007;**25**:2677–2684.
5. Klug, M.G., M.H. Soonpaa, G.Y. Koh, and L.J. Field, Genetically selected cardiomyocytes from differentiating embryonic stem cells form stable intracardiac grafts. *The Journal of Clinical Investigation*, 1996;**98**:216–224.
6. Vulliet, P.R., M. Greeley, S.M. Halloran, K.A. MacDonald, and M.D. Kittleson, Intra-coronary arterial injection of mesenchymal stromal cells and microinfarction in dogs. *Lancet*, 2004;**363**:783–784.
7. Dvir, T. et al., Prevascularization of cardiac patch on the omentum improves its therapeutic outcome. *Proceedings of the National Academic Science USA*, 2009;**106**:14990–14995.
8. Fujimoto, K.L., K. Tobita, W.D. Merryman, J.J. Guan, N. Momoi, D.B. Stolz, M.S. Sacks, B.B. Keller, and W.R. Wagner, An elastic, biodegradable cardiac patch induces contractile smooth muscle and improves cardiac remodeling and function in subacute myocardial infarction. *Journal of the American College of Cardiology*, 2007;**49**:2292–2300.

9. Simpson, D., H. Liu, T.H.M. Fan, R. Nerem, and S.C. Dudley, A tissue engineering approach to progenitor cell delivery results in significant cell engraftment and improved myocardial remodeling. *Stem Cells*, 2007;**25**:2350–2357.

10. Wei, H.J. et al., Porous acellular bovine pericardia seeded with mesenchymal stem cells as a patch to repair a myocardial defect in a syngeneic rat model. *Biomaterials*, 2006;**27**:5409–5419.

11. Chen, Q.Z., S.E. Harding, N.N. Ali, A.R. Lyon, and A.R. Boccaccini, Biomaterials in cardiac tissue engineering: Ten years of research survey. *Materials Science and Engineering R-Reports*, 2008;**59**:1–37.

12. Jawad, H., N.N. Ali, A.R. Lyon, Q.Z. Chen, S.E. Harding, and A.R. Boccaccini, Myocardial tissue engineering: A review. *Journal of Tissue Engineering and Regenerative Medicine*, 2007;**1**:327–342.

13. Zimmermann, W.H. et al., Engineered heart tissue grafts improve systolic and diastolic function in infarcted rat hearts. *Nature Medicine*, 2006;**12**:452–458.

14. Christman, K.L., H.H. Fok, R.E. Sievers, Q. Fang, and R.J. Lee, Fibrin glue alone and skeletal myoblasts in a fibrin scaffold preserve cardiac function after myocardial infarction. *Tissue Engineering*, 2004;**10**:403–409.

15. Landa, N., L. Miller, M.S. Feinberg, R. Holbova, M. Shachar, I. Freeman, S. Cohen, and J. Leor, Effect of injectable alginate implant on cardiac remodeling and function after recent and old infarcts in rat. *Circulation*, 2008;**117**:1388–1396.

16. Dai, W., L.E. Wold, J.S. Dow, and R.A. Kloner, Thickening of the infarcted wall by collagen injection improves left ventricular function in rats: A novel approach to preserve cardiac function after myocardial infarction. *Journal of the American College of Cardiology*, 2005;**46**:714–719.

17. Chen, Q.Z., A. Bismarck, U. Hansen, S. Junaid, M.Q. Tran, S.E. Harding, N.N. Ali, and A.R. Boccaccini, Characterisation of a soft elastomer poly(glycerol sebacate) designed to match the mechanical properties of myocardial tissue. *Biomaterials*, 2008;**29**:47–57.

18. Cwajg, J.M., E. Cwajg, S.F. Nagueh, Z.X. He, U. Qureshi, L.I. Olmos, M.A. Quinones, M.S. Verani, W.L. Winters, and W.A. Zoghbi, End-diastolic wall thickness as a predictor of recovery of function in myocardial hibernation: Relation to rest-redistribution T1-201 tomography and dobutamine stress echocardiography. *Journal of the American College of Cardiology*, 2000;**35**:1152–1161.

19. Stuckey, D.J., C.A. Carr, D.J. Tyler, and K. Clarke, Cine-MRI versus two-dimensional echocardiography to measure in vivo left ventricular function in rat heart. *NMR in Biomedicine*, 2008;**21**:765–772.

20. Kim, R.J., E. Wu, A. Rafael, E.L. Chen, M.A. Parker, O. Simonetti, F.J. Klocke, R.O. Bonow, and R.M. Judd, The use of contrast-enhanced magnetic resonance imaging to identify reversible myocardial dysfunction. *New England Journal of Medicine*, 2000;**343**:1445–1453.

21. Piegat, A., M. El Fray, H. Jawad, Q.Z. Chen, and A.R. Boccaccini, Inhibition of calcification of polymer-ceramic composites incorporating nanocrystalline TiO_2. *Advances in Applied Ceramics*, 2008;**107**:287–292.

22. Carr, C.A. et al., Bone marrow-derived stromal cells home to and remain in the infarcted rat heart but fail to improve function: An in vivo cine-MRI study. *American Journal of Physiology Heart and Circulatory Physiology*, 2008;**295**:H533–H542.

23. Stuckey, D.J., C.A. Carr, D.J. Tyler, E. Aasum, and K. Clarke, Novel MRI method to detect altered left ventricular ejection and filling patterns in rodent models of disease. *Magnetic Resonance in Medicine*, 2008;**60**:582–587.

24. Chen, Q.Z. et al., An elastomeric patch derived from poly(glycerol sebacate) for delivery of embryonic stem cells to the heart. *Biomaterials*, 2010. Published online, DOI: 10.1016/j.biomaterials. 2010.01.108.

25. Wang, Y., Y.M. Kim, and R. Langer, In vivo degradation characteristics of poly(glycerol sebacate). *Journal of Biomedical Material Research A*, 2003;**66**:192–197.

26. Schakenraad, J.M., M.J. Hardonk, J. Feijen, I. Molenaar, and P. Nieuwenhuis, Enzymatic activity toward poly(L-lactic acid) implants. *Journal of Biomedical Materials Research*, 1990;**24**:529–545.

27. Nahrendorf, M. et al., Serial cine-magnetic resonance imaging of left ventricular remodeling after myocardial infarction in rats. *Journal of Magnetic Resonance Imaging*, 2001;**14**:547–555.

28. Jawad, H., A.R. Boccaccini, N.N. Ali, and S.E. Harding, Assessment of cellular toxicity of TiO_2 nanoparticles for cardiac tissue engineering applications. In: *Nanotoxicology*, 2011;**5**:372–380.

29. Radisic, M., H. Park, T.P. Martens, J.E. Salazar-Lazaro, W. Geng, Y. Wang, R. Langer, L.E. Freed, and G. Vunjak-Novakovic, Pre-treatment of synthetic elastomeric scaffolds by cardiac fibroblasts improves engineered heart tissue. *Journal of Biomedical Materials Research A*, 2008;**86**:713–724.

30. Hench, L.L. and J.M. Polak, Third-generation biomedical materials. *Science*, 2002;**295**;1014–1017.

31. MacNeil, S., Progress and opportunities for tissue-engineered skin. *Nature*, 2007;**445**:874–880.

32. Zheng, M.H., C. Willers, L. Kirilak, P. Yates, J. Xu, D. Wood, and A. Shimmin, Matrix-induced autologous chondrocyte implantation (MACI): Biological and histological assessment. *Tissue Engineering*, 2007;**13**:737–746.

33. Macchiarini, P. et al., Clinical transplantation of a tissue-engineered airway. *Lancet*, 2008;**372**:2023–2030.

34. Kempen, D.H., M.J. Yaszemski, A. Heijink, T.E. Hefferan, L.B. Creemers, J. Britson, A. Maran, K.L. Classic, W.J. Dhert, and L. Lu, Non-invasive monitoring of BMP-2 retention and bone formation in composites for bone tissue engineering using SPECT/CT and scintillation probes. *Journal of Controlled Release*, 2009;**134**:169–176.

35. Hwang do, W. et al., Real-time in vivo monitoring of viable stem cells implanted on biocompatible scaffolds. *European Journal of Nuclear Medicine and Molecular Imaging*, 2008;**35**:1887–1898.

36. Kim, K., C.G. Jeong, and S.J. Hollister, Non-invasive monitoring of tissue scaffold degradation using ultrasound elasticity imaging. *Acta Biomaterialia*, 2008;**4**:783–790.

37. Terrovitis, J.V. et al., Magnetic resonance imaging of ferumoxide-labeled mesenchymal stem cells seeded on collagen scaffolds-relevance to tissue engineering. *Tissue Engineering*, 2006;**12**:2765–2775.

38. Nitzsche, H., H. Metz, A. Lochmann, A. Bernstein, G. Hause, T. Groth, and K. Mader, Characterization of scaffolds for tissue engineering by benchtop-MRI. *Tissue Engineering Part C Methods*, 2009;**15**(3):513–521.

39. Hartman, E.H., J.A. Pikkemaat, J.W. Vehof, A. Heerschap, J.A. Jansen, and P.H. Spauwen, In vivo magnetic resonance imaging explorative study of ectopic bone formation in the rat. *Tissue Engineering*, 2002;**8**:1029–1036.

40. Poirier-Quinot, M., G. Frasca, C. Wilhelm, N. Luciani, J.C. Ginefri, L. Darrasse, D. Letourneur, C. Le Visage, and F. Gazeau, High resolution 1.5T magnetic resonance imaging for tissue engineering constructs: A non invasive tool to assess 3D scaffold architecture and cell seeding. *Tissue Engineering Part C Methods*, 2009;**16**(2):185–200.

Further Readings

Braybrook, J.H., *Biocompatibility Assessment of Medical Devices and Material*. Braybrook: Wiley VCH, Weinheim, Germany 1996.

Von Recum, A.F., *Handbook of Biomaterials Evaluation*. Von Recum: London, UK: Taylor & Francis, 1999.

CHAPTER 21

REGULATION OF MEDICAL DEVICES

LEARNING OBJECTIVES

After a careful study of this chapter, you should be able to do the following:

1. Understand the roles of regulations and standards
2. Be aware of regulatory authorities of five countries/regions with the most advanced medical device regulations
3. Be aware of what medical devices are
4. Describe the classification of medical devices
5. Describe your possible future roles in the field of biomedical engineering

21.1   REGULATIONS VERSUS STANDARDS

Regulations represent legal rules, established by government authorities, that dictate what procedures can be performed and how they should or should not be performed. In the case of tissue engineering, this can include how a biomaterial is fabricated, measured, and tested. Regulations are mandatory and legally obligatory, with penalties in place for any breaches, as determined by audits or legal investigations. In general, regulations normally apply to medical devices, rather than specific materials that contribute to their fabrication. Why do we need regulations? Basically, they have been put in place to protect the health and welfare of patients being treated in clinical settings, in this context, for tissue reconstruction strategies. Table 21.1 lists five most dominant regulatory authorities.

Standards are guidelines referred to by legislation, which provide guidelines on technical procedures and are usually produced by private or public, nongovernmental organizations. While standards are in principle voluntary, they can be mandated in a regulation by a government and thus can become legally binding.

Table 21.1
Five Regulatory Authorities

Title	Regions/Countries	Websites
European Commission on Health and Consumers	European Union	http://ec.europa.eu/dgs/health_consumer/index_en.htm
Food and Drug Administration (FDA)	USA	http://www.fda.gov/
Medical Devices Bureau of Health Canada	Canada	http://www.hc-sc.gc.ca/index-eng.php
Ministry of Health, Labor and Welfare (MHLW)	Japan	http://www.mhlw.go.jp/english/index.html
Therapeutic Good Administration (TGA)	Australia	http://www.tga.gov.au/

21.2   MEDICAL DEVICES

21.2.1   Definition of Medical Devices

Although each regulatory authority has its own definition of medical devices, the term "medical devices" is defined as:

> Any instrument, apparatus, implement, machine, appliance, implant, in vitro reagent or calibrator, software, material, or other similar or related articles, intended by the manufacture to be used, alone or in combination, for human beings for one or more of the specific purposes of (Figure 21.1):

- Diagnosis
- Prevention
- Monitoring

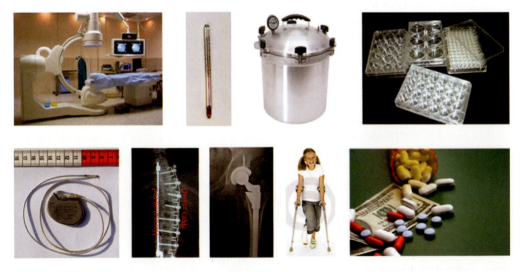

Figure 21.1
Examples of medical devices.

- Treatment
- Investigation
- Supporting or sustaining life
- Control of conception
- Disinfection of medical devices [1].

Hence, medical devices are not just those that are implantable or those that are used in medical study, diagnosis, or monitoring, as most of us would assume.

21.2.2   Biomaterials in the Legal Context

In a regulatory sense, a biomaterial is a component of a medical device, and thus can represent any material used in a medical device. In a regulatory sense, "bio" in biomaterial means "biomedical." As introduced in *Chapter 1*, in the scientific field of biomaterials, and the related fields of tissue engineering and regenerative medicine, a biomaterial is defined as "a substance that has been engineered to take a form which, alone or as part of a complex system, is used to direct, by control of interactions with components of living systems, the course of any therapeutic or diagnostic procedure" [2]. In other words, biomaterials directly interact with tissues, most commonly in implantable devices used for treatment or diagnostic purposes.

21.2.3   Classification of Medical Devices in the Legal Field

Medical devices are classified by government regulatory authorities based on their complexity and level of control necessary to assure their safety and effectiveness. Each country or region defines these categories in different ways.

21.2.3.1   Classification in Canada and EU   Four classes of medical devices are based on the level of control necessary to ensure the safety and effectiveness of the device:

- Class I: The lowest potential risk, not requiring a license
- Class II: Requires a declaration from the manufacturer of the safety and effectiveness of a device
- Class III and IV: A greater potential risk, subject to in-depth scrutiny

Canadian classes of medical devices generally correspond to the *European Council Directive (ECD) 93/42/EEC* (Table 21.2).

21.2.3.2   Classification in the United States   The classification here is based on the level of control necessary to ensure the safety and effectiveness of the device:

- Class I: General controls
- Class I devices present minimal potential for harm to the user and are subject only to general controls.
- Class II: General controls with special controls
- Class III: General controls and *premarket approval (PMA)*

In general, implants of biomaterials fall into FDA classes II and III.

21.2.3.3   Classification of TGA   In Australia a higher classification is given to devices with increasing degree of invasiveness, depending on which tissue the device is applied to (e.g., Class III corresponds to chronic implantable devices). In a regulatory sense, a

Table 21.2

Some Accepted Classifications of Medical Devices

Authorities	Classes			
TGA (Australia)	I		IIa, IIb	III
FDA (USA)	I	II	III	
ECHC (Europe)	I	IIa	IIb	III
Health Canada	I	II	III	IV
General description	Noninvasive and/ or transient use (e.g., dermal)	Minimally invasive, short term (e.g., eyes and ear canal)	Short- to medium-term contact with blood, oral/ nasal mucosae	Medium- to long-term contact, chronic implants, control systems
Restrictions	General	General and specific	General control and PMAs	
Health risk	Low	Low/moderate	Moderate/high	High
Examples	Surgical instruments, mechanical barriers	Contact lenses, ultrasound probes	Orthopedic implants, dialysis machines	Pacemakers, perfusion pumps, vascular stents

biomaterial is a component of a medical device [1], and thus a biomaterial can describe materials used in a medical device; on its own, a transplantable biomaterial may fall into a higher class, depending on its complexity and for which tissue type it is used.

21.3   PRECLINICAL TESTING

Guidelines for preclinical testing of biomaterials allow for those that are newly developed, or are modifications of an existing material or device component (Table 21.3). Generally, completely new biomaterials will go through strict PMA, while materials used in existing medical devices will be assessed to a more relaxed level.

21.4   CLINICAL TRIALS

Clinical trials of a new or modified medical treatment (in our case, a new or existing biomaterial, or material component of a biomedical device) are divided into four phases.

21.4.1   Phase I Trials: Is the Treatment Safe?

Researchers test an experimental drug or treatment on a small group of people (20–80) for the first time to evaluate its safety, determine a safe dosage range, and identify side effects. At this stage, the primary goal is to make the most basic determination of whether the device is harmful or not.

21.4.2   Phase II Trials: Is the Treatment Effective?

Once a device has proven not to be harmful according to Phase I testing outcomes, researchers then assess whether or not the device is capable of performing the intended

Table 21.3

Preclinical Evaluation Guidelines

Use of Material in the Device	Testing of Biomaterial Required	Reference to Other Users	Reference to Guarantee or Literature
No change in material	No	Not necessary	Not necessary
Material is used in a similar application	No	Yes	Yes
Material is used in other devices, but different applications	Limited testing to show applicability	Yes	Yes
Same material, but change in sterilization procedure	Yes, show that sterilization does not change material properties	May be	May be
Same material, but change in manufacturing procedure	Yes, show that manufacturing procedure does not change material properties	Not applicable	Not applicable
New material	Extensive tests required. May require clinical trials and/or PMA[a]	Not applicable	Not applicable

[a] *PMA, premarket approval.*

function. In Phase II trials, an experimental treatment is given to a larger group of people (100–300) to evaluate its effectiveness and also to confirm that it is still safe. The primary goal is essentially to prove the effectiveness.

21.4.3 Phase III Trials: How Does the Treatment Compare?

As mentioned in *Chapter 20*, it is not adequate simply to consider a device in terms of whether the risks to the patient are greater if the device is used or not. To change an existing treatment protocol involves complex legislative processes, as well as time-consuming and costly medical training. If a new medical device is not better than the existing one, there is no point to introduce the new product.

In Phase III trials, the experimental treatment is given to large groups of people (1000–3000) to confirm its effectiveness, monitor side effects, compare it to commonly used treatments, and collect information that will allow the experimental drug or treatment to be used safely. In short, in Phase III, the primary goal is to prove *better than existing*.

21.4.4 Phase IV Trials: Postmarket Surveillance

In Phase IV trials, longer-term studies provide additional information including the risks, benefits, and optimal usage after a device or treatment has been used widely and routinely for periods of years to decades. Many treatments only show drawbacks after years of clinical application. Many antibiotics, for example, have long-term side effects. Tetracyclines cause teeth discoloration in the fetus as they develop in infancy (Figure 21.2). For this same reason, tetracyclines are contraindicated for use in children under 8 years of age. In regard to biomaterials, there have been extreme cases of harm caused by long-term effects, such as beer drinker's cardiomyopathy and cancer caused

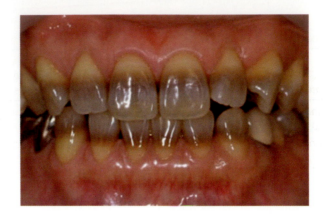

Figure 21.2
Tetracycline teeth.

by chromium ions released into drinking water. These cases emphasize the need for regulation of biomaterials testing.

21.5   DEVELOPMENT OF MEDICAL DEVICES AND POSSIBLE CAREER OPPORTUNITIES

Knowledge of materials science and engineering is not only useful in the processing and manufacture of medical devices. It can also form the basis of other career opportunities in medical device development. Biomaterials development is currently a growth area, and there is a demand for innovation in this field, which requires input from all branches of science, medicine, clinical and biological sciences. The ability to integrate with areas in tissue engineering makes this area of medical device development a highly rewarding career option, which can directly impact human lives. Engineers with a practical knowledge of medical practices and basic biological principles are readily sought and integrated with scientists and clinical practitioners. This is especially evident in countries whose governments support new technologies to drive innovation in medical and surgical treatments.

The development of medical devices involves a series of phases and steps (Table 21.4), including research and development (R&D), manufacture, testing and evolution, legal approval, and clinical application. As a materials scientist/engineer working in a technical or management capacity, you may find yourself in any of the following types of organizations:

- Research Institutes
  - Materials science
  - Biomedical engineering
  - Cross-disciplinary research
- Hospitals and/or clinical laboratories
- Manufacturers and service providers:
  - Biotechnology companies
  - Medical and surgical device manufacturers
  - Pharmaceutical companies
- Specialist consultancies
- Standardization organizations
- Government regulatory authorities

Table 21.4

Development of a Medical Device

Conception and Development	Manufacture	Packing and Labeling	Advertising	Sale	Use	Disposal
Researcher and manufacturer (following standards)			Vendor		User and public	
Premarket regulation			Placing-on-market regulation		Postmarket surveillance/ vigilance	

21.6   CHAPTER HIGHLIGHTS

1. Regulations are the legal aspect. Standards are the technical aspect.
2. Five regulatory authorities: TGA, HC, EuroC, Japan, and FDA.
3. Medical devices: Anything manufactured with medical purposes.
4. Classification of medical devices: Biomaterial implants fall in higher classes.
5. Four phases of clinical trials
6. Career opportunities

ACTIVITIES

Watch the biographical film *Erin Brockovich*.

SIMPLE QUESTIONS IN CLASS

1. Which of following organizations can set mandatory and legally obligatory rules?
   a. International Organization for Standardization (ISO)
   b. Food and Drug Administration (FDA)
   c. ASTM International (American Society for Testing and Materials)
   d. Therapeutic Good Administration (TGA)
2. In general, the regulations are for _____, rather than for _____.
   a. Biomaterials, ... all materials
   b. Medical devices, ... materials
   c. Materials, ... medical devices
   d. Biomaterials, ... medical devices
3. Medical devices are classified based on the level of control necessary to assure the safety and effectiveness of the device. Which class of medical devices has the greatest potential risk and is subject to in-depth scrutiny?
   a. Class I
   b. Class II
   c. Class III
   d. Class IV
4. Medical devices are classified based on the level of control necessary to assure the safety and effectiveness of the device. Which class of medical devices has the lowest potential risk and does not require a license?
   a. Class I
   b. Class II

    c. Class III

    d. Class IV

5. In _____ trials, researchers test a new medical device on a small group of people (20–80) for the first time to _____.

    a. Phase I, … evaluate safety.

    b. Phase II, … see if it has therapeutic effect.

    c. Phase III, … compare the new device with the existing ones.

    d. Phase IV, … evaluate the long-term effect of the medical device.

6. In Phase II trials, the experimental study of a new medical device is performed on a larger group of people (100–300) to _____.

    a. Evaluate its safety

    b. Compare the new device with the existing ones

    c. See if it has therapeutic effect

    d. Evaluate the long-term effect of the medical device

PROBLEMS AND EXERCISES

1. Discuss the relationship between standards and regulations.
2. Discuss the difference in the concepts of biomaterials used in the scientific and legal community.
3. Discuss the three classes of medical devices in the FDA system, in terms of the level of control necessary to ensure the safety and effectiveness of the device.
4. Describe the scale and major objective of phase I clinical trial.
5. Describe the scale and major objective of phase II clinical trial.
6. Describe the scale and major objective of phase III clinical trial.
7. Describe the scale and major objective of phase IV clinical trial.
8. Compare the clinical objectives of four phases of clinical trials, and discuss the rationales behind the objectives.

BIBLIOGRAPHY

References

1. Von Recum, A.F. ed., *Handbook of Biomaterials Evaluation: Scientific, Technical and Clinical Testing of Implant Materials*, 2nd edn. London, U.K.: Taylor & Francis, 1999.
2. Statement of Aims and scope, *Biomaterials*, 2011. http://www.journals.elsevier.com/biomaterials/ Accessed July 17, 2014.

Websites

http://www.cctec.cornell.edu/events/mddbootcamp/presentations/Preclinical%20_Hartman.pdf.
http://ec.europa.eu/dgs/health_consumer/index_en.htm.
http://www.fda.gov/downloads/Drugs/GuidanceComplianceRegulatoryInformation/Guidances/ucm074957.pdf.
http://www.hc-sc.gc.ca/index-eng.php.
http://www.mhlw.go.jp/english/index.html.
http://www.tga.gov.au/.

Further Reading

Von Recum, A.F. ed., *Handbook of Biomaterials Evaluation: Scientific, Technical and Clinical Testing of Implant Materials*, 2nd edn. London, U.K.: Taylor & Francis, 1999.

INDEX

A

ACE, *see* Angiotensin-converting enzyme (ACE) inhibitors
Acorn CorCap™ heart mesh (knitted poly(ethylene terephthalate)), 476
Acrylate polymers
    activators, 303
    bone cements, 301–303
    carboxylic acid, 300
    liquid monomer, 301–302
    PMMA, 300–301
    polyacrylate, 300–301
    shrinkage level, 301–303
    total hip replacement, 301–302
Acute coronary syndrome, 468
Acute rheumatic fever (ARF), 471
Adipose-derived stem cells, 552
Adult stem cells, 543–544
Aluminum oxide/alumina (Al_2O_3)
    CoCrMo alloys and PTFE, 189
    corrosion resistance and biocompatibility, 188–189
    CrCoMo-on-UHMWPE, 190
    hip joint structure, 189–190
    implant material, 193
    load-bearing sites, 195
    mechanical properties, 188
    replacement, hip, 189, 191
    wear of joints minimization, 191–193
    Young's modulus, 196
American Dental Association (ADA), 137
Amphiphile phospholipids, 529, 531
Anatomy
    cardiac muscle, 577
    digestive system, 500
    female and male reproductive systems, 512
    lymphatic system, 497
    respiratory system, 490–491
Androgen insensitivity syndrome, 513
Angina, chronic condition, 468
Angiotensin-converting enzyme (ACE) inhibitors, 473

Animal models
    abdominal, 666
    cardiovascular implants, 665–666
    dental applications, 666
    implantable devices, 665
    neurology, 666
    ophthalmology, 666
    orthopedics, 666
    otology, 666
    respiratory system, 666
    urogenital tract, 667
    wound healing, 667
Aorta and coronary arteries, 465–467
Apatite
    A–WGC, 222
    bone minerals, 214–215
    phosphate minerals, 214
Apatite–wollastonite glass-ceramics (A–WGC), 222
ARF, *see* Acute rheumatic fever (ARF)
Arteries, veins and capillaries, 462, 464–465
Articulations and articular cartilage, 431–432
Artificial blood vessels
    aorta prostheses and PTFE, 304–305
    aorta repair/replacement, 439
    bypass surgery, 482
    PTFE applications, 258, 260
Artificial bone
    antagonistic mechanical properties (strength–toughness), 397
    biomimetic techniques, 398
    description, 397
    highly hierarchical composite structure, 397–398
Artificial esophagus, 504–505
Artificial liver support system, 506–507
Artificial sphincters, inflatable polymer cuff, 504–505
Autografting, 237, 428–429, 475, 592
Autologous grafting, bypass surgery, 473–474
Autologous skeletal myoblasts, 549
A–WGC, *see* Apatite–wollastonite glass-ceramics (A–WGC)

(
B
II

C

1,380   1
B